D1235044

DUNCAN'S DICTIONARY FOR NURSES

DUNCAN'S DICTIONARY FOR NURSES

HELEN A. DUNCAN, R.N., M.A.

Springer Publishing Company, Inc., New York

Foreword

This new dictionary is a complete, up-to-date reference work for nurses at all levels. Prepared by a nurse, it will be useful not only to professional nurses, but also to students of nursing, practical nurses, and paramedical personnel.

One of the basic values of this dictionary is that it defines many terms relevant to the nursing field, but not found in medical dictionaries or in their condensed versions for nurses. Of course, it also includes the definitions of medical terms that nurses must and do use in their work.

Definitions of the nearly 11,000 terms have been kept simple, clear, and direct, and include commonly used synonyms. Many prefixes and suffixes, along with their definitions are listed in alphabetical order; thus the meaning of a complex word can be quickly determined by looking up the definitions of its component parts in the regular listing. In addition, it includes terms from disciplines related to nursing to the extent that nurses use these terms in their practice.

Acknowledgments

Acknowledgment is made for permission to use some definitions and illustrations from *Livingstone's Dictionary for Nurses,* published by E. & S. Livingstone, Ltd., Edinburgh and London. Some illustrations have been taken or adapted from Avice Kerr's *Orthopedic Nursing Procedures,* second edition, and from *Clinical Coordination of Anatomy and Physiology* by Martha Pitel and Mildred Schellig. Both of these books were published by Springer Publishing Company, Inc.

Pronunciation

The system of pronunciation used has deliberately been kept simple. Words that the nurse might have difficulty pronouncing are broken down into their component syllables and, when necessary, respelled phonetically. The accented syllable is indicated by a slanting mark at its termination. (′).

Vowels

Vowels are usually pronounced long or short, and are given the ordinary English pronunciation. When short, they are unmarked and are pronounced as follows:

a as in fast or father	*o* as in for or hot
e as in bed	*u* as in but
i as in fit	

When long, they are given a long mark and are pronounced as follows:

ā as in tame	*ō* as in over
ē as in he	*ū* as in use
ī as in time	

The final syllables of words that end with *a* are usually pronounced as though the word ended with *ah,* as for example, coma (kō′-mah). Those that end with *y* are usually pronounced as though they ended with a short *i,* as for example, chemistry (kem′-is-tri).

Consonants

Consonants ordinarily take the common English language

pronunciation. When this is not the case, the word is re-spelled phonetically, for example:

c may be pronounced as *s* or *k* as in cicatrix (sik′-a-triks)
ch is usually pronounced as *k* as in psychosis (sī-kō′-sis)
g may be pronounced as *j* as in pharyngeal (far-in′-jē-al)
ph may be pronounced as *f* as in pharyngeal (far-in′-jē-al)
psy may be pronounced as sī as in psychosis (sī-kō′-sis)

Abbreviations Used in Definitions

adj.	adjective
adv.	adverb
cf.	compare [Latin, *confer*]
e.g.	for example [Latin, *exempli gratia*]
i.e.	that is [Latin, *id est*]
n.	noun
opp.	opposite to
per se	as such
q.v.	which see [Latin, *quod vide*]
pl.	plural
sing.	singular
syn.	synonym
v.	verb
v.i.	intransitive verb
v.t.	transitive verb

A

A,Å: Abbreviation for Angstrom unit (*q.v.*).

a-: Denotes absence, separation, away from, without, not. a- before a consonant; changes to an- before a vowel.

AA: Abbreviation for (1) achievement age; (2) Alcoholics Anonymous.

aa: Abbreviation for *ana*. Sign meaning of each; used in prescription writing.

AAIN: Abbreviation for American Association of Industrial Nurses.

ab-: Denotes absent, away from, off, negative, separation, departure from.

abacterial (ā-bak-tē′-ri-al): Without bacteria; free from bacteria.

abarognosis (ab-ar-og-nō′-sis): Lack or loss of the ability to estimate weight.

abarticulation (ab′-ar-tik-ū-lā′-shun): 1. The dislocation of a joint. 2. A synovial or freely movable joint; *e.g.*, the hip. See **diarthrosis**.

abasia (a-bā′-zi-a): Inability to walk, or unsteadiness of gait, due to motor incoordination.—abasic, adj.

abdomen (ab′-do-men): The belly. The largest body cavity; lies between the thorax from which it is separated by the diaphragm, and the pelvis; is enclosed by a wall made up of muscles, the vertebral column and the two ilia; contains the viscera (*q.v.*); is lined with a serous membrane, the peritoneum, which is also reflected over most of the organs as a covering. ACUTE A., term for a pathological condition within the belly that requires immediate surgery. PENDULOUS A., occurs when the anterior wall relaxes and the abdomen sags or hangs down. SCAPHOID A., describes an A. in which the anterior wall 'caves in.'—abdominal, adj. See **regions, abdominal**.

abdomin-, abdomino-: Denotes the abdomen.

abdominocentesis (ab-dom-i-nō-sen-tē′-sis): Surgical puncture of the abdominal wall for the aspiration of fluid from the abdominal cavity.

abdominohysterectomy (ab-dom′-i-nō-his-ter-ek′-to-mi): Operation for the removal of the uterus through an incision in the abdominal wall.

abdominopelvic (ab-dom′-i-nō-pel′-vik): Pertaining to the abdomen and pelvis or pelvic cavity.

abdominoperineal (ab-dom′-i-nō′-per-in-ē′-al): Pertaining to the abdomen and the perineum. A. EXCISION OF THE RECTUM, an operation in which the part of the bowel above a cancerous growth in the rectum is brought out of the abdominal wall as a permanent colostomy, and the growth is removed via the perineum.

abdominoscopy (ab-dom-i-nos′-ko-pi): Examination or inspection of the abdomen and/or its viscera, either externally by the usual methods or internally by endoscopy, or both.

abduce (ab-dūs′): Abduct (*q.v.*).

abducens (ab-dū′-senz): Term applied to structures that draw a part away from the median line of the body, or that cause this to happen; *e.g.*, A. muscle, nerve.

abduct (ab-dukt′): To draw away from the midline of the body or from an adjoining part. Abduce. Opp. to adduct.—abduction, n.

abduction (ab-duk′-shun): 1. The drawing away of a part from the midline of the body or of one part from an adjoining part. Opp. to adduction. 2. The act of turning outward.

abductor (ab-duk′-tor): A muscle which, on contraction, draws a part away from the median line of the body; or a nerve supplying such a muscle. Opp. to adductor.

aberration (ab-er-rā′-shun): A deviation from normal. MENTAL A., a mild mental abnormality. SPHERICAL A., imperfect focus of light rays by a lens.—aberrant, adj.

abiosis (ab-i-ō′-sis): Without life.

abirritant (ab-ir′-rit-ant): 1. Relieving or lessening irritation. 2. An agent that relieves or lessens irritation.

ablactation (ab-lak-tā′-shun): 1. Stoppage of the flow of milk. 2. Weaning a child.

ablatio (ab-lā′-shē-ō): Ablation; removal; detachment. A. PLACENTAE, premature detachment of the placenta. A. RETINAE, detachment of the retina.

ablation (ab-lā′-shun): Removal; detachment. In surgery, removal or amputation of a part.

ablepharia (ab-lef-ā′-ri-a): Congenital absence of the eyelids; may be total or partial.

ablepsia (ab-lep′-si-a): Blindness.

ablution (ab-lū′-shun): Washing or cleansing, especially of the body.

ablutomania (ab-lū-tō-mān′-i-a): Abnormal interest in washing, bathing, or cleansing.

abnormal (ab-nor′-mal): Not normal; irregular; different from the usual.—abnormality, n.

abocclusion (ab-ō-kloo′-zhun): Descriptive of dentition in which the upper and lower teeth do not meet.

aboiement (a-bwah-mon′): The involuntary uttering of abnormal sounds, usually barking.

abort (a-bort′): 1. To terminate before full development. 2. To check a disease process in its early stages. 3. To terminate a pregnancy before the fetus is viable.

aborticide (a-bor′-ti-sīd): 1. Destruction of the fetus in the uterus. 2. A drug or agent that is capable of destroying a fetus in the uterus.

abortifacient (ab-or-ti-fā′-shent): 1. Causing abortion. 2. Drug or agent that causes expulsion of a non-viable fetus.

abortion (a-bor′-shun): 1. Abrupt termination of a process. 2. Expulsion from uterus of product of conception before it is viable, *i.e.,* before the end of the 28th week. ACCIDENTAL A., one due to an accident. ARTIFICIAL A., one brought on intentionally. COMPLETE A., the entire contents of the uterus are expelled. CRIMINAL A., an illegal intentional evacuation of the uterus. HABITUAL A., repeated successive abortions; preferable term is recurrent abortion. INCOMPLETE A., part of the fetus or placenta is retained within the uterus. INDUCED A., artificial A. INEVITABLE A., one which has advanced to a stage where termination of the pregnancy cannot be prevented. JUSTIFIABLE A., one performed to save the life of the mother. MISSED A., early signs and symptoms of pregnancy disappear and the fetus dies but is not expelled for some time. See **carneous mole.** SEPTIC A., one associated with uterine infection and rise in body temperature. THERAPEUTIC A., intentional termination of a pregnancy which is a hazard to the mother's life. THREATENED A., slight blood loss per vaginum while cervix remains closed. TUBAL A., tubal pregnancy that dies and is expelled from the fimbriated end of the fallopian tube.—abortive, adj.

abortus fever: See **brucellosis.**

aboulia (a-boo′-li-a): Abulia (*q.v.*).

abrachia (a-brăk′-i-a): Congenital absence of the arms.

abrasion (a-brā′-zhun): Superficial injury to skin or mucous membrane from scraping or rubbing; excoriation.—abrade, v.t.; abrasive, adj.; abrasive, n.

abreaction (ab-re-ak′-shun): In psychoanalysis, an emotional reaction resulting from recall of a repressed idea or memory; may come about from talking to the analyst or under the influence of light anesthesia. See **narcoanalysis.** Syn., catharsis.

abruptio (ab-rup′-shē-ō): A tearing away; separation. A. PLACENTAE; premature separation of the placenta from the wall of the uterus.

abscess (ab′-ses): Localized collection of pus formed by the disintegration of tissue as a result of action by pyogenic organisms. May be acute or chronic. ALVEOLAR A., at the root of a tooth. BRODIE'S A., chronic osteomyelitis (*q.v.*) occurring without previous acute phase; most often seen in young adults. COLD A., one occurring in the course of such chronic inflammation as may be due to the tubercle bacillus; usually slow growing and accompanied by little inflammation. PSOAS A., a cold abscess in the psoas muscle resulting from disease, usually tuberculosis of the lower dorsal or lumbar vertebrae.

abscission (ab-sish′-un): The cutting off of a part by surgery.

absolute (ab′-sōl-ūt): Unlimited; unconditional. A. ALCOHOL, alcohol which contains less than 1 percent of water. A. VALUES, numbers as opposed to percentages, often said of cell types in a blood count.

absorb (ab-sorb′): 1. To suck up, draw up, take in or imbibe, as a gas or fluid. 2. To take in through the skin, as certain rays. 3. The incorporation by body cells or tissues of substances from the blood or lymph.

absorbefacient (ab-sor-be-fā′-shent): Causing absorption; an agent or medication that promotes or causes absorption.

absorbent (ab-sor′-bent): 1. Having the power to absorb (*q.v.*). 2. Any agent or substance that has the power to absorb.

absorption (ab-sorp′-shun): 1. The assimilation, incorporation, or taking up of one substance by another, *e.g.,* liquids by solids, or gases by liquids or solids. 2. The passage of a substance through a body surface or membrane into the body fluids or tissues. 3. The taking up of heat by the body.

abstract (ab′-strakt): In pharmacology, a preparation made from the soluble principle of a drug, or its fluidextract (*q.v.*), evaporated to twice the original strength of the drug, and to which lactose is usually added. A. THINKING, the use of concepts and ideas independent of concrete objects.

abulia (a-boo'-li-a): Abnormal lack of ability to exercise will power; indecision or hesitancy in making decisions. Characteristic of certain psychoses and neuroses.

a.c.: Abbreviation for *ante cibum,* meaning before meals.

acapnia (a-kap'-ni-a): A condition of diminished carbon dioxide content of the blood; sometimes used when hypocapnia is meant. —acapnial, adj.

acardia (a-kar'-di-a): Congenital absence of the heart.

acariasis (ak-a-rī'-a-sis): Any disease caused by an acarid (*q.v.*).

acarid (ak'-a-rid): A mite; a member of the order *Acarina* (*q.v.*).

Acarina (ak-a-rī'-na): An order of *Arachnida* (*q.v.*); includes mites and ticks.

acarophobia (ak-ar-ō-fō'-bi-a): 1. Morbid dread of small organisms such as mites, ticks. 2. The delusion that the skin is infested with worms, mites, ticks or other small crawling organisms.

Acarus (ak'-ar-us): A genus including many species of ticks and mites. The term is often loosely used to designate any mite. A. SCABIEI (*Sarcoptes scabiei*) or itch mite is a human parasite that causes scabies (*q.v.*).

acatalepsy (a-kat'-a-lep-sē): Lack of understanding; dementia; impairment of the mind.—acataleptic, adj.

acatamathesia (a-kat-a-ma-thē'-zi-a): Lack or loss of ability to understand or comprehend, particularly speech.

acataphasia (a-kat-a-fā'-zi-a): Lack of power to express connected thought or to formulate sentences correctly.

accident: Any unexpected unfortunate occurrence, particularly one causing bodily injury. CEREBROVASCULAR A., one that occurs within the cerebrum, *e.g.,* cerebral hemorrhage; abbrev. CVA. A. PRONE, in psychiatry, susceptible to accidents due to psychological causes.

accommodation (a-kom-mō-dā'-shun): Adjustment or adaptation of an organ or a part to changing circumstances, particularly the automatic adjustment of the lens of the eye so that a distinct image is always obtained, regardless of the nearness or distance of the object being viewed.

accouchement (a-koosh'-mon): Delivery in childbirth. Confinement.

accoucheur (a-koo-sher'): A male obstetrician (*q.v.*).

accoucheuse (a-koo-shuz'): A midwife or female obstetrician.

accretion (a-krē'-shun): 1. An increase in substance or deposit around a central object. 2. Accumulation of foreign matter in a space or cavity. 3. Adherence or growing together of parts normally separate.

Ace bandage: See **bandage.**

acephalous (a-sef'-a-lus): Without a head.

acetabulum (as-et-ab'-ū-lum): A cup-like socket on the external aspect of the innominate bone, into which the head of the femur fits to form the hip joint.—acetabula, pl.; acetabular, adj.

acetate (as'-e-tāt): Any salt of acetic acid.

acetic acid (a-sē'-tik): The acid present in vinegar. In weak solution, antidote for alkaline poisons. Has several other uses in medicine.

acetoacetic acid (as-ē'-tō-as-ē'-tik as'-id): Syn., diacetic acid. A monobasic keto acid. Produced at an interim stage in the oxidation of fats in the human body. In some metabolic upsets, *e.g.,* acidosis and diabetes mellitus, it is present in excess in the blood and escapes in the urine. (It changes to acetone if urine is left standing.) The excess acid in the blood can produce coma.

Acetobacter (a-sēt-ō-bak'-ter): A genus of aerobic, rod-shaped bacteria, important in the production of vinegar.

acetone (as'-e-tōn): A colorless, inflammable liquid with characteristic sweetish odor and acrid taste; found in minute quantities in normal urine and in larger amounts in diabetic urine. Made commercially for use as a solvent. A. BODIES, intermediate products of fat metabolism which become greatly increased in the blood and urine in diabetes mellitus, pregnancy, starvation, after anesthesia and in other conditions of disturbed metabolism. Also called ketone bodies.

acetonemia (as-e-tō-nē'-mi-a): Acetone bodies in the blood.—acetonemic, adj.

acetonuria (as-e-tō-nū'-ri-a): Excess acetone bodies in the urine which give it a peculiar, sweet smell. Occurs in diabetes, carcinoma, fevers and some digestive disorders.— acetonuric, adj.

acetylcholine (as-et-il-kō'-lēn): Chemical substance released from autonomic nerve endings to activate muscle, secretory glands, and other nerve cells. Important in the transmission of nerve impulses across the synapse between one nerve fiber and another. The fibers that release this chemical are described as cholinergic.

achalasia (ak-a-lā′-zi-a): Failure to relax; often refers to sphincter muscles. CARDIAC A., contraction of the sphincter muscle between the esophagus and stomach, with consequent dilatation of the esophagus.

ache (āk): A continuous pain as differentiated from one that is sudden, spasmodic or intermittent; may be described according to severity, ranging from dull to severe, or according to location; *e.g.,* headache.

achievement (a-chēv′-ment): Accomplishment. A. AGE, a figure obtained by test; expresses the level of an individual's educational achievement as compared to that of the average child of the same chronological age. A. QUOTIENT, a figure obtained by dividing the achievement age by the mental age; indicates the state of progress in learning. A. TEST, a standardized test used to measure a person's skill or knowledge in one or more fields of work or study.

Achilles (a-kil′-ēz): Mythical Greek warrior whose entire body was invulnerable to injury with the exception of his heel. A. TENDON, the tendinous termination of the soleus and gastrocnemius muscles; is inserted into the calcaneus. A. JERK, the motor response to striking the A. TENDON.

achillorrhaphy (ak-il-or′-a-fi): The operation of stitching the Achilles tendon.

achillotomy (ak-il-ot′-o-mi): Subcutaneous division of the Achilles tendon.

achlorhydria (a-klor-hī′-dri-a): The absence of free hydrochloric acid in the stomach. Occurs in pernicious anemia, gastric cancer, gastritis, pellagra, and sprue.—achlorhydric, adj.

acholia (a-kōl′-i-a): Absence of bile.—acholic, adj.

acholuria (a-kol-ū′-ri-a): Absence of bile pigment from the urine. See **jaundice**.—acholuric, adj.

achondroplasia (a-kon-drō-plā′-zi-a): Arrested growth of the long bones; a congenital, often familial condition that results in dwarfism. The intellect is not usually impaired. Syn., fetal rickets.—achondroplastic, adj.

achoresis (ak-ō-rē′-sis): Permanent diminution of the capacity of a hollow organ, such as the stomach or bladder.

achromatic (a-krō-mat′-ik): 1. Free from color. 2. Lacking normal pigment. 3. Not readily colored by staining agents.

achromatopsia (a-krō-ma-top′-si-a): Color blindness.

achromatosis (a-krō-ma-tō′-sis): Absence or deficiency of natural pigmentation, as in the iris or the skin.

achromia (a-krō′-mi-a): Absence of color. Also achroma.

achylia (a-kī′-li-a): Absence of chyle (*q.v.*).—achylic, adj.

achymia (a-kī′-mi-a): Deficiency or imperfect formation of chyme.

acid: Any substance that in solution gives rise to an excess of hydrogen ions. Identified by (1) turning blue litmus paper red; (2) being neutralized by an alkali with the formation of a salt. (In popular jargon, any substance with a sour taste.)

acidaminuria (as-id-am-i-nū′-ri-a): The presence of an excess of amino acids in the urine.

acid-base balance: A normal equilibrium, or ratio, between the acid and base elements of the blood and body fluids. When the blood is in acid-base balance, the pH of the serum remains at 7.35 to 7.45. See **acidosis, alkalosis.**

acidemia (as-id-ē′-mi-a): Abnormal acidity of the blood, giving increased hydrogen ions, and a below normal pH (*q.v.*). See **acidosis**.—acidemic, adj.

acid-fast: A term used in bacteriology to describe an organism which, when stained, does not become decolorized when subjected to dilute acids, *e.g.,* tubercle bacillus (*Mycobacterium tuberculosis*), leprosy bacillus (*Mycobacterium leprae*), smegma bacillus (*Mycobacterium smegmatis*).

acid-forming foods: Those that predominantly produce an acid ash when metabolized. They include eggs, meat, fish, poultry, breads, cereals, pastries, puddings, cranberries, plums, prunes. Syn., acidogenic.

acidify (a-sid′-i-fī): 1. To become acid. 2. To render acid.

acid intoxication: Severe acidosis causing a toxic condition of the body. May be due to accumulation of acid products resulting from faulty or incomplete oxidation of fats, or by acids introduced into the body from without.

acidity (a-sid′-it-i): The state of being acid or sour. The degree of acidity can be determined and interpreted on the pH scale, pH 6.9 denoting a very weak acid and pH 1 a caustic acid.

acidogenic (as-id-ō-jen′-ik): Producing acid, particularly in the urine.

acidophil(e) (a-sid′-ō-fil; a-sid′-ō-fīl): 1. A cell or tissue that stains readily with an acid dye. 2. A microorganism that grows well in an acid medium.

acidophilus milk (as-i-dof′-i-lus): Milk that

has been fermented by *Lactobacillus acidophilus*; sometimes used to change intestinal flora.

acidosis (as-id-ō′-sis): Depletion of the body's alkali reserve, with resulting disturbance of the acid-base balance. May be secondary to some other condition; seen in diabetes mellitus, nephritis, epilepsy, starvation, cyclic vomiting, diarrhea, and toxemias. Acidemia. See **ketosis.**—acidotic, adj.

acid phosphatase (fos′-fa-tāz): An enzyme found in many tissues and fluids of the body, including the liver, spleen, pancreas, kidney, blood plasma, red blood cells, seminal fluid. In cancer of the prostate gland the serum A.P. is elevated.

acid stomach: A condition due to the formation of excessive acid in the stomach or to an acid residue left in the stomach by certain foods; marked by heartburn, belching, and pain in the upper part of the abdomen.

aciduria (as-id-ū′-ri-a): Excretion of an acid urine. Current research suggests there may be some association with mental subnormality.

acini (as′-in-i): Minute saccules or alveoli lined or filled with secreting cells, found in various glands and organs; they cluster around a narrow lumen like grapes on a stem; several A. combine to form a lobule. Term commonly applied to the saclike termini of the small tubular passages in the lungs; sometimes used as a synonym for alveoli.—acinus, sing.; acinous, acinar, adj.

acme (ak′-me): 1. In illness, the time of greatest intensity of a symptom or symptoms. 2. The crisis or critical stage of a disease.

acne, acne vulgaris (ak′-ne vul-gar′-is): A skin condition common in both sexes during adolescence, in which blackheads (comedones) are associated with a papular and pustular eruption of the pilosebaceous follicles. Usual sites are the face, neck, and upper parts of chest and back. There are many types and degrees of severity. Syn., common acne, acne simplex. Individual predispositions include seborrhea (*q.v.*), dyspepsia, constipation, endocrine imbalance; tends to be worse in women at menstruation. A. ROSACEA, nowadays called 'rosacea' is a pronounced erythema of the brow, cheeks, and nose, resulting from dilatation of subcutaneous capillary vessels. Seen mostly in adults and is aggravated by hot drinks, alcoholic drinks, and rich or fried foods.

acneiform (ak-ne′-i-form): Resembling acne.

acomia (a-kō′-mi-a): Baldness.

acoria (a-kō′-ri-a): Continual hunger due to loss of the sensation of satiety; the appetite may not be large but the patient never feels that he has had enough to eat.

acousma (a-koos′-ma): An auditory hallucination in which one hears such nonverbal sounds as buzzing, ringing, hissing.

acoustic (a-koo′-stik): Pertaining to: (1) the sense or organs of hearing; (2) the science of sound.

acquired (a-kwīrd′): Not inherited; resulting from learning, experience, or other influences originating outside the organism after birth. A. IMMUNITY, any type of immunity that is not inherited. See **immunity.** A. REFLEX, same as conditioned reflex(*q.v.*).

acr-, acro-: Denotes an extremity of the body.

acral (ak′-ral): Pertaining to or affecting the peripheral parts of the body; *e.g.*, ears, fingers, toes.

acrid (ak′-rid): Bitter, burning, irritating, pungent.

acroarthritis (ak-rō-arth-rī′-tis): Inflammation of the joints of the hands or feet.

acrocephalia (ak-rō-sef-ā′-li-a): Acrocephaly (*q.v.*).

acrocephaly (ak-rō-sef′-a-li): A congenital malformation whereby the top of the head is more or less pointed, due to premature closure of the coronal, sagittal, and lambdoid sutures.—acrocephalic, acrocephalous, adj.

acrocephalosyndactyly (ak-rō-sef-a-lō-sin-dak′-til-i): A congenital malformation consisting of a pointed top of head, with webbed hands and feet. Acrocephalosyndactylism. See **syndactyly.**

acrocyanosis (ak-rō-sī-a-nō′-sis): Cyanosis of the extremities. Often associated with chilblains when the skin may be bluish or reddish and mottled; usually due to a vasomotor disturbance. In infants, the extremities are blue and cold while the cheeks and trunk are pink; usually due to faulty cardiopulmonary function; tends to clear with warmth.—acrocyanotic, adj.

acrodynia (ak-rō-din′-i-a): Painful reddening of the extremities such as occurs in pink disease (*q.v.*).

acrogeria (ak-rō-jer′-i-a): Premature aging of the skin of the hands and legs with loosening and wrinkling; tends to run in families.

acromacria (ak-rō-mak′-ri-a): Spider fingers; arachnodactyly (*q.v.*).

acromania (ak-rō-mā′-ni-a): A violent form of mania characterized by excessive motor activity and sometimes by muteness.

acromegaly (ak-rō-meg′-a-li): A not uncommon disease, characterized by enlargement of the hands, face and feet. Occurs in adult life and is due to disturbed function of the pituitary gland.—acromegalic, adj.

acromioclavicular (ak-rō-mi-ō-kla-vi′kū-lar): Pertaining to the acromion process of the scapula and the clavicle.

acromion (ak-rō′-mi-on): The point or summit of the shoulder; the triangular process at the extreme outer end of the spine of the scapula. It articulates with the clavicle.—acromial, adj.

acromphalus (a-krom′-fa-lus): 1. The center of the navel. 2. Undue projection of the navel.

acromyotonia (ak-rō-mī-ō-tō′-ni-a): Myotonia (*q.v.*) of the hand or foot resulting in spastic deformity.

acronyx (ak′-rō-niks): An ingrowing nail.

acroparesthesia (ak-rō-par-es-thē′-zi-a): Tingling or numbness of one or more of the extremities, particularly the hands and fingers. Sometimes there is pain, pallor, or cyanosis.

acrophobia (ak-rō-fō′-bi-a): Morbid fear of being at a height.

acroscleroderma (ak-rō-skler-ō-der′-ma): Hardening and thickening of the skin of the extremities; usually symmetrical; can cause deformity; occurs most often in women.

acrotic (a-krot′-ik): 1. Pertaining to the surface, especially to the glands of the skin. 2. Without pulse.

acrotism (ak′-rō-tizm): Extremely weak or absent pulse.

acrylics (a-kril′-iks): A group of thermoplastic substances used in making prostheses. —acrylic, adj.

ACTH: Adrenocorticotropic hormone. See **corticotropin.**

acting out: In psychiatry, the neurotic gratification of a repressed or unfulfilled wish by compulsive behavior, usually involving another person.

actinism (ak′-tin-izm): The chemical action of spectral rays.—actinic, adj. The actinic dermatoses are skin conditions in which the integument is abnormally sensitive to ultraviolet light, *e.g.,* xeroderma pigmentosum.

actinobiology (ak′-tin-ō-bī-ol′-ō-ji): The study of the effects of radiation on living organisms.

actinodermatitis (ak-tin-ō-der-ma-tī′-tis): Irritation of the skin resulting from exposure to the sun or other rays.

Actinomyces (ak-tin-ō-mī′-sēz): A genus of parasitic fungus having a radiating mycelium. Also called 'ray fungus.' Some of the antibiotic drugs are produced from fungi of this genus.

actinomycosis (ak-tin-ō-mī-kō′-sis): An infrequent, infectious disease of man and some animals (cattle, horses, swine); caused by the Actinomyces that usually enters the body through dental caries or infected gums; characterized by formation of deep subcutaneous nodules or tumors that are first livid and hard, then suppurate and rupture forming fistulous tracts that discharge a thick, oily pus containing yellow granules. Sites most often affected are jaw, lung, and intestine. Man may become infected by handling diseased animals or through a human bite. Syn., lumpy jaw.—actinomycotic, adj.

actinotherapy (ak-tin-ō-ther′-a-pi): Treatment by nonionizing (especially ultraviolet and infrared) radiations, similar to those in natural sunlight, but produced by artificial means.

action: The activity or function of any part of the body. ANTAGONISTIC A., performed by those muscles that limit the movement of an opposing group. Also, counteraction of the effect of one drug by another. BUFFER A., (1) prevents change in the reaction of *p*H; (2) prevents jarring. COMPULSIVE A., performed by an individual at the supposed instigation of another's dominant will, but against his own. CUMULATIVE A., suddenly increased intensity of reaction to a drug after several doses. IMPULSIVE A., that resulting from a sudden urge rather than the will. REFLEX A., a specific involuntary motor or secretory response to a sensory stimulus. SEXUAL A., coitus, cohabitation. SPECIFIC A., that brought about by certain agents in a particular disease; *e.g.,* salicylates in acute rheumatism. SPECIFIC DYNAMIC A., the stimulating effect upon the metabolism produced by the ingestion of food, especially proteins, causing the metabolic rate to rise above basal levels. SYNERGISTIC A., that brought about by (1) cooperation of two or more muscles, neither of which could bring about the action alone; (2) the activity of one drug in increasing the effect of another.

activator: A substance which renders something else active. A term often used in connection with hormones and enzymes, *e.g.,* secretin, an intestinal hormone, activates the pancreas; enterokinase, an intestinal enzyme, activates trypsinogen. An enzyme activator is called 'coenzyme' or 'kinase.'—activate, v.

active: 1. Energetic, as A. treatment; not passive (*q.v.*). 2. Due to an intrinsic as distinguished from a passive force, as A. hyperemia (*q.v.*) and A. immunity (*q.v.*). A. MOVEMENTS, those produced by the patient using his neuromuscular mechanism. A. PRINCIPLE, one that gives a complex drug its chief value; *e.g.,* atropine in belladonna.

activities of daily living: Term used in rehabilitation nursing; the activities normally performed by the individual himself for his health and comfort; *i.e.,* eating, dressing, toileting, bathing, exercising. Abbrev. ADL.

acuity (a-kū′-it-i): Sharpness, clearness, keenness, distinctness. AUDITORY A., ability to hear clearly and distinctly. Tests include the use of tuning fork, whispered voice and audiometer. In infants, simple sounds, *e.g.,* bells, rattles, cup and spoon are utilized. VISUAL A., extent of visual perception; dependent on the clarity of retinal focus, integrity of nervous elements and cerebral interpretation of the stimulus. Usually tested by Snellen's letters. See **Snellen's test types.**

acupuncture (ak-ū-punk′-tūr): The insertion or introduction of needles or fine, hollow tubes into tissue for the purpose of counter-irritation, or to withdraw fluid as a therapeutic measure or for diagnostic tests. See **Southey's tubes.**

acus (ā′-kus): A needle, particularly a surgical needle.

acute (a-kūt′): Short and severe; not long drawn out and chronic. A. DILATATION OF THE STOMACH, sudden enlargement of this organ due to paralysis of the muscular wall. See **paralytic ileus.** A. HEART FAILURE, cessation or impairment of heart action, in previously undiagnosed heart disease, or in the course of another disease. A. YELLOW ATROPHY, acute, diffuse necrosis of the liver; icterus gravis; malignant jaundice.

acyanotic (a-sī-an-ot′-ik): Without cyanosis.

acyesis (a-sī-ē′-sis): 1. Absence of pregnancy. 2. Sterility in the female.—acyetic, adj.

acystia (a-sis′-ti-a): Congenital absence of the urinary bladder.—acystic, adj.

AD: Abbreviation for right ear.

ad-: Denotes to, toward, before, near, adjacent. May change to ac- before c, k, or q; af- before f; ag- before g· al- before l; ap-

before p; as- before s; at- before t.

-ad: Denotes toward, in the direction of.

adactylia (a-dak-til′-i-a): Congenital absence of fingers or toes, or both. Also adactylism, adactyly.

Adam's apple: Common name for the laryngeal prominence in the front of the neck, especially in the adult male, formed by the junction of the two wings of the thyroid cartilage.

Adams-Stokes disease: A disease condition characterized by sudden attacks of unconsciousness; associated with heart block. Also called Adams-Stokes syndrome.

adaptability (ad-apt-a-bil′-i-ti): The ability to adjust mentally and physically to circumstances.

adaptation (ad-ap-tā′-shun): 1. Mental and physical adjustment to the environment 2. Any beneficial change made to meet environmental change. 3. The action of the eye in adjusting to variations in the intensity of light.—adaptable, adj.

addict (ad′-ikt): One who is unable to resist indulgence in some habit, such as the use of drugs or alcohol.—addict, v.t., v.i.; addiction, n.

addiction (a-dik′-shun): A state in which habitual use of a physical substance such as alcohol or a drug has created a strong psychological dependence that cannot be controlled; withdrawal of the substance causes severe distress symptoms.

addisonism (ad′-i-son-izm): 1. A symptom complex sometimes seen in persons with pulmonary tuberculosis; includes weight loss, weakness, pigmentation of the skin, but not due to disease of the adrenal gland and not severe enough to be classified as Addison's disease. 2. Temporary dysfunction of the adrenal cortex.

Addison's disease: Deficient secretion from the adrenal cortex, causing electrolytic upset, diminution of blood volume, lowered blood pressure, marked anemia, hypoglycemia, great muscular weakness, gastrointestinal upsets, and bronzelike pigmentation of the skin; usually caused by tuberculosis. [Thomas Addison, English physician, diagnostician and teacher. 1793-1860.]

adduct (ad-dukt′): To draw toward the midline of the body or toward a neighboring part. Opp. to abduct.—adduction, n.

adduction (ad-duk′-shun): 1. The drawing of a part of the body toward the midline, or of a part toward an adjacent part. Opp. to abduction. 2. The act of turning inward.

adductor (ad-duk′-tor): Any muscle which moves a part toward the median axis of the body. Opp. to abductor.

aden-, adeno-: Denotes gland, glands.

adenectomy (ad-en-ek′-to-mi): 1. Surgical removal of a gland. 2. Surgical removal of an adenoid growth.

adenitis (ad-en-ī′-tis): Inflammation of a gland or lymph node. CERVICAL A., inflammation of lymph nodes in the neck. HILAR A., inflammation of bronchial lymph nodes.

adenocarcinoma (ad-en-ō-kar-sin-ō′-ma): A malignant growth of glandular tissue.— adenocarcinomatous, adj.; adenocarcinomata, pl.

adenofibroma (ad-en-ō-fī-brō′-ma): See fibroadenoma.

adenoid (ad′-e-noid): 1. Resembling a gland. 2. In the plural, usually refers to overgrowth of lymphoid tissue in the nasopharynx.

adenoidectomy (ad-e-noid-ek′-to-mi): Surgical removal of adenoid tissue from the nasopharynx.

adenolymphocele (ad-en-ō-lim′-fō-sēl): A cyst in a lymph node.

adenolymphoma (ad-en-ō-lim-fō′-ma): An adenoma of a lymph gland.

adenoma (ad-en-ō′-ma): A tumor of glandular tissue, usually benign.—adenomatous, adj.; adenomata, pl.

adenomatome (ad-en-ō′-ma-tōm): A scissors-like instrument for removing adenoids.

adenomyoma (ad-en-ō-mī-ō′-ma): A tumor, usually benign, composed of muscle and glandular elements, *e.g.,* an A. of the uterosacral ligaments is composed of smooth muscle in which islands of aberrant endometrium are found.—adenomyomatous, adj.; adenomyomata, pl.

adenomyosis uteri (ad-en-ō-mī-ō′-sis ū′-te-rī): A general enlargement of the uterus due to overgrowth of the myometrium, in which there is a benign invasion of the endometrium.

adenopathy (ad-en-op′-a-thi): Any disease of a gland, especially a lymphatic gland.— adenopathic, adj.

adenosclerosis (ad-en-ō-skler-ō′-sis): Hardening of a gland with or without swelling, usually due to replacement by fibrous tissue or calcification.—adenosclerotic, adj.

adenosine triphosphate (a-den′-ō-sēn): A chemical substance found in living cells, chiefly in striated muscle. During muscle contraction it breaks down and releases energy needed for muscle activity. Abbreviated ATP.

adenotonsillectomy (ad-en-ō-ton-sil-ek′-to-mi): Surgical removal of the adenoids and tonsils.

adenovirus (ad-en-ō-vī′-rus): Many types have been isolated. Some cause upper respiratory infection, others pneumonia, others tumors, others epidemic keratoconjunctivitis.

ADH: Antidiuretic hormone (*q.v.*).

adhesion (ad-hē′-zhun): Abnormal union of two parts, often after inflammation; a band of fibrous tissue which joins such parts. In the abdomen it may cause intestinal obstruction; in joints it restricts movement; between two surfaces of pleura it prevents complete pneumothorax.—adherent, adj.; adherence, n.; adhere, v.t., v.i.

adiaphoresis (a-dī-a-for-ē′-sis): Deficiency or absence of visible perspiration.—adiaphoretic, adj.

adiaphoretic (a-dī-a-for-et′-ik): 1. Pertaining to or characterized by absence or deficiency of visible perspiration. 2. An agent that causes reduction of or prevents sweating.—adiaphoresis, n.

adipocele (ad′-i-po-sēl): A hernia in which the sac contains fat or fatty tissue. Lipocele.

adipoma (ad-i-pō′-ma): A tumor made up of fat or fatty tissue. Lipoma.

adipose (ad′-i-pōz): Fat; fatty; of a fatty nature; pertaining to fat.

adiposis (ad-i-pō′-sis): Obesity; corpulence; fatness; abnormal deposit of fat in the body as a whole or in any of its parts.

adiposity (ad-i-pos′-it-i): Excessive accumulation of fat in the body.

adiposogenital dystrophy (ad-i-pō-sō-jen′-i-tal dis-trō-fi): A syndrome in which there is increase in body fat accompanied by underdevelopment of genital organs and changes in secondary sex characteristics, loss of sexual power, loss of hair. Thought to be due to a disorder of the pituitary gland or hypothalamus.

adiposuria (ad-i-pō-sū′-ri-a): Fat in the urine. Lipuria.

adipsia (a-dip′-si-a): Absence of the sensation of thirst; avoidance of taking fluid by mouth.

aditus (ad′-it-us): In anatomy, an entrance or opening to an organ or part.

adjustment: 1. The mechanism by which the tube of a microscope is raised or low-

ered thereby bringing the lens into focus.
2. In psychology, the relationship between an individual, his inner self, and the environment.

adjuvant (ad'-joo-vant): A substance included in a prescription to aid the action of other drugs. A. THERAPY, supportive measures in addition to main treatment.

ADL: Abbreviation for activities of daily living (*q.v.*).

Adler's theory(ad'-ler):Holds that neuroses arise as compensations for feelings of inferiority, either social or physical. [Alfred Adler, Austrian psychiatrist. 1870-1937.]

ad lib: Abbreviation for *ad libitum,* meaning at pleasure, without restraint, as much as desired.

adnexa (ad-nek'-sa): Structures which are in close proximity to a part; appendages or accessory parts. A. OCULI, the lacrimal apparatus and other appendages of the eye. A. UTERI, the ovaries, uterine tubes and uterine ligaments.

adnexitis (ad-nek-sī'-tis): Inflammation of the adnexa uteri. See **adnexa.**

adolescence (ad-ō-les'-sens): The age between the beginning of puberty and full maturity; youth.—adolescent, adj.; n.

adoral (ad-ōr'-al): Near or toward the mouth.

adrenal (ad-rē'-nal): 1. Near the kidney. 2. A small body or gland, one of which lies above each kidney. Consists of an inner part, the medulla, which secretes norepinephrine and an outer part, the cortex, which secretes substances called corticoids (*q.v.*) that are essential to life; the cortex also secretes some sex hormones. Total effect of the cortical secretions includes growth and weight changes, basal metabolism regulation, neuromuscular activity, gastrointestinal function, maintenance of body fluid balance, reproduction. Functionally, the A. glands are closely related to the pituitary and other endocrine glands.

adrenalectomy (ad-rē-nal-ek'-to-mi): Removal of an adrenal gland for tumor or for treatment of hypertension, malignant disease of breast, etc. If bilateral, requires replacement administration of cortical hormones.

Adrenalin: Trade name for epinephrine (*q.v.*).

adrenaline (ad-ren'-a-lin): Epinephrine (*q.v.*).

adrenergic (ad-ren-er'-jik): Term applied to sympathetic nerves which liberate an epinephrine-like substance called sympathin from their terminations. Opp. to cholinergic (*q.v.*).

adrenocorticotropic (ad-rēn-ō-kor-ti-kō-trōp'-ik): Having a hormonic effect on the cortex of the adrenal gland. See **corticotropin.** Also adrenocorticotrophic.

adrenogenital syndrome (ad-rēn-ō-jen'-it-al-sin²drōm):Virilism in the female resulting from overproduction of androgens; may be due to hyperplasia, adenoma, or carcinoma. In female children is usually evident at birth and represented by pseudohermaphrodism; in male children not usually evident until the child is three or four years of age and is represented by precocious sexual development.

adrenolytic (ad-rē-nō-lit'-ik): 1. That which antagonizes or inhibits the action or secretion of epinephrine. 2. Having a depressing effect on the sympathetic (adrenergic) nerve fibers.

adsorbents (ad-sorb'-ents): Solids which attract gases or dissolved substances to their surfaces, as a film. Charcoal adsorbs gases and acts as a deodorant. Kaolin adsorbs bacterial and other toxins, hence used in food poisoning.

adsorption (ad-sorp'-shun): The process by which a gas or liquid is collected and concentrated at the surface of another substance.

adulteration (a-dul-ter-ā'-shun): The addition of an impure, cheap, or inferior substance to another substance with a deliberate attempt to alter that substance and to deceive the user; the usual implication is that the original substance is thereby rendered less effective, less desirable, weaker, or cheaper.—adulterant, n.

advancement: In surgery, an operation in which a muscle or tendon is severed and reattached farther forward. Specifically, the operation to remedy strabismus; the muscle tendon opposite to the direction of the squint is detached and sutured to the sclera anteriorally.

adventitia (ad-ven-tish'-i-a): The external coat of an organ or structure, especially of an artery or vein.—adventitious, adj.

Aedes (ā-ē'-dēz): A genus of mosquitoes. A. AEGYPTI is the principal vector of yellow fever and dengue.

AEG: Air encephalography. See **pneumoencephalography.**

-aemia: See **-emia.**

aer-, aero-: Denotes: (1) Air, atmosphere; (2) gas; (3) relationship to aviation.

aeration (ā-er-ā′-shun): 1. Exposing to or supplying with air. 2. Charging a fluid with gas or air. 3. The process, which occurs within the lungs, whereby the CO₂ in the blood is exchanged for O₂.—aerate, v.; aerated, adj.

aeremia (ā-er-ēm′-ia): An air embolism; the presence of air in the blood.

Aerobacter: An organism of which two species are closely related to *Escherichia coli* and are frequently found in the gastrointestinal tract of man as well as in water, food, milk, soil, and sometimes infections. (See **Escherichia.**)

aerobe (ā′-er-ōb): A microorganism that requires oxygen from the air to maintain life.—aerobic, adj.

aeroembolism (ā-er-ō-em′-bol-izm): A condition that occurs particularly in aviators; caused by rapid ascent to great heights. Nitrogen bubbles form in the blood and spinal fluid; symptoms include rash, pain in the joints and lungs, itching, urticaria, neuritis, paresthesia, sometimes paralysis and coma.

aerogenous (ā-er-oj′-en-us): 1. Gas producing. 2. Descriptive of organisms that produce gas; *e.g.*, Welch's bacillus (*q.v.*).

aerogram (ā′-er-ō-gram): An x-ray picture of a hollow organ or structure after it has been filled with air or a gas.

aeromedicine (ā-er-ō-med′-i-sin): Aviation medicine (*q.v.*).

aeroneurosis (ā-er-ō-nū-rō′-sis): A chronic functional psychoneurosis, occurs in aviators; caused by prolonged periods of anoxia and stress; characterized by gastric distress, insomnia, worry, loss of self-confidence, and various other physical and emotional symptoms.

aero-otitis media (ā-er-ō-ō-ti′-tis mē′-di-a): Inflammation of the middle ear due to trauma caused by the rapid descent of an aircraft from a high altitude.

aerophagy (ā-er-of′-a-ji): Air swallowing, followed by belching and distention of the stomach and colon; a habit associated with nervous or digestive disorders. Also aerophagia.

aerophobia (ā-er-ō-fō′-bi-a): 1. Abnormal dread of fresh air or drafts of air. 2. Abnormal dread of being up in the air, as of flying.

Aeroplast: A spray-on dressing for burns, wounds, surface lesions.

aerosol (ā′-er-ō-sol): Atomized particles suspended in a gas or the air. They may be used: (1) as inhalation therapy; (2) to sterilize the air; (3) in mosquito and insect control; (4) as a deodorant.

Aesculapius (es-kū-lā′-pi-us): The mythical god of medicine.

aesthesio-: See **esthesio-**

afebrile (a-feb′-ril): Without fever.

affect (af′-ekt): A feeling evoked by a stimulus; may be directed toward anything. In psychiatry, that aspect of the mind that is concerned with emotions or mood. The term is often used interchangeably with emotion.—affective, adj.

affection (a-fek′-shun): Any abnormal physical or mental state or condition.

affective psychosis (a-fek′-tiv sī-kō′-sis): A psychosis in which the predominant disturbance is in the person's emotions and mood or feeling tone.

afferent (af′-er-ent): Conveying to or toward a center; term used to designate nerves, blood vessels and lymphatics that perform this function. A. NERVE, a bundle of nerve fibers that carry impulses from the periphery to the central nervous system; receptors connect directly to them. Often synonymous with sensory nerve.

affinity (a-fin′-i-ti): 1. Attraction; in chemistry, the attraction between substances, *e.g.*, oxygen and hemoglobin. 2. Common relationship.

afflux (af′-luks): The rush of blood or other body fluid to a part, causing congestion.

affusion (af-fū′-zhun): The act of pouring water on the body or a part of it; usually to reduce fever or nervousness.

afibrinogenemia (a-fī-brin-ō-jen-ē′-mi-a): A rare congenital or acquired disease characterized by decreased fibrinogen in the circulating blood. More correctly, hypofibrinogenemia.—afibrinogenemic, adj.

African trypanosomiasis (af′-rik-an trī-pan-ō-sōm-ī′-a-sis): An acute, infectious, highly fatal disease, particularly of tropical Africa; caused by the *Trypanosoma gambiense;* transmitted to man by the bite of a tsetse fly which has become infected by having previously bitten an infected man or animal. Often called African sleeping sickness.

afterbirth: The placenta, cord and membranes which are normally expelled from the uterus after childbirth.

aftercare: Denotes the care given during convalescence and rehabilitation, after conclusion of treatment.

11 agoraphobia

afterimage: A visual impression of an object which persists after the object has been removed. This is called 'positive' when the image is seen in its natural bright colors; 'negative' when the bright parts become dark, while the dark parts become light.

afterpains: The cramplike pains felt after childbirth, particularly by multiparae, due to contraction and retraction of the uterine muscle fibers.

Ag: Chemical symbol for silver.

agalactia (a-ga-lak′-shi-a): Non-secretion or imperfect secretion of milk after childbirth.—agalactic, adj.

agammaglobulinemia (a-gam-a-glob-ūl-in-ēm′-i-a): Absence of gamma globulin in the blood, with consequent inability to produce immunity to infection.—agammaglobulinemic, adj.

agar, agar-agar (a′-gar): A gelatinous substance obtained from certain seaweeds. It is used as a bulk-increasing laxative and in bacterial culture media.

age: 1. The amount of time which has passed since an individual was born. 2. A particular period of human life; e.g., middle age. 3. To produce, artificially, the effects of age; e.g., to age wine. 4. To grow old. ACHIEVEMENT A., the expression, in years, of a child's intellectual development as compared with his chronological age. CHRONOLOGICAL A., the actual number of years the individual has lived. MENTAL A., the figure which expresses the mental ability of an individual as compared with that of the average child of the same chronological age; it is determined by standardized tests. PHYSIOLOGICAL A., the term applied to A. as assessed from appearance and behavior.

agenesis (a-jen′-e-sis): 1. Incomplete and imperfect development of an organ or part. 2. Congenital absence of an organ or part.—agenetic, adj.

agent: A person, substance, or force that acts, or is capable of acting on something else, thereby producing an effect. CATALYTIC A., a substance that enhances or speeds a reaction without itself being affected.

ageusia (a-gŭ′-si-a): Absence, loss, or impairment of the sense of taste.

agglutination (a-gloo′-tin-ā′-shun): 1. A phenomenon characterized by the clumping of bacteria or red blood cells distributed in a fluid, apparently effected by the specific immune antibodies called 'agglutinins,' that develop in the blood of a previously infected or sensitized person. 2. The union of surfaces in the healing of a wound.—agglutinate, v.t., v.i.

agglutinins (a-gloo′-tin-inz): Specific factors present in sera which agglutinate or clump organisms or particulate protein matter. See **antibodies.**

agglutinogen (a-gloo-tin′-ō-jen): A factor that stimulates production of a specific agglutinin, used in the production of immunity; e.g., dead bacteria as in vaccine, particulate protein as in toxoid.

aggressin (a-gres′-in): A metabolic substance believed to be produced by certain bacteria to enhance their aggressive action against their host.

aggression (a-gresh′-un): An attitude of animosity or hostility, or an assaultive action, usually resulting from frustration or a feeling of inferiority.—aggressive, adj.

agitated depression (aj′-i-tā-ted dē-presh′-un): Marked restlessness, continual activity, despondency and apprehension. Often involutional.

agitation (aj-i-tā′-shun): Excessive chronic restlessness with constant purposeless physical activity, sometimes with mental disturbance.

agitographia (aj-i-tō-graf′-i-a): A condition in which the patient writes with excessive speed and unconsciously omits words or parts of words. Often associated with agitophasia (q.v.).

agitophasia (aj-i-tō-fā′-zē-a): A condition in which the patient speaks with excessive speed and unconsciously omits, slurs, or distorts words or parts of words.

aglossia (a-glos′-i-a): Congenital absence of the tongue.

aglutition (a-gloo-tish′-un): Difficulty in swallowing or inability to swallow; dysphagia.

agnail (ag′-nāl): Hangnail.

agnathia (ag-nā′-thi-a): A developmental anomaly characterized by absence or imperfect development of the lower jaw.—agnathus, agnathy, n.; agnathous, adj.

agnosia (ag-nō′-zi-a): Inability to recognize sensory impressions, due to organic brain disorder. Several varieties are identified according to the sense organ involved; e.g., auditory, optic, olfactory.—agnostic, adj.

agonist (ag′-on-ist): Muscle that shortens to perform a movement. See **antagonist.**

agoraphobia (ag-or-a-fō′-bi-a): Morbid fear of being alone in large open places.—agoraphobic, adj.

agranulocyte (a-gran′-ū-lō-sīt): A nongranular leucocyte.—agranulocytic, adj.

agranulocytosis (a-gran-ū-lō-sī-tō′-sis): An acute, serious condition characterized by marked reduction or complete absence of granulocytes or polymorphonuclear leucocytes, fever, and ulceration of mucous surfaces, especially those of the gastrointestinal tract. May result from: (1) toxic reaction to the sulfonamides, antithyroid drugs, gold salts and certain synthetic preparations; (2) excessive irradiation of the bone marrow.—agranulocytotic, adj.

agraphia (a-graf′-i-a): Inability to express thoughts in writing, due to a central lesion; writing is characterized by omissions, repetitions, incorrect use of words, and faulty grammar.—agraphic, adj.

agromania (ag-rō-mā′ni-a): Abnormal desire to live in solitude or in the country.

ague (āg′-ū): 1. Old name for malaria. 2. A malarial type of fever that occurs intermittently, accompanied by shivering, chills, and sweating. FACIAL A., tic douloureux (*q.v.*).

AHA: Abbreviation for the American Hospital Association (*q.v.*).

ailment (āl′-ment): An illness, disease, or complaint.

ailurophobia (ā-loo-rō-fō′-bi-a): Abnormal fear of cats.

air: The colorless, odorless, tasteless gaseous mixture which surrounds the earth. It consists of approximately 4 parts nitrogen to one part of oxygen, contains small amounts of such other substances as carbon dioxide, argon, ozone, neon, ammonia, krypton, and xenon, and variable amounts of water vapor. Also called atmosphere (*q.v.*). A. BED, a rubber mattress inflated with air. COMPLEMENTAL A., the extra air that can be drawn into the lungs by deep inspiration. A. HUNGER, inspiratory and expiratory distress characterized by sighing and gasping; due to anoxia. RESIDUAL A., that which still remains in the alveoli of the lung after forced expiration. STATIONARY A., that which remains after normal expiration. SUPPLEMENTAL A., the extra air that can be expired without effort. A. SICKNESS, altitude sickness (*q.v.*). A. SWALLOWING, aerophagia (*q.v.*). TIDAL A., that which passes in and out of the lung in normal breathing.

airway: 1. Any natural passageway for air. 2. Any one of several kinds of devices for maintaining a clear and unobstructed passageway for air to enter and leave the lungs; often used during general anesthesia.

akathisia (ak-a-thiz′-i-a): Inability to sit still. A state in which the patient feels a distressing inner restlessness that results in motor restlessness.

akinetic (a-kīn-et′-ik): Without movement. A. EPILEPSY, epileptic fits where instead of a tonic and clonic phase the patient is limp, the whole body remaining flaccid until consciousness returns. A. CATATONIA occurs in schizophrenia. A. MUTISM, sustained periods of unconsciousness in which the patient appears to be relaxed and asleep, but he can only be roused for a few moments; occurs in tumors of third ventricle, midbrain, and thalamus.—akinesia, n.

akr-, akro-: See **acr-**.

ala (ā′-la): Any wing-like process.—alae, pl.; alar, adj.

alalia (a-lā′-li-a): Lack of the power of speech; may be caused by impairment of the organs of speech or by a central lesion, or it may be of psychic origin.

alar (ā′-lar): 1. Wing-like. 2. Pertaining to the armpit.

alastrim (al-as′-trim): A tropical disease believed to be a less virulent form of smallpox; may be confused with chickenpox. Variola minor.

Albee's operation (al′-bēz): Produces ankylosis of the hip. Upper surface of head of femur is removed, and corresponding edge of acetabulum. A. BONE GRAFT, operation for spinal fixation. Spinous processes of diseased area are exposed and split. Graft from tibia is placed in raw area. [Fred Houdlett Albee, New York surgeon. 1876-1945.]

Albers-Schönberg disease: A spotty calcifying of the bones, which fracture spontaneously. 'Marble bones.' Syn., osteopetrosis. [Heinrich Ernst Albers-Schönberg, German surgeon. 1865-1921.]

albinism (al′-bin-ism): A recessive genetic condition in which the inability to produce melanin results in lack of pigmentation of the skin, hair, and eyes.

albino (al-bī′-nō): A person affected with albinism (*q.v.*); strictly speaking, a male person so affected.—albiness, f.; albinotic, adj.

albumin (al-bū′-min): Also albumen. A variety of protein found in animal and vegetable matter. It is soluble in water and coagulates on heating. SERUM A., the chief protein of blood plasma and other serous fluids. Lactalbumin is the albumin found in milk.—albuminous, albuminoid, adj.

albuminemia (al-bū-min-ē′-mi-a): The presence of an abnormal amount of albumin in the blood plasma.

albuminometer (al-bū-min-om′-et-er): A graduated test tube in a special stand for estimating quantity of albumin in a fluid.

albuminuria (al-bū-min-ū′-ri-a): The presence of albumin in the urine. Temporary albuminuria may occur in fevers, pregnancy, or after exercise; it usually clears up completely after the cause is removed. It may also be the result of renal impairment caused by kidney disorders, malignant hypertension, congestive heart failure. CHRONIC A. leads to hypoproteinemia (*q.v.*). ORTHOSTATIC or POSTURAL A. is an abnormality of little importance in which A. depends on the upright posture, and is absent in the urine secreted during sleep (the morning specimen).—albuminuric, adj.

albumose (al′-bū-mōs): An early product of proteolysis during gastric digestion. It resembles albumin but is not coagulated by heat.

albumosuria (al-bū-mō-sū′-ri-a): The presence of an albumose in the urine.—albumosuric, adj.

alcohol (al′-ko-hol): A colorless, volatile, flammable liquid produced by fermentation of carbohydrates. The principal constituent of wines and spirits. Taken in small amounts it is a stimulant; in larger amounts it is a depressant. It enhances the action of barbiturates and tranquilizers. Medicinal uses include local application as an antiseptic or astringent; internal use as a cardiac stimulant and for its euphoric effect; as a base for tinctures; to preserve anatomical specimens. As a food, alcohol furnishes about 100 calories of heat per ounce. ABSOLUTE A., contains at least 99% pure alcohol; occasionally used by injection for relief of trigeminal neuralgia and other intractable pain. DENATURED A., has had some substance added to make it unfit for internal use. ETHYL A., ordinary alcohol; made from grain. ISOPROPYL A., used for rubbing and as a disinfectant; not for internal use. METHYL A., made by distilling wood; for external use only. WOOD A., methyl A. RUBBING A., a rubefacient; not for internal use. A. PSYCHOSIS, see **Korsakoff's syndrome.**

alcoholic (al-ko-hol′-ik): 1. Pertaining to or containing alcohol. 2. One who habitually uses alcoholic beverages to excess. A. PSYCHOSES, a group of mental disorders caused by poisoning with alcohol; associated with brain damage; includes delirium tremens, Korsakoff's psychosis, and often hallucinosis.

Alcoholics Anonymous: A fellowship of people previously addicted to alcohol. Their main aim is curing others of alcoholism.

alcoholism (al′-ko-hol-izm): 1. Alcohol poisoning. 2. The overuse of alcohol to the extent that it is uncontrollable. May be acute or chronic. In its chronic form it causes severe disturbances of the nervous and digestive systems.

alcoholuria (al-ko-hol-ū′-ri-a): Alcohol in the urine. Basis of one test for fitness to drive a car after drinking alcohol.

aldehyde (al′-de-hīd): Any of a large class of substances that are formed by the oxidation of alcohol and that contain the chemical group -CHO.

aldosterone (al-dos′-ter-ōn): A potent adrenocortical steroid which, by renal control, regulates electrolyte metabolism; hence described as a 'mineralocorticoid.' Secretion is regulated by the renin-angiotensin system. It increases excretion of potassium and conserves sodium and chloride.

aldosteronism: A condition of eltrolyte balance ;caused by excessive secretion of aldosterone; marked by alkalosis and possibly tetany.

Aldrich's syndrome: A condition caused by a sex-linked recessive trait that is transmitted to a male by an unaffected female; characterized by thrombocytopenic purpura, chronic eczema, chronic suppurative otitis media, anemia and unusual susceptibility to infection; most affected subjects die early in life.

Aleppo boil: See **leishmaniasis.**

alethia (a-lē′-thi-a): A constant dwelling on past events; inability to forget.

aleukemic (a-lū-kē′-mik): See **leukemia.**

aleukia (a-lū′-ki-a): Lack of or abnormal decrease in the number of white blood cells, or of blood platelets.

alexia (a-leks′-i-a): Word blindness; a type of aphasia with loss of ability to interpret the significance of printed or written words, but without loss of visual power or intelligence. Due to a brain lesion.—alexic, adj.

algae (al′-jē): A large group of simple, unicellular marine plants, including seaweed and fresh water plants, varying in size from microscopic to many feet in length. Some are useful as food, others in the preparation of medicinal substances. Algae collect on the top of sand filters and are effective in screening out bacteria thus helping in the purification of water.

algesia (al-jē'-zi-a): Excessive sensitivity to pain; hyperesthesia (*q.v.*).—algesic, adj. Opp. to analgesia.

algesimeter (al-jē-sim'-e-ter): An instrument which registers the degree of sensitivity to pain.

-algia: Denotes pain.

algid (al'-jid): 1. Cold. 2. Condition after a severe attack of fever, especially malaria, with collapse, extreme coldness of the body, suggesting a fatal termination. During this stage the rectal temperature may be high.

alginates (al'-jin-ātz): Seaweed derivatives which, when applied locally, encourage the clotting of blood. They are available in solution and in specially impregnated gauze.

algophily (al-gof'-i-li): Sexual perversion characterized by a morbid love of inflicting, experiencing, or thinking about pain.

algophobia (al-gō-fō'-bi-a): Morbid dread of witnessing or experiencing pain.

algor (al'-gor): Coldness; rigor; a chill. A. MORTIS, the gradual cooling of the body after death.

alienation (ā-li-en-ā'-shun): In psychiatry, mental illness.

alienist (ā'-li-en-ist): One skilled in the treatment of mental disorders; a psychiatrist (*q.v.*). In legal medicine, one qualified to testify in court as an expert concerning mental responsibility.

alignment (a-līn'-ment): Arranging in a straight line, as bones after a fracture. Also alinement.

aliment (al'-i-ment): Food.

alimentary (al-i-ment'-a-ri): Pertaining to food. A. CANAL or TRACT, the passage down which the food goes during the process of digestion; it begins at the mouth and ends at the anus; the structures forming it are the mouth, pharynx, esophagus, stomach, small intestine, colon and rectum. A. SYSTEM, the alimentary canal and those organs connected with it that are concerned with digestion and absorption of food and the elimination of residual waste.

alimentation (al-i-men-tā'-shun): The act of nourishing with food; feeding.

aliquot (al'-i-kwat): Part contained by the whole an integral number of times. The sample withdrawn from a 24-hour urine specimen.

alkalemia (al-kal-ē'-mi-a): An increase in the alkalinity of the blood which normally has a *p*H of 7.4. See **alkalosis.**—alkalemic, adj.

alkali (al'-kal-ī): Any one of a class of soluble bases which neutralize acids to form salts and combine with fats to form soaps. Alkaline solutions turn red litmus blue.— alkalis, pl. A. RESERVE, a biochemical term denoting the amount of buffered alkali (normally bicarbonate) available in the blood for the neutralization of acids formed in or introduced into the body. When the alkali reserve falls, acidosis results; when it rises above normal, alkalosis results.

alkaline (al'-kal-īn): 1. Possessing the properties of or pertaining to an alkali. 2. Containing an excess of hydroxyl over hydrogen ions.

alkaline ash diet: A diet consisting of foods that produce an alkaline ash when metabolized; includes fruits, vegetables, milk and some other proteins.

alkaline reserve: The amount of alkaline compounds, chiefly sodium bicarbonate, present in the body fluids and capable of neutralizing acids.

alkalinuria (al-kal-in-ūr'-i-a): Alkalinity of urine.—alkalinuric, adj.

alkaloid (al'-kal-oid): Resembling an alkali. A name often applied to a large group of organic bases found in the leaves, seeds, bark, and other parts of plants and which possess important physiological actions. Morphine, quinine, caffeine, atropine and strychnine are well-known examples of alkaloids.—alkaloidal, adj.

alkalosis (al-kal-ō'-sis): Excess of alkali or reduction of acid in the body. Develops from a variety of causes such as overdosage with alkali, excessive vomiting or diarrhea, and hyperventilation. See **hyperpnea.** Results in neuromuscular excitability expressed clinically as tetany (*q.v.*).

alkaptonuria (al-kap-ton-ūr'-i-a): The presence of homogenistic acid in the urine, resulting from only partial oxidation of phenylalanine and tryosine; the urine turns brown on standing.

allantiasis (al-an-tī'-a-sis): Sausage poisoning; botulism.

allantois (al-an'-tō-is): A tubular diverticulum of the posterior part of the yolk sac of the embryo, passing into the body stalk, thus taking part in the formation of the umbilical cord and, later, the placenta.— allantoic, allantoid, adj.

allelomorphs (a-lē'-lō-morfs): Inherited

characteristics which are alternative and contrasting (typical of artificial selection), such as tallness or shortness. Also, the genes on which these characteristics depend. The basis of Mendel's law of dominants and recessives.—allelomorphic, adj.; allelomorphism, n.

allergen (al′-er-jen): Any agent capable of producing a state or manifestation of allergy; may be protein or nonprotein, *e.g.,* foods, drugs, animal hair or fur, pollens, dust, fungi, bacteria.—allergenic, adj.; allergenicity, n.

allergy (al′-er-ji): A hypersensitive reaction to a particular allergen (*q.v.*) or a foreign substance (which is harmless to the great majority of individuals), following initial sensitizing contact, as in hay fever, asthma, urticaria, vasomotor rhinitis, reactions to drugs, and contact dermatitis. It is due to an antigen-antibody reaction, though the antibody formed is not always demonstrable.—allergic, adj. See **anaphylaxis** and **sensitization.**

allochiria (a-lō-kī′-ri-a): An abnormality of tactile sensibility under test, wherein the patient refers a given stimulus to the other side of the body. Also allocheiria.

all-or-none law: States that when a nerve fiber or muscle fiber is stimulated it responds to its fullest extent or not at all.

allotriophagy (a-lot-ri-of′-a-ji): The eating of injurious or usually non-edible substances. Pica.

allotropism (a-lot′-rō-pizm): The existence of an element in two or more distinct forms each having its own distinct characteristics. —allotrope, n.; allotropic, adj.

alopecia (al-ō-pē′-shi-a): Baldness which can be congenital, premature or senile. A. AREATA, a patchy baldness, usually of a temporary nature. Cause unknown, but shock and anxiety are common precipitating factors. Exclamation mark hairs are diagnostic. A. CICATRISATA, syn., pseudopelade; progressive, irreversible A. of the scalp in which tufts of normal hair occur between many bald patches. Folliculitis decalvans is an A. of the scalp characterized by pustulation and scars.

Exclamation mark hair

alteregoism (awl-ter-ē′-go-izm): Having an interest only in those persons whose situation is similar to one's own.

alternating pressure mattress: See **pulsating mattress.**

alt. hor.: Abbreviation for *alternis horis,* meaning every other hour.

altitude sickness: Occurs during airplane flights at high altitudes, due to lessened oxygen pressure; symptoms include headache, lassitude, fatigue, sleepiness, sometimes depression.

alveolitis (al-vē-ō-lī′-tis): Inflammation of an alveolus.Term sometimes used instead of pyorrhea.

alveolus (al-vē′-o-lus): In anatomy, a term used to designate a small cavity or a saclike dilatation; a tooth socket; an air vesicle of the lung; or a gland follicle or acinus. —alveoli, pl.; alveolar, adj.

Alzheimer's disease: A form of presenile dementia caused by atrophy of the prefrontal lobes of the brain, due to hyaline degeneration of medium and smaller cerebral blood vessels; usually occurs in patients under fifty. [Alois Alzheimer, German physician. 1864-1915.]

A.M.: Abbreviation for *ante meridian,* meaning before noon.

AMA: Abbreviation for American Medical Association (*q.v.*). Organized in 1847; devoted to the promotion and improvement of medicine and public health; official publication is the *Journal of the American Medical Association,* abbreviated *JAMA.*

amalgam (a-mal′-gam): An alloy of mercury. DENTAL A., used for filling teeth; contains mercury, silver and tin.

amastia (a-mas′-ti-a): Congenital absence of the breasts.

amaurosis (am-aw-rō′-sis): Partial or total blindness, particularly that which occurs without apparent disease or lesion of the eye; often temporary.

amaurotic familial idiocy: A form of familial subnormality of unknown cause but thought to be due to a congenital defect in the metabolism of fats; characterized by progressive degeneration of the nervous system with convulsions, ataxia, spasticity, weakness of extremities, lack of mental development, progressive blindness due to optic atrophy. Tay-Sachs disease.

ambi-: Denotes both, on both sides.

ambidextrous (am-bi-deks′-trus): Able to use both hands equally well.—ambidexter, adj.; ambidexterity, n.

ambiopia (am-bi-ō′-pi-a): Diplopia (*q.v.*).

ambivalence (am-biv′-al-ens): 1. Coexistence of contradictory and opposing emotions toward one person or object at the same time; *e.g.,* love and hate. 2. The conflict caused by an incentive that is at once positive and negative.—ambivalent, adj.

ambivalent (am-biv'-al-ent): 1. Pertaining to or characterized by ambivalence (*q.v.*). 2. A normal type of personality varying between introversion and extroversion (*q.v.*).

amblyopia (am-bli-ō'-pi-a): Defective vision when there is no detectable disease of the eye or error in refraction.—amblyopic, adj.

amboceptor (am-bo-sep'-tor): The antibody developed in immune serum which, in association with complement, causes lysis of the specific bacteria or other antigen to which the host has been sensitized. See **antibodies.**

ambulant (am'-bū-lant): Able to walk.

ambulatory (am'-bū-la-tor-i): Mobile. Walking about. A. TREATMENT, method of treatment which insists on keeping the patient on his feet as much as possible.

ameba (am-ē'-ba): An elementary unicellular protozoon that moves by extruding pseudopodia (*q.v.*), is capable of ingestion, absorption, respiration, excretion, and reproduction by simple fission. *Entamoeba histolytica* is one form parasitic to man, causing amebic dysentery. Also amoeba. —amebae, amebas, amoebae, pl.; amebic, amoebic, adj.

amebiasis (am-ē-bī'-a-sis): Infestation of the large intestine by the protozoon *Entamoeba histolytica,* where it causes ulceration by invasion of the mucosa. This results in passage per rectum of necrotic mucous membrane and blood, hence the term "amebic dysentery." If the amebae enter the portal circulation they may cause liver necrosis (hepatic abscess). Diagnosis is by isolating the ameba in the stools. Also amoebiasis.

amebic (a-mē'-bik): Pertaining to, resembling, or caused by an ameba. Also amoebic.

amebicide (am-ē'-bi-sīd): An agent that

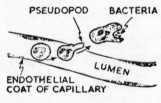

PSEUDOPOD   BACTERIA

ENDOTHELIAL
COAT OF CAPILLARY

LUMEN

**Ameboid movement of white
blood cells**

kills amebae.—amebicidal, adj.

ameboid (am-ē'-boid): Resembling an ameba in shape or in mode of movement; *e.g.,* white blood cells.

amelanotic (a-mel-a-not'-ik): Without pigment.

amelia (a-mē'-li-a): Congenital absence of a limb or limbs. COMPLETE A., absence of both arms and legs.

amelioration (a-mē-li-or-ā'-shun): Reduction of the severity of symptoms. Improvement in the general condition.

amenorrhea (a-men-ō-rē'-a): Absence of the menses. PRIMARY A., Failure of menstruation to become established at puberty. SECONDARY A., absence of the menses after they have once commenced.—amenorrheal, adj.

amentia (a-men'-shi-a): Congenital mental subnormality; to be distinguished from "dementia."

American Hospital Association: Organized in 1899 and devoted chiefly to promoting and maintaining high standards of care in hospitals in the United States. *Hospitals* is its official publication.

American Journal of Nursing: The official publication of the American Nurses' Association; abbreviated *AJN;* published monthly. The American Journal of Nursing Company also assumes responsibility for the publication of *Nursing Outlook, Nursing Research,* and (in cooperation with the National Library of Medicine) the *International Nursing Index.*

American Nurses' Association: Founded in 1908 after having been affiliated for 12 years with an association that also included Canadian nurses. It is the official organization for graduate nurses in the U.S.; its official publication is the *American Journal of Nursing.* Its purposes are to promote the professional and educational advancement of nurses, bring nurses into contact with each other, disseminate information about nursing.

American Nurses' Foundation: A separate organization established by the American Nurses' Association in 1955. It promotes and conducts nursing research and disseminates research findings.

American Red Cross: See Red Cross, International Red Cross.

ametria (a-mē'-tri-a): Congenital absence of the uterus.

ametropia (a-met-rō'-pi-a): Defective sight due to imperfect refractive power of the eye that prevents images from focusing properly on the retina.—ametropic, adj., ametrope, n.

Amigen (am'-i-jen): Protein nutrients for intravenous injection.

amines (am'-ēns): Name given to organic compounds that contain the amino group (NH_2). They are derived from ammonia; important in biochemistry.

amino acids (am'-i-nō, a-mē'-nō): Organic acids in which one or more of the hydrogen atoms are replaced by the amino group, NH_2. They are the end product of protein hydrolysis and from them the body resynthesizes its protein. Ten cannot be elaborated in the body and are therefore essential in the diet—arginine, histidine, isoleucine, leucine, lysine, methionine, phenylalanine, threonine, tryptophan and valine. The others are designated nonessential A.A.

amino-aciduria (am-i-nō-as-i-dū'-ri-a): Increase in urinary secretion of amino acids.

amitosis (a-mĭ-tō'-sis): Multiplication of a cell by direct fission.—amitotic, adj.

ammonia (a-mō'-ni-a): A colorless, volatile, alkaline gas with a pungent odor, formed by decomposition of nitrogenous matter. Highly soluble in water; widely used for cleaning purposes. AROMATIC SPIRIT OF A., solution of ammonia, water and aromatic oils; has fleeting action as a circulatory and respiratory stimulant; used in cases of fainting.

amnesia (am-nē'-zi-a): Partial or complete loss of memory for past experiences; memory is not destroyed, for the experiences may be recalled without relearning when the patient recovers from the amnesia. May be caused by concussion, electroshock, dementia, hysteria, senility, alcoholism. ANTEROGRADE A., loss of memory for recent events. RETROGRADE A., loss of memory for events that occurred before the incident that caused the amnesia.—amnesic, adj.

amniocentesis (am-ni-ō-sen-tē'-sis): Removal of a small amount of amniotic fluid from its sac by aspiration through the abdominal wall for diagnostic purposes. Analysis of the chromosomes or enzyme production of the fetal cells can determine as many as 35 disorders of the fetus's body chemistry that may lead to mental or physical retardation and sometimes death; e.g., mongolism or the presence of a deforming virus infection such as German measles. The liquor contains increased hemoglobin products in Rhesus incompatability.

This kind of prenatal diagnosis is currently available only in the larger medical centers.

amniography (am-ni-og'-ra-fi): X-ray of the gravid uterus after the amniotic sac has been injected with an opaque medium; outlines the umbilical cord and placenta. Used as a diagnostic aid when placenta previa is suspected.—amniogram, n.; amniographical, adj.; amniographically, adv.

amnion (am'-ni-on): The innermost membrane enclosing the fetus and containing the amniotic fluid (liquor amnii). It ensheaths the umbilical cord and is connected with the fetus at the umbilicus. Also called the bag of waters.—amnionic, amniotic, adj.

amnioscopy (am-ni-os'-ko-pi): Inspection of the amniotic sac using an optical instrument (amnioscope).—amnioscopic, adj.; amnioscopically, adv.

amniotic fluid infusion: Escape of amniotic fluid into the maternal circulation.

amniotome (am'-ni-o-tōm): An instrument for rupturing the fetal membranes.

amniotomy (am-ni-ot'-o-mi): Surgical rupture of the fetal membranes to induce or expedite labor.

amok (a-mok'): A wild, frenzied, maniacal manner of behavior that threatens harm to others.

amorphous (a-mor'-fus): Having no regular shape; formless.—amorphia, amorphism, n.

amor sui: Love of self; vanity.

ampere (am'-peer): The unit of intensity of an electric current.

amph-, amphi-: Denotes around, on both sides, both.

amphetamines (am-fet'-a-mēnz): A group of chemical substances that stimulate the cerebral cortex of the brain; highly addicting. Sometimes used in therapy and often misused by both adults and adolescents to produce euphoria and control fatigue.

amphiarthrosis (am-fi-arth-rō'-sis): A slightly movable joint. The articulating surfaces are separated by fibrocartilage.—amphiarthroses, pl.

amphitrichate (am-fi-trī'-kāt): Describing a microorganism that has a flagellum or flagella at both ends.

amphoteric (am-fō-ter'-ik): Having two opposite characteristics; said especially of a substance that reacts as either an acid or a base.

ampule (am'-pūl): A small, hermetically sealed glass vial containing a single sterile dose of a drug. Also ampul, ampoule.

ampulla (am-pool′-a): Any flask-like dilatation. A. OF VATER, the enlargement formed by the union of the common bile duct with the pancreatic duct where they enter the duodenum. [Abraham Vater, German anatomist. 1684-1751.]—ampullae, pl.; ampullar, ampullary, ampullate, adj.

amputation (am-pū-tā′-shun): Removal of an appending part, generally by surgery; e.g., breast, limb.

amputee (am-pū-tē′): A person who has had one or more limbs amputated.

amylase (am′-i-lās): Any enzyme which converts starches into sugars. PANCREATIC A., amylopsin (q.v.). SALIVARY A., ptyalin (q.v.).

amyloid (am′-i-loid): 1. Starchlike. 2. A waxlike protein complex that has some starchlike qualities; may be deposited in tissues in certain pathological states. See **amyloidosis.**

amyloidosis (am-i-loid-ō′-sis): A disease in which amyloid is formed and deposited in body tissues or organs, especially the liver and kidney. It may occur in the terminal phase of any toxic condition of long duration. Also amyloid degeneration.

amylolysis (am-i-lol′-is-is): The digestion of starch.—amylolytic, adj.

amylopsin (am-i-lop′-sin): A pancreatic enzyme, which, in an alkaline medium, converts insoluble starch into soluble maltose.

amylose (am′-i-lōs): Polysaccharide (q.v.).

amylum (am′-i-lum): Starch.

amyluria (am-i-lū′-ri-a): Starch in the urine.

amyocardia (a-mī-ō-kar′-di-a): Weakness of the heart muscle.

amyotonia (a-mī-ō-tō′-ni-a): Myatonia. Lack or loss of muscle tone.

amyotrophic lateral sclerosis: See **sclerosis.**

amyotrophy (a-mi-ot′-rō-fi): Progressive muscle wasting or atrophy. Also amyotrophia.—amyotrophic, adj.

ANA: Abbreviation for the American Nurses' Association (q.v.).

ana-: Denotes up, upward, back, backward, excessive, again.

anabasis (an-ab′-a-sis): A stage of worsening in a disease.

anabolic (an-a-bol′-ik): Pertaining to or promoting anabolism. A. COMPOUND, a chemical substance that causes a synthesis of body protein.

anabolism (an-ab′-ōl-izm): The constructive phase of metabolism during which nutritive

substances are utilized to form body substance.—anabolic, adj.

anachlorhydria (an-a-klor-hī′-dri-a): Lack of hydrochloric acid in the gastric juice.

anacholia (an-a-kō′-li-a): Decrease in the secretion of bile.

anacidity (an-as-id′-it-i): Lack of normal acidity, especially in the gastric juice. See **achlorhydria.**

anaclitic (an-a-klit′-ik): Depending on others; refers especially to the infant. A. DEPRESSION, that which occurs in all aspects of an infant's development following its separation from its mother or mother surrogate.

anacrotism (an-ak′-rot-izm): An oscillation in the ascending curve of a sphygmographic pulse tracing, occurring in aortic stenosis.—anacrotic, adj.

anacusis (an-a-kū′-sis): Absence or loss of hearing. Also anacusia, anacousia, anakusis.

anaerobe (an-ā′-er-ōb): A microorganism which will not grow in the presence of molecular oxygen. When this is strictly so, it is termed an 'obligatory A.' The majority of pathogens are indifferent to atmospheric conditions and will flourish in the presence or absence of oxygen and are therefore termed 'facultative anaerobes.'—anaerobic, adj.

anal (ā′-nal): Pertaining to, or relating to the anus. A. EROTICISM, deriving sexual pleasure from anal functions. A. FISSURE, a crack or slit in the mucous membrane at the margin of the anus. A. FISTULA, an abnormal opening onto the skin or mucous membrane near the anus; it may or may not communicate with the rectum. A. PHASE, the period in a child's development, usually from one to three years of age, when he is intensely interested in the process and products of defecation.

analeptic (an-a-lep′-tik): Restorative. Most analeptics stimulate the central nervous system. 'Household' analeptics include smelling salts, cordials, whisky and brandy.

analgesia (an-al-jē′-zi-a): Loss of painful impressions without loss of consciousness. —analgesic, analgetic, adj.

analgesic (an-al-jē′-zik): 1. Insensible to pain. 2. Alleviating pain. 3. A drug that relieves pain. Syn., anodyne.

analgia (an-al′-ji-a): Without pain.—analgic, adj.

analogous (an-al′-o-gus): Similar in function, but not in origin.—analogue, n.

analysand (an-al′-i-sand): That which is

being analyzed; one who is under psycho-analysis.

analysis (an-al′-i-sis): In chemistry, a term used to denote the determination of the composition of a compound substance. In psychiatry, psychoanalysis (*q.v.*).—analyses, pl.; analytic, adj.; analytically, adv.

analyst (an′-a-list): A person experienced in performing analyses. In psychiatry, a psychoanalyst (*q.v.*).

anamnesis (an-am-nē′-sis): 1. The act of remembering or recalling to mind. 2. That which is recollected. 3. A medical history of a patient.

ananastasia (an-an-a-stā′-zi-a): Lack or loss of ability to stand up or to arise from a sitting position; due to abulia (*q.v.*).

anandria (an-an′-dri-a): Lack or loss of virility or masculinity.

anaphase (an′-a-fāz): A phase in mitosis (*q.v.*).

anaphia (an-ā′-fi-a): Loss or lack of the sense of touch.—anaptic, adj.

anaphoresis (an-a-for-ē′-sis): Absence or reduction of secretion of sweat.

anaphrodisia (an-af-rō-diz′-i-a): Lack or loss of sexual impulse.

anaphrodisiac (an-af-rō-diz′-i-ak): An agent that diminishes sexual desire. Also antaphrodisiac.

anaphylactin (an-a-fil-ak′-tin): An agent that is thought to be responsible for producing a state of anaphylaxis (*q.v.*).

anaphylactogen (an-a-fil-ak′-to-jen): A substance that induces a state of anaphylaxis.

anaphylactoid (an-a-fil-ak′-toid): Pertaining to or resembling anaphylaxis.

anaphylaxis (an-a-fil-ak′-sis): A hypersensitive state of the body to a foreign protein (*e.g.,* horse serum) so that the injection of a second dose after ten days brings about an acute reaction which may be fatal; in lesser degree it produces breathlessness, pallor, shock in varying degrees, and collapse. In mild cases, symptoms include fever, reddening of the skin, itching and hives.—anaphylactic, adj. See **allergy** and **sensitization.**

anaplasia (an-a-plāz′-i-a): Loss of the distinctive characteristics of a cell, with reversion to a more primitive type, often associated with proliferative activity as in cancer.—anaplastic, adj.

anarithmia (an-a-rith′-mi-a): Loss of ability to count and/or use numbers correctly, thought to be due to a brain lesion.

anarthria (an-ar′-thri-a): Loss of ability to pronounce words distinctly, due to muscle

dysfunction; thought to result from a brain lesion.

anasarca (an-a-sark′-a): Serous infiltration of the subcutaneous connective tissue and serous cavities; generalized edema; dropsy.—anasarcous, adj.

anastomosis (an-as-to-mō′-sis): 1. The intercommunication of the branches of two or more arteries or veins. 2. In surgery, the establishment of an intercommunication between two hollow organs, vessels or nerves.—anastomoses, pl.; anastomotic, adj.; anastomose, v.i., v.t.

anatherapeusis (an-a-ther-a-pū′-sis): Treatment by steadily increasing doses of a medication.

anatomist (a-nat′-o-mist): One who specializes in the study of anatomy or who performs dissections.

anatomy (a-nat′-o-mi): The science that deals with the structure and composition of the body; it is largely based on dissection.—anatomical, adj.; anatomically, adv.

anatoxin (an-a-toks′-in): Syn., toxoid (*q.v.*).

anatripsis (an-a-trip′-sis): The use of rubbing or friction as a treatment. May or may not include the simultaneous application of a medicament.

anazoturia (an-a-zō-tūr′-i-a): Less than the normal amount of nitrogenous substances in the urine.

anchyl-: See **ankyl-.**

ancon (ang′-kon): The elbow joint.—ancones, pl.; anconoid, adj.

anconitis (ang-kō-nī′-tis): Inflammation of the elbow joint.

ancyl-: See **ankyl-.**

Ancylostoma (an-si-los′-tō-ma): A genus of nematodes, including the hookworms.

ancylostomiasis (an-si-lōs-tō-mī′-a-sis): Hookworm disease (*q.v.*).

andr-, andro-: Denotes man, male; having the characteristics of a man.

androgen (an′-drō-jen): Any substance that stimulates development and preservation of the secondary male characteristics; usually a hormone such as testosterone (*q.v.*). When given to females these substances have a masculinizing effect.—androgenic, androgenous, adj.

androgynus (an-droj′-i-nus): An individual with both male and female characteristics. Also androgyne. See **hermaphrodite.**—androgynous, adj.; androgynism, n.

andromania (an-drō-mā′-ni-a): Nymphomania (*q.v.*).

androphobia (an-drō-fō′-bi-a): A morbid dislike or fear of men or of the male sex.—androphobic, adj.

androsterone (an-dros′-ter-ōn): An androgenic hormone found in the urine; also prepared synthetically.

anemia (a-nē′-mi-a): Term applied to a large group of disorders that result from deficiency in the number of red blood cells or their hemoglobin content, or both. Types are differentiated on the basis of cause, hereditary factors, size, shape and hemoglobin content of the red blood cells, response to therapy, etc. Also classified as primary when due to disease of the blood or blood-producing organs; secondary when it is the result of another pathological condition such as cancer, bleeding ulcers, etc. Clinical features include pallor, easy fatigue, breathlessness on exertion, giddiness, palpitation, loss of appetite, gastrointestinal disorders and amenorrhea. ADDISONIAN A., pernicious A. COOLEY'S A., thalassemia (*q.v.*). HEMOLYTIC A., a type characterized by excessive destruction of the red blood cells. See **acholuric jaundice.** IRON DEFICIENCY A., by far the commonest type; due to insufficient intake of iron because of inadequate or ill-balanced diet, or impaired absorption, or to increased bodily needs as in pregnancy, or to excessive loss as in hemorrhage. MACROCYTIC A., a group of anemias characterized by abnormally large red blood cells of which the commonest causes are deficiency of either vitamin B$_{12}$ or folic acid. See **Banti's disease.** PERNICIOUS A., a chronic disorder primarily of middle and old age due to atrophy of the stomach mucosa and its consequent failure to produce a factor necessary for the absorption of vitamin B$_{12}$, and treated by regular and lifelong injections of the vitamin. SICKLE CELL A., a hereditary and familial type of A., peculiar to Negroes; the red cells acquire a characteristic crescent or sickle shape; sometimes accompanied by pain and leg ulcers.

anemophobia (an-e-mō-fō′-bi-a): Abnormal fear of wind or draughts of air.

anencephalia (an-en-sef-ā′-li-a): Congenital absence of the brain. A term used in connection with fetal monsters. The condition is incompatible with life. Also anencephaly.—anencephalous, anencephalic, adj.

anepia (an-ēp′-i-a): Lack of ability to speak.

anergy (an′-er-ji): 1. Lethargy; inactivity; sluggishness. 2. Decreased sensitivity to specific antigens. Also anergia.—anergic, adj.

anesthesia (an-es-thēz′-i-a): Loss of sensation in a part of the body or the whole of it. May be caused by introduction of a drug, trauma, disease, or hypnosis. GENERAL A., loss of sensation with loss of consciousness. In LOCAL A. the nerve conduction is blocked and painful impulses fail to reach the brain. SPINAL A., may be caused by (1) injection of an anesthetic into the spinal subarachnoid space; (2) a lesion of the spinal cord.

anesthesiologist (an-es-thēz-i-ol′-o-jist): A physician who specializes in anesthesiology (*q.v.*).

anesthesiology (an-es-thēz-i-ol′-o-ji): The science of anesthetics, their administration and effects.

anesthetic (an-es-thet′-ik): 1. A drug that produces anesthesia. 2. Causing anesthesia. 3. Insensible to stimuli. GENERAL A., a drug that produces general anesthesia (*q.v.*) by inhalation or injection. LOCAL A., a drug that causes local insensibility to pain when injected into the tissues or applied topically.

anesthetist (an-es′-the-tist): One who administers anesthetics.

anesthetization (an-es-thet-i-zā′-shun): The act of producing insensibility to pain through the administration of an anesthetic (*q.v.*).—anesthetize, v.t.

aneuria (a-nū′-ri-a): Lack of nervous energy.—aneuric, adj.

aneurin(e) (an-ū′-rin): Thiamine or vitamin B$_1$. See **thiamine.**

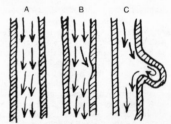

Development of aneurysm
A. normal B. weakness in wall of artery C. aneurysm

aneurysm (an′-ūr-izm): Permanent local dilatation of a blood vessel, most commonly the aorta, due to fault in the wall through defect, disease or injury, producing a pulsating swelling over which a murmur may be heard. ARTERIOVENOUS A., an abnormal direct connection between an artery and a vein, usually following an injury. CIRSOID A., a tangled mass of pulsating blood vessels, appearing as a subcutaneous tumor, usually on the scalp. FALSE A., one in which all the coats of the vessel rupture and the blood is retained by the surrounding tissues.

angi-, angio-: Denotes a vessel(s), particularly a blood vessel.

angiectasis (an-ji-ek′-ta-sis): Abnormal dilatation of blood vessels.—angiectatic, adj. See **telangiectasis.**

angiitis (an-ji-ī′-tis): Inflammation of a blood or lymph vessel.—angiitic, adj.

angina (an-jī′-na): A sense of suffocation, choking, or constriction; or a disease characterized by spasmodic suffocative attacks. LUDWIG′S A., a severe, acute, purulent infection of the floor of the mouth, particularly around the submaxillary gland, usually caused by streptococcus; may originate with a dental infection. See **cellulitis.** A. PECTORIS, severe but temporary paroxysmal attack of cardiac pain which may radiate to shoulder or arm, accompanied by feeling of suffocation and impending death. Results from cardiac ischemia; usually caused by cardiac disease, but may be precipitated by exercise or emotional stress. VINCENT′S A., an infection of the mouth, particularly the gums, but may extend to the tonsils and pharynx; caused by a spirochete and bacillus in synergism. Necrosis of the gingiva is one of its main features. Seen mostly in adolescents. Also trench mouth. —anginal, anginoid, adj.

angiocardiogram (an-ji-ō-kar′-di-ō-gram): Film demonstrating the heart and great vessels after intravenous injection of opaque medium.

angiocardiography (an-ji-ō-kar-di-og′-ra-fi): Demonstration of heart and great vessels by means of injection of opaque medium into cardiac circulation.—angiocardiographic, adj.; angiocardiographically, adv.

angiocarditis (an-ji-ō-kar-dī′-tis): Inflammation of the great vessels and the heart.

angiocholecystitis (an-ji-ō-kōl-ē-sis-tī′-tis): Inflammation of bile ducts and gall bladder.

angiodermatitis (an-ji-ō-der-ma-tī′-tis): Inflammation of the blood vessels of the skin.

angiography (an-ji-og′-ra-fi): Demonstration of the arterial system by means of injection of opaque medium.—angiogram, n.; angiographic, adj.; angiographically, adv.

angiokeratoma (an-ji-ō-ker-a-tō′-ma): A skin disease characterized by thickening of the epidermis and appearance of wart-like elevations.

angiolipoma (an-ji-ō-lip-ō′-ma): An angioma that contains fat; seen mostly in subcutaneous tissue.

angiolith (an′-ji-ō-lith): A calculus in the wall of a blood vessel.

angiology (an-ji-ol′-o-ji): The science dealing with blood and lymphatic vessels. —angiological, adj.; angiologically, adv.

angiolymphitis (an-ji-ō-lim-fī′-tis): Lymphangitis (q.v.).

angioma (an-ji-ō′-ma): An innocent tumor formed of blood vessels. See **hemangioma, lymphangioma.** CAVERNOUS A., A tumor of erectile connective tissue in which the larger spaces are filled with blood.—angiomatous, adj.; angiomata, pl.

angiomalacia (an-ji-ō-ma-lā′-shi-a): Softening of the blood vessel walls.

angiomegaly (an-ji-ō-meg′-a-li): Enlargement of one or more blood vessels, particularly when it occurs in the eyelid.

angioneurosis (an-ji-ō-nū-rō′-sis): A condition caused by injury or disease of the nerves of the vasomotor system.

angioneurotic edema (an-ji-ō-nū-rot′-ik ē-dē′-ma): A condition characterized by sudden development of local lesions resembling urticaria, accompanied by swelling of subcutaneous and submucous tissues. One form is thought to be due to allergy, usually food allergy; another is considered to be hereditary and may be fatal; in some cases the cause is unknown. May involve the face, hands or genitals, and mucous membrane of the mouth and throat; edema of the glottis may be fatal. Occasionally, forms part of the picture in anaphylaxis and penicillin sensitization.

angioplasty (an′-ji-ō-plas-ti): Plastic surgery of blood vessels.—angioplastic, adj.

angiosarcoma (an-ji-ō-sar-kō′-ma): A malignant tumor arising from blood vessels and containing many fine blood or lymph vessels.—angiosarcomatous, adj.; angiosarcomata, pl.

angiosclerosis (an-ji-ō-skler-ō′-sis): Hardening of the blood vessel walls; usually involves arteries, veins, and capillaries.

angiospasm (an′-ji-ō-spazm): Constricting spasm of a blood vessel.

angiostenosis (an-ji-ō-sten-ō′-sis): Narrowing of the lumen of a vessel; usually refers to a blood vessel.

angiotensin (an-ji-ō-ten′-sin): A polypeptide formed by the action on a plasma substrate of the enzyme renin (q.v.) found in the kidney cortex. A potent vasoconstrictor substance, and has been synthesized. Formerly called angiotonin or hypertensin.

angor (ang'-or): A feeling of extreme distress or anguish. Angina (*q.v.*). A. ANIMI, a deep sense of impending doom; common in angina pectoris.

Angström unit: An internationally adopted unit of measurement, used primarily to express electromagnetic wavelengths. Equals 0.0000001 of a millimeter; 1/10,000 of a micron; 1/254,000,000 of an inch. [A. J. Angström, Swedish physicist. 1814-1874.]

anhapia (an-hā'-fi-a): Anaphia (*q.v.*).

anhedonia (an-hē-dō'-ni-a): The inability to experience happiness.

anhidrosis (an-hī-drō'-sis): Absence or deficiency of sweat secretion.—anhidrotic, adj.

anhidrotic (an-hīd-rot'-ik): 1. Reducing perspiration. 2. An agent that reduces perspiration.

anhydremia (an-hīd-rēm'-i-a): Decreased fluid content of the blood.—anhydremic, adj.

anhydrous (an-hīd'-rus): Entirely without water, dry.

anicteric (an-ik'-ter-ik): Without jaundice.

anile (ā'-nīl): Infirm, particularly in reference to old women. Old-womanish.—anility, n.

aniline (an'-i-lin): An oily compound obtained from the dry distillation of coal and much used in the preparation of dyes for medical as well as industrial uses.

anima (an'-i-ma): In psychiatry, the inner being or personality as contrasted with the persona or outer character of a person. See **persona.**

animate (an'-i-mat): Having life.

anion (an'-ī-on): A negatively charged ion that is attracted to and moves toward the positively charged anode during electrolysis (*q.v.*).

aniridia (an-i-rid'-i-a): Lack or defect of the iris; usually congenital and usually bilateral. Also called irideremia.

anis-, aniso-: Denotes irregular or unequal.

anischuria (an-is-kū'-ri-a): Incontinence of urine.

aniseikonia (an-i-sī-kō'-ni-a): A visual defect in which the retinal image of an object is different in the two eyes.

anisochromatic (an-i-sō-krō-mat'-ik): Not of uniform color throughout.

anisocoria (an-i-sō-kō'-ri-a): Inequality in the diameter of the pupils.

anisocytosis (an-i-sō-sī-tō'-sis): Inequality in the size of cells that are normally uniform, especially red blood cells.

anisodactyly (an-i-sō-dak'-ti-li): Unequal length in corresponding digits.—anisodactylous, adj.

anisognathous (an-i-sog'-na-thus): Having jaws of unequal size with the upper one usually being the larger.

anisomastia (an-i-sō-mas'-ti-a): Inequality in the size of the breasts.

anisomelia (an-i-sō-mē'-li-a): A condition of inequality between two paired limbs.

anisometropia (an-i-sō-me-trō'-pi-a): A difference in the refractive power of the two eyes, usually correctable by ordinary lenses.

anisopiesis (an-i-sō-pī-ē'-sis): Inequality of arterial blood pressure in different parts of the body as registered by a sphygmomanometer.

anisuria (an-i-sū'-ri-a): A condition marked by changes in the amount of urine excreted, alternating between polyuria and oliguria.

ankle (ang'-kl): A synovial hinge joint, the distal ends of the tibia and fibula articulating with the talus (astragalus); the joint between the lower leg and the foot. A. CLONUS, a series of rapid muscular contractions of the calf muscle when the foot is dorsiflexed by pressure upon the sole. A. JERK, contraction of calf muscles causing extension of the foot, elicited by tapping the tendon of Achilles.

ankyl-, ankylo-: Denotes: (1) crooked, curved; (2) stiff, immobile, constricted or closed because of adhesion.

ankyloblepharon (ang-ki-lō-blef'-a-ron): Adhesion of the ciliary edges of the eyelids to each other.

ankylocolpos (ang-ki-lō-kol'-pos): Imperforation of the vagina due to adhesion of the vaginal walls.

ankylodactylia (ang-ki-lō-dak-til'-i-a): A deformity in which two or more fingers or toes are in adhesion with each other.

ankyloglossia (ang-ki-lō-glos'-i-a): Tongue-tie.

ankylosis (ang-ki-lō'-sis): Stiffness or fixation of a joint.—ankylose, v.t., v.i.; ankylosed, adj.

Ankylostoma: Ancylostoma (*q.v.*).

ankylostomiasis: Ancylostomiasis (*q.v.*).

annular (an'-ū-lar): Ring-shaped. A. LIGAMENTS, surround adjoining parts and bind them together; *e.g.*, A. L. of the wrist and of the ankle.

annulus (an'-ū-lus): A ring or ring-like structure. Also anulus.

ano-: Denotes: (1) anus; (2) upper or upward, *e.g.*, anoopsia.

anoci-association (a-nō-si-a-sō-si-ā'-shun):

A method of preventing or minimizing surgical shock by allaying the patient's anxiety, fear, or apprehension through the use of sedatives and hypnotics previous to anesthesia, and by measures that reduce postoperative discomfort.

anode (an'-ōd): The positive pole or terminus of an electric source such as the galvanic battery.—anodal, anodic, adj.

anodmia (an-od'-mi-a): Anosmia (*q. v.*).

anodontia (an-ō-don'-shi-a): Absence of the teeth; may be congenital or, in an older person, due to removal.

anodyne (an'-ō-dīn): A remedy that relieves pain. Analgesic.

anodynia (an-ō-din'-i-a): Absence of pain.

anomaly (a-nom'-a-li): That which is unusual, abnormal or uncomforming; that in which there is marked deviation from the normal in form, structure, or location.—anomalous, adj.

anomia (an-ō'-mi-a): Inability to name objects or persons. Same as nominal aphasia.

anonychia (an-ō-nik'-i-a): Absence of a nail or nails.

anoopsia (an-ō-op'-si-a): Strabismus in which there is a tendency for the eye to turn upward.

Anopheles (a-nof'-e-lēz): A genus of mosquito. The females are the host of the malarial parasite, and their bite is the means of transmitting the disease to man. See **malaria.**

anophoria (an-o-fō'-ri-a): The condition in which one eye turns upward because its visual axis rises above that of the other eye which is normal. Also anopia, anotropia, hyperphoria.

anophthalmia (an-of-thal'-mi-a): A congenital anomaly characterized by the absence of one or both eyes.

anopsia (an-op'-si-a): Suppression of or inability to use the vision; may result from failure to use the eyes due to long confinement in a dark place, from cataract, or from refractive errors of high degree.

anorchid (an-or'-kid): A male with congenital absence of testes in the scrotum; may be unilateral or bilateral. Also anorchis, anorchus.

anorectal (ā-nō-rek'-tal): Pertaining to the anus and rectum, as a fissure (*q. v.*).

anorectic (an-ō-rek'-tik): 1. Appetite depressant. 2. Pertaining to anorexia.

anorexia (an-ō-reks'-i-a): Loss or deficiency of appetite for food. A. NERVOSA, hysterical aversion to food leading to atrophy of the stomach, emaciation and, in women, amenorrhea.—anorexic, anorectic, adj.

anorthography (an-or-thog'-ra-fi): Loss of ability to express oneself correctly in writing; agraphia (*q. v.*).

anorthopia (an-or-thō'-pi-a): A distortion of vision in which straight lines appear as bent or curved lines.

anoscopy (a-nos'-ko-pi): Examination of the lower rectum and the anus by means of an anoscope.

anosmia (an-oz'-mi-a): Absence of the sense of smell; may result from a lesion of the olfactory nerve, an obstruction in the nasal passages, cerebral disease involving the olfactory center, or there may be no apparent cause.—anosmic, anosmatic, anosmous, adj.

anostosis (an-os-tō'-sis): Defective formation or ossification of bone.

anovesical (ā-nō-ves'-i-kal): Pertaining to both the anus and the urinary bladder.

anovular (an-ov'-ū-lar): Not pertaining to, associated with, or coincidental with ovulation. A. BLEEDING is uterine bleeding that has not been preceded by ovulation.

anoxemia (an-oks-ē'-mi-a): Literally, no oxygen in the blood. More correctly, hypoxemia (*q. v.*); less than the physiologically normal amount of oxygen in the blood.—anoxemic, adj.

anoxia (an-ok'-si-a): Literally, no oxygen in the tissues. More correctly, hypoxia (*q. v.*); less than the normal physiological amount of oxygen in the organs or tissues, or failure of the tissues to utilize sufficient oxygen.—anoxic, adj.

ansa: An anatomical term used to describe any loop-like structure.

antacid (ant-as'-id): 1. Neutralizing or counteracting an acid. 2. Any substance that neutralizes or counteracts acidity, *e.g.,* that of the gastric juice.

antagonism (an-tag'-o-nizm): Active opposition; a characteristic of some drugs, muscles and organisms.—antagonistic, adj.

antagonist (an-tag'-o-nist): 1. A muscle that relaxes to allow its agonist (*q. v.*) to perform a movement. 2. Any agent that opposes or nullifies the action of another agent.

ante-: Denotes before, with reference to time or place.

antebrachium (an-tē-brā'-kē-um): The arm between the elbow and the wrist; the forearm.

ante cibum (antē sī'-bum): Before meals. Abbreviated a.c.

antecubital (an-tē-kū'-bi-tal): In front of the elbow.

anteflexion (an-tĕ-flek′-shun): The bending forward of an organ. Commonly applied to the position of the uterus. Opp. to retroflexion.

antehypophysis (an-tĕ-hī-pof′-i-sis): The anterior lobe of the pituitary body.

antemetic (ant-ĕ-met′-ik): Antiemetic (*q.v.*).

ante mortem (an-tĕ mor′-tem): Before death. Opp. to post mortem.—antemortem, adj.

antenatal (an-tĕ-nā′-tal): Pertaining to any event or condition that occurs or exists in the embryo or the mother during the period between conception and delivery of the child, normally 40 weeks or 280 days.

antepartum (an-tĕ-par′-tum): Before birth. More generally confined to the three months preceding full-term delivery.

antepyretic (an-tĕ-pī-ret′-ik): Before the onset of fever. (Not to be confused with antipyretic.)

anterior (an-tĕ′-ri-or): In front of; the front surface of; ventral.—anteriorly, adv. A. CHAMBER OF THE EYE, the space between the posterior surface of the cornea and the A. surface of the iris; contains aqueous humor (*q.v.*). A. TIBIAL SYNDROME, severe pain and inflammation over A. tibial muscle group, with inability to dorsitlex the foot.

anterior poliomyelitis: Poliomyelitis (*q.v.*).

antero-: Denotes before, in front of.

anterograde (an′-ter-ō-grăd): Proceeding or extending forward. A. AMNESIA, see **amnesia.**

anteroinferior (an′-ter-ō-in-fē′-ri-or): In front and below.

anterolateral (an′-ter-ō-lat′-er-al): Pertaining to the front and one side.

anteromedian (an-ter-ō-mē′-di-an): In front of and toward or on the midline.

anteroposterior (an′-ter-ō-pos-tē′-ri-or): Passing from before backwards. Relating to both front and back.

anterosuperior (an′-ter-ō-sūp-ĕr′-i-or): In front and above.

anteversion (an-tĕ-ver′-zhun): The forward tilting or displacement forward, without bending, of the whole of an organ or part. Opp. to retroversion.—anteverted, adj.; antevert, v.t., v.i.

anthelmintic (ant-hel-min′-tik): 1. Destructive to intestinal worms. 2. Any remedy for the destruction or elimination of intestinal worms.

anthracemia (an-thra-sē′-mi-a): Anthrax septicemia; the presence of *Bacillus anthracis* in the blood stream.—anthracemic, adj.

anthracia (an-thrā′-shi-a): A condition

characterized by the formation of carbuncles.

anthracosis (an-thra-kō′-sis): Black pigmentation of lungs due to inhalation of carbon particles; causes chronic inflammation. A form of pneumoconiosis (*q.v.*).—anthracotic, adj.

anthrax (an′-thraks): An acute, contagious disease of cattle and sheep which may be transmitted to man through a skin abrasion, inhalation, or ingestion, causing a malignant pustule. Causative organism is *Bacillus anthracis.* Preventive measures include prophylactic immunization of cattle and man. See **woolsorter's disease.**

anthropology(an-thrō-pol′o-ji): The study of mankind in all its aspects. Divided into various branches, such as criminal, cultural and physical anthropology.—anthropological, adj.; anthropologically, adv.

anthropophobia (an-thrō-pō-fō′-bi-a): A morbid dread of human society or companionship.

anthropozoonosis (an-thrō-pō-zō-ō-nō′-sis): A disease which may affect either animal or man and may be transmitted from one species to the other.

anti-: Denotes against, effective against, opposed to, counter.

antiagglutinin (an-ti-ag-gloo′-tin-in): A specific antibody that has the power of neutralizing or destroying the action of the corresponding agglutinin.

antianaphylaxis (an-ti-an-a-fil-aks′-is): A state of insusceptibility or immunity. A state in which anaphylaxis is avoided by injecting small but progressively increasing amounts of the antigen to which the subject is sensitive. Also anergy, desensitization.

antianemic (an-ti-an-ēm′-ik): 1. Any agent that prevents, counteracts, or relieves anemia. 2. Relieving or preventing anemia.

antiantibody (an-ti-an′-ti-bod-i): A substance that is formed in the body after the injection of an antibody which the substance is intended to counteract.

antibacterial (an-ti-bak-tĕr′-i-al): 1. Destroying bacteria or preventing their growth and reproduction. 2. An agent that destroys bacteria or interferes with their growth or reproduction.

antibechic (an-ti-bek′-ik): 1. Relieving cough. 2. An agent that relives cough.

antibiosis (an-ti-bī-ōs′-is): An association between organisms which is harmful to one of them. Opp. to symbiosis.—antibiotic, adj.

antibiotic (an-ti-bī-ot′-ik): 1. Pertaining to

antibiosis (*q.v.*). 2. Destructive to life. 3. Antibacterial substances, originally derived from fungi, molds or bacteria; many are now produced synthetically. Some are active against only certain bacteria, fungi, or viruses; others are active against a wider range of microorganisms. Some are effective when given by injection or orally; others are rarely used internally because of their high toxicity but are effective applied topically. BROAD-SPECTRUM A., one which is effective against many different microorganisms.

antibodies (an′-ti-bod-ēz): Specific protein substances in the blood that destroy or render inactive certain foreign substances, particularly bacteria and their products. May be developed naturally or in response to a specific antigen that has been introduced into the body parenterally or otherwise; may be transferred to the fetus in utero; may develop as a result of a subclinical infection with the specific agent, thus producing immunity to the specific disease. They cause agglutination, flocculation, inactivation or lysis of the antigen. A. include agglutinins, amboceptors, antienzymes, antitoxins, bacteriolysins, cytotoxins, hemolysins, opsonins and precipitins.

antibromic (an-ti-bro′-mik): 1. Counteracting unpleasant odors. 2. A deodorizer.

anticardium (an-ti-kar′-di-um): The epigastrium; the 'pit of the stomach.'

anticheirotonus (an-ti-kī-rot′-o-nus): A spasmodic flexion of the thumb, often seen before or during an epileptic seizure.

anticholagogue (an-ti-kōl′-a-gog): Any agent or process that interferes with the secretion of bile by the liver.

anticholinergic (an-ti-kōl-in-er′-jik): Inhibitory to the action of a parasympathetic nerve by interfering with the action of acetylcholine, a chemical by which such a nerve transmits its impulses at neural or myoneural junctions.

anticoagulant (an-ti-kō-ag′-ū-lant): An agent that prevents or retards clotting of the blood. Small amount made in the human body. Uses are: (1) to obtain specimens suitable for pathological investigation and chemical analyses when whole blood or plasma is required instead of serum; the anticoagulant usually is oxalate; (2) to obtain blood suitable for transfusion, the anticoagulant usually being sodium citrate; (3) as a therapeutic agent in the treatment of coronary thrombosis, phlebothrombosis, etc.

anticonceptive (an-ti-kon-sep′-tiv): Contraceptive.

anticonvulsant (an-ti-kon-vul′-sant): 1. Relieving or preventing convulsions. 2. An agent that stops or prevents convulsions.—anticonvulsive, adj.

anticus (an-tī′-kus): Anterior; in front of.

antidepressant (an-ti-dē-pres′-ant): 1. Preventing or reducing depression. 2. A drug or other agent that reduces or prevents depression.

antidiabetic (an-ti-dī-a-bet′-ik): Literally, 'against diabetes.' Used to describe therapeutic measures in diabetes mellitus, *e.g.*, the hormone insulin (*q.v.*).

antidiarrheal (an-ti-dī-a-rē′-al): 1. Preventing or alleviating diarrhea. 2. An agent that prevents or checks diarrhea.

antidinic (an-ti-din′-ik): 1. Relieving dizziness. 2. An agent that relieves dizziness.

antidiphtheritic (an-ti-dif-ther-it′-ik): Against diphtheria. Describes preventive measures such as immunization; therapeutic measures; serum used to give passive immunity.

antidiuretic (an-ti-dī-ū-ret′-ik): 1. Reducing the secretion of urine. 2. An agent that reduces the volume of urine secreted. A. HORMONE, secreted by the posterior pituitary gland; abbrev. ADH. See **diabetes**.

antidote (an′-ti-dōt): An agent that counteracts or neutralizes the action of a poision.

antiemetic (an-ti-ē-met′-ik): 1. Against emesis (*q.v.*). 2. Any agent that prevents nausea and vomiting.

antienzyme (an-ti-en′-zīm): A substance that exerts a specific inhibiting effect on an enzyme. Antienzymes are found in the digestive tract where they prevent digestion of its lining, and in the blood where they act as antibodies (*q.v.*).

antiepileptic (an-ti-ep-i-lep′-tik): Name given to drugs that reduce the frequency of epileptic attacks.

antifebrile (an-ti-feb′-ril): 1. Against fever. 2. Any agent that reduces or allays fever.

antifungal (an-ti-fung′-al): Any agent that destroys or inhibits the growth of fungi.

antigalactic (an-ti-ga-lak′-tic): 1. Reducing the secretion of milk. 2. Any drug or agent that tends to diminish the secretion of milk. Also, antigalactagogue.

antigen (an′-ti-jen): Any substance, usually protein, which under favorable conditions can stimulate the production of antibodies (*q.v.*).—antigenic, adj.

antihemophilic globulin (an-ti-hē-mō-fil′-ik

antihemorrhagic

glob′-ū-lin): A factor involved in blood-clotting; it is deficient in persons with hemophilia (q.v.).

antihemorrhagic (an-ti-hem-o-raj′-ik): 1. Preventing hemorrhage. 2. Any drug or agent that prevents hemorrhage. A. VITAMIN, vitamin K (q.v.).

antihidrotic (an-ti-hī-drot′-ik): Anhidrotic (q.v.)

antihistamines (an-ti-hist′-a-mēnz): Drugs that suppress some of the effects of released histamine (q.v.); widely used in treatment of hay fever, uticaria, angioneurotic edema, and some forms of pruritus. Because of their antiemetic properties, are used to prevent motion and radiation sickness. Side effects include drowsiness.—antihistaminic, adj. and n.

antihydropic (an-ti-hī-drop′-ik): 1. Relieving or reducing dropsy. 2. An agent used to treat dropsy.

antihypertensive (an-ti-hī-per-ten′-siv): 1. Counteracting hypertension. 2. Any drug or agent that lowers blood pressure in hypertensive patients.

antihypnotic (an-ti-hip-not′-ik): 1. Preventing sleep. 2. An agent that prevents or hinders sleep.

anti-immune (an-ti-i-mūn′): Preventing the development of immunity.

anti-infective (an-ti-in-fek′-tiv): 1. Counteracting infection. 2. Any agent that counteracts or prevents infection. See vitamin A.

antiketogenic (an-ti-kē-tō-jen′-ik): Inhibiting the formation of ketone bodies.

antilepsis (an-ti-lep′-sis): 1. Treatment of a disease by application of a remedy to a healthy part; called treatment by derivation or revulsion. 2. Support; e.g., a bandage.—antileptic, adj.

antilethargic (an-ti-le-thar′-jik): 1. Preventing or hindering sleep. 2. An agent that counteracts lethargy.

antilithic (an-ti-lith′-ik): 1. Counteracting the formation of stones or calculi. 2. An agent that helps prevent the formation of stones or calculi or that aids in their dissolution.

antiluetic (an-ti-loo-et′-ik): Any agent that prevents or cures syphilis (lues).

antilysin (an-ti-lī′-sin): An antibody that opposes the activity of a lysin thereby protecting the cells against the effects of the lysin (q.v.).

antilysis (an-til′-i-sis): The prevention or inhibition of lysis (q.v.).

antilyssic (an-ti-lis′-ik): Preventing or checking rabies.

antimalarial (an-ti-ma-lā′-ri-al): 1. Preventing or alleviating malaria. 2. Any measure taken to prevent or suppress malaria.

antimetabolite (an-ti-me-tab′-o-līt): Compound which is sufficiently similar to the chemicals needed by a cell to be incorporated into the nucleoproteins of that cell. In so doing, it prevents further development of the cell. The best known examples at present are the folic acid antagonists, aminopterin and amethopterin, given orally in the treatment of acute leukemia.

antimetropia (an-ti-me-trō′-pi-a): An ocular condition in which the two eyes present different refractive errors; e.g., one may be hypermetropic and the other myopic.

antimicrobic (an-ti-mī-krō′-bik): 1. Opposing or not believing the theory that microorganisms may be pathogens. 2. Acting to check or prevent the growth or action of microbes. 3. An agent that destroys or inhibits the growth or multiplication of microorganisms.

antimitotic (an-ti-mī-tot′-ik): 1. Inhibiting mitosis. 2. An agent that inhibits or prevents reproduction of a cell by mitosis.

antimycotic (an-ti-mī-kot′-ik): 1. Destructive to fungi. 2. An agent that destroys fungi.

antinarcotic (an-ti-nar-kot′-ik): 1. Preventing or relieving the effects of a narcotic drug (q.v.). 2. A drug or agent that counteracts the stupor produced by a narcotic drug.

antineoplastic (an-ti-nē-ō-plas′-tik): Inhibiting or preventing the growth of a neoplasm or the development and proliferation of malignant cells.

antineuritic (an-ti-nū-rit′-ik): 1. Relieving or preventing neuritis. 2. Any agent that prevents neuritis; specially applied to vitamin B complex (q.v.).

antiodontalgic (an-ti-ō-don-tal′-jik): 1. An agent that relieves or prevents toothache. 2. Relieving or preventing toothache.

antiotomy (an-ti-ot′-o-mi): Surgical removal of the tonsils.

antiovulatory (an-ti-ov′-ū-la-to-ri): Suppressing or inhibiting ovulation.

antioxidant (an-ti-oks′-id-ant): Any substance that delays the process of oxidation.

antiparasitic (an-ti-par-a-sit′-ik): 1. Destructive to parasites. 2. Any agent that destroys parasites or inhibits their growth.

antipathy (an-tip′-a-thi): Incompatability; aversion; distaste; dislike. In medicine, the mutual antagonism between two diseases. —antipathic, adj.

antipellagra (an-ti-pel-ag′-ra): 1. Against

pellagra. 2. Pertaining to the nicotinic acid portion of vitamin B complex (*q.v.*).

antiperiodic (an-ti-pēr-i-od′-ik): 1. Preventing the periodic recurrence of symptoms or of a disease. 2. An agent that prevents the periodic return of a disease or its symptoms, *e.g.*, quinine in malaria.

antiperistalsis (an-ti-per-i-stal′-sis): A reversal of the normal peristaltic action, *i.e.*, the peristaltic wave proceeds from below upward.—antiperistaltic, adj.

antiphlogistic (an-ti-flō-jis′-tik): 1. Relieving or reducing inflammation. 2. Any agent that relieves or reduces inflammation.

antiplastic (an-ti-plas′-tik): Unfavorable to the healing process, especially granulation and scar formation.

antiprothrombin (an-ti-prō-throm′-bin): An anticoagulant present in the blood that acts to prevent conversion of prothrombin into thrombin.

antipruritic (an-ti-proo-rit′-ik): 1. Any agent that relieves or prevents itching. 2. Having the action of preventing or relieving itching.

antipurpuric (an-ti-pur′-pū-rik): Against purpura. Pertaining to vitamin P (hesperidin) (*q.v.*).

antipyic (an-ti-pī′-ik): 1. Preventing suppuration. 2. An agent that prevents or inhibits the formation of pus.

antipyogenic (an-ti-pī-ō-jen′-ik): Antipyic (*q.v.*).

antipyretic (an-ti-pī-ret′-ik): 1. Reducing or relieving fever. 2. Any agent that reduces or relieves fever.—antipyresis, n.

antipyrotic (an-ti-pī-rot′-ik): 1. Useful in relieving pain and promoting healing of burns. 2. An agent used to allay pain in the treatment of burns.

antirabic (an-ti-rā′-bik): 1. Preventive or curative of rabies. 2. Any agent that prevents or cures rabies.

antirachitic (an-ti-rak-it′-ik): 1. Preventing or curing rickets. 2. Any agent used to prevent or cure rickets. 3. Pertaining to vitamin D (*q.v.*).

antirheumatic (an-ti-roo-mat′-ik): 1. Any agent that prevents or relieves rheumatism. 2. Preventing or relieving rheumatism.

antiscorbutic (an-ti-skor-bū′-tik): 1. Any agent that prevents or cures scurvy. 2. Preventing or curing scurvy. 3. Pertaining to vitamin C (*q.v.*).

antisecretory (an-ti-sē-crēt′-o-ri): 1. Preventing or inhibiting secretion. 2. Any agent that prevents or inhibits secretion.

antisepsis (an-ti-sep′-sis): 1. The prevention of sepsis (*q.v.*) by any or all of the following actions: destroying the microorganisms that produce infection; preventing their access to the site of potential infection; or inhibiting their growth and multiplication. Introduced into surgery in 1880 by Lord Lister who used carbolic acid. 2. The use of methods or agents to prevent the development of sepsis.

antiseptic (an-ti-sep′-tik): Any substance or agent that inhibits the growth and multiplication of microorganisms which produce infection or disease. It may also destroy them, but not necessarily. Term often used loosely for germicide (*q.v.*) or bactericide (*q.v.*).—antiseptic, adj.

antisepticism (an-ti-sep′-ti-sizm): The systematic use of agents or methods to prevent the development of sepsis (*q.v.*).—antisepticize, adj.

antiserum (an-ti-sēr′-um): A serum (from man or animal) that contains specific antibody or antibodies against a specific bacterium or other antigenic agent; the specific antibodies may be produced by infection with the specific bacterium or toxin, or by immunization through repeated injection of the specific bacterium or toxin into the tissues or blood. Useful in creating passive immunity (*q.v.*) or in treating such diseases as diphtheria, tetanus, meningitis.

antisialagogue (an-ti-sī-al′-a-gog): 1. Inhibiting salivation. 2. An agent that inhibits or arrests the secretion of saliva.

antisialic (an-ti-sī-al′-ik): 1. Antisialagogue (*q.v.*). 2. Checking the flow of saliva.

antisocial (an-ti-sō′-shal): Against society. A term used to denote a psychopathic state in which the individual cannot accept the obligations and restraints imposed by a community on its members.—antisocialism, n.

antispasmodic (an-ti-spaz-mod′-ik): 1. Relieving spasm. 2. Any agent or measure used to relieve muscle spasm.

antispastic (an-ti-spas′-tik): Antispasmodic (*q.v.*).

antistalsis (an-ti-stal′-sis): Reverse peristalsis (*q.v.*).

antistatic (an-ti-stat′-ik): Any measures taken to prevent or deal with the collection of static electricity.

antisterility (an-ti-ster-il′-it-i): Pertaining to vitamin E (*q.v.*).

antistreptolysin (an-ti-strep-tol′-i-sin): An inhibitor of streptolysin (*q.v.*). A raised A. titer in the blood is indicative of recent streptococcal infection.

antisudorific (an-ti-sūd-or-if′-ik): 1. Reducing or preventing excessive perspiration.

2. An agent that reduces or prevents excessive perspiration. Also antisudoral.

antisyphilitic (an-ti-sif-i-lit′-ik): 1. Any measures taken or agents used to combat syphilis. 2. Effective against syphilis..

antitabetic (an-ti-ta-bet′-ik): 1. Counteracting or preventing tabes dorsalis. 2. An agent effective in lessening the symptoms of tabes dorsalis (*q.v.*).

antithermic (an-ti-ther′-mik): 1. Cooling; acting to reduce body temperature. 2. An agent that lowers the body temperature. Syn., antipyretic (*q.v.*).

antithrombin (an-ti-throm′-bin): A. or antithrombins are substances occurring naturally in the blood, *e.g.*, heparin, or are given therapeutically, and which inhibit clotting by preventing reaction between thrombin (*q.v.*) and fibrinogen (*q.v.*).—antithrombotic, adj.

antithrombotic (an-ti-throm-bot′-ik): Any measures that prevent or relieve thrombosis.

antithyroid (an-ti-thī′-roid): 1. Any agent or drug used to reduce the activity of the thyroid gland; *e.g.*, thiouracil. 2. Counteracting the influence of the thyroid gland.

antitoxic (an-ti-tok′-sik): Antidotal; counteracting or neutralizing the action of a toxin. ANTITOXIC SERA, the serum of horses which have been immunized by injections of pathogenic bacterial toxins, such as tetanus and gas gangrene. Such serum contains antibodies or antitoxins, and after injection confers a temporary immunity against the original toxin. The therapeutic use of antitoxic sera declined after the discovery of the sulphonamides and antibiotics.

antitoxin (an-ti-tok′-sin): An agent that neutralizes a given toxin. It is elaborated in the body in direct response to the invasion by bacteria or a toxin, or to the injection of a small dose of treated toxin.—antitoxic, adj.

antitrismus (an-ti-triz′-mus): Inability to close the mouth due to muscle spasm.

antituberculin (an-ti-tū-ber′-kū-lin): An antibody developed within the body after the injection of tuberculin (*q.v.*).

antituberculotic (an-ti-tū-ber-kū-lot′-ik): 1. Effective against tuberculosis. 2. An agent that is effective against tuberculosis.

antitumorigenic (an-ti-tū-mor-i-jen′-ik): 1. Preventing or inhibiting the growth of a tumor. 2. An agent that prevents or inhibits the growth of a tumor.

antitussive (an-ti-tus′-iv): 1. Relieving or suppressing cough. 2. Any measure or agent that supresses cough.

antivenin (an-ti-ven′-in): An antiserum (*q.v.*) obtained from an animal immunized against the venom of a particular snake or insect and containing antitoxin to that venom. Used as an antidote in cases of poisoning by snake bite.

antiviral (an-ti-vī′-ral): Acting against viruses.

antivitamin (an-ti-vīt′-a-min): A substance that interferes with the absorption or utilization of a vitamin.

antivivisection (an-ti-viv-i-sek′-shun): Opposition to the use of living animals for experimentation or the manufacture of antisera.

antrectomy (an-trek′-to-mi): 1. Excision of the walls of an antrum, particularly the mastoid antrum. 2. Excision of the pyloric antrum of the stomach.

antritis (an-trī′-tis): Inflammation of an antrum, particularly the antrum of Highmore.

antrobuccal (an-trō-buk′-al): Pertaining to the maxillary antrum and the mouth. A. FISTULA can occur after extraction of an upper molar tooth, the root of which has protruded into the floor of the antrum.

antrostomy (an-tros′-to-mi): An incision into an antrum for the purpose of drainage.

antrotomy (an-trot′-o-mi): The operation of cutting into an antrum.

antrum (an′-trum): A closed or nearly closed cavity, especially in a bone, e.g., the antrum of Highmore in the superior maxillary bone. [Nathaniel Highmore, British physician. 1613-1685.] The term is also used to describe the pyloric end of the stomach when it is partially shut off from the fundus, during digestion, by the contraction of the pyloric sphincter.—antral, adj.

anulus (an′-ū-lus): See **annulus**.

anuresis (an-ū-rē′-sis): Failure to excrete urine. May be due to either lack of secretion or obstruction in the urinary passages.

anuria (a-nū′-ri-a): Absence of secretion of urine. See **suppression**.—anuric, adj.

anus (ā′-nus): The end of the alimentary canal, at the extreme termination of the rectum. It is formed of a sphincter muscle which relaxes to allow fecal matter to pass through. ARTIFICIAL A., one produced surgically in some higher part of the bowel in cases of obstruction through any cause.

IMPERFORATE A., one which has no opening; atresia ani. It is often due to a congenital defect.—anal, adj.

anvil (an′-vil): The incus, the middle of the three small bones of the middle ear. Likened to an anvil in shape.

anxiety (ang-zī′-e-ti): Feelings of fear, apprehension and dread. See **neurosis**. A. NEUROSIS, A. STATE, a neurosis characterized by recurrent acute A. attacks (panics). The attacks consist of all the signs and symptoms of fear, leading up to fear of impending collapse and sometimes death.

anydremia (an-i-drē′-mi-a): Anhydremia (*q.v.*).

AORN: Abbreviation for Association of Operating Room Nurses.

aorta (ā-or′-ta): The main artery of the body. ASCENDING A., that portion which arises in the left ventricle of the heart and, passing upward, joins the heart to the arch of the A. ARCH OF THE A., passes antero-posteriorly over the heart's base, joining the ascending to the descending A. DESCENDING A., is that portion which extends downward from the arch to the division, at the level of the fourth lumbar vertebra, into the right and left common iliac arteries. The portion above the diaphragm is called the THORACIC A., and the portion below the diaphragm is called the ABDOMINAL A.—aortal, aortic, adj.

aortarctia (ā-or-tark′-shi-a): Narrowing or stenosis of the aorta.

aortectasia (ā-or-tek-tā′-zi-a): Dilatation of the aorta.

aortic (ā-or′-tik): Pertaining to the aorta. A. ANEURYSM, see **aneurysm**. A. INCOMPETENCE, A. regurgitation resulting usually from rheumatic or syphilitic disease and allowing reflux of blood from aorta back into the left ventricle. A. MURMUR, abnormal heart sound heard over the A. area; a systolic murmur alone is the murmur of A. stenosis; a diastolic, the murmur of A. incompetence. A. PLEXUS, important network of sympathetic nerves, extending from the celiac (solar) plexus over the anterolateral aspect of the aorta and downwards to the hypogastric plexus. A. STENOSIS, narrowing of A. valve occurring as a result of rheumatic heart disease. A. VALVE, formed of three semilunar cusps at exit of left ventricle and beginning of the aorta.

aortitis (ā-or-tī′-tis): Inflammation of the aorta.

aortogram (ā-or′-to-gram): See **arteriogram**.

aortography (ā-or-tog′-raf-i): See **arteriography**.—aortographic, adj.; aortographically, adv.

aortomalacia (ā-or-tō-mal-ā′-shi-a): Softening of the walls of the aorta.

aortosclerosis (ā-or-tō-skler-ō′-sis): Sclerosis of the aorta.

aortostenosis (ā-or-tō-sten-ō′-sis): Narrowing of the aorta.

aortotomy (ā-or-tot′-o-mi): Incision into the aorta.

ap-, aph-, apo-: Denotes away from, off, detached, separate, formed from, related to.

apandria (ap-an′-dri-a): Morbid aversion to males.

apastia (a-pas′-ti-a): Abstention from food when it occurs as a symptom of neurological or psychological disorder.

apathy (ap′-a-thi): Want of feeling or emotion; indifference; insensibility. In psychiatry, abnormal listlessness and lack of activity.—apathic, apathetic, adj.

apepsia (a-pep′-si-a): Lack of or imperfect gastric digestion of food.

apepsinia (a-pep-sin′-i-a): Absence of pepsin or pepsinogen in the gastric juice.

aperient (a-pêr′-i-ent): A mild laxative.

aperistalsis (a-per-i-stal′-sis): Absence of peristaltic movement in the bowel. Characterizes the condition of paralytic ileus (*q.v.*).—aperistaltic, adj.

aperture(ap′-er-tûr): An opening or orifice.

apex (ā′-peks): In anatomy, a term used to designate the top of a body or organ or the pointed end of a cone-shaped or pyramidal structure; *e.g.*, the heart, lungs. Also applied to the terminal end of a tooth. A. BEAT, in a heart of normal size the A. beat (systolic impulse) can be seen or felt in the 5th left intercostal space in the midclavicular line. It is the lowest and most lateral point at which an impulse can be detected and provides a rough indication of the size of the heart. A. OF THE HEART, blunt, narrow end enclosing mainly the left ventricle; it rests on the diaphragm. A. OF THE LUNG, that portion nearest shoulder level.—apical, adj.; apices, pl.

Apgar score: The numerical expression of a newborn infant's condition, being the sum of points given for heart rate, crying power, muscle tone, plantar reflex and skin color, the assessments being made at one minute and five minutes after birth. [Virginia

30

Apgar, American anesthesiologist. 1909-.]

aphagia (a-fā′-ji-a): Inability to swallow.—aphagic, adj.

aphakia (a-fā′-ki-a): Absence of the crystalline lens.—aphakic, adj.

aphalangia (a-fa-lan′-ji-a): Congenital absence of a finger or toe or of one or more phalanges of a finger or toe.

aphasia (a-fā′-zi-a): Loss or impairment of the ability to use words to express one's ideas, or impairment of the ability to comprehend spoken or written language. Aphasia is organic, being caused by a brain lesion. There are many recognized varieties. MOTOR A., loss of ability to articulate, although understanding remains. SENSORY A., loss of power to recognize the meaning of written or spoken words or phrases.—aphasic, adj.

aphemia (a-fē′-mi-a): Motor aphasia (*q.v.*). Loss of ability to articulate words.

aphephobia (af-e-fō′-bi-a): Morbid dread of physical contact with other persons or of being touched by another.

aphonia (a-fō′-ni-a): Loss of voice from a cause other than a cerebral lesion. May be due to organic causes such as disease or injury of the larynx, or to psychic causes.—aphonic, adj.

aphonogelia (a-fō-nō-jē′-li-a): Inability to laugh out loud.

aphrasia (a-frā′-zi-a): Inability to speak or to use connected phrases in speaking. A. PARANOICA, voluntary and stubborn silence in the mentally ill.

aphrodisiac (af-rō-diz′-i-ak): 1. Exciting or arousing the sexual impulse. 2. A drug or agent that stimulates or arouses the sexual impulse.

aphrodisiomania (af-rō-diz′-i-ō-mā′-ni-a): Excessive and abnormal sexual interest. Erotomania.

aphronesia (a-fro-nē′-si-a): Dementia; silliness; foolishness.

aphthae (af′-thē): Small whitish or grayish ulcerous areas, usually surrounded by a ring of erythema, found on mucous membrane of the mouth, sometimes also of the gastrointestinal tract. Caused by various fungi and bacteria. Characteristic of such diseases as thrush, sprue, aphthous stomatitis (*q.v.*). BEDNAR'S A., whitish ulcerous spots on the posterior part of the hard palate, seen in young children. CACHECTIC A., an often fatal disease characterized by lesions under the tongue and such severe constitutional symptoms as enlargement and degeneration of liver and spleen.—aptha, sing.; aphthous, adj.

apical (āp′-i-kal): Pertaining to or located at the apex of a structure.

apicoectomy (ap-ik-ō-ek′-to-mi): Excision of the root of a tooth.

apicolysis (ap-ik-ol′-i-sis): The operation of stripping the parietal pleura from the upper chest wall to ensure collapse of the lung apex when it contains a tuberculous cavity.

aplasia (a-plā′-zi-a): Incomplete development of an organ or tissue; absence of growth.

aplastic (a-plas′-tik): 1. Without structure or form. 2. Incapable of forming new tissue.

apnea (ap-nē′-a): A transitory cessation of breathing as seen in Cheyne-Stokes respiration (*q.v.*). It is due to lack of the necessary CO_2 tension in the blood for stimulation of the respiratory center.—apneic, adj.

apocrine (ap′-ō-krin): Designating a type of glandular secretion that contains some of the protoplasm of the cells that elaborate it. A. GLANDS, modified sweat glands, especially in the axillae, genital and perineal regions; they produce both sweat and a solution that, after puberty, is responsible for body odor.

apodemialgia (a-pō-dē-mi-al′-ji-a): A morbid longing to leave one's home; wanderlust.

apodia (a-pō′-di-a): Congenital absence of one or both feet.—apodal, adj.

apogee (ap′-ō-jē): The climax or crisis of a disease, or the period of greatest severity of a disease.

aponeurosis (ap-ō-nū-rō′-sis): A broad glistening sheet of tendon-like tissue which serves to invest and attach muscles to each other, and also to the parts which they move.—aponeuroses, pl.; aponeurotic, adj.

aponeurositis (ap-ō-nū-rō-sī′-tis): Inflammation of an aponeurosis.

apophysis (a-pof′-i-sis): A projection, protuberance or outgrowth. Usually used in connection with bone.—apophyses, pl.; apophyseal, apophysial, adj.

apoplexy (ap′-ō-pleks-i): Stroke. Sudden unconsciousness usually caused by cerebral embolism, hemorrhage or thrombosis. There is stertorous breathing, incontinence of urine and feces and a varying degree of hemiplegia (*q.v.*).—apoplectic, apoplectiform, adj.

aposia (a-pō′-zi-a): 1. Absence of the sensation of thirst. 2. Reluctance to taking fluid by mouth.

apositia (ap-ō-sish′-i-a): Disgust for and aversion to food.

apothecaries' system (a-poth′-e-kar-ēz): A

system of weights and measures in which weights are given in grains, scruples, drams, ounces and pounds. Capacity is given in minims, fluidrams, fluidounces, gills, pints, and quarts.

appendage (a-pen'-dij): A subordinate, attached or suspended part of an organ or structure; usually less important in function and smaller than the main structure.

appendectomy (a-pen-dek'-to-mi): 1. Surgical removal of the vermiform appendix (*q.v.*). 2. Surgical removal of an appendage.

appendicectomy (ap-en-di-sek'-to-mi): Appendectomy (*q.v.*).

appendices epiploicae (a-pen'-di-sēz ep-i-plō'-i-sē): Peritoneum-covered tabs of fat that are attached to the tenia (*q.v.*) of the colon.

appendicitis (a-pen-di-sī'-tis): Inflammation of the vermiform appendix (*q.v.*), chronic or acute; usually sudden in onset with pain over the entire abdomen but which later localizes in the lower right side.

appendicolithiasis (a-pen-di-kō-li-thī'-a-sis): A condition marked by the presence of stones in the vermiform appendix.

appendicostomy (a-pen-di-kos'-to-mi): An operation in which the appendix is brought to the surface and an opening made into it. This admits a catheter via which the large bowel can be irrigated.

appendix (a-pen'-diks): An appendage. A. VERMIFORMIS, a worm-like appendage of the cecum; about the thickness of a pencil and may be from two to six inches long, ending in a blind extremity. Usually extends downward in the right iliac region but its position is variable. Apparently functionless. Frequently referred to as the vermiform appendix.—appendices, pl.; appendiceal, appendicular, adj.

apperception (ap-er-sep'-shun): Clear perception of a sensory stimulus, in particular where there is identification or recognition.—apperceptive, adj.

appestat (ap'-e-stat): The center in the brain, probably in the hypothalamus, that controls the appetite.

appetite (ap'-e-tit): A normal desire to satisfy a natural physical or mental need; specifically, the desire to eat.

applicator (ap'-li-kā-tor): An instrument for applying local remedies, often consisting of a slender rod of wood or metal to which a cotton pledget has been attached.

apposition (ap-o-zish'-un): 1. The approximation or bringing together of two surfaces or edges. 2. Side by side.

apraxia (a-praks'-i-a): Loss of ability to perform purposeful movements or to execute acts that were hitherto done more or less automatically, *e.g.*, tying shoelaces, when there is no paralysis. Due to a brain lesion.—apraxic, apractic, adj.

aproctia (a-prok'shi-a): Absence or imperforation of the anus; a congenital anomaly.

aprosexia (ap-rō-seks'-i-a): Inability to fix the attention or to concentrate, arising from such causes as mental deficiency or deficient hearing or vision.

aprosody (a-prōs'-o-di): The absence, in one's speech, of the normal rhythm and variations in stress and tone.

apsychia (ap-sik'-i-a): Temporary loss of consciousness; *e.g.*, fainting.

APT: Alum-precipitated diphtheria toxoid; a diphtheria prophylactic used mainly for immunization of children.

aptitude (ap'-ti-tūd): Natural ability or acquired facility in performing certain tasks, either mental or physical. In psychology, potential rather than developed ability or facility for learning a certain kind of performance; *e.g.*, musical aptitude. A. TEST, one which permits evaluation of a person's potential for performance in tasks which may or may not have similarity to the test tasks.

aptyalia (ap-tī-ā'-li-a): Absence or diminished secretion of saliva. Also aptyalism.

apyrexia (ā-pī-reks'-i-a): Absence of fever.—apyrexial, apyretic, adj.

AQ: Achievement quotient (*q.v.*).

aq: Abbreviation for *aqua,* meaning water.

aqua (ak'-wa): Water. A. DESTILLATA, distilled water. A. FORTIS, nitric acid. A. MENTHAE PIPERITAE, peppermint water.

aquapuncture (ak-wa-pungk'-tūr): The hypodermic injection of water as a placebo, for counterirritation, or for any other purpose.

aqueduct (ak'-we-dukt): A canal in an organ or structure for the passage of fluid. A. OF SYLVIUS, the canal connecting the 3rd and 4th ventricles of the brain; aqueductus cerebri. [Francois Sylvius de la Boe, French anatomist. 1614-1672.]

aqueous (ā'kwē-us): Watery. A. HUMOR, the watery, transparent fluid contained in the anterior and posterior chambers of the eye.

arachidonic acid (ar-ak-i-don'-ik as'-id): One of the essential fatty acids. Found in small amounts in human and animal liver and organ fats. A growth factor.

Arachnida (a-rak'-ni-da): A class of Arthropoda, comprising mites, ticks, spiders, scorpions.

arachnidism (a-rak'-ni-dizm): Systemic poisoning resulting from the bite of a spider.

arachnitis (a-rak-ni'-tis): Inflammation of the arachnoid membrane.

arachnodactyly (a-rak'-nō-dak'-til-i): A congenital abnormality resulting in long, slender, curved fingers, often called 'spider' fingers.

arachnoid (a-rak'-noid): Resembling a spider's web, denoting specifically the arachnoidea, a delicate membrane enveloping the brain and spinal cord, lying between the pia mater internally and the dura mater externally; the middle serous membrane of the meninges.—arachnoidal, adj.

arachnoidea (a-rak-noid'-ē-a): See **arachnoid**.

arachnoidism (a-rak'-noid-izm): Poisoning by a spider bite.

arachnoiditis (a-rak-noid-ī'-tis): Arachnitis (q.v.).

arachnophobia (a-rak-nō-fō'-bi-a): Morbid fear of spiders.

arbor: In anatomy, a structure or part that is tree-like in appearance. A. ALVEOLARIS, the branched terminal end of an air passage in the lung. A. VITAE, (1) the tree-like outline of white substance seen on section of the cerebellum; (2) the pattern of folds and ridges seen in the mucous membrane of the uterine cervix.

arborization (ar-bor-ī-zā'-shun): An arrangement resembling the branching of a tree. Characterizes both ends of a neuron, i.e., the dendrons and the axon as it supplies each muscle fiber.

arboviruses (ar-bo-vī'-rus-es): An abbreviation for viruses transmitted by arthropods. Members of the mosquito-borne group cause yellow, dengue and Rift valley fevers in man. The sandfly transmits sandfly fever. The tick-borne group cause various fevers that can give rise to encephalitis complex. Also called arborviruses.

arc (ark): REFLEX A., in anatomy, the pathway over which a nerve impulse travels in producing a reflex action; i.e., the afferent nerve that carries the impulse to a nerve center, the nerve center, the efferent nerve that carries the impulse to a peripheral organ or structure, and the organ or structure that produces the reflex action.

arch: A curve or loop; a curved or bow-like structure. A. OF THE AORTA, the curved part between the ascending and descending aorta. A. OF THE FOOT, (1) transverse, along the line of the tarsometatarsal joints; (2) inner longitudinal, formed by the cal-

caneus, talus, navicular, three cuneiforms and the first three toes; (3) outer longitudinal, formed by the calcaneus, cuboid and the fourth and fifth toes. PALMAR A., the arch formed by the union of the radial and ulnar arteries in the palm. PLANTAR A., that formed by the anastomosis of the plantar and dorsalis pedis arteries in the foot. PUBIC A., that formed by the convergence of the rami of the ischium and pubis on each side; it is immediately below the symphysis pubis. ZYGOMATIC A., that formed by the malar and temporal bones.

archoptosis (ar-kō-tō'-sis): Prolapse of the rectum.

archorrhagia (ar-kō-rā'-jē-a): Hemorrhage from the rectum.

archorrhea (ar-kō-rē'-a): A liquid discharge from the rectum.

arcuate (ar'-kū-āt): Bow-shaped or arched.

arcus senilis (ar'-kus sen-il'-is): An opaque, grayish-white ring around the edge of the cornea, seen in old people.

areflexia (a-rē-flek'-si-a): The state of being without reflexes.

areola (ar-ē'-o-la): 1. The pigmented area around a part, e.g., the nipple; or around an area, e.g., around certain lesions on the skin. 2. The part of the iris immediately surrounding the pupil. 3. A minute interstice or space in a tissue. SECONDARY A., a dark circle of pigmentation which surrounds the primary areola of the nipple in pregnancy.—areolar, adj.

areolitis (ar-ē-ō-lī'-tis): Inflammation of the areola of the nipple.

argentum (ar-jen'-tum): Silver. Symbol is Ag.

arginase (ar'-jin-ās): An enzyme found in the liver, kidney and spleen. It splits arginine into ornithine and urea.

arginine (ar'-jin-ēn): One of the essential amino acids (q.v.). It is obtained from animal and vegetable proteins and must be supplied in the diet.

arginosuccinicaciduria (ar-ji-nō-suk-sin-ik-as-i-dū'-ri-a): The presence of arginosuccinic acid in the urine. Due to an inborn error in metabolism and currently associated with mental retardation.

argon (ar'-gon): An inert, gaseous element present in small quantity, 0.94 per cent, in the atmosphere. It is used in gas-filled electric bulbs.

Argyll Robertson pupil (ar-gīl' rob'-ert-son): One which reacts to accommodation, but not to light. Diagnostic sign in certain diseases including neurosyphilis. [D. M. C. L.

Argyll Robertson, Scottish physician. 1837-1909.]

argyria (ar-jir'-i-a): A permanent grayish or bluish discoloration of tissues resulting from long administration of silver salts. Argyrosis. Argyrism.

ariboflavinosis (a-rī'-bō-flā-vin-ōs-is): A deficiency state caused by lack of riboflavin and other members of the vitamin B complex. Characterized by cheilosis, seborrhea, angular stomatitis, glossitis, and photophobia.

arithmomania (ar-ith-mō-mā'-ni-a): A psychoneurosis characterized by an obsession with numbers and unnecessary, incessant counting.

arm: In common usage, the upper extremity from the shoulder to the wrist. In anatomy, the part of the upper extremity from the shoulder to the elbow, as distinguished from the forearm.

armamentarium (ar-ma-men-tā'-rē-um): Word used to describe the entire equipment of a medical practitioner or institution; includes instruments, books, medicines, appliances, etc.

aromatic (ar-ō-mat'-ik): A medicinal substance having a fragrant, spicy aroma, often of vegetable origin, used as a stimulant. —aromatic, adj.

arrectores pilorum (ar-ek'-tor-ēz pī-lōr'-um): Minute, internal, plain, involuntary muscles attached to hair follicles, which, under the influence of terror or cold, contract and thus erect the follicles, causing 'gooseflesh.'

arrest: The sudden stoppage or cessation of a physiological function or of the course of a disease. CARDIAC A., complete cessation of the heart beat. EPIPHYSEAL A., arrest of the growth of the long bones by premature fusion of the diaphysis and epiphysis.

arrhenoblastoma (a-rēn-ō-blas-tō'-ma): A relatively rare malignant tumor of the ovary that may result in production of androgen and consequent masculinization.

arrhythmia (a-rith'-mi-a): Any deviation from the normal rhythm, *e.g.,* of the heart beat. SINUS A., increase of the pulse beat on inspiration, decrease on expiration. Appears to be normal in some children.

arsenic (ar'-sen-ik): A metallic element. Formerly widely used in medicine; now largely replaced by penicillin. Its toxic potential is high. —arsenical, adj.

arsenicals (ar-sen'-i-kals): Drugs containing arsenic, formerly much used but now largely replaced by antibiotics.

artefact: See **artifact.**

arteri-, arterio-: Denotes artery, arteries.

arteriarctia (ar-te-ri-ark'-shi-a): Vasoconstriction; reducing the caliber of an artery or arteries.

arteriectasia (ar-te-ri-ek-tā'-si-a): Vasodilation; increasing the caliber of an artery or arteries.

arteriectomy (ar-te-ri-ek'-to-mi): Excision of an artery or, more usually, part of an artery.

arteriogram (ar-tē'-ri-ō-gram): Film demonstrating arteries after injection of opaque medium.

arteriography (ar-tē-ri-og'-raf-i): 1. Graphic recording of the pulse. 2. Demonstration of the arterial system by means of injection of opaque medium. —arteriographic, adj.; arteriographically, adv.

arteriole (ar-tē'-ri-ōl): A small artery, particularly one joining an artery to a capillary.

arteriolith (ar-tē'-ri-ō-lith): A calculus in an arterial wall or in a thrombus.

arteriomalacia (ar-tē-ri-ō-ma-lā'-shi-a): Softening of the walls of an artery or arteries.

arteriopathy (ar-tē-ri-op'-ath-i): Any disease of an artery or arteries. —arteriopathic, adj.

arterioplasty (ar-tē-ri-ō-plas'-ti): Plastic surgery applied to an artery. Term often used to denote an operation for the reconstruction of an artery after an aneurysm. —arterioplastic, adj.

arteriorrhagia (ar-tē-ri-ō-rā'-ji-a): Hemorrhage from an artery.

arteriorrhaphy (ar-tē-ri-or'-a-fi): 1. Suture of an artery. 2. A plastic procedure on an artery, such as obliteration of an aneurysm.

arteriosclerosis (ar-tē-ri-ō-skler-ō'-sis): Degenerative changes in the arteries; primarily a thickening of the walls with loss of elasticity. CEREBRAL A., A. involving the arteries of the brain. CORONARY A., that involving the coronary arteries. A. OBLITERANS, A. in which the lumen of the artery is obscured by the proliferation of the inner lining. SENILE A., occurs as a natural process during aging. —arteriosclerotic, adj.

arteriostenosis (ar-tē-ri-ō-sten-ō'-sis): A temporary or permanent decrease in the size of the lumen of an artery or arteries.

arteriotomy (ar-tē-ri-ot'-o-mi): Incision of an artery.

arteriovenous (ar-tē'-ri-ō-vēn-us): Pertaining to both an artery and a vein.

arterioversion

arterioversion (ar-tē-ri-ō-ver'-shun): A turning back or eversion of the walls of the cut ends of an artery to arrest hemorrhage.

arteritis (ar-te-rī'-tis): Inflammation of an artery. See **endarteritis, periarteritis.**—arteritic, adj.

artery (ar'-te-ri): A vessel carrying blood from the heart to the various tissues. The internal endothelial lining provides a smooth surface to prevent clotting of blood. The middle layer of plain muscle and elastic fibers allows for distension as blood is pumped from the heart. The outer, mainly connective tissue layer prevents overdistension. The lumen is largest nearest to the heart; it gradually decreases in size.—arterial, adj. A. FORCEPS, hemóstatic (*q.v.*) forceps.

arthr-, arthro-: Denotes joint(s).

arthral (ar'-thral): Relating or pertaining to a joint.

arthralgia (ar-thral'-ji-a): Pain in a joint, especially when there is no inflammation. Syn., arthrodynia.—arthralgic, adj.

arthrectomy (ar-threk'-to-mi): Excision of a joint.

arthritis (ar-thrī'-tis): Inflammation of a joint, often accompanied by pain, swelling, stiffness and structural changes. May be caused by a variety of factors including infection, neurological disorders, metabolic disturbances, neoplasms, bursitis, acromegaly, trauma. ACUTE A., A. marked by pain, heat, redness, swelling; may be due to gout, rheumatism, gonorrheal infection, trauma. ACUTE RHEUMATIC A., rheumatic fever. A. DEFORMANS, rheumatoid A., usually begins in the fingers and is progressive, resulting in deformity. A. DEFORMANS JUVENILIS, Still's disease (*q.v.*). See **Perthes' disease.** A. DEFORMANS NEO-PLASTICA, osteitis fibrosa (*q.v.*). A. NODOSA (A. URATICA), gout.—arthritic, adj.

arthrocele (ar'-thrō-sēl): 1. A swollen joint. 2. A hernia of the synovial membrane into the joint capsule.

arthrocentesis (ar-thrō-sen-tē'-sis): A puncture of a joint cavity for the purpose of withdrawing fluid.

arthrochondritis (ar-thrō-kon-drī'-tis): Inflammation of the cartilages within and around a joint.

arthroclasia (ar-thrō-klā'-zi-a): Breaking down of an ankylosed joint to produce a wider range of movement. Arthroclasis.

arthrodesis (ar-throd'-e-sis): The fixation or stiffening of a joint by surgical means.

arthrodia (ar-thrō'-di-a): A joint permitting gliding movement.—arthrodial, adj.

arthrodynia (ar-thrō-din'-i-a): Pain in a joint. See **arthralgia.**—arthrodynic, adj.

arthro-endoscopy (ar-thrō-end-os'-kop-i): Visualization of the interior of a joint using an endoscope (*q.v.*).—anthro-endoscopic, adj.; arthro-endoscopically, adv.

arthrogram (ar'-thrō-gram): An x-ray film demonstrating a joint.

arthrography (ar-throg'-raf-i): X-ray of a joint, sometimes after injection of air or radiopaque material.—arthrographic, adj.; arthrographically, adv.

arthrolith (ar'-thrō-lith): A calculus or 'stone' within a joint.

arthrology (ar-throl'-o-ji): The science that deals with joints, their diseases and treatment.

arthrolysis (ar-throl'-i-sis): The operation of restoring mobility to an ankylosed joint by breaking up adhesions.

arthroncus (ar-throng'-kus): Swelling or tumor of a joint.

arthroneuralgia (ar-thrō-nū-ral'-ji-a): Neuralgia of a joint.

arthropathy (ar-throp'-ath-i): Any joint disease.—arthropathic, adj.

arthroplasty (ar'-thrō-plas-ti): Plastic surgery on a joint; the repair or re-formation of a joint by surgical means.

Arthropoda (ar-throp'-o-da): A large group of invertebrate animals (over 700,000 species) whose members are characterized by segmented bodies, a hard outer shell, and paired jointed appendages. Includes the spiders and insects. Many species are important in medicine because they are parasites, vectors of disease, or troublesome pests whose bites and stings produce varying physiological reactions.

arthrosclerosis (ar-thrō-skler-ō'-sis): Stiff-

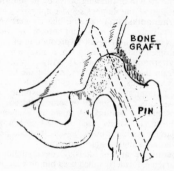

Arthrodesis of hip

ening of a joint(s), particularly in the aged.

arthroscope (ar'-thrō-skōp): An instrument used for the visualization of the interior of a joint cavity. See **endoscope.**—arthroscopic, adj.

arthroscopy (ar-thros'-kop-i): The act of visualizing the interior of a joint with an arthroscope.—arthroscopic, adj.

arthrosis (ar-thrō'-sis): 1. A joint or articulation. 2. Degeneration or disease of a joint. See **amphiarthrosis, diarthrosis, pseudoathrosis, synarthrosis, synchondrosis.**

arthrosteitis (ar-thros'-tē-ī'-tis): Inflammation of the bone of a joint.

arthrostomy (ar-thros'-tō-mi): The surgical establishment of an opening into a joint, usually for the purpose of drainage.

arthrosynovitis (ar-thrō-sin-ō-vī'-tis): Inflammation of the synovial membrane of a joint.

arthrotomy (ar-throt'-o-mi): Incision into a joint.

articular (ar-tik'-ū-lar): Pertaining to a joint or articulation. Applied to cartilage, surface, capsule, etc.

articulate (ar-tik'-ū-lāt): 1. To join together, as in a joint. 2. Articulated; jointed. 3. To enunciate words and sentences distinctly.

articulated (ar-tik'-ū-lāt-ed): The state of being joined together. In anatomy, the connection of separate parts in such a way as to permit motion.

articulation (ar-tik-ū-lā'-shun): 1. The junction of two or more bones; a joint. 2. Enunciation of speech.—articular, adj.

articulo mortis (ar-tik'-ū-lō mor'-tis): At the instant of death.

artifact (ar'-ti-fakt): 1. Any artificial product resulting from a physical or chemical agency. 2. An unnatural change in a structure or tissue. Also artefact.

artificial (ar-ti-fish'-al): Imitated by art; not natural; made or invented or performed by man. Applied to anus, eye, feeding, heart, insemination, kidney, limb, pneumothorax, respiration, ventilation.

arytenoid (ar-i-tē'-noid): Shaped like a funnel or the mouth of a pitcher. A. CARTILAGES, found one on either side, forming the posterior wall of the upper rim of the larynx. Their function is to regulate the tension in the vocal cords.

AS: Abbreviation for left ear.

asbestos (as-bes'-tos): A fibrous, incombustible, mineral substance; does not conduct heat. Used to make protective clothing for industry; small spicules may cause hyperkeratotic papules (asbestos corns or warts) on hands of workers.

asbestosis (as-bes-tō'-sis): Fibrosis of the lungs resulting from the prolonged inhalation of fine asbestos dust and fibrils. See **pneumoconiosis.**

ascariasis (as-kar-ī'-a-sis): Infestation with worms of the genus Ascaris (*q.v.*). The bowel is most often affected, but in the case of round worms, infestation may spread to the stomach, liver and lungs. Also ascaridiasis, ascaridosis, ascariosis.

ascaricide (as-kar'-is-īd): An agent that is lethal to worms of the genus Ascaris.

Ascaris (as'-kar-is): A genus of nematode worms to which belong the round worm (*Ascaris lumbricoides*) and the threadworm (*Enterobius vermicularis*).—ascarides, pl.

Aschheim-Zondek test: A test for pregnancy using an immature mouse. [Selmar Aschheim, German gynecologist. 1878- Bernhard Zondek, German gynecologist in Israel. 1891- .]

Aschoff's node: A flat white mass of Purkinje fibers found in all mammalian hearts at the base of the interatrial septum and forming the beginning of the atrioventricular bundle of His. [Ludwig Aschoff, German pathologist. 1866-1942.]

Aschoff's nodules: Nodules made up of collections of cells and leukocytes, seen in the interstitial tissues of the heart in patients with rheumatic myocarditis.

ascites (as-sī'-tēz): Accumulation of free serous fluid in the peritoneal cavity. Causes include cirrhosis of the liver, tumor, tuberculous peritonitis, interference in venous circulation, cardiac or renal failure. Syn., hydroperitoneum, abdominal dropsy.—ascitic, adj.

Ascomycetes (as-kō-mī-sē'-tēz): A group of fungi; includes yeasts, blue molds, mildews, ergot, truffles.

ascorbic acid (a-skor'-bik): Vitamin C (*q.v.*). Essential element of diet; not stored in the body so needs to be supplied regularly. Used as a dietary supplement in anemia and to promote wound healing.

ASD: Abbreviation for atrial septal defect (*q.v.*).

-ase: Denotes: (1) enzyme; (2) destroying substance.

asemia (a-sē'-mi-a): Inability to communicate by the usual means; *i.e.,* the patient cannot produce or comprehend spoken or written language, signs, etc. A form of aphasia. Syn., asymbolia.—asemic, adj.

asepsis (a-sep′-sis): The state of being free from living pathogenic organisms.—aseptic, adj., ascepticize, v.

aseptic technique: A precautionary method used in any procedure where there is a possibility of introducing organisms into the patient's body. Every article used must have been sterilized.

asexual (a-seks′-ū-al): Without sex or without reference to sex. A. REPRODUCTION, reproduction without sexual union.

asexualization (a-seks′-ū-al-ī-zā′-shun): Castration or sterilization of an individual.

asiderosis (a-sid-er-ō′-sis): Iron deficiency.

-asis: Denotes affected with, state or condition.

asocial (a-sō′-shul): Unable or unwilling to conform to the social demands of the environment; selfish; withdrawn from normal social intercourse.

aspergillosis (as-per-jil-ō′-sis): Infection caused by any species of *Aspergillus* (*q.v.*), characterized by formation of granulomatous lesions in the skin, ear, sinuses, lungs, and sometimes in the meninges and bones. More likely to occur in people who handle grain or seeds. See **bronchomycosis.**

Aspergillus (as-per-jil′-us): A genus of fungi, found in soil, manure, and on various grains; includes many species of molds, some of which are pathogenic.

aspermia (a-sperm′-i-a): Inability to form or to ejaculate semen, or absence of sperm in the semen.

aspersion (as-per′-shun): The sprinkling of water on the body or on an affected part; a procedure used in hydrotherapy.

asphyxia (as-fiks′-i-a): Suffocation; local or systemic lack of oxygen and increase in carbon dioxide in the blood as a result of interruption of breathing. This occurs when not enough oxygen is taken in or when the tissues are unable to utilize what is taken in; *e.g.*, in drowning, poisoning by a gas such as carbon monoxide or by a substance such as cyanide. BLUE A. or A. LIVIDA, a condition of the newborn when the color is deep blue but there is good muscle tone and responsiveness to stimuli. WHITE A. or A. PALLIDA, more serious condition of the newborn; the skin is pale and there is flaccidity and unresponsiveness to stimuli.

aspiration (as-pi-rā′-shun): 1. The act of drawing in the breath; inspiration. 2. The withdrawal of fluids from a body cavity by means of a suction or siphonage apparatus.

A. PNEUMONIA, inflammation of lung from inhalation of foreign body, usually fluid or food particles.—aspirate, v.t.

aspirator (as′-pi-rā-tor): An apparatus for collecting material by suction, specifically for withdrawing fluid or gas from a cavity for diagnostic or therapeutic purposes.

assay (a′-sā): The use of physical, chemical, or biological methods to analyze, test, or examine a substance to determine its purity or the relative proportion of its constituents.—assay, v.

assimilation (as-sim-i-lā′-shun): The process whereby the already digested foodstuffs are absorbed and utilized by the tissues. The constructive phase of metabolism. Syn., anabolism.—assimilable, adj.; assimilate, v.t., v.i.

association (as-sō-si-ā′-shun): A union or close relationship of ideas, things, or persons. In psychology, A. OF IDEAS, the principle by which ideas, emotions, and movements are connected so that their succession in the mind occurs; one idea calls up another that was previously linked with it. A. AREAS, areas in the cortex of the brain whose function is not known; it is assumed they serve some sort of integrative function. A. TEST, the subject responds immediately with another word when the examiner speaks a word; the nature of the response and the time it takes for the response are used in diagnosis. FREE A., ideas arising spontaneously when censorship is removed.

astasia (as-tā′-zi-a): Inability to stand erect due to muscle incoordination which is not of physical origin. A. ABASIA, hysterical inability to stand or walk while other use of legs is normal.

asteatosis (as-tē-a-tō′-sis): Lack or deficiency of secretion by the sebaceous glands. A. CUTIS, a skin condition characterized by dryness, scaliness and sometimes fissures; causes include nervous system disorders, senility, contact with irritants such as chemicals, detergents.

astereognosis (a-stē-rē-og-nō′-sis): Loss of the power to recognize the shape and consistency of objects by touching them.

asteroid (as′-ter-oid): Star-shaped.

asthenia (as-thē′-ni-a): Weakness, debility; lack or loss of strength, particularly muscle strength. ASTHENIC TYPE, see **Kretschmer's personality types**. The term often forms part of combination words; *e.g.*, neurasthenia.

asthenopia (as-the-nō'-pi-a): 1. Poor vision. 2. Eyestrain or speedy tiring of the eyes, usually due to weakness of visual organ or muscles and attended by headache, sometimes pain in the eyes.

asthma (az'-ma): A disease characterized by recurrent paroxysmal attacks of difficulty in breathing which may be accompanied by wheezing, cough, sense of suffocation or constriction of the chest. Occurs most frequently in children or during the first four decades of life. Many cases are due to inhalation or ingestion of substances to which the patient is hypersensitive. A family history of asthma is often present. BRONCHIAL A., attack of breathlessness associated with bronchial obstruction or spasm. Characterized by expiratory wheeze. CARDIAC A., paroxysmal dyspnea in left ventricular failure. STATUS ASTHMATICUS, repeated attacks of asthma without any period of freedom between spasms. —asthmatic, adj.

astigmatism (a-stig'-ma-tizm): Defective vision caused by inequality of one or more of the refractive surfaces of the eye, usually the corneal, so that the light rays do not converge to a single point on the retina. May be congenital or acquired. Syn., astigmia.—astigmatic, astigmic, adj.

astomia (a-stō'-mi-a): A congenital anomaly characterized by absence of the mouth.—astomatous, astomous, adj.

astr-, astro-: Denotes star(s), the heavens.

astragalus (as-trag'-a-lus): The ankle bone or talus upon which the tibia rests.—astragalar, adj.

astraphobia (as-tra-fō'-bi-a): Morbid fear of lightning and thunder.

astringent (as-trin'-jent): An agent that contracts organic tissue, thus lessening secretion, arresting hemorrhage, diarrhea, etc.—astringency, n. astringe, v.t.; astringent, adj.

astrocyte (as'-trō-sīt): A star-shaped cell, particularly a neuroglial cell. See **neuroglia**.

astrocytoma (as-trō-sī-tō'-ma): A relatively common, slow growing tumor of the central nervous system, formed from astrocytes (*q.v.*).

astroglia (as-trog'-li-a): Neuroglia (*q.v.*) that is composed of astrocytes.

astrophobia (as-trō-fō'-bi-a): Morbid fear of the stars and of celestial space.

asyllabia (a-sil-lā'-bi-a): A form of aphasia in which one recognizes individual letters of the alphabet but cannot form them into syllables or comprehend them when combined to form syllables.

asylum (a-sī'-lum): Old term for a mental hospital.

asymbolia (a-sim-bō'-li-a): Inability to recognize such symbols of communication as words, gestures, signs, etc. Asemia (*q.v.*).

asymmetry (ā-sim'-et-ri): Lack of similarity of the organs or parts on each side.

asymptomatic (a-simp-to-mat'-ik): Symptomless.

asynergy (a-sin'-er-jē): Failure of organs or parts which normally work together to do so.

asystole (a-sis'-to-lē): Imperfect, incomplete, or no contraction of the ventricles of the heart during systole (*q.v.*).

atactic (a-tak'-tik): Ataxic. See **ataxia**.

atactilia (a-tak-til'-i-a): Loss of ability to recognize impressions received through the sense of touch.

ataractic (at-a-rak'-tik): An agent that helps to relieve anxiety thus providing emotional equilibrium and tranquility without causing drowsiness. Syn., tranquilizer, neuroleptic.

ataraxia (at-a-rak'-si-a): A state of tranquility or calmness in which neither consciousness or mental faculties are interfered with.—ataractic, adj.

atavism (at'-a-vizm): The reappearance of an hereditary trait which has skipped one or more generations.—atavic, atavistic, adj.

ataxia, ataxy (a-taks'-i-a, a-taks'-i): Defective muscular control resulting in jerky and irregular movements, due to a lesion in the central nervous system. LOCOMOTOR ATAXIA, the disordered gait and loss of sense of position in the lower limbs, which occurs in tabes dorsalis (*q.v.*).—atactic, ataxic, adj.

atelectasis (at-e-lek'-ta-sis): 1. Imperfect expansion of the lungs at birth. 2. Collapse or airless state of an adult lung, partial or complete, due to occlusion of a bronchus or bronchiole caused by inspiration of a foreign object, tumor, aneurysm, mucous plug, certain drugs, a disease such as tuberculosis. Also a complication following abdominal surgery.—atelectatic, adj.

atherogenic (ath-e-rō-jen'-ik): Capable of producing atheroma.—atherogenesis, n.

atheroma (ath-e-rō'-ma): 1. Deposition of hard yellow plaques of lipoid material in the intimal layers of the arteries; the primary lesion in atherosclerosis (*q.v.*). May be related to high level of cholesterol in the blood. Of great importance in the coronary arteries in predisposing to coronary thrombosis. 2. A sebaceous cyst; see under **cyst.** —atheromatous, adj.

atherosclerosis (ath-er-ŏ-skler-ŏ′-sis): Arteriosclerosis coexisting with atheroma (*q.v.*).—atherosclerotic, adj.

atherosis (ath-er-ŏ′-sis): Atherosclerosis (*q.v.*).

athetosis (ath-e-tŏ′-sis): A condition marked by purposeless, involuntary, repeated, sinuous, writhing movements of the fingers and hands, toes and feet; sometimes involving most of the body. Generally due to a brain lesion. Seen chiefly in children in whom it is usually congenital; in older patients it is usually associated with cerebrovascular disease.—athetoid, athetotic, adj.

athlete's foot: See **tinea.**

athlete's heart: Lay term for a hypertrophic or dilated heart that is supposed to be the result of repeated overexertion.

athrepsia (a-threp′-si-a): Marasmus. Term used particularly in reference to children who suffer from progressive physical weakness and emaciation resulting from malnutrition.—athreptic, adj.

athrombia (a-throm′-bi-a): Lack of or defect in the clotting of the blood.

athyroidism (a-thī′-roid-izm): Lack of thyroid secretion because of absence or dysfunction of the gland. May be congenital or acquired; when congenital it produces cretinism (*q.v.*); when acquired in maturity it produces myxedema (*q.v.*).

atlas: The first cervical vertebra which supports the head; so called because the Greek hero, Atlas, was supposed to carry the earth on his shoulders. It articulates with the occipital bone above and the second cervical vertebra (axis) below.—atloid, adj.

atmosphere (at′-mos-fēr): See **air.**—atmospheric, adj. A. exerts a pressure of approximately 15 lb. per sq. in. at sea level; this increases below and decreases above sea level. It is also affected by humidity, moist air being lighter than dry air.

atom (at′-om): The smallest particle of an element capable of existing individually and of taking part in a chemical reaction without losing its identity. Over 100 different atoms have been recognized; in combination with one or more atoms of the same or another element, make up all

the known kinds of matter. Consists of a central, positively-charged nucleus which contains practically all of the mass of the atom, and surrounding negatively-charged electrons which move in an orbit around the nucleus.—atomic, adj.

atomic (a-tom′-ik): Pertaining to an atom. A. WEIGHT, the weight of an atom of a substance compared with that of an atom of hydrogen.

atomization (at-om-ī-zā′-shun): A mechanical process whereby a liquid is divided into a fine spray.—atomizer, n.

atonic (a-ton′-ic): Without tone; weak.—atonia, atony, atonicity, n.

atopic (a-top′-ik): 1. Pertaining to atopy (*q.v.*). 2. Out of place; displaced.

atopy (at′-op-i): Allergy which is hereditary. Term covers diseases such as hay fever, asthma, urticaria, and eczema where there is a clear family history of these conditions. —atopic, adj.

ATP: Adenosine triphosphate (*q.v.*).

atremia (a-trē′-mi-a): 1. Absence of tremor. 2. An hysterical condition in which the patient is unable to walk although the movements of walking can be performed without discomfort while lying down.

atresia (a-trē′-zi-a): Imperforation or closure of a normal body opening or canal, usually a congenital malformation.—atresic, atretic, adj.

atrial (ā′-tri-al): Pertaining to an atrium. A. FIBRILLATION, chaotic cardiac irregularity without any semblance of order; the fibers of the atria contract rapidly and convulsively, independently of each other and of the contractions of the ventricles; commonly associated with mitral stenosis and nodular toxic goiter, but also with other diseases of the heart; sometimes seen in general toxic conditions. A. FLUTTER, rapid, regular cardiac rhythm caused by an irritable focus in atrial muscle and usually associated with organic heart disease; speed of atrial beats may be between 200 and 400; ventricles usually respond to every second beat, but may be slowed by carotid sinus pressure.

atrial septal defect: Continued patency of the foramen ovale (*q.v.*) after birth.

atrichia (a-trik′-i-a): Lack or loss of hair. Syn., atrichosis.—atrichous, adj.

atrioventricular (ā-tri-ŏ-ven-trik′-ū-lar): Pertaining to the atria and the ventricles of the heart. Applied to a node, tract, and valves. Syn., auriculoventricular.

atrium (ā'-tri-um): Either of the two upper chambers of the heart; they receive blood from the veins and force it into the ventricles. See **auricle.**—atria, pl.; atrial, adj.

atrophy (at'-rō-fi): Wasting, emaciation, diminution in size and function of an organ or part that had previously reached mature size. May result from a pathological condition or a physiologic cause such as aging or disuse.—atrophied, atrophic, adj. ACUTE YELLOW A., massive necrosis of the liver associated with severe infection, toxemia of pregnancy, or ingested poisons. MUSCULAR A., affects principally the skeletal muscles; may result from interruption of nerve supply, disuse, or pathology of muscle tissue. PROGRESSIVE MUSCULAR A., a chronic disease marked by progressive wasting of the muscles, beginning with those in the upper extremities.

ATS: Antitetanus serum. Contains tetanus antibodies. Produces artificial passive immunity. A test dose must be given first. Can cause anaphylaxis.

ATT: Antitetanus toxoid. Contains treated tetanus toxins. Produces artificial active immunity. Does not cause anaphylaxis.

attendant: A nonprofessional person who performs many different kinds of services in assisting the professional nurse to care for the sick.

attenuation (a-ten-ū-ā'-shun): A bacteriological process by which organisms are rendered less virulent by exposure to an unfavorable environment such as drying, heating, or being passed through another organism. They can then be used in the preparation of vaccines.—attenuant, attenuated, adj.; attenuate. v.t., v.i.

attitude: 1. A settled mode of thinking. 2. Posture; position of the body or limbs, particularly a position assumed in illness or abnormal mental states such as catatonia (q.v.).

attraction: The force or influence existing mutually between particles or masses which causes them to be drawn toward each other. CAPILLARY A., the force which causes a fluid to be drawn into and to rise in a tube of fine caliber.

atypical (ā-tip'-i-k'l): Not typical; unusual, irregular; not conforming to type, e.g., A. pneumonia.

audi-, audio-, audito-; Denotes: (1) sound; (2) hearing.

audile (aw'-dil): 1. Relating to hearing. 2. Denoting a person with a type of mental imagery which recalls auditory impressions more readily than visual or motor.

audiogram (aw'-di-ō-gram): A chart showing acuity of hearing as measured by the audiometer (q.v.).

audiology (aw-di-ol'-o-ji): The science dealing with hearing.—audiological, adj.; audiologically, adv.

audiometer (aw-di-om'-et-er): A precision instrument for measuring the activity and range of hearing. It generates pure tones over a wide range of pitch and intensity.—audiometric, adj.; audiometry, audiometrist, n.

audition (aw-dish'-un): 1. The act of hearing. 2. Perception of sound.

auditory (aw'-dit-ō-ri): Pertaining to the sense or organs of hearing. A. AREA, that portion of the temporal lobe of the cortex which interprets sound. A. MEATUS, the canal between the pinna and the eardrum. A. NERVES, the eighth pair of cranial nerves. A. OSSICLES, the three tiny bones stretching across the cavity of the middle ear—malleus, incus and stapes. A. TUBE, eustachian tube (q.v.).

Auerbach's plexus (ow'-er-bakh): A plexus of autonomic nerve fibers situated between the longitudinal and circular fibers of the muscular coat of the stomach and intestines; the myenteric plexus. [Leopold Auerbach, German neuropathologist. 1828-1897.]

aura (aw'-ra): A premonition; a peculiar sensation or warning, recognized by the patient, of an impending convulsion or seizure such as occurs in epilepsy. May be auditory, optic, kinesthetic, epigastric, etc. in nature.

aural (awr'-al): 1. Pertaining to the ear. 2. Pertaining to an aura.

auricle (aw'-ri-k'l): 1. The pinna or flap of the external ear. 2. An appendage to the cardiac atrium. 3. Commonly used mistakenly for atrium (q.v.).—auricular, adj.

auricular (aw-rik'-ū-lar): Pertaining to (1) an auricle; (2) the ear. A. FIBRILLATION, A. FLUTTER, see **atrial fibrillation, atrial flutter.**

auriculoventricular: See **atrioventricular.**

auripuncture (aw-ri-pungk'-tur): Puncture of the tympanic membrane (q.v.).

auris (aw'-ris): The ear.

auriscope (aw'-ris-kōp): An instrument for examining the ear, usually incorporating both magnification and electric illumination. A kind of otoscope.

auscultation (aws-kul-tā′-shun): A method of listening to the body sounds for diagnostic purposes, particularly the heart, lungs, and fetal circulation. It may be (1) immediate, by placing the ear directly against the body; (2) mediate, by the use of a stethoscope.—auscultatory, adj.; auscult, auscultate, v.

aut-, auto-: Denotes: (1) self, the same one; (2) self-regulating; (3) self-caused, self-induced.

autism (aw′-tizm): 1. Schizophrenic (q.v.) syndrome in childhood. 2. A state of morbid self-absorption in which one is dominated by self-centered thoughts that are wishful, symbolic, delusional or hallucinatory and not modified by logic or rational processes.

autistic (aw-tis′-tik): Morbidly self-centered thinking, governed by the wishes of the individual; wishful thinking (phantasy), in contrast to reality thinking. Occurs in schizophrenia (q.v.).—autism, n.

autoagglutination (aw-tō-a-gloo-tin-ā′-shun): Agglutination of an individual's red blood corpuscles by his own serum, in the absence of a specific antibody.

autoantibody (aw-tō-an′-ti-bod-i): An antibody formed in an individual and which reacts against other antigenic substances in the same individual.

autoantigen (aw-tō-an′-ti-jen): Something within the body capable of initiating the production of autoantibody.

autoclave (aw′-tō-klāv): 1. An apparatus for high-pressure steam sterilization. 2. To sterilize in an autoclave.

autodigestion (aw-tō-di-jest′-chun): Self-digestion of body tissues by their own secretions. Autolysis (q.v.).

autoeroticism (aw-tō-e-rot′-i-sizm): Sensual self-gratification obtained by self-manipulation or from looking at one's erogenous zones such as the mouth, anus, genitals. See **erotogenic.**

autogenous (aw-toj′-e-nus): Self-generated; endogenous; originating within the body and not acquired from any outside source. Applied to bone graft, skin graft, etc. A. VACCINE, one prepared from the bacteria from the patient's own infection. Also autogenetic, autogenic.

autograft (aw′-tō-graft): A graft in which the tissue is taken from another part of the body which is to receive it.

autohypnosis (aw-tō-hip-nō′-sis): Self-induced hypnosis.

autoimmunization (aw′-tō-im-mū-nī-zā′-shun): Immunization obtained by having an attack of a disease or by processes occuring naturally in the body. See **Hashimoto's disease.**

autoinfection (aw-tō-in-fek′-shun): Infection arising from an organism already present within the body or transferred from one part of the body to another by fingers, etc.

autointoxication (aw-tō-in-tok′-si-kā-shun): Poisoning from faulty metabolic products elaborated within the body, or from some uneliminated toxin generated within the body.

autolysis (aw-tol′-i-sis): Autodigestion (q.v.) which occurs if digestive ferments escape into surrounding tissues.—autolytic, adj.

automatic (aw-tō-mat′-ik): That which is performed without the influence of the will; spontaneous; non-volitional acts; involuntary acts.

automatism (aw-tom′-a-tizm): Performance of involuntary acts without intention or purpose, often without knowledge that they are taking place. Occurs in somnambulism, hysterical and epileptic states.

autonomic (aw-tō-nom′-ik): Independent; self-governing. A. NERVOUS SYSTEM (A.N.S.), that part of the peripheral nervous system which is made up of nerve cells and fibers that cannot be controlled by will. In common usage the term is applied to all nerves and ganglia not included in the central nervous system. It is divided into the parasympathetic and sympathetic portions and controls the functioning of glands, smooth muscle tissue and the heart.

autophagia (aw-tō-fā′-ji-a): The biting of one's own flesh; occurs sometimes in dementia.

autophilia (aw-tō-fil′-i-a): Narcissism; self-love to a pathological degree.

autophobia (aw-tō-fō′-bi-a): Morbid fear of one's self or of being alone.

autoplasty (aw′-tō-plas-ti): Replacement or repair of injured or diseased tissues by a graft of healthy tissues from another area of the same body.—autoplastic, adj.; autoplast, n.

autopsy (aw′-top-si): The examination of the organs of a dead body for the purpose of determining the cause of death or of studying the pathological conditions of the organs. Syn., postmortem examination, necropsy.

autosome (aw′-tō-sōm): One of the ordinary chromosomes equally distributed among the germ cells.

autosuggestion (aw-tō-sug-jest′-yun): 1.

41   **azotemia**

Self-suggestion; uncritical acceptance of ideas arising in the individual's own mind. Occurs in hysteria. 2. The technique of trying to improve health or change behavior by constant repetition of certain phrases; e.g., 'Every day in every way I am getting better and better.'

autotherapy (aw-tō-ther′-a-pi): 1. Treatment by administration of filtrates of the patient's own secretions. 2. Cure of disease without medical supervision; self-cure.

autotoxicosis (aw-tō-tok-si-kō′-sis): Autointoxication (q.v.).

autotransfusion (aw-tō-trans-fū′-zhun): The infusion into the patient of the actual blood lost by hemorrhage, especially when it occurs into the abdominal cavity as in ruptured ectopic pregnancy or ruptured spleen. Also called autoreinfusion.

autovaccine (aw-tō-vak′-sēn): Autogenous vaccine (q.v.).

aux-, auxe-, auxo-: Denotes: (1) growth, enlargement; (2) accelerating, stimulating.

auxotherapy (awk-sō-ther′-a-pi): Substitution therapy; e.g., organotherapy or hormonotherapy (q.v.).

A-V: Abbreviation for atrioventricular or atriovenous. A-V BLOCK, a type of heart block in which the impulse between the atria and the ventricles of the heart is either slowed down or blocked.

avascular (a-vas′-kū-lar): Bloodless; not vascular; i.e., without blood vessels. May be normal, as in cartilaginous tissue, or pathological. A. NECROSIS, death of bone from deficient blood supply following injury or disease. It is often a precursor of osteoarthritis.—avascularize, v.t., v.i.; avascularity, n.

avascularization (a-vas-kū-lar-ī-zā′-shun): The act of expelling blood from a part as by application of elastic bandage or by posture.

aversion (a-ver′-zhun): A method of treatment by deconditioning. Effective in some forms of addiction and abnormal behavior.

aviation medicine: The branch of medicine that is concerned with physiological, pathological, and emotional conditions or disturbances resulting from travel in an airplane.

aviation physiology: That branch of physiology that is concerned with physiological changes that occur during various activities at high altitudes; e.g., flying in an airplane or space vehicle, mountain climbing.

aviator's disease: A condition marked by headache, drowsiness, vasomotor and other disturbances; sometimes seen in aviators.

aviator's ear: Aero-otitis media (q.v.).

avian (ā′-vi-an): Pertaining to birds. A. TUBERCLE BACILLUS, resembles other types of tubercle bacilli but attacks primarily birds including chickens and ducks; seldom causes disease in man.

avidin (av′-i-din): An antivitamin; a specific protein found in raw egg-white. It interferes with the absorption of biotin (q.v.), thus producing biotin deficiency.

avirulent (a-vir′-ū-lent): Without virulence (q.v.).

avitaminosis (ā-vīt-a-min-ō′-sis): Any disease resulting from a deficiency of one or more vitamins in the diet; includes such disease conditions as scurvy, beri-beri, and rickets.

avulsion (a-vul′-shun): A forcible wrenching away, as of a limb, nerve, or polypus. PHRENIC A., tearing of the phrenic nerve, paralyzing one side of the diaphragm; a procedure used to obtain rest for a tuberculous base of lung.

axilla (ak-sil′-a): The armpit.—axillae, pl.; axillary, adj.; applied to nerves, blood vessels and lympthatics.

axion (ak′-sē-on): The brain and spinal cord.

axis (aks′-is): 1. The second cervical vertebra. 2. An imaginary line passing through the center. 3. The median line of the body. —axial, adj.

axon (aks′-on): That process of a nerve cell conveying impulses away from the cell body and toward the next nerve; the essential part of the nerve fiber and a direct prolongation of the nerve cell. Also called axis-cylinder, axis-cylinder process, neuraxon, neurite.—axonal, adj.

axonotmesis (ak-son-ot-mē′-sis): Peripheral degeneration as a result of damage to the axons of a nerve. The internal architecture is preserved and recovery depends upon regeneration of the axons, and may take many months (about an inch a month is the usual speed of regeneration). Such a lesion may result from pinching, crushing, or prolonged pressure.

azoospermia (a-zō-ō-sperm′-i-a): Sterility in the male through absence of motile spermatozoa in the semen.

azote (az′-ōt): Nitrogen.

azotemia (az-ō-tē′-mi-a): The presence of pathological amounts of nitrogenous products, principally urea, in the blood. Seen in such conditions as circulatory or renal failure, gastrointestinal hemorrhage, dehydration. Uremia (*q.v.*).—azotemic, adj.

azoturia (az-ō-tū′-ri-a): The presence of excessive amounts of urea or other nitrogenous products in the urine.—azoturic, adj.

azygos (az′-i-gos): Occurring singly, not paired. A. VEINS, three unpaired veins of the abdomen and thorax which empty into the inferior vena cava.

B

Babinski's reflex: Movement of the great toe upward (dorsiflexion) instead of downward (plantar flexion), and fanning of the other toes, on stroking the outer border of the sole of the foot. Seen in disease or injury to the upper motor neurons on the homolateral side in organic but not hysteric hemiplegia. Babies exhibit dorsiflexion, but after learning to walk they show the normal plantar flexion. Also called Babinski's great toe sign. [Joseph François Felix Babinski, French neurologist. 1857-1932.]

baccate (bak'-āt): Resembling a berry.

Bacillaceae (bas-i-lā'-sē-ē): A large family of spore-forming organisms commonly found in soil. Most are harmless to man but a few cause serious infections, *e.g.*, *Bacillus anthracis* (anthrax), *Clostridium tetani* (tetanus), *Clostridium welchii* (gas gangrene).

bacillary dysentery (bas'-i-lar-i dis'-en-ter-i): A severe form of enteritis marked by abdominal pain, severe diarrhea, sometimes bloody stools. Caused by a bacteria of the *Shigella* genus. Especially prevalent in tropical climates.

bacille Calmette Guérin: A vaccine prepared from bovine tubercle bacilli; intended for use in producing active immunity to tuberculosis in children and young adults. Originally given by mouth, now subcutaneously. Abbreviation, BCG.

bacillemia (bas-i-lēm'-i-a): The presence of bacilli in the blood.—basillemic, adj.

bacillosis (bas-i-lō'-sis): A general infection caused by bacilli.

bacilluria (bas-i-lū'-ri-a): The presence of bacilli in the urine.—bacilluric, adj.

Bacillus bas-il'-us): A term now restricted to a genus of rod-shaped microorganisms of the family Bacillaceae (*q.v.*), consisting of aerobic, gram-positive cells that produce endospores; the majority are motile by means of flagella. These organisms are saprophytes; their spores are common in soil and dust. B. ANTHRACIS causes anthrax in man and animals.

bacillus (bas-il'-us): A general term loosely employed to designate any rod-shaped microorganism.—bacilli, pl.; bacillary, adj.

backbone: The spinal or vertebral column.

backflow: The flowing of a current or substance in a direction opposite to that it usually takes, *e.g.*, regurgitation.

bacteremia (bak-ter-ē'-mi-a): The presence of bacteria in the circulating blood. Also bacteriemia.—bacteremic, adj.

bacteria (bak-tē'-ri-a): One-celled, plantlike microorganisms, a great many varieties of which are found in man's environment; the majority are not disease producing. Structurally, there is a protoplast, containing cytoplasmic and nuclear material (not seen by ordinary methods of microscopy) within a limiting cytoplasmic membrane, and a supporting cell wall. Other structures such as flagella, fimbriae and capsules may also be present. Individual cells may be spherical (cocci), straight or curved rods (bacilli), or spiral (spirilla); they may form chains or masses, and some show branching with mycelium (*q.v.*) formation. They may produce various pigments including chlorophyll. Reproduction is chiefly by simple binary (*q.v.*) fission. Some live on dead organic matter and so are saprophytes; others live in living tissue and so are parasites. Each variety has its own requirements as to nourishment, light, moisture, pH, etc. Some are pathogenic to man and animals; some cause plant diseases.—bacterium, sing.; bacterial, adj.

bacterial resistance: The resistance which some organisms, particularly pathogenic organisms, develop for a drug to which they were originally susceptible.

bactericide (bak-tēr'-i-sīd): Any agent which destroys bacteria.—bactericidal, adj.; bactericidally, adv.

bacteriocidin (bak-tēr-i-ō-sī'-din): Antibody which kills bacteria.

bacteriologist (bak-tēr-i-ol'-ō-jist): One who studies and is skilled in the science of bacteriology.

bacteriology (bak-tēr-i-ol'-ō-ji): The science and study of bacteria.—bacteriological, adj.; bacteriologically, adv.

bacteriolysin (bak-tēr-i-ol'-i-sin): A specific antibody (*q.v.*), produced in the blood after an infection with an organism and which is capable of destroying the invading organism by lysis.—bacteriolytic, adj.

bacteriolysis (bak-tēr-i-ol'-i-sis): The disin-

tegration and dissolution of bacteria.—
bacteriolytic, adj.

bacteriophage (bak-tēr′-i-ō-fāj): A filterable virus parasitic on bacteria.

bacteriophobia (bak-tēr-i-ō-fō′-bi-a): Morbid fear of bacteria or disease-producing organisms.

bacteriosis (bak-tēr-i-ō′-sis): Any disease caused by bacteria.

bacteriostasis (bak-tēr-i-ō-stā′-sis): Arrest or hindrance of bacterial growth.—bacteriostatic, adj.

bacteriostat (bak-tēr′-i-ō-stat): An agent that prevents or inhibits the growth of bacteria.

bacteriotherapy (bak-tēr′-i-ō-ther′-ap-i): Treatment of disease by introduction of bacteria into the blood stream, *e.g.*, malaria in the treatment of neurosyphilis.—bacteriotherapeutic, adj.

bacteriotoxemia (bak-tēr′-i-ō-tok-sē′-mi-a): The presence of bacterial toxins in the circulating blood.

bacteriotoxin (bak-tēr-i-ō-tok′-sin): A toxin that is produced by bacteria or one that is toxic to bacteria.

bacteriuria (bak-tēr-i-ū′-ri-a): The presence of bacteria in the urine. Also bacteruria.—bacteriuric, adj.

bag: A pouch or sac. B. OF WATERS, the membranous sac that contains the amniotic fluid and the fetus. COLOSTOMY B., one worn over the stoma after a colostomy. In obstetrics, a silk or rubber B. that is inserted into the uterine cavity and then inflated to induce labor or dilate the cervix; common types are Barnes and Voorhees.

bagassosis (bag-a-sō′-sis): A respiratory disorder caused by inhalation of the dust of cane sugar waste that remains after the sugar is extracted. Also baggascosis.

baker's itch: Contact dermatitis (*q.v.*) resulting from handling sugar or flour; probably allergic.

baking soda: Sodium bicarbonate (*q.v.*).

balance: In physiology, the harmonious relation between the parts and organs of the body and their functions. ACID-BASE B., a normal equilibrium or ratio between the acid and base elements of the blood and body fluids; expressed by the symbol *p*H. FLUID B., term commonly used to express the concept of both water balance and electrolyte balance in the body. NITROGEN B., balance between the intake and output of nitrogen; *negative nitrogen balance* occurs when more nitrogen is lost than is taken into the body; may happen in such condi-

tions as burns, starvation, fevers, malnutrition. *Positive nitrogen b.* occurs when more nitrogen is taken into than is lost from the body. WATER B., that between the amount of water taken into and excreted from the body. ELECTROLYTE B. is associated with WATER B., since the electrolytes are the ions present in body water; term refers to the concentrations of ions of electrolytes in the interstitial fluid and the blood plasma, which are normally essentially the same.

balanitis (bal-a-nī′-tis): Inflammation of the glans penis, often associated with phimosis.

balanoposthitis (bal-an-ō-pos-thī′-tis): Inflammation of the glans penis and prepuce.

balanus (bal′-an-us): The glans of the penis or clitoris.

Balkan frame: A frame, usually made of wood or iron pipes, fitted over a bed and to which weights and pulleys are attached; used to suspend immobilized fractured limbs and provide for continuous traction.

ball-and-socket joint: A joint in which the round head of one bone fits into a cavity of another bone permitting full freedom of movement or circumduction (*q.v.*), *e.g.*, the shoulder or hip joint.

ballismus (ba-liz′-mus): The occurrence of violent, quick, jerking, or twisting movements, caused by contraction of arm or leg muscles and seen in chorea. May be bilateral; when it occurs in only one side it is called hemiballism. Also ballism.

ballistocardiograph (ba-lis-tō-kar′-di-ō-graf): An apparatus for estimating the volume of cardiac output by recording the movement of the body resulting from the contraction of the ventricles and ejection of blood into the aorta. The record of this movement is called a ballistocardiogram.

ballistophobia (ba-lis-tō-fō′-bi-a): Morbid fear of missiles.

ballooning (ba-loon′-ing): Distending a body cavity by the introduction of air or other agent to facilitate its examination or for therapeutic purposes.

ballottement (ba-lot-mon′): Testing for a floating object, especially used to diagnose pregnancy. A finger is inserted into the vagina and the uterus is pushed forward; if a fetus is present it will fall back again, bouncing in its bath of fluid. RENAL B., palpation of the kidney by pushing it suddenly and firmly forward from the back with one hand while the other hand is pressed firmly into the abdominal wall.

balm (bahm): A healing or soothing medication, usually an ointment. Syn., balsam (*q.v.*).

balneotherapy (bal-nē-ō-ther′-ap-i): The treatment of disease by the use of baths, *e.g.,* hot, cold, or salt water baths. Also balneotherapeutics.

balsam (bawl′-sam): A pharmaceutical preparation containing resinous substances; used topically for its healing and soothing qualities.

bandage (ban′-dij): A piece of cloth or other material, of varying size and shape, applied to some part of the body to hold a dressing or splint in place; support, compress or immobilize a part; prevent or correct a deformity; or to aid in the arrest of hemorrhage. Depending on its purpose and the part to which it is applied, B.'s are made of gauze, muslin, flannel, elastic webbing, rubber, adhesive plaster or moleskin, paper, cohesive material which adheres to itself but not to any other substance, and wide-mesh material impregnated with such substances as plaster of paris, waterglass, chalk, dextrin, starch, etc., which harden

or solidify after application. Shapes of bandages are: ROLLER, a continuous strip of material of varying length and width, which has been tightly wound; TRIANGULAR, half of a piece of material 36 to 40 inches square; CRAVAT, a triangular B. folded upon itself several times until the desired width is obtained; TAILED, made of several strips of material which are joined to each other only in the middle third; HANDKERCHIEF, a large square of material, sometimes with ties to hold it in place. Bandages are also classified according to the way they are applied: CIRCULAR, applied in several circular turns about a part; OBLIQUE, several slanting turns about a part, but the turns do not overlap; SPIRAL, several turns about a part, each one higher on the part than the previous one and overlapping it by about two-thirds; SPIRAL REVERSE, a spiral B. in which the roll of material is given a half-twist at each turn so that the inside of the roll becomes the outside, thus the B. is made to fit a part that is not uniform in size throughout; FIGURE-OF-EIGHT,

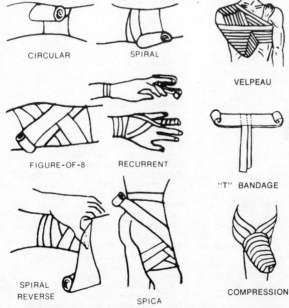

Bandage terminology

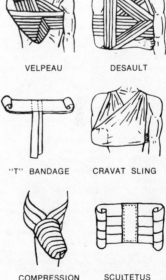

Types of bandages

a series of turns, each one crossing the previous one at midpoint and then encircling a part above or below the crossing so that the finished B. describes a figure eight; SPICA, a type of spiral B. in which the turns are folded regularly upon themselves in the form of the letter V, a maneuver which helps make the B. fit such parts as the shoulder, groin, foot; RECURRENT, a series of turns starting in the middle of the area to be covered and then proceeding to either side with each turn overlapping and coming back to the starting point, used for such areas as the tip of a finger, the head, or an amputation stump. ACE B., trade mark for a roller bandage made of elastic material and frequently used to make firm, continuous pressure on a part. BARTON'S B., a figure-of-eight B. used to support a fractured lower jaw. CAPELINE B., a spica B. applied in the form of a cap or hood to cover the head, shoulder, amputation stump. COMPRESSION B., one applied firmly enough to compress a part but not shut off the blood supply. DEMIGAUNTLET B., covers the hand but not the fingers. DESAULT'S B. binds the elbow to the side, used for fractured clavicle. ESMARCH'S B., a rubber B. applied to a limb from the distal end upward, used to expel blood from a part to be operated upon. SCULTETUS B., a many-tailed B. for chest or abdomen. SUSPENSORY B., one applied like a sling to support a part, *e.g.*, the scrotum. VELPEAU'S B., one which binds the arm to the chest with the hand resting on the opposite shoulder, used for fractured clavicle. T-B., two strips of material joined like the letter T, used for holding perineal dressings in place.

Bandl's ring (band'-l): A ridge that can be felt at the junction of the isthmus and the fundus of the uterus; develops in abnormally prolonged labor and interferes with the expulsion of the fetus. [Ludwig Bandl, German obstetrician. 1842-1892.]

bandy leg: Bowleg.

bank: 1. In medicine, a place for storage of such materials as whole blood, plasma, bone, skin, cornea, or other human tissue, to be used therapeutically, often in reparative surgery. 2. A reserve supply of certain human tissue or blood to be used therapeutically in another person, *e.g.*, eye B., blood B.

Banti's disease: Now more often regarded as a clinical syndrome rather than a disease. Characterized by gastrointestinal bleeding, anemia, leukopenia, and thrombocytopenia. There is increased pressure in the portal veins. [Guido Banti, Italian physician. 1852-1925.]

barba (bar'-ba): The beard or the hair of the head.

Barbados leg (bar-bā'-dōz): See **elephantiasis.**

barber's itch or **rash:** See **sycosis.**

barbiturates (bar-bit'-ū-rātz): A large group of synthetic compounds derived from barbituric acid and widely used for their hypnotic or sedative effects. Small changes in the basic structure result in the formation of rapid-, medium-, or long-acting drugs, and a wide range is now available. Continued use may lead to tolerance and dependence, hence addiction. Action is potentiated in the presence of alcohol. Overdosage may lead to profound narcosis, respiratory depression, and death. Allergic skin conditions may develop in some patients.

barbotage (bar-bo-tazh'): A method of spinal anesthesia; a small amount of solution from a syringe is injected into the subarachnoid space and the plunger partially withdrawn, allowing the cerebrospinal fluid to mix with the remaining fluid in the syringe. Part of this mixture is then injected and the plunger partially withdrawn again. This process may be repeated several times before all of the medication in the syringe has been injected.

baresthesia (bar-es-thē'-zi-a): The pressure sense.

Barlow's disease: Syn., infantile scurvy (*q.v.*). [Thomas Barlow, English physician. 1845-1945.]

Barnes' bag: See **bag.**

baromacrometer (bar-ō-mā-krom'-e-ter): An instrument for measuring the length and weight of the newborn.

barospirator (bar-ō-spī'-rā-tor): A machine for producing artificial respiration, *e.g.*, the Drinker respirator (*q.v.*).

barotalgia (bar-ō-tal'-ji-a): Pain in the middle ear caused by a difference in the air pressure in it and in the surrounding atmosphere.

barotitis (bar-ō-tī'-tis): Inflammation of the middle ear caused by changes in atmospheric pressure.

barotrauma (bar-ō-traw'-ma): Injury due to a change in atmospheric or water pressure, *e.g.*, ruptured eardrum.

Barré-Guillain syndrome (bar-rā'gē-yan'): A neurologic syndrome; cause unknown but thought to be due to a virus; symptoms include pain, tenderness and weakness of muscles; the chief laboratory finding is an increase in the protein content of the cerebrospinal fluid without an accompanying increase in the cell count.

barrel chest: The enlarged, rounded thorax seen in persons with chronic emphysema.

barren (bar'-en): Sterile, particularly in reference to the female.

barrier (bar'-ē-er): An obstruction, obstacle, blocking agent. BLOOD-BRAIN B., the mechanism which prevents certain substances such as bacteria or their toxins, or drugs, from passing from the blood to the cerebrospinal fluid or brain. PLACENTAL B., the tissue in the placenta which prevents certain substances from passing from the mother's blood to that of the fetus. B. NURSING, a method of preventing the spread of infection from an infected patient to others in the area by the use of isolation technique (q.v.).

bartholinitis (bar-tol-in-ī'-tis): Inflammation of Bartholin's glands (q.v.).

Bartholin's glands (bar'-to-linz): Two small bean-shaped mucus-secreting glands situated on either side of the vaginal orifice at the base of the labia minora; they open onto the surface by means of a single long duct and are of clinical importance because they frequently become infected, particularly with the gonococcus organism. [Caspar Bartholin, Danish anatomist. 1655-1738.]

Bartonella fever: Non-protozoal hemolytic anemia. Occurs in several forms; endemic in Peru. Syn., Oroya fever, Carrion's disease. Probably transmitted by sandflies. Also bartonellosis.

baruria (bar-ū'-ri-a): The condition in which the urine has an abnormally high specific gravity.

basal ganglia (bā'-sal gan'-gli-a): Four small islands of grey matter located in the white matter at the base of the cerebrum. The lentiform nucleus, comprising globus pallidus and putamen, together with the caudate nucleus, make up the corpus striatum, which with the claustrum is called the B.G. Concerned with modifying and coordinating voluntary muscle movement. Site of degeneration in Parkinson's disease. See **paralysis.**

basal metabolic rate: The rate at which energy is expended by an individual during digestive, physical, and emotional rest, as estimated by measuring the amount of O_2 intake and CO_2 output during a specified time period. Abbreviated BMR.

basal metabolism test: A test for measuring the basal metabolic rate (q.v.).

basal narcosis (nar-kō'-sis): The preanesthetic administration of narcotic drugs which reduce fear and anxiety, induce sleep and thereby minimize postoperative shock.

base (bās): 1. The lowest part. 2. The main part of a compound. 3. In chemistry, the substance which combines with an acid to form a salt.—basal, basic, basilar, adj.

basement membrane: A thin, delicate, transparent layer of tissue underlying the epithelium of mucous membranes and glands.

basilic (ba-sil'-ik): Prominent. B. VEIN, a large vein on the inner side of the arm. The MEDIAN B. VEIN, at the bend of the elbow, is generally chosen for venipuncture.

basocyte (bā'-sō-sīt): A basophil or leukocyte cell.

basocytopenia (bā-sō-sīt-ō-pē'-ni-a): Basophilic leukopenia or a decrease in the proportion of basophils in the blood.

basocytosis (bā-sō-sī-tō'-sis): Basophilic leukocytosis or an abnormal increase in the proportion of basophilic leukocytes in the blood.

basophil(e) (bā'-sō-fil): 1. A substance, cell, or tissue that stains well with basic dyes. 2. A polymorphonuclear leukocyte distinguished by the presence of large granules which stain intensely with basic dyes and have a relatively lightly staining nucleus; they make up approximately 0.5% of the leukocytes in the circulating blood. Their function is unknown; they increase in numbers in such pathological conditions as Hodgkin's disease, smallpox, chickenpox, myelotic leukemia.

basophilia (bā-sō-fil'-i-a): 1. Increase of basophils in the circulating blood. 2. A condition in which red blood cells show basophilic-staining granules; seen in leukemia, advanced anemia, malaria, lead poisoning and some other toxic states.

basophobia (bā-sō-fō'-bi-a): Morbid fear of walking.

bath: 1. The apparatus or place used for bathing. 2. The immersion of all or any part of the body into water or other substance, or the application of a spray, jet, or vapor from a fluid, for cleansing purposes or therapy. The term is modified according to (a) temperature, e.g.., cold, contrast, hot, tepid; (b) medium used, e.g., mud, sand, water, wax; (c) medicament added, e.g., potassium permanganate, saline, sulfur; (d) function of medicament, e.g., astringent, disinfectant; (e) part bathed, e.g., arm, sitz bath; (f) environment, e.g., bed. See **hydrotherapy, balneotherapy.**

bathophobia (bath-ō-fō'-bi-a): An exaggerated fear of deep places or of looking down into deep places.

battered baby syndrome: A baby with swollen and bruised portions of body. Radiographically there is subperiosteal new bone at ends of long bones and fracture separation of cartilaginous epiphyses.

battered child syndrome: The result of deliberate trauma inflicted on a young child by custodians; includes any or all of the following conditions: bruises of the skin, multiple fractures, hematomata, malnutrition, retarded growth and development, bone deformities.

baunscheidtism (bawn'-shīt-izm): A method of producing counterirritation by acupuncture (q.v.) using an instrument with several needles; the skin may be rubbed with an irritant such as croton oil or oil of mustard before the treatment, or the needles dipped into an irritant before use. Named for its inventor, Karl Baunscheidt.

Bazin's disease: Erythema induratum. A chronic, recurrent disorder, involving the skin of the legs of women. There are deep-seated nodules which later ulcerate. [Antoine Pierre Ernest Bazin, French dermatologist. 1807-1878.]

BCG: Abbreviation for bacille Calmette Guérin (q.v.).

b.d.: Abbreviation for bis die, twice a day.

bead (bēd): A small, usually spherical projection. RACHITIC BEADS, a series of small, rounded prominences at the points where the ribs join their cartilages; sometimes seen in rickets; also rachitic rosary.

bearing down: 1. A pseudonym for the expulsive pains in the second stage of labor. 2. A feeling of weight and descent in the pelvis associated with uterine prolapse or pelvic tumor.

beat (bēt): A throb or pulsation as of the blood in the heart or an artery. APEX B., see **apex.** DROPPED B., refers to loss of an occasional ventricular beat as occurs in extrasystole (q.v.). ECTOPIC B., one which does not originate in the sinus node. PREMATURE B., an extrasystole. See **pulse.**

bechic (bek'-ik): 1. A cough remedy. 2. Acting to control coughing.

bed: A couch or other article of furniture to sleep or rest in or on. The term generally is used to include the frame, springs, mattress and bed linen. AIR B., one with an inflatable mattress, usually rubber. ANESTHETIC B., one which is prepared to receive a patient who has had a general anesthetic; also called ETHER B. GATCH B., one with a crank mechanism to permit raising and lowering of the head to knees. ROCKING B., one with a motor attachment which causes it to rock at a regular rate; used as a means of artificial respiration. WATER B., one with a rubber mattress partly filled with water; used to prevent bedsores.

bed board: A board placed beneath the mattress to give support to certain areas of the body; often used in cases of low back pain.

bedbug: A blood-sucking insect of the genus Cimex; small, wingless, reddish-brown in color, hard and smooth in appearance, and with a distinctive odor. They live and lay eggs in cracks and crevices of furniture and walls, and can survive long periods without food. They are nocturnal in habit, and an irritating substance in their saliva causes their bites to produce wheals with a central hemorrhagic point. They apparently are not vectors of disease but their bites leave a route for secondary infection. See **Cimex.**

bedpan: A special, appropriately shaped receptacle used to receive fecal and urinary waste from patients who are bedfast.

bedrail: A device which is fastened to the side of the bed to prevent the patient from falling or getting out of bed.

bedrest: 1. A device used for propping a patient up in bed. 2. Continuous confinement to bed for the purpose of rest.

bedsore (bed'-sōr): Decubitus ulcer (q.v.).

Beer's knife: Delicate instrument with triangular blade used in cataract operations for incision of cornea preparatory to removal of lens. [Georg Joseph Beer, Austrian ophthalmologist. 1763-1821.]

behavior (bē-hāv'-yor): In general sense, conduct. As a psychological term, means response of an organism to its situation in relation to its environment. B. THERAPY, see **aversion.** B. REFLEX, one acquired through training or repetition. INCONGRUOUS B., B. that is inconsistent with the individual's usual behavior.

behaviorism (bē-hāv'-yor-izm): Psychological term that denotes an approach to psychology through the study of responses and reactions, i.e., objective, observable behavior, rather than through such subjective phenomena as ideas or emotions. Developed by John B. Watson, American psychologist [1878-1958].

bejel (bej'-el): An endemic, non-venereal disease found in Arabs of the Near and Middle East, mostly in children; the causative organism is indistinguishable from that which causes syphilis.

bel: A term used to express a unit of sound intensity. See **decibel.**

belch: 1. An eructation (q.v.). 2. To eructate, or allow gas from the stomach to escape noisily through the mouth.

'belle indifference': The incongruous lack of emotion or anxiety despite incapacitating symptoms, commonly shown by patients with hysteria. First noted by Janet (1893). [Pierre Marie Felix Janet, French psychiatrist, 1859-1947.]

Bellocq's sound or cannula (bel'-oks, kan-ū'-la): A curved tube used for plugging the posterior nares in epistaxis.

Bell's mania: Acute delirious mania. A severe psychosis combining delirium with the gross psychomotor activity of mania; may lead to death through exhaustion. Was almost invariably fatal before the introduction of electrotherapy. [Luther V. Bell, American physician. 1806-1862.]

Bell's palsy: Pain and paralysis of the muscles of facial expression, due to a lesion of the seventh cranial nerve; of unknown cause. Results in distortion of the face. [Charles Bell, Scottish anatomist and surgeon. 1774-1842.]

belly: 1. The abdomen. 2. The fleshy, prominent part of a muscle. B. BUTTON, the navel or umbilicus.

Bence Jones protein: Protein bodies appearing in the urine of persons suffering from disease of the bone marrow, e.g., myelomatosis (q.v.). Their characteristic quality is that on heating the urine, they are precipitated out of solution at 50° to 60° C; they redissolve on further heating to boiling point and reprecipitate on cooling. [Henry Bence Jones, London physician. 1814-1873.]

bends: Decompression sickness. Cramps that often attack a person who goes too quickly from a place of abnormal atmospheric pressure to one of normal pressure; observed in aviators and divers. See **caisson disease.**

Benedict's solution (ben'-ē-dikts sol-ū'-shun): A solution of copper sulphate which is easily reduced, producing color changes. Used to detec⁺ 'he presence of sugar.

benign (be-nīn): Innocent; mild; non-re-

current. A term used to denote the opposite of malignant.

benzene (ben'-zēn): A colorless, inflammable liquid obtained from coal tar. Extensively used as a solvent. Its chief importance in medicine is in industrial toxicology. Continued exposure to it results in leukopenia, anemia, and purpura.

beriberi (ber'-ē-ber'-ē): A deficiency disease caused by lack of thiamine (vitamin B_1). Occurs mainly in those countries where the staple diet is polished rice; also occurs in areas where there is famine for any length of time and in such places as crowded prisons when the diet is inadequate; rare in the U.S. The symptoms are pain from neuritis, paralysis, muscular wasting, chronic constipation, progressive edema, mental deterioration and, finally, heart failure.

bestiality (bês-ti-al'-i-ti): Sexual relations between human and animal.

beta rays (bā'-ta): Streams of matter that are emitted from radioactive bodies with great velocity; their penetrating power is greater than that of alpha rays (q.v.).

Betz cells: Giant cells of the cerebral cortex in the area anterior to the rolandic fissure.

bezoar (be'-zōr): A ball or concretion found in the alimentary tract of certain animals and sometimes in the stomach of man, particularly in psychiatric patients; usually made up of ingested hair and vegetable fibers. In olden days thought to have magical therapeutic value, and still used in some parts of the world as a medicament.

bi-, bin-: Denotes: (1) two, twice; (2) between, affecting two similar parts, double (chemistry); (3) life, living organism or tissue.

bibulous (bib'-ū-lus): Absorbent; spongy.

bicameral (bī-kam'-er-al): Consisting of two chambers or hollows; term often used to describe an abscess which is divided into two cavities by a septum.

bicarbonate (bī-kar'-bon-āt): A salt of carbonic acid. BLOOD B., that in the blood, indicating the alkali reserve. Also called plasma B.

bicaudate (bī-kaw'-dāt): Having two tails.

bicellular (bī-sel'-ū-lar): Composed of two cells.

bicephalus (bī-sef'-a-lus): Having two heads. Dicephalus.

biceps (bī'-seps): A muscle possessing two heads or points of origin, e.g., the flexor biceps in front of the humerus.—bicipital, adj.

bichloride (bī-klō'-rīd): A compound, particularly a salt, in which the molecules contain two equivalents of chlorine to one of another element. B. OF MERCURY, a corrosive antiseptic, formerly much used both as a germicide and as an antisyphilitic; highly toxic.

biconcave (bī-kon′-kăv): Concave or hollow on both surfaces.

biconvex (bī-kon′-veks): Convex on both surfaces.

bicornuate (bī-kor′-nū-āt): Having two horns, generally applied to a double uterus or a single uterus possessing two horns. Also bicornate.

bicuspid (bī-kus′-pid): Having two cusps or points. B. TEETH, the premolars. B. VALVE, the mitral valve between the left atrium and ventricle of the heart.

b.i.d.: Abbreviation for *bis in die*, twice a day.

bidet (bi′-dā): A low-set, trough-like basin or sitz bath in which the perineum can be immersed while the legs are outside and the feet on the floor. Can have attachments for douching the vagina or rectum.

biduous (bid′-ū-us): Lasting or remaining for two days.

bifid (bī′-fid): Divided into two parts. Cleft. Forked.

bifocal (bī-fō′-kal): Having two foci; term used especially in reference to eyeglasses that have a lens that corrects for near vision set into a lens that corrects for distant vision.

biforate (bī-fō′-rāt): Having two perforations or openings.

bifurcation (bī-fur-kā′-shun): A division or forking into two branches, or the site where such division occurs, *e.g.*, the B. of an artery.—bifurcate, adj.; v.t., v.i.

bigeminal (bī-jem′-i-nal): Paired; double. B. PULSE, two rapid pulse beats followed by a pause before the next pair of beats.

bilateral (bī-lat′-er-al): 1. Having two sides. 2. Pertaining to both sides of a structure or the body.—bilaterally, adv.

bile (bīl): A bitter, alkaline, viscid, greenish-yellow to golden brown, slightly antiseptic fluid secreted by the liver and stored in the gallbladder from which it is released into the duodenum via the common bile duct and where it aids digestion by emulsifying fats, stimulating peristalsis, and preventing putrefaction. It contains water, mucin, lecithin, cholesterol, B. salts and the pigments bilirubin and biliverdin. B. DUCTS, the hepatic and cyctic, which join to form the common B. duct. B. SALTS, emulsifying agents—sodium glycocholate and taurocholate.—bilious, biliary, adj.

Bilharzia (bil-har′-zi-a): Syn., Schistosoma (*q.v.*).

bilharziasis (bil-hār-zī′-a-sis): Syn., Schistosomiasis (*q.v.*).

biliary (bil′i-ar-i): Pertaining to bile, the bile ducts, or the gallbladder. B. COLIC, excruciating, paroxysmal pain in the upper right quadrant of the abdomen and referred to the shoulder, due to smooth muscle spasm arising in the bile passages; often caused by pressure of a stone in the gallbladder or its passage through the ducts. B. FISTULA, an abnormal track conveying bile to the surface or to some internal organ.

bilious (bil′-yus): 1. Pertaining to bile. 2. Pertaining to excess of bile. 3. A popular non-medical word signifying a digestive upset, often with headache and constipation, and attributed to excess secretion of bile.

bilirubin (bi-li-roo′-bin): The pigment that gives bile its orange color; it is a waste product from the breakdown of hemoglobin.

bilirubinemia (bi-li-roo-bin-ēm′-i-a): The presence of more bilirubin in the blood than the slight amount normally found there.

bilirubinura (bi-li-roo-bin-ūr′-i-a): The presence of more bilirubin in the urine than the slight amount normally found there.

biliuria (bi-li-ū′-ri-a): The presence of bile or bile salts in the urine.—biliuric, adj.

biliverdin (bi-li-ver′-din): The green pigment of bile formed by oxidation of bilirubin.

bilobate (bī-lō′-bāt): Having two lobes.

bilobular (bī-lob′-ū-lar): Having two little lobes or lobules.

bimanual (bī-man′-ū-al): 1. Pertaining to

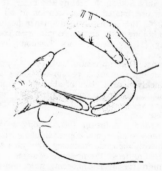

Bimanual examination

both hands. 2. Performed with both hands, *e.g.,* in gynecology, the method of examining internal genital organs with one hand on the abdomen and the finger or fingers of the other hand in the vagina.

bimaxillary (bī-mak′-sil-ar-i): 1. Pertaining to both jaws. 2. Affecting both jaws.

binary (bī′-na-ri): Made up or consisting of two things; characterized by two. In chemistry, a compound made up of two elements. In anatomy, dividing or separating into two. B. FISSION, reproduction of cells by division into two approximately equal parts.

binaural (bin-aw′-ral): Pertaining to, or having, two ears. Applied to a type of stethoscope (*q.v.*).

binauricular (bin-aw-rik′-ū-lar): 1. Pertaining to both auricles. 2. Affecting both auricles.

binder (bīnd′-er): A broad bandage, applied snugly about the abdomen or breasts, usually after childbirth or operation.

Binet's test (bē′-nā): A series of graded intelligence tests in which an individual's intelligence level (mental age) is compared with his chronological age. Also called Binet-Simon test. [Alfred Binet, French psychologist. 1857-1911.]

binocular (bin-ok′-ū-lar): 1. The use of both eyes in vision. 2. Pertaining to both eyes. 3. Describing an optical instrument requiring both eyes for its use.

binotic (bin-ot′-ik): Pertaining to both ears; binaural.

binovular (bin-ov′-ū-lar): Derived from two separate ova. B. twins may be of different sexes. See **uniovular**.

bio-: Denotes: (1) life; (2) living organism or tissue.

bio-assay (bī-ō-as′-sā): Assessing the potency or strength of a substance by comparison of the effects it has on living organisms, *e.g.,* animals, with the effects of a standardized preparation. Syn., biological assay.

biochemistry (bī-ō-kem′-is-tri): The study of chemical changes occurring within living tissues; physiological chemistry.—biochemical, adj.

biogenesis (bī-ō-jen′-e-sis): 1. The origin of living organisms. 2. Term used to describe the theory that living organisms can be produced only by organisms already living; opp. to the theory of spontaneous generation.—biogenetic, adj.

biologicals (bī-ō-loj′-i-kals): Complex medicinal preparations, prepared from living organisms or their products, *e.g.,* antigens, antitoxins, sera, vaccines.

biologist (bī-ol′-ō-jist): A person who is an expert in, or who specializes in, biology.

biology (bī-ol′-ō-ji): The science of life, dealing with the structure, function and organization of all living things.—biologic, biological, adj.; biologically, adv.

biolysis (bī-ōl′-i-sis): The breaking down of organic matter by the chemical action of such living organisms as bacteria.

biophysics (bī-ō-fiz′-iks): The branch of knowledge that deals with (1) the physics of living organisms; (2) the applications of the principles and methods of physics to the problems of living organisms.

biopsy (bī′-op-si): 1. Observation of a living subject or of tissue taken from a living body, as opposed to a postmortem observation. 2. Term used to describe the removal of tissue from a living body for microscopic examination to establish diagnosis. ASPIRATION or NEEDLE B., examination of tissue removed by a hollow needle. PUNCH B., the material to be examined is removed by a punch. SPONGE B., the material to be examined is obtained by laying a sponge over a lesion or a membrane. STERNAL B., bone marrow to be examined is removed from the sternum by puncture or aspiration. SURFACE B., examination of tissue removed from a surface by scraping, used especially to diagnose cancer of the uterine cervix.

biotherapy (bī-ō-ther′-a-pi): The treatment of disease with a living microorganism or the product of a living microorganism.

biotin (bī′-o-tin): One of the members of the vitamin B complex. Small amounts are found in many plant and animal foods. It is synthesized from ingested foods in the intestine; antibiotics interfere with this process. Eggwhite in quantity (raw) interferes with its absorption. Presumed essential to man. Sources are yeast, liver, kidney, egg yolk, milk.

biotripsis (bī-ō-trip′-sis): Wearing away or eroding of the skin, seen mostly in the elderly.

bipara (bip′-a-ra): A woman who has given birth to two children at two different labors.

biparietal (bī-pa-rī′-et-al): Pertaining to both parietal bones.

biparous (bip′-ar-us): Producing two offspring at one birth.

biped (bī′-ped): 1. Any animal with two feet, as man. 2. Two-footed.

biopolar (bī-pō′-lar): Having two poles. B. NERVE CELL, a nerve cell with two processes.

birth: The act of expelling the young from

the mother's body; delivery; being born. B. CANAL, the cavity or canal of the pelvis through which the baby passes during labor. B. CERTIFICATE, a legal document given on registration, within a specified period after birth, listing date and place of birth, name and sex of child, names of parents, other pertinent information. B. CONTROL, the prevention or regulation of conception by any means; contraception. B. INJURY, any injury occurring during parturition, *e.g.,* fracture of a bone, subluxation of a joint, injury to a peripheral nerve, intracranial hemorrhage. B. TRAUMA, see **trauma.** PREMATURE B., one occurring after the seventh month of pregnancy, but before term.

birthmark: A hemangioma or other blemish present on the skin at birth; nevus (*q.v.*).

bisect (bī'-sekt): To divide into two parts.— bisection, n.

bisexual (bī-seks'-ū-al): 1. Having the interests and characteristics of both sexes. 2. Having gonads of both sexes; hermaphrodite. 3. Relating to both sexes. 4. Consisting of both sexes. 5. In psychiatry, responsive to both sexes.

bis in die: Twice a day. Abbreviated b.i.d. or b.d.

bismuth (biz'-muth): A greyish metal. Various preparations formerly much used internally for their antisyphilitic, antidiarrheal, antiacid, antiseptic and astringent actions; externally for their protective actions.

bistoury (bis'-tū-ri): A long narrow knife, straight or curved, used for cutting from within outwards in the opening of a hernial sac, an abscess, sinus or fistula.

Bitot's spots or patches (bē-tō): Shiny, gray, triangular spots, seen at the sides of the cornea,and associated with vitamin A deficiency. Also called xerosis corneae. [Pierre Bitot, French physician. 1822-1888.]

bitters: Bitter tasting medicinal substances that are used as tonics or stomachics (*q.v.*).

bituminosis (bī-too-mi-nō'-sis): A form of pneumoconiosis caused by inhalation of soft-coal dust.

black death: An extremely virulent form of the plague that ravaged Europe and Asia in the 14th century. Named for the hemorrhagic, blackening spots which formed on the skin.

blackhead: See **comedo.**

black lung, black lung disease: Pneumoconiosis (*q.v.*). So called by coal miners because the inhalation of coal dust blackens the lungs and slowly destroys the lung tissues.

blackout: A condition characterized by failure of vision and unconsciousness of short duration, caused by sudden reduction in the amount of blood reaching the brain and retina.

blackwater fever: A malignant form of malaria (*q.v.*) occurring in the tropics, especially Africa. There is great destruction of red blood cells, and this causes a very dark colored urine.

bladder: A membranous sac that serves as a receptacle or reservoir for a fluid or gas. ILEAL B., see **ileoureterostomy.** IRRITABLE B., sensitivity of the bladder accompanied by constant desire to urinate. NERVOUS B., describing the condition when one has a constant desire to urinate but cannot completely empty the bladder. RECTAL B., term used to describe the result of surgery in which the ureters are transplanted to the rectum. STAMMERING B., describes the condition when the stream of urine is interrupted several times during voiding. URINARY B., the muscular bag in the pelvis that serves as a reservoir for urine. See **gallbladder.**

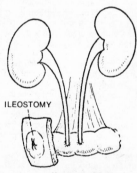

ILEOSTOMY

Ileal bladder

Blalock-Taussig operation: An anastomosis between the subclavian artery and the pulmonary artery; most often performed on a child affected with tetralogy of Fallot; helps increase the blood flow through the lungs and reduces cyanosis by supplying more oxygen to the tissues. [Alfred Blalock, American surgeon, 1899-. Helen Taussig, American pediatrician. 1898- .]

blood

bland: Mild, nonirritating, soothing.

blast: An immature stage in cell development before the distinctive characteristics of the particular cell appear. Often used as a word termination to describe a particular kind of cell, *e.g.,* neuroblast.

blast-, blasto-: Denotes bud, budding; used particularly in relation to a primitive cell or element in the early stage of development of the embryo.

-blast: Denotes an embryonic or formative cell.

blastoderm (blas'-tō-derm): A delicate, membranous lining of the zona pellucida of the fertilized ovum. The rudimentary structure from which the embryo is formed.

blastoma (blas-tō'-ma): A true tumor; a tumor originating from embryonal cells. Syn., blastocytoma.—blastomatous, adj.

blastomyces (blas-tō-mī'-sēz): Yeast-like organism of the genus Blastomyces.—blastomycetes, pl.

blastomycosis (blas-tō-mī-kō-sis): Granulomatous and suppurative inflammation characterized by formation of multiple abscesses in skin and subcutaneous tissues, sometimes also affecting the viscera and bones. Caused by infection with an organism of the genus Blastomyces.—blastomycotic, adj.

blastula (blas'-tū-la): The stage of development at which an embryo consists of one or several layers of cells around a central fluid-filled cavity.

bleb: A large blister. See **blister, bulla, vesicle.**

bleeder: One who is subject to frequent loss of blood, as one suffering from hemophilia (*q.v.*).

bleeding time: The time required for the spontaneous arrest of bleeding from a skin puncture: under controlled conditions this forms a clinical test. Not to be confused with clotting time (*q.v.*).

blennophthalmia (blen-of-thal'-mi-a): Catarrhal conjunctivitis.—blennophthalmic, adj.

blennorrhagia (blen-o-rā'-ji-a): 1. A copious mucous discharge. 2. Gonorrhea.

blennorrhea (blen-ō-rē'-a): Syn., blennorrhagia (*q.v.*).—blennorrheal, adj.

bleph-, blephar-, blepharo-: Denotes eyelid.

blepharitis (blef-a-rī'-tis): Inflammation of the eyelids, particularly the edges.—blepharitic, adj.

blepharoblennorrhea (blef-a-rō-blen-ō-rē'-a): Conjunctivitis accompanied by a purulent discharge.

blepharon (blef'-a-ron): The eyelid; palpebra.—blephara, pl.

blepharopachynsis (blef-a-rō-pa-kin'-sis): Abnormal thickening of an eyelid.

blepharophimosis (blef-a-rō-fi-mō'-sis): Abnormal narrowing of the slit between the eyelids.

blepharoplasty (blef'-a-rō-plas-ti): Plastic repair of an eyelid. Sometimes done for cosmetic purposes to remove wrinkles and bulges caused by hereditary factors or aging.

blepharoplegia (blef-ar-ō-plē'-ji-a): Paralysis of an eyelid.

blepharoptosis (blef-a-rō-tō'-sis): Drooping of an upper eyelid. See **ptosis.**—blepharoptotic, adj.

blepharospasm (blef'-a-rō-spazm): Spasm of the muscles in the eyelid. Excessive winking.—blepharospastic, adj.

blepharostenosis (blef-a-rō-ste-nō'-sis): Abnormal narrowing of the slit between the eyelids.

blindness: Loss or lack of ability to see; may be due to disorder of the organ of sight or to a lesion in the central nervous system. COLOR B., a term loosely applied to any deviation from the normal ability to distinguish hues accurately. CONCUSSION B., that caused by violent explosion, gunfire, etc. DAY B., hemeralopia (*q.v.*). FUNCTIONAL B., occurs without any disorder of the organ of sight. NIGHT B., nyctalopia (*q.v.*). PSYCHIC B., inability to recognize known objects due to a lesion in the central nervous system.

blind spot: The spot at which the optic nerve leaves the retina. It is insensitive to light.

blister: Separation of the epidermis from the dermis by a collection of fluid, usually serum or blood. See **vesicle.** FEVER B., herpes simplex (*q.v.*) of the lip.

block: 1. An obstruction or stoppage. 2. An obstruction in the path of a nerve or muscle impulse. 3. Regional anesthesia. HEART B., see under **heart block.** NERVE B., producing anesthesia in a specific location by injecting an anesthetic near the nerve that supplies that area. SADDLE B., an anesthetized area, shaped like a saddle, produced in caudal anesthesia (*q.v.*).

blood: The red, viscid fluid filling and circulating through the heart and blood vessels; supplies nutritive material to, and carries waste away from, the body tissues. Consists of plasma, a clear straw-colored fluid with particles or corpuscles immersed in it. Corpuscles (blood cells) are of two varieties: (1) red (also called erythrocytes) are nonnucleated, biconcave disks, present in normal blood in amounts ranging from 4,000,000 to 6,000,000 per cu mm; they transport oxygen from the lungs to the tissues and carry carbon dioxide away from the tissues; (2) white cells, or leukocytes, are nucleated, granular, motile cells; the range in normal blood is from 5,000 to 10,000 per cu mm with definite percentages of each of several types; they protect the body by destroying invading organisms. Also present are minute cell fragments called platelets or thrombocytes which are important in the clotting mechanism; the normal range is 200,000 to 500,000 per cu mm. ARTERIAL B., aerated blood which carries oxygen to tissues. DEFIBRINATED B., that in which the fibrin has been removed by agitation and which therefore does not clot. LAKED B., that in which the red cells are hemolysed. OCCULT B., that which is not visible; its presence is determined by chemical tests. VENOUS B., that which has transported oxygen to the tissues and has picked up carbon dioxide which is being carried back to the lungs. WHOLE B., that from which none of its elements has been removed. B. BANK, see **bank.**

blood-brain barrier: See **barrier.**

blood casts: Casts that contain red blood corpuscles, formed in the renal tubules and found in the urine in certain kidney diseases.

blood corpuscles: Blood cells. See **blood erythrocyte, leukocyte, platelet.**

blood count: Calculation of the number of red or white cells per cubic millimeter of whole blood, using a hemocytometer. DIFFERENTIAL B.C., an estimate of the relative number of each of the various types of white cells in a cubic millimeter of blood.

blood crossmatching: A technique used for determining the compatibility of bloods, done before transfusion. See **blood groups.**

blood culture: After withdrawal of blood from a vein, it is incubated in a suitable medium, at an optimum temperature, so that any contained organisms can multiply and so be isolated and identified under the microscope. See **bacteremia** and **septicemia.**

blood groups: All human blood belongs to one of four major groups (also called types), A, B, AB, and O, the division being based upon the presence of specific antigens (agglutinogens) in the red cells, and of specific antibodies (agglutinins) in the ser-

um. The cells of groups A, B, and AB contain the corresponding agglutinogens, A, B, and AB; O contains none. The serum of A blood contains beta agglutinins, B contains alpha agglutinins, O contains both alpha and beta, and AB contains neither. If incompatible bloods are mixed (e.g., A and B), the agglutinins in the serum of one type will cause agglutination (clumping) of the red cells of the other type, and this may lead to a severe, sometimes fatal reaction in the patient. Since O blood cells contain no agglutinogens, it can safely be given to persons with any type of blood and thus is known as the universal donor. Since AB blood contains no agglutinins, it can safely receive A, B, and O blood and thus is known as the universal recipient. In addition to classification into the four major groups, blood is also classified according to the presence or absence of an hereditary factor known as the Rh (Rhesus) factor. Blood which contains this factor is called Rh positive and that which does not is called Rh negative. If an Rh negative person is given Rh positive blood in transfusion, antibodies develop in the recipient's blood and, in the event of a second transfusion, will cause agglutination of red cells and a severe reaction in the patient. This factor is responsible for the development of erythroblastosis fetalis which results when the fetus receives the Rh positive factor from the father and has an Rh negative mother. Some of the Rh positive factor enters the mother's blood stream via the placenta; her blood builds up antibodies against this substance and they enter the fetus's circulation (again via the placenta) where they cause agglutination of the red cells.

bloodletting: Venesection (q.v.).

blood nitrogen urea: Nitrogen in the form of urea found in whole blood or serum. See **blood urea, urea.**

blood plasma: The liquid portion of whole blood. Composed of over 90 percent water, 6 to 8 percent protein substances, mineral salts, foodstuffs, waste products, clotting agents, antibodies, and hormones.

blood platelets: Small, circular or oval colorless disks found in the circulating blood, averaging about 250,000 in 1 cu mm of blood. Important in the clotting of blood because they release thrombokinase which, in the presence of calcium, reacts with prothrombin to form thrombin. Syn., thrombocyte.

blood poisoning: Septicemia (q.v.).

blood pressure: The pressure exerted on the blood vessel walls, measured in millimeters by a sphygmomanometer. SYSTOLIC P., the highest point registered on the apparatus when the heart muscle is at the maximum contraction; the normal adult range is likely to be between 110 and 145 mm. DIASTOLIC P., the lowest point registered on the apparatus when the left ventricle is in a state of relaxation; the normal adult range is likely to be between 60 and 80 mm. ARTERIAL P., that in the arteries. VENOUS P., that in the veins.

blood sedimentation rate: Also called erythrocyte sedimentation rate (ESR). The rate, determined by laboratory test, at which red blood cells settle to the bottom of a special glass test tube. The sedimentation rate is increased in infections and conditions in which cell destruction occurs. The test is useful in diagnosing and following such illnesses as rheumatic fever, arthritis, and myocarditis.

blood serum: The fluid which exudes when blood clots; it is plasma minus the clotting agents.

bloodshot: Congestion of blood in the small vessels of a localized area, as occurs, *e.g.*, in the conjunctiva when the small vessels dilate and become visible.

blood smear: A drop of blood, placed on a glass slide and then spread and stained for microscopic examination.

blood substitute: A substance such as human plasma, serum albumin, dextran, gum acacia, or gelatin, given by transfusion in cases of hemorrhage or shock.

blood sugar: The amount of glucose in the circulating blood; varies within the normal limits of 80 to 120 mg per ml of blood serum, or 70 to 105 mg per ml of whole blood. This level is controlled by various enzymes and hormones, the most important single factor being insulin (*q.v.*). See **hyperglycemia, hypoglycemia.**

blood transfusion: The intravenous replacement of lost or destroyed blood by compatible citrated human blood. Also used for severe anemia with deficient blood production and for treatment of shock or severe infections. Fresh blood from a donor or stored blood from a blood bank may be used. It can be given 'whole,' or with some plasma removed ('packed-cell' transfusion). If incompatible blood is given severe reaction follows. See **blood groups.**

blood types: See **blood groups.**

blood typing: The determination of an individual's blood group by laboratory tests. See **blood groups, blood crossmatching.**

blood urea: The amount of urea (*q.v.*) in the blood; varies within the normal range of 20 to 40 mg per 100 ml of blood. The level is virtually unaffected by the amount of protein in the diet when the kidneys, which are the main organs of excretion of urea, are normal. When they are diseased, the blood urea quickly rises. See **uremia.**

blood vessels: The tubes which transport the blood throughout the body; arteries, veins, capillaries.

blotch: A spot or blemish, or an abnormally pigmented or reddened area on the skin or a membrane.

blue baby: The appearance produced by some congenital heart defects which allow the arterial and venous blood to become mixed. The appearance, by contrast, of a newborn child suffering from temporary anoxia is described as 'blue asphyxia.' B. BABY OPERATION, a procedure designed to ameliorate the lack of adequate oxygenation of an infant's blood caused by the tetralogy of Fallot (*q.v.*).

Blue Cross: A type of group health insurance that pays all or part of a member's hospital expenses.

Blue Shield: A type of group health insurance that pays part or all of a member's doctor bills.

BMR: Basal metabolic rate (*q.v.*).

body: 1. The trunk or frame of a person and the structures it contains as differentiated from the head and extremities. 2. The largest or principal part of an organ, *e.g.*, the body of the uterus. 3.Any mass of material. B. IMAGE, the image in an individual's mind of his own body. Distortions of this occur as a result of affective disorders, parietal lobe tumors, or trauma. B. MECHANICS, the application of the principles of kinesiology (*q.v.*) to body activities so as to correlate actions of the various parts and thus prevent injuries and problems related to posture. B.TEMPERATURE, that of the healthy body; 98.6°F when taken by mouth, usually one degree higher by rectum.

Boeck's disease (beks): A form of sarcoidosis (*q.v.*). [Caesar P. M. Boeck, Norwegian pathologist. 1845-1917.]

Boerhaave's glands (boor′-hav-ez): The sweat glands, first described by Boerhaave. [Hermann Boerhaave, Dutch physician. 1668-1738.]

boil: A furuncle (*q.v.*).

boloscope (bō′-lo-skōp): An instrument for locating metallic foreign bodies in tissues.

bolus

bolus (bō′-lus): 1. A large pill. 2. A soft, pulpy mass of masticated food ready to swallow.

bone: 1. The hard, connective tissue forming the skeleton. 2. Any distinct piece of the skeleton. B. TISSUE may be either compact or cancellous. About one third of the total weight is accounted for by the organic matter of the fibrous tissue and the remaining two thirds by the inorganic mineral matter deposited in it. There are 206 named bones in the body; they make up about one-seventh of the body weight. In children the proportion of organic matter is greater, giving a tendency to bend rather than break; in elderly people the mineral content is in greater proportion, causing the bones to become brittle.—bony, adj. B. CONDUCTION, usually refers to conduction of sound waves through the skull to the hearing receptors in the ear by means of a hearing device applied to the exterior of the skull. B. GRAFT, transplantation of a piece of bone from one part of the body to another, or from one person to another. Used to repair bone defects, afford support, or to supply osteogenic tissue. See **cancellous, compact, marrow.**

booster dose: A later dose given to enhance the effect of an initial or previous dose; usually applied to antigens given for the purpose of producing specific antibodies.

borborygmus (bor-bo-rig′-mus): Rumbling or gurgling noises caused by the movement of flatus in the intestines.—borborygmi, pl.

Bordetella pertussis (bor-de-tel′-la per-tus′- is): The organism that causes whooping cough. See **pertussis.**

boric acid: A common mild antiseptic, used in the form of a solution, ointment, or powder for surface application to skin and mucous membranes of the eye, ear, nose, bladder, etc. Serious and fatal accidents have occurred from internal use. Also boracic acid.

Bornholm disease: Epidemic pleurodynia (q.v.) probably caused by a virus through contact infection. There is severe diaphragmatic pain. Named for a Danish island. See **fibrositis.**

boron (bo′-ron): The active substance in boric acid (q.v.).

Borrelia (bor-rē′-li-a): A genus of spirochetes; among the many species are the organisms that cause various types of relapsing fever.

boss: 1. A rounded projection or eminence as on a bone or tumor. 2. The projection of the spine in kyphosis (q.v.).

botany (bot′-a-ni): The science of plants.—botanic, adj.

botryoid (bot′-rē-oid): Like a bunch of grapes in appearance.

botulin (bot′-ū-lin): A very active toxin that affects the nervous system; sometimes found in imperfectly preserved or canned non-acid vegetables or meat such as sausage; causes botulism (q.v.); is produced by an anaerobic organism *Clostridium botulinum,* widely distributed in soil and the intestines of domestic animals.

botulism (bot′-ū-lizm): A severe type of food poisoning caused by botulin (q.v.). Characterized by sudden onset, vomiting, abdominal pain, malaise, dry mouth, dizziness, muscular weakness, cyanosis, and ocular and pharyngeal paralysis, within 24 to 72 hours after eating food contaminated by the *Clostridium botulinum.* Often fatal.

bougie (boo′-zhē): A flexible, slender cylindrical instrument of varying sizes, shapes and materials; used to explore or dilate a canal such as the anus, urethra, or esophagus, to dilate a stricture of a canal or structure such as the cardiac sphincter, to induce labor, or as a guide for the passage of other instruments.

bouillon (boo′-e-yaw): A broth prepared from animal flesh. Used as a food and as a culture medium for bacteria.

bovine (bō′-vēn): Pertaining to the cow or ox. The bovine type of the tubercle bacillus (*Mycobacterium tuberculosis*) may infect the bones, glands, and joints in human beings.

bowel (bow′-el): The intestine; the gut. SMALL B., the first 23 ft. of the intestine, the first 10 or 11 in. of which is the duodenum; the next two-fifths is the jejunum and the remaining three-fifths the ileum. LARGE B. measures 6 ft. in length but is larger in diameter than the small intestine and has other distinguishing features such as the structure of its lining membrane. See **colon.**

bowleg: The outward curving or arching of the leg, or both legs, at and/or below the knee; genu varum.

Bowman's capsule: The expanded beginning of a renal tubule in the kidney. It and the tuft of capillaries that it surrounds make up a malpighian corpuscle.

Boyle's law: At any stated temperature, a given mass of gas varies in volume inversely in proportion to the pressure exerted upon it. [Robert Boyle, English physicist. 1627-1691.]

BP: Abbreviation for blood pressure.

brachi-, brachio-: Denotes the arm.

brachial (brā′-ki-al): Pertaining to the arm. Applied to vessels in this region and a nerve plexus at the root of the neck.

brachialgia (brā-ki-al′-ji-a): Pain in the arm.

brachium (brā′-ki-um): 1. The arm, especially from the shoulder to the elbow. 2. Any arm-like appendage.—brachia, pl.; brachial, adj.

brachy-: Denotes short, shortness.

brachydactylia (brak-i-dak-til′-i-a): Abnormal shortness of the fingers and/or the toes.

Bradford frame: A canvas and metal device used for immobilizing the spine or pelvis, resting the trunk or back muscles, or preventing deformity in patients with certain fractures, dislocations or diseases of the spinal or pelvic bones. Consists of a tubular steel frame with two canvas slings allowing a 4- to 6-inch gap to facilitate use of the bedpan. [Edward H. Bradford, American orthopedic surgeon. 1848–1926.]

brady-: Denotes: (1) slow; (2) dull.

bradycardia (brad-i-kar′-di-a): Slow rate of heart contraction, resulting in a slow pulse rate. In febrile states, for each degree rise in body temperature, the expected increase in pulse rate is ten beats per minute. When the latter does not occur, the term 'relative B.' is used.

bradykinesia (brad-i-kī-nē′-si-a): Excessive slowness of movement.

bradylalia (brad-i-lā′-li-a): Abnormal slowness of speech, due to a lesion in the central nervous system.

bradylexia (brad-i-lek′-si-a): Abnormal slowness of reading due to a brain disorder.

bradypnea (brad-ip-nē′-a): Abnormal slowness of breathing.

Braille (brāl): A kind of writing and printing used for the blind; the letters are made up of points or dots that the blind person can feel.

brain: The encephalon; that part of the cen-

tral nervous system contained in the cranial cavity. It consists of the cerebrum, cerebellum, pons varolii, midbrain (mesencephalon) and medulla oblongata. B. CENTER, a group of nerve cells in a circumscribed area of the brain that are concerned with the regulation of a certain function, *e.g.,* sight, hearing, speech, etc. B. STEM, all of the brain except the cerebrum and the cerebellum, *i.e.,* the midbrain, pons, and medulla oblongata.

brainwashing: A kind of mental conditioning in which stress and mental torture are used to force a captive person to accept a set of beliefs that are contrary to his former beliefs but in accord with those of his captor.

brain waves: Rhythmic fluctuations in the electric current set up in the cortex of the brain by brain action. They may be recorded by electroencephalography.

bran: The husk of grain. The coarse outer part of cereals, especially wheat, high in roughage and the vitamin B complex.

branchial (brang′-ki-al): 1. Pertaining to gills. 2. Pertaining to the fissures or clefts which occur on each side of the neck of the human embryo, and which enter into the development of the nose, ears, and mouth. B. CYST, a swelling in the neck arising from such embryonic remnants.

brandy: An alcoholic liquid distilled from wine. Contains about 50% alcohol.

brash: A burning sensation in the stomach caused by excessive acidity and often accompanied by belching of sour, burning fluid. Syn., heartburn, pyrosis.

break-bone fever: See **dengue.**

breast: The anterior upper part of the thorax; the mammary gland. B. AMPUTATION, mastectomy (*q.v.*). B. BONE, the sternum. B. PUMP, an apparatus operated by hand or electricity, for removing milk from the breast. FUNNEL B., deformity caused by abnormal depression of the sternum. CHICKEN B., or PIGEON B., deformity re-

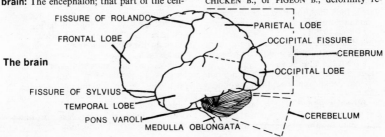

The brain

FISSURE OF ROLANDO

FRONTAL LOBE

FISSURE OF SYLVIUS

TEMPORAL LOBE

PONS VAROLI

MEDULLA OBLONGATA

PARIETAL LOBE

OCCIPITAL FISSURE

CEREBRUM

OCCIPITAL LOBE

CEREBELLUM

sulting from prominent sternum, often caused by rickets (*q.v.*).

breath: The air inhaled and exhaled during respiration. B. SOUNDS, those which can be heard with a stethoscope during respiration.

breathe: The act of alternately inhaling air into and exhaling air from the lungs.

breathing: The act of inhaling and exhaling air. ASTHMATIC B., harsh breathing accompanied by a wheezing sound, especially on expiration. COGWHEEL B., jerky B. COSTAL B., that accomplished chiefly by the intercostal muscles. DIAPHRAGMATIC B., that accomplished chiefly by movements of the diaphragm. Also called ABDOMINAL B. MOUTH B., HABITUAL B. through the mouth rather than the nose. PERIODIC B., Cheyne-Stokes respiration (*q.v.*). STERTOROUS B., characterized by a snoring sound on expiration.

breech (brēch): The buttocks (*q.v.*). B. PRESENTATION, the position of the fetus during labor in which the buttocks instead of the head presents at the uterine orifice.

bregma (breg′-ma): The junction of the coronal and sagittal sutures; the anterior fontanel.—bregmata, pl.; bregmatic, adj.

brewer's yeast: A rich source of vitamin B complex; the dried pulverized cells of a yeast (*Saccharomyces cerevisiae*); so called because it is used in the brewing process.

bridge: A structure that joins two parts or organs. B. OF NOSE, the upper part of the external nose, formed by union of the nasal bones. In dentistry, a device bearing one or more artificial teeth which is anchored to the natural teeth.

Bright's disease: Inflammation of the kidney. Nephritis (*q.v.*). Term is frequently used to describe various diseases of the kidney, especially nephrosis and nephritis, in which albumin appears in the urine. [Richard Bright, English physician. 1789-1858.]

Brill's disease: A mild form of typhus fever, rare in the U.S. Also called sporadic typhus. [Nathan Edwards Brill, American physician. 1860-1925.]

brim: The edge or margin of a part. B. OF THE PELVIS, the bony ring that divides the true from the false pelvis.

brisement forcé (brēz′-maw for-sā′): The forcible breaking up of anything, as of bony ankylosis.

Broadbent's sign: Visible retraction of the left side and back, in the region of the eleventh and twelfth ribs, synchronous with each heart beat and due to adhesions between the pericardium and diaphragm. See **pericarditis**. [William Henry Broadbent, English physician. 1835-1907.]

broad ligament: Lateral ligament; double fold of parietal peritoneum which hangs over the uterus and outstretched fallopian tubes, forming a lateral partition across the pelvic cavity.

broad-spectrum: A term used to describe an agent, particularly an antibiotic, that is effective against a wide variety of microorganisms.

Broca's area (brok′-a): The motor center for speech; situated at the commencement of the sylvian fissure in the left hemisphere of the cerebrum. Injury to this center results in inability to speak. [Pierre Paul Broca, French surgeon. 1824-1880.]

Brodie's abscess: See **abscess**. [Sir Benjamin Collins Brodie, English surgeon. 1783-1862.]

bromhidrosis (brōm-hid-rō′-sis): A profuse, fetid perspiration, especially associated with the feet, groin, axillae. Syn., fetid perspiration, osmidrosis.—bromhidrotic, adj. Also bromidrosis.

bromides (brō′-mīdz): A small group of drugs, compounds of bromine and another element, that have a mild depressant action on the central nervous system. Used for sedation and hypnosis; also used extensively in epilepsy before phenobarbital was introduced. Eliminated slowly; may cumulate and cause toxic condition. Skin eruptions are common. Have long been used as sedatives, but since their value is questionable, this use is decreasing.

brominism (brō′-min-izm): Chronic poisoning due to continued or excessive use of bromides. Also bromism.

bromoderma (brō-mō-der′-ma): Skin eruption resembling acne caused by use of bromine or its compounds. Often a symptom of brominism (*q.v.*).

bromomania (brō-mō-mā′-ni-a): Psychosis or delirium caused by overuse of bromides.

Bromsulphalein (brōm-sul′-fa-lin): A preparation of sulfobromophthalein, a dye used in liver function tests; it is injected intravenously. Normally 80% of the dye is removed by the liver and the rest by other organs; in pathological conditions, when the liver is not functioning properly, it removes less of the dye which then remains in the blood.

bronch-, bronchi-, bronchio-, broncho-: Denotes bronchus, bronchiole.

bronchadenitis (brong′-kad-e-nī′-tis): Inflammation of the bronchial glands. Also broncho-adenitis.

bronchi (brong′-kī): The two tubes into which the trachea (windpipe) divides at its lower end; they serve to convey air into the lungs.—bronchus, sing., bronchial, adj.

bronchial (brong′-kē-al): Pertaining to the bronchi. B. ASTHMA, see **asthma.** B. TUBES, subdivisions of the bronchi after they enter the lungs. B. PNEUMONIA, see **bronchopneumonia.** B. TREE, the trachea, bronchi and all their branching structures.

bronchiarctia (brong-ki-ark′-shi-a): Bronchiostenosis (*q.v.*).

bronchiectasis (brong-ki-ek′-ta-sis): Chronic dilatation of the bronchi or bronchioles, characterized by productive cough, profuse expectoration of mucopurulent material, fetid breath, and enlargement of the air passages. Usually follows infection such as bronchopneumonia with lobular collapse (which may have occurred in infancy). May lead to greatly limited ventilatory capacity and recurrent infection of the lungs, cerebral abscess, or amyloid disease.—bronchiectatic, adj. Also bronchiectasia.

bronchiole (brong′-ki-ōl): One of the minute subdivisions of the bronchi which terminate in the alveoli or air sacs of the lungs.—bronchiolar, adj.

bronchiolitis (brong-kē-ō-lī′-tis): Inflammation of the bronchioles. Also called capillary bronchitis and bronchopneumonia (*q.v.*).—bronchiolitic, adj.

bronchitis (brong-kī′-tis): Inflammation of the bronchial mucous membrane; may be primary or secondary, acute or chronic. ACUTE B., occurs chiefly in young children or elderly persons; usually an extension of infection following a common cold, upper respiratory infection, measles, or influenza. CHRONIC B., occurs chiefly in older persons; may follow acute B., develop gradually, or be secondary to another condition such as sinusitis; tends to recur and to be worse in cold, foggy weather; can cause right-sided heart failure, especially when associated with gross emphysema. See **cor pulmonale.**—bronchitic, adj.

bronchoblennorrhea (brong-kō-blen-ō-rē′-a): Expectoration of copious mucopurulent sputum, often seen in chronic bronchitis.

bronchocele (brong′-kō-sēl): 1. A circumscribed swelling or dilatation of a bronchus. 2. A goiter.

bronchocephalitis (brong-kō-sef-a-lī′-tis): Whooping cough. (See **pertussis.**)

bronchoconstrictor (brong-kō-kon-strik′-tor): Any agent that causes constriction of the bronchi thus decreasing the caliber of the pulmonary air passages.

bronchodilator (brong-kō-dī′-lā-tor): Any agent that causes dilatation of the bronchi thus increasing the caliber of the pulmonary air passages.

bronchogenic (brong-kō-jen′-ik): Arising from a bronchus. Also bronchiogenic.

bronchogram (brong′-kō-gram): Radiological picture of the bronchial tree rendered radiopaque.

bronchography (brong-kog′-raf-i): Preparation of x-ray film after introduction of radiopaque substance into the bronchial tree.—bronchographic, adj.; bronchographically, adv.

broncholith (brong′-kō-lith): A stone or concretion in a bronchus or bronchial tube.

bronchomycosis (brong-kō-mī-kō′-sis): General term used to cover a variety of fungus infections of the bronchi and lungs, *e.g.*, pulmonary moniliasis, aspergillosis (*q.v.*). —bronchomycotic, adj.

bronchophony (brong-kof′-o-ni): Abnormal voice sounds as heard through the stethoscope when applied over consolidated lung tissue.

bronchopleural fistula (brong-kō-ploo′-ral fis′-tūl-a): Pathological communication between the pleural cavity and a bronchus.

bronchopneumonia (brong-kō-nū-mō′-ni-a): Inflammation of the bronchi and lungs; small areas of the lungs are consolidated and coalesce but do not have a lobar or lobular distribution; usually begins at the termini of bronchioles and alveoli and usually in both lungs. Caused by a number of microorganisms. May occur as a primary infection in infants and the aged, in whom it is relatively common, but may also be secondary to measles, whooping cough, upper respiratory infections and debilitating diseases.—bronchopneumonic, adj.

bronchopneumonitis (brong-kō-nū-mō-nī′-tis): Bronchopneumonia (*q.v.*).

bronchopulmonary (brong′-kō-pul′-mon-ar-i): Pertaining to the bronchi and the lungs.—bronchopulmonic, adj.

bronchorrhea (brong-kō-rē′-a): An excessive discharge from the bronchial mucous membrane.—bronchorrheal, adj.

bronchoscope (brong′-kō-skōp): A type of endoscope (*q.v.*) used for examining the interior of the bronchi, removal of a foreign body, biopsy, etc.—bronchoscopic, adj.; bronchoscopy, n.; bronchoscopically, adv.

bronchosinusitis (brong-kō-sī-nus-ī′-tis): A simultaneous infection of the bronchi and the paranasal sinuses.

bronchospasm (brong′-kō-spazm): Sudden, temporary constriction of the bronchial tubes due to contraction of involuntary plain muscle in their walls.—bronchospastic, adj.

bronchospirometer (brong-kō-spī-rom′-eter): An instrument for measuring the capacity of one lung.—bronchospirometric, adj.; bronchospirometry, n.

bronchostenosis (brong-kō-ste-nō′-sis): Narrowing of a bronchus.—bronchostenotic, adj.

bronchotomy (brong-kot′-ō-mi): A surgical incision into the larynx, trachea, or a bronchus.

bronchotracheal (brong-kō-trā′-kē-al): Pertaining to bronchi and trachea.

bronchus (brong′-kus): One of the two tubes into which the trachea divides; one enters each lung where it divides and subdivides.—bronchi, pl.

brontophobia (bron-tō-fō′-bi-a): Abnormal fear of thunder.

brossage (brō-sazh′): Brushing with a stiff brush to remove granulations, especially from the everted eyelids in cases of trachoma.

brow: The forehead; the region of the supraorbital ridge. B. PRESENTATION, the position of the fetus during labor in which the brow presents at the uterine orifice making normal delivery almost impossible.

brownian movement or motion: The peculiar, random, dancing movements exhibited by finely divided particles in solution; often seen in microscopic viewing of bacteria in suspension.

Brucella (broo-sel′-la): A genus of bacteria causing brucellosis (undulant fever in man; contagious abortion in cattle). B. ABORTUS is the bovine strain, B. MELITENSIS the goat strain, both transmissible to man via infected milk. [David Bruce, British pathologist and bacteriologist. 1855-1931].

brucellosis (broo-sel-lō′-sus): A generalized infection in man resulting from one of the species of Brucella (*q.v.*), characterized by recurrent attacks of fever and mental depression, headache, malaise, anemia, weight loss, weakness, sweating, constipation. Rarely transmitted from man to man, but spreads from animal to animal and animal to man. Known by many names including Malta fever, undulant fever, Mediterranean fever, abortus fever.

Brudzinski's sign: Either of two reflexes seen in patients with meningitis. 1. Neck sign; immediate flexion of knees and hips on raising head from pillow. 2. Leg sign; when one leg is flexed onto the abdomen, the other knee and leg tend to flex also. [Josef von Brudzinski, Polish physician. 1874-1917.]

bruise (brooz): A discoloration of the skin due to an extravasation of blood into the underlying tissues; there is no abrasion of the skin. A contusion.

bruit (broo′-ē): A sound or murmur heard on auscultation, especially an abnormal one.

bruxism (bruks′-izm): Grinding of the teeth, especially during sleep.

bruxomania (bruks-ō-mā′-ni-a): Grinding of the teeth during waking hours; a neurotic habit.

Bryant's traction: Skin traction (*q.v.*) is applied to the lower limbs, the legs are then

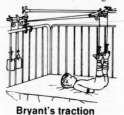

Bryant's traction

suspended vertically (from an overhead beam), so that the buttocks are lifted just clear of the bed. Used for fractures of the femur in children. [Sir Thomas Bryant, English surgeon. 1828-1914.]

BSR: Blood sedimentation rate. See **erythrocyte sedimentation rate.**

BTU: Abbreviation for British thermal unit; the amount of heat required to raise the temperature of one pound of water one degree Fahrenheit.

bubo (bū′-bō): An inflammatory swelling of a lymph node, especially in the groin or axilla, due to absorption of infective material, often proceeding to suppuration. A feature of soft sore (chancroid), lymphogranuloma inguinale, and plague.—bubonic, adj.

bubonic plague (bū-bon′-ik plāg): An acute, infectious, frequently fatal disease caused by the *Pasteurella pestis,* characterized by chills, fever, and formation of buboes. Common in the Orient. This was the black death of the Middle Ages.

bucca (buk'-a): The cheek.

buccal (buk'-al): Pertaining to the cheek or mouth.

buccinator (buk'-si-nā-tor): One of the cheek muscles.

buccula (buk'-ū-la): Double chin.

Buck's extension: An apparatus for obtaining extension of a fractured lower extremity; consists of a weight and pulley and adhesive straps. [Gurdon Buck, American surgeon. 1807-1877.]

budding (bud'-ing): Asexual reproduction by division into two unequal parts.

Buerger's disease (ber'-gers): Thromboangiitis obliterans (*q.v.*). Obliterative vascular disease of peripheral vessels. B. EXERCISES were designed to treat this condition. The legs are placed alternately in elevation and dependence. [Leo Buerger, American physician. 1879-1943.]

buffer: 1. A chemical substance which, when present in a solution, causes resistance to *p*H change (*q.v.*) when acids or alkalis are added. Sodium bicarbonate is one of the chief buffers of the blood and tissue fluids. 2. A substance which tends to offset the reaction of another agent when given in conjunction with it.

bulb: 1. A rounded, globular part of a vessel or tube. 2. Old name for the medulla oblongata.—bulbar, bulbous, adj.

bulbar: Pertaining to the medulla oblongata. See **paralysis** and **poliomyelitis.**

bulbospinal (bul-bō-spī'-nal): Pertaining to the medulla oblongata and the spinal cord, particularly to the nerve fibers which connect them.

bulbourethral (bul-bō-ū-rē'-thral): Applied to two racemose glands (Cowper's) which open into the bulb of the urethra.

bulimia (bū-lim'-i-a): Excessive appetite, usually experienced soon after a meal. Seen in some cerebral lesions, diabetes mellitus and psychotic states.—bulimic, adj.

bulkage (bulk'-ij): A material such as agar which increases the volume of the intestinal content thereby stimulating peristalsis.

bulla (bul'-la): A large watery blister. A bleb. In dermatology, bulla formation is characteristic of the pemphigus group of dermatoses, but occurs sometimes in other diseases of the skin, *e.g.,* in impetigo, in dermatitis herpetiformis, etc.—bullae, pl.; bullate, bullous, adj.

Buller's shield: A watchglass enclosed within a frame of adhesive plaster, to protect one eye when the other is infected. [Frank Buller, Canadian ophthalmologist. 1844-1905.]

BUN: Abbreviation for blood urea nitrogen.

bundle of His: Syn., atrioventricular bundle. Neuromuscular fibers that arise at the atrioventricular node, pass along the interventricular septum to be distributed throughout the ventricular walls. They transmit the impulse for ventricular contraction; failure to do so produces heart block (*q.v.*). [Wilhelm His, German physician. 1863-1934.]

bunion (bun'-yun): Syn., hallux valgus. A deformity of the head of the metatarsal bone at its junction with the great toe. Friction and pressure of shoes at this point cause the bursa to become inflamed and enlarged thus causing enlargement of the joint and lateral displacement of the great toe. The prominent bone with its bursa is called a bunion. TAILOR'S B., inflammation and enlargement of the head of the fifth metatarsal bone.

buphthalmos (boof-thal'-mos): A condition of infants in which there is an increase in intraocular fluid with consequent increase in the size of the eyeball. Also called congenital glaucoma.

buret, burette (bū-ret'): A graduated glass tube fitted with a stopcock, used for measuring liquids and for delivering an accurately measured amount of a liquid.

Burkitt's tumor: Primary malignant lymphoma of the jaw in African children residing in a geographical belt of high sunshine, endemic malaria, and mosquito-borne virus diseases. [Denis Burkitt. Contemporary surgeon, Uganda.]

burn: 1. A lesion of the tissues due to chemicals, dry heat, electricity, flame, friction, or radiation; classified in three degrees, viz., erythema, vesiculation, or deeper destruction. 2. In chemistry, to oxidize. 3. To feel the sensation of heat.

burping (burp'-ing): Belching.

bursa (bur'-sa): A fibrous sac lined with synovial membrane and containing a small quantity of synovial fluid. Bursae are found between (1) tendon and bone; (2) skin and bone; (3) muscle and muscle. Their function is to facilitate movement without friction between these surfaces.—bursae, pl.

bursectomy (bur-sek'-to-mi): The surgical removal of a bursa (*q.v.*).

bursitis (bur-sī'-tis): Inflammation of a bursa; may be acute or may develop slowly after repeated injuries or strain. Characterized by pain, swelling and tenderness. Prominent locations are the shoulder; the elbow, as in miner's, student's, or tennis elbow; the prepatellar bursa, as in housemaid's knee; and the metatarsophalangeal joint where it becomes the cause of a bunion.

buttock (but'-ok): One of the two fleshy projections posterior to the hip joints. Formed mainly of the gluteal muscles.

butyric (bū-tir'-ik): Relating to butter. B. ACID, occurs naturally in butter, cod liver oil, sweat, feces, urine, and other substances; has an unpleasant odor; is a product of the putrefaction of protein.

byssinosis (bis-in-ō'-sis): A chronic industrial disease of the lungs occurring in workers in cotton mills and due to inhalation of cotton dust. A form of pneumoconiosis (*q.v.*).

C

C: Abbreviation for centigrade.

c̄: Abbreviation for *cum,* meaning with.

CA: Chronological age.

cachet (kash-ā′): A flat capsule formed of rice paper, enclosing any bitter powdered drug which is to be taken orally.

cachexia (ka-kek′-si-a): A term denoting a state of constitutional disorder, malnutrition, general ill health, and wasting away of body tissue. The chief signs are pale mucous membranes, anemia, emaciation, sallow unhealthy skin, and heavy lusterless eyes. —cachectic, adj.

cachinnation (kak-i-nā′-shun): Hysteric or immoderate laughter without any apparent cause; often seen in schizophrenia.

cacomelia (kak-o-mē′-li-a): Congenital deformity of a limb or limbs.

cacosmia (kak-oz′-mi-a): 1. A foul odor. 2. A hallucination of an odor, particularly of putrefaction.

cadaver (ka-dav′-er): A corpse or dead body.—cadaveric, cadaverous, adj.

caduceus (ka-dū′-sē-us): Insignia of the medical corps of the U.S. Army. Consists of the wand of Hermes or Mercury entwined with two serpents. The insignia of the medical profession is the staff of Aesculapius which has one serpent twined about it.

caesarean: See **cesarean.**

caffeinism (kaf′-ē-in-izm): Poisoning induced by excessive use of coffee or other caffeine-containing preparations. Symptoms include insomnia, irritability, palpitation and dyspepsia.

Caffey's disease: A type of hyperostosis (*q.v.*) of infants in which there is swelling of the tissues over the affected bone, fever, irritability, and periods of exacerbation and remission. Also called infantile cortical hyperostosis.

cage: THORACIC C., the bony structure that encloses the organs of the thorax (*q.v.*); is made up of the sternum, ribs, and part of the vertebral column.

caisson disease (kā′-son); 'Decompression illness.' The bends. It results from sudden reduction in atmospheric pressure, *e.g.,* divers on returning to surface, airmen ascending to great heights. Due to bubbles of nitrogen which are released from solution in the blood; symptoms vary according to the site of these. The condition is largely preventable by proper and gradual decompression technique.

calcaneodynia (kal-kā-nē-ō-din′-i-a): Pain in the heel, especially when standing or walking.

calcaneus (kal-kā′-nē-us): The heel bone, largest of the tarsal bones. The os calcis. Also calcaneum.

calcareous (kal-kā′-rē-us): Pertaining to or containing lime or calcium; of a chalky nature.

calcariuria (kal-kā-ri-ū′-ri-a): The presence of calcium salts in the urine.

calcemia (kal-sē′-mi-a): An excessive amount of calcium in the blood.

calciferol (kal-sif′-er-ol): Synthetic vitamin D. This, or natural vitamin D, is essential for the uptake and utilization of calcium. Given in rickets and to prevent hypocalcemia in celiac disease, and in parathyroid deficiency and lupus vulgaris.

calciferous (kal-sif′-er-us): Containing calcium, lime, or chalk.

calcification (kal-sif-i-kā′-shun): The hardening of an organic substance by a deposit of calcium salts within it. May be normal as in bone or pathological as in arteries.

calcium (kal′-si-um): A soft, white metallic element, essential for the formation and maintenance of bone; 2 percent of body weight is calcium, of which 97 percent is in the bones and teeth. Its deposition in the bones is controlled by the parathyroid gland and its utilization by bone is dependent on vitamin D (*q.v.*). It is a vital electrolyte in the blood, especially in relation to clotting, and to neuromuscular activity. Several of its salts are used in medicine.

calciuria (kal-si-ū′-ri-a): The presence of calcium in the urine.

calculogenesis (kal-kū-lō-jen′-e-sis): The formation of calculi.

calculus (kal′-kū-lus): An abnormal concretion composed chiefly of mineral substances and formed usually in the passages that transmit secretions, or in the cavities that act as reservoirs for them. Commonly called 'stones.' ARTHRITIC C., a deposit of urates in or around a joint. BILIARY C., one formed in a bile duct or gallbladder; a gallstone. RENAL C., one formed in the kidney. URINARY C., one formed in any part of the urinary tract.—calculi, pl.; calculous, calculary, adj.

calf (kaf): The muscular portion at the back of the leg below the knee, formed principally by the bellies of the soleus and gastrocnemius muscles. C. BONE, the fibula.—calves, pl.

caliber (kal'-i-ber): The diameter of a round structure such as a tube or canal.

califacient (kal-i-fā'-shent): An agent that produces a feeling of warmth in the part to which it is applied.

caligo (ka-lī'-gō): Dimness or obscurity of vision.

caliper (kal'-i-per): 1. A two-pronged instrument for measuring the diameter of a round body; used chiefly in measuring pelvic diameters. 2. A two-pronged instrument with sharp points which are inserted into the lower end of a fractured long bone to exert traction directly on the bone.

calisthenics (kal-is-then'-iks): Systematic light exercises to preserve health, develop muscles and gracefulness; 'setting-up' exercises.

callomania (kal-ō-mā'-ni-a): A type of mania in which the person has delusions of personal beauty.

callosity (kal-os'-i-ti): A local hardening of the skin caused by pressure or friction. The epidermis becomes hypertrophied. Most commonly seen on the feet and palms of the hands.

callus (kal'-us): 1. A callosity (*q.v.*). 2. The partly calcified tissue which forms about the ends of a broken bone, which ultimately accomplishes repair of the fracture. When this is complete the bony thickening is known as 'permanent C.'—callous, adj.

calor (kal'-or): Heat; one of the classic local signs of inflammation.

caloric (kal-or'-ik): Pertaining to: (1) heat; (2) calories.

caloric test: A test for assessing vestibular function. When a normal ear is irrigated with hot water, there is rotary nystagmus toward that ear; if irrigated with cold water, there is rotary nystagmus toward the opposite ear. In vestibular disease, there is no nystagmus with either hot or cold water irrigation of an affected ear.

calorie (kal'-ō-rē): The term usually designates the small calorie which is the amount of heat required to raise the temperature of 1 gram of water 1°C. Usually written with a small 'c' and may be abbreviated to cal.; sometimes called gram calorie. The large

calorie is the amount of heat required to raise the temperature of 1 kilogram of water 1°C, thus it is 1000 times as large as the small calorie; usually written with a capital 'C,' may be abbreviated to Cal.; sometimes called kilogram calorie; is used in the study of metabolism. Also calory.

calorific (kal-ō-rif'-ik): Heat-producing. C. VALUE, the number of calories produced by a given amount of food, *e.g.*, 1 gram of protein and carbohydrate each liberate 4 calories, 1 gram of fat liberates 9 calories.

calorimeter (kal-ō-rim'-e-ter): An apparatus for measuring heat production. The respiration C. is used for determining the body's basal metabolic rate by measuring the gaseous exchange within the lungs.

calvarium (kal-vā'-ri-um): The vault of the skull; the skullcap. Also calvaria.

calvities (kal-vish'-i-ēz): Baldness.

calyx (kā'-liks): In anatomy one of the cuplike extensions of the renal pelvis, into which the pyramids of the renal medulla project.—calyces, pl.

camera (kam'-er-a): In anatomy, a cavity, chamber, or ventricle.

camisole (kam'-i-sōl): A canvas shirt with long sleeves, used to restrain violent or irrational patients; a straight jacket.

canal (ka-nal'): In anatomy, a relatively narrow tube, channel, duct, or passage in bone or tissue.

canaliculus (kan-a-lik'-ū-lus): 1. A minute capillary passage. 2. Any small canal, such as the passage leading from the edge of the eyelid to the lacrimal sac, or one of the numerous small canals that lead from the Haversian canals and terminate in the lacunae of bone.—canaliculi, pl.; canalicular, adj.; canaliculization, n.

cancellous (kan'-sel-us): Resembling latticework; light and spongy; like a honeycomb. Underlying the compact bone in epiphyses, sternum, ribs, vertebrae, and diploë of the skull there is C. bone, the interstices of which are filled with red bone marrow.

cancer (kan'-ser): A general term that covers many malignant growths in many parts of the body. The growth is purposeless, parasitic, and flourishes at the expense of the human host. The cause is unknown; it is not contagious; it is not believed to be hereditary. It is considered curable if discovered early and if all cancer cells are removed by surgery or destroyed by radiation. Characteristics are the tendency to cause local destruction, to spread by metastasis, to recur after removal, and to cause toxemia. Carcinoma refers to malignant tumors of the skin or mucous membrane, sarcoma to tumors of connective tissue.—cancerous, adj.

cancericidal (kan-ser-i-sī′-dal): Destructive to the cells of cancer.

cancerophobia (kan-ser-ō-fō′-bi-a): Extreme fear of cancer.

cancrum oris (kan′-krum or′-is): Gangrenous stomatitis (*q.v.*), occurring in malnourished children; also seen in such debilitating conditions as leukemia, Hodgkin's disease, and severe cases of measles, tuberculosis, malaria or kala-azar. Also noma.

Candida (kan′-di-da): A genus of fungi. Yeast-like cells that form some filaments. Widespread in nature. *Candida (Monilia* or *Oidium)* *albicans* is a commensal of the mouth, throat, vagina, gut and skin of man. Becomes pathogenic in some physiological and pathological states. May produce infections such as thrush, vulvovaginitis, balanoposthitis and pulmonary disease.

candidiasis (kan-di-dī′-a-sis): Infection with a fungus of the genus Candida. Syn., moniliasis, thrush. Characterized by formation of pseudomembranes on mucous surfaces, skin lesions that resemble eczema, sometimes granulomata. Skin and local infections are usually benign; systemic infections, which usually involve the kidney, may be fatal.

canicola fever (kan-i-kō′-la): Infection of man by the *Leptospira canicola* from rats, dogs, pigs, foxes, mice, voles and possibly cats. There is high fever, headache, conjunctival congestion, jaundice, severe muscular pains, rigors and vomiting. As the fever abates in about one week, the jaundice disappears. See **Weil's disease.**

canine (kān′-īn): Resembling a dog. C. TEETH, four in all, two in each jaw, situated between the incisors and the premolars. Those in the upper jaw are popularly known as the 'eye teeth,' those on the lower jaw as the 'stomach teeth.'

canker (kang′-ker): An ulceration occurring chiefly on the lips, mouth, and inside of the cheek.

cannabis (kan′-a-bis): The flowering tops of hemp plants. Seldom used in modern medicine. C. SATIVA, popularly known as bhang, hashish or marihuana, is used illegally as snuff, in cigarettes and in intoxicating drinks for its euphoric effects which resemble those of opium. It is habituating. C. INDICA, Indian hemp, was once used as a sedative in nervous disorders; it is a narcotic.

cannula (kan′-ū-la): A hollow tube for the introduction or withdrawal of fluid from the body. In some patterns the lumen is fitted with a sharp-pointed trocar to facilitate insertion. It is withdrawn when the C. is *in situ.*—cannulae, pl.

canthitis (kan-thī′-tis): Inflammation of the tissues at the canthus (*q.v.*).

canthus (kan′-thus): The angle formed by the junction of the eyelids. The inner one is known as the 'nasal C.' or the medial palpebral commissure, and the outer one as the 'temporal C.' or the lateral palpebral commissure.—canthal, adj.; canthi, pl.

capeline (kap′-e-lin): See under **bandage.**

capillary (kap′-i-lar-i): 1. Hair-like. 2. Any tiny thin-walled vessel, forming part of a network which facilitates rapid exchange of substances between the contained fluid and the surrounding tissues. BILE C. begins in a space in the liver and joins others, eventually forming a bile duct. BLOOD C. unites an arteriole and a venule. C. FRAGILITY refers to an abnormal case of rupture of the blood capillaries. LYMPH C. begins in the tissue spaces throughout the body and joins others, eventually forming a lymphatic vessel.

capillus (ka-pil′-lus): A hair, specifically of the head.—capilli, pl.

capistration (kap-i-strā′-shun): Phimosis (*q.v.*).

capitate (kap′-i-tāt): 1. Head-shaped; having a rounded extremity. 2. One of the eight carpal bones, so called because it has a head-shaped process.

capitellum (kap-it-el′-um): Capitulum humeri. See **capitulum.**

capitulum (ka-pit′-ū-lum): A small, rounded head or prominence on a bone by which it articulates with another bone. C. HUMERI, the small, rounded protuberance on the lower, outer end of the humerus; it articulates with the head of the radius. Also capitellum.

capsitis (kap-sī′-tis): Inflammation of the capsule that encloses the crystalline lens.

capsule (kap′-sūl): 1. The ligaments which surround a joint. 2. A gelatinous or rice paper container for noxious drugs. 3. The outer membranous covering of certain organs, such as the kidney, liver, spleen, adrenals.—capsular, adj.

capsulectomy (kap-sū-lek′-to-mi): Surgical excision of a capsule. Refers to a joint or lens; less often to the kidney.

capsulitis (kap-su-lī'-tis): Inflammation of a capsule. Sometimes used as a synonym for the condition commonly called frozen shoulder (*q.v.*).

capsulotomy (kap-su-lot'-o-mi): Incision of a capsule, usually referring to that surrounding the crystalline lens of the eye.

caput (kap'-ut): 1. A general term applied to the superior extremity of an organ or part. 2. The superior extremity of the body; the head. C. SUCCEDANEUM, a serous effusion overlying the scalp periosteum on an infant's head. Due to pressure during labor; disappears in a few days.

carbhemoglobin (karb-hē-mō-glō'-bin): The compound formed when carbon dioxide unites with hemoglobin; about 8-10% of the carbon dioxide in the blood is in this form.

carbohemia (kar-bō-hēm'-i-a): An excessive amount of carbon dioxide in the blood. Also carbonemia.

carbohydrate (kar-bō-hī'-drāt): An organic compound containing carbon, hydrogen and oxygen, the latter two usually in the proportion to form water. Formed in nature by photosynthesis in plants. Carbohydrates are heat producing; they include starches, sugars and cellulose and are classified in three groups—monosaccharides, disaccharides and polysaccharides. They make up about half our daily intake of food; that which is not oxidized is stored as glycogen or converted into fat and stored.—See **calorific.**

carbohydraturia (kar-bō-hī-dra-tū'-ri-a): The presence of one or more carbohydrates in the urine.

carbolic acid (kar-bol'-ik as'-id): Phenol (*q.v.*).

carbolism (kar'-bōl-izm): Poisoning with phenol (carbolic acid).

carbolize (kar'-bōl-īz): To treat or impregnate with phenol (carbolic acid).

carboluria (kar-bōl-ū'-ri-a): Green or dark colored urine due to excretion of carbolic acid, as occurs in carbolic acid poisoning. —carboluric, adj.

carbon: A non-metallic element present in all organic compounds. C. DIOXIDE, a tasteless, colorless gas; a waste product of many forms of combustion and metabolism, excreted by the lungs. When dissolved in a fluid, carbonic acid is formed; a specific amount of this in the blood produces inspiration; in cases of insufficiency, inhalations of C.D. act as a respiratory stimulant. It is also mixed with O_2 in anesthetic gases to stimulate respiration. In its solid form—C.D. snow—it is used as an escharotic and refrigerant. C. MONOXIDE, an insidious, colorless, odorless gas, present in illuminating gas, the exhaust of combustion motors and the products of incomplete combustion of wood and coal. It forms a stable compound with hemoglobin, thus robbing the body of its oxygen-carrying mechanism; signs of hypoxia ensue. C. TETRACHLORIDE, a colorless liquid with an odor similar to chloroform. Used chiefly as a solvent and detergent. In medicine used as an anthelmintic against tapeworm and other intestinal parasites, sometimes in combination with chenopodium oil; highly toxic; previous fasting and subsequent purging is necessary.

carbonate (kar'-bon-āt): 1. To charge with carbon dioxide. 2. Any salt of carbonic acid.—carbonated, adj.

carbon dioxide: See under **carbon.**

carbonic acid: A solution of carbon dioxide in water; often called carbonated water.

carbon monoxide: See under **carbon.**

carbonuria (kar-bo-nū'-ri-a): An excess of carbon dioxide or other carbon compounds in the urine.

carboxyhemoglobin (kar-bok-si-hē-mō-glō'-bin): A stable compound formed by the union of carbon monoxide and hemoglobin; the red blood cells thus lose their respiratory function, as occurs in carbon monoxide poisoning.

carbuncle (kar'-bung-k'l): An acute, circumscribed, painful, suppurative inflammation (usually caused by a staphylococcic organism) involving several hair follicles and surrounding subcutaneous tissue, forming an extensive slough with several discharging sinuses. Frequently occurs on the back of the neck and most often in men; diabetics are particularly susceptible.—carbuncular, adj.

carcin-, carcino-: Denotes cancer.

carcinogen (kar'-si-nō-jen): Any cancer-producing substance or agent, *e.g.,* friction, injury, pressure, coal tar and its products, prolonged exposure to heat, sun or radiation.—carcinogenic, adj.; carcinogenicity, n.

carcinogenesis (kar-si-nō-jen'-e-sis): The production or origin of cancer.—carcinogenetic, adj.

carcinoid (kar'-si-noid): A circumscribed tumor, usually benign and usually occurring in the gastrointestinal tract. C. SYNDROME, a condition in which a c. of the gut or occasionally a carcinoma of the lung secretes 5-Hydroxytryptomine; characterized by flushing of the face, diarrhea, and right heart failure.

carcinolytic (kar-si-nō-lit′-ik): Destructive of carcinoma cells or pertaining to such destruction.

carcinoma (kar-si-nō′-ma): A malignant new growth derived from epithelial and glandular tissues, which tends to infiltrate into surrounding tissues and to spread by metastasis; the cells resemble those of the tissue where the growth is found. Syn., cancer (*q.v.*).—carcinomatous, adj.; carcinomata, pl. C. IN SITU, asymptomatic condition; cells resembling cancer cells grow from the cervical basal layer and eventually involve the whole epithelium so that its layers can no longer be recognized; often applied to such condition in the uterine cervix; also called preinvasive cancer.

carcinomatophobia (kar-si-nō-ma-tō-fō′-bi-a): Morbid fear of carcinoma.

carcinomatosis (kar-si-nō-ma-tō′-sis): A condition in which cancer is widespread throughout the body. Also carcinosis.

carcinosarcoma (kar-si-nō-sar-kō′-ma): A tumor which has the characteristics of both carcinoma and sarcoma.

cardi-, cardia-, cardio-: Denotes: (1) the heart; (2) heart action.

cardia (kar′-di-a): The esophageal opening into the stomach.

-cardia: Denotes the heart or heart action.

cardiac (kar′-di-ak): 1. Pertaining to the heart. 2. Pertaining to the cardia. 3. A person who has heart disease. 4. An agent or drug which acts especially on the heart. C. ARREST, complete cessation of the heart's activity. C. ASTHMA, see **asthma.** C. ATROPHY, fatty degeneration of the heart muscle. C. BED, one which can be manipulated so that the patient is supported in a sitting position. C. CATHETERIZATION, a long plastic catheter is inserted into an arm vein and passed along to the right atrium, ventricle, and pulmonary artery for (1) recording pressure in these areas; (2) introducing contrast medium prior to x-ray and high-speed photography. Especially useful in the diagnosis of congenital heart defects. C. COMPENSATION, the maintenance of effective circulation, in cases of cardiac disease or disorder, by some mechanism such as hypertrophy of the muscle. C. CYCLE, the period from the beginning of one heart beat to the beginning of the next; includes systole, diastole, and rest period. C. DECOMPENSATION, inability of the heart to maintain normal circulation; symptoms are dyspnea, cyanosis and edema. C. EDEMA,

gravitational dropsy. C. FAILURE, sudden fatal stoppage of the heart's action. C. INSUFFICIENCY, inability of the heart to function normally. C. TAMPONADE, compression of the heart; can occur in surgery or result from penetrating wounds or puncture of the heart which result in hemorrhage into the pericardium. EXTERNAL C. MASSAGE, done for cardiac arrest. With the patient on his back on a firm surface, the lower portion of sternum is depressed 1½ to 2 inches each second.

cardialgia (kar-di-al′-ji-a): 1. Literally, pain in the heart. 2. A painful sensation in the 'pit of the stomach,' often called heartburn.

cardiataxia (kar-di-a-tak′-si-a): Irregularity of heart action due to incoordination of the contractions.

cardiectasis (kar-di-ek′-ta-sis): Dilatation of the heart.

cardiectomy (kar-di-ek′-to-mi): Surgical removal of the cardiac end of the stomach.

cardinal (kar′-di-nal): Primary or fundamental, as cardinal symptoms—temperature, pulse, respiration.

cardiocele (kar′-di-ō-sēl): The protrusion of the heart from its cavity through an opening in the diaphragm or a wound.

cardiocentesis (kar-di-ō-sen-tē′-sis): Surgical puncture of the heart.

cardiocirrhosis (kar-di-ō-sir-rō′-sis): Cirrhosis of the liver accompanied by heart disease.

cardioclasis (kar-di-ok′-la-sis): Rupture of the heart.

cardiodynia (kar-di-ō-din′-i-a): Pain in the heart.

cardiogenesis (kar-di-ō-jen′-e-sis): The development of the heart in the embryonic stage of life.

cardiogenic (kar-di-ō-jen′-ik): 1. Pertaining to the development of the heart. 2. Developing or having its origin in the heart, *e.g.,* the shock in coronary thrombosis.

cardiogram (kar′-di-ō-gram): A recording of the movements of the heart, traced by a cardiograph (*q.v.*).

cardiograph (kar′-di-ō-graf): An instrument for recording graphically the force and form of the heart beat.—cardiographic, adj.; cardiographically, adv.

cardioinhibitor (kar-di-ō-in-hib′-i-tor): An agent that slows or restrains the action of the heart.—cardioinhibitory, adj.

cardiolith (kar′-di-ō-lith): A stone or concretion in the heart tissue.

cardiologist (kar-di-ol′-ō-jist): One who specializes in the study and treatment of heart diseases.

cardiology (kar-di-ol′-o-ji): That branch of medicine that deals with the heart, its functions and diseases.

cardiomalacia (kar-di-ō-mā-lā′-shi-a): Softening of the heart muscle.

cardiomegaly (kar-di-ō-meg′-a-li): Enlargement of the heart.

cardiomyoliposis (kar-di-ō-mī-ō-lī-pō′-sis): Fatty degeneration of the heart muscle.

cardiomyopathy (kar-di-ō-mī-op′-a-thi): A disorder of heart muscle; acute, sub-acute, or chronic; cause may be obscure; may be associated with endocardial or pericardial pathology.—cardiomyopathic, adj.

cardiomyotomy (kar-di-ō-mī-ot′-o-mi): Operation of incising constricting muscle at the junction of the esophagus and the stomach to relieve dysphagia in cardiospasm (*q.v.*).

cardiopalmus (kar-di-ō-pal′-mus): Palpitation of the heart.

cardiopathy (kar-di-op′-a-thi): Heart disease.—cardiopathic, adj.

cardiophobia (kar-di-ō-fō′-bi-a): Morbid fear of heart disease.

cardioptosis (kar-di-ō-tō′-sis): Downward displacement of the heart.

cardiopulmonary (kar-di-ō-pul′-mon-a-ri): Pertaining to heart and the lungs. C. BYPASS, used in open heart surgery. The heart and lungs are excluded from the circulation and replaced by a pump-oxygenator.—cardiopulmonic, adj.

cardiorator (kar′-di-ō-rā-tor): An apparatus for visual recording of the heart beat.

cardiorenal (kar-di-ō-rē′-nal): Pertaining to the heart and kidney.

cardiorespiratory (kar-di-ō-res-pī′-ra-to-ri): Pertaining to the heart and the respiratory system.

cardiorrhaphy (kar-di-or′-a-fi): The procedure of suturing the heart muscle.

cardiorrhexis (kar-di-ō-rek′-sis): Rupture of the heart.

cardiosclerosis (kar-di-ō-skle-rō′-sis): Hardening of the heart muscle.

cardioscope (kar′-di-ō-skōp): An instrument fitted with a lens and illumination, for examining the inside of the heart.—cardioscopic, adj.; cardioscopically, adv.

cardiospasm (kar′-di-ō-spazm): Spasm of the cardiac sphincter between the esophagus and the stomach, causing retention within the esophagus thus giving rise to pain and sometimes regurgitation. Usually no pathological change is found.

cardiothoracic (kar-di-ō-thō-ras′-ik). 1. Pertaining to the heart and thoracic cavity. 2. A specialized branch of surgery.

cardiothyrotoxicosis (kar-di-ō-thī-rō-tok-si-kō′-sis): Toxic hyperthyroidism accompanied by cardiac involvement.

cardiotomy (kar-di-ot′-o-mi): 1. Surgical incision of the heart. 2. An operation in which the cardiac sphincter is cut in order to reduce stricture of the esophagus.

cardiovalvulitis (kar-di-ō-val-vū-lī′-tis): Inflammation of the heart valves.

cardiovascular (kar′-di-ō-vas′-kū-lar): Pertaining to the heart and blood vessels.

cardioversion (kar-di-ō-ver′-shun): Restoring the heart's normal rhythm by applying an electric countershock to control fibrillation.

carditis (kar-dī′-tis): Inflammation of the heart. A word seldom used without the corresponding prefix, *e.g.*, endo-, myo-, pan-, peri-.

caries (kār′-i-ēz): Inflammatory decay of bone or teeth, usually associated with pus formation. SPINAL C., Pott's disease (*q.v.*).—carious, adj.

carina (kar-īn′-a): Any keel-like structure.

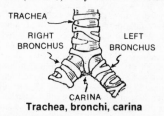

Trachea, bronchi, carina

Most frequently refers to the C. TRACHEAE, a ridge across the base of the trachea where it separates to form the two bronchi.—carinal, adj.

carminative (kar-min′-a-tiv): 1. Having the power to relieve flatulence and associated colic. 2. An agent that helps to prevent the formation of gas and is capable of causing gas to be expelled from the gastrointestinal tract.

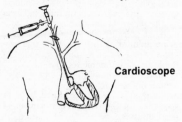

Cardioscope

cast

carneous (kar'-nē-us): Fleshy. C. MOLE, see **mole.**

carnophobia (kar-nō-fō'-bi-a): Morbid aversion to meat as food.

carotene (kar'-ō-tēn): A yellow pigment, found in carrots, tomatoes and other vegetables and fats, which can be converted into vitamin A by the liver. A provitamin.

carotid (kar-ot'-id): The principal artery on each side of the neck. At the bifurcation of the common C. into the internal and external C. there are: (1) the C. BODIES, a collection of chemoreceptors which, being sensitive to chemical changes in the blood, protect the body against lack of O₂; (2) the C. SINUS, a collection of receptors sensitive to pressure changes; increased pressure causes slowing of the heart beat and lowering of blood pressure.

carpal tunnel syndrome: Pain, numbness and tingling in the area of distribution of the median nerve in the hand. Due to compression as the nerve passes through the fascial band. Most common in middle-aged women. Nocturnal.

carphology (kar-fol'-o-ji): Involuntary picking at the bedclothes; an extremely grave symptom seen in great exhaustion, high fevers, delirium. Syn., floccillation.

carpometacarpal (kar'-pō-met-a-kar'-pal): Pertaining to the carpal and metacarpal bones, the joints between them, and the ligaments joining them.

carpopedal (kar-pō-pē'-dal): Pertaining to the wrist and foot or to the hands and feet. C. SPASM, spasm of hands and feet in tetany, provoked by pressure applied to the principal nerves and vessels of the upper arm (Trousseau's sign).

carpoptosis (kar-pop-tō'-sis): Wristdrop.

carpus (kar'-pus): The wrist, consisting of eight small bones.—carpal, adj.

carrier (kar'-i-er): A healthy animal or human host who harbors a pathogenic or potentially pathogenic microorganism in the absence of discernible disease and serves as a possible source of infection. ACTIVE C., one who becomes a C. after recovering from the disease.

car sickness: A form of motion sickness (q.v.).

cartilage (kar'-til-ij): Gristle; a tough connective tissue, characterized by firmness and nonvascularity. There are three main varieties: (1) HYALINE C., a semi-transparent substance of a pearly-bluish color possessing considerable elasticity. (2) YELLOW ELASTIC C. possesses a network of yellow elastic fibers, branching and anastomosing in all directions; it is a true C. found, for example, in the external ear. (3) WHITE FIBROCARTILAGE consists of dense white fibrous tissue of great strength and rigidity. It forms the intervertebral disks. ENSIFORM C., the xiphoid process of the sternum. EPIPHYSEAL C., that present between the ends and shafts of the long bones in children. It allows growth in length.—cartilaginous, adj.

caruncle (ka-rung'-k'l): A red, fleshy projection; that at the inner corner of eye being a lacrimal C. URETHRAL C. is a small bright red growth at the entrance to the female urethra. It is very painful and bleeds readily on being touched. CARUNCULAE MYRTIFORMES, the tag-like ends left after rupture of the hymen during coitus. —caruncular, carunculate, carunculated, adj.

cary-, caryo-: Same as kary-, karyo- (q.v.).

caseation (kā-zē-ā'-shun): The formation of a soft, cheese-like mass, as occurs in tuberculosis.—caseous, adj.

case: C. HISTORY, a biography of a patient's physical and pathological experiences, collected for scientific purposes; sometimes obtained by interview, sometimes collected over the years; includes the history of the present condition for which he is being treated. C. RECORD, all of the data that accumulated about a patient's history, disease, treatment, etc. during his hospital stay; it is placed in the permanent files of the hospital and is admissible as evidence in court. C. STUDY, a method of learning about various diseases and their treatment; frequently employed in schools of nursing.

casein (kā'-sē-in): A protein formed when milk enters the stomach. Coagulation occurs, due to the action of rennin on the caseinogen in the milk, splitting it into two proteins, one being casein. The casein combines with calcium and a clot is formed.

caseinogen (kā-sē-in'-ō-jen): A protein in milk which is converted into casein by the action of rennin in the stomach.

cast: 1. Fibrous material and exudate which has been molded to the form of the cavity or tube in which it has collected, and this can be identified under the microscope. It is also classified according to its constitution; bloody, epithelial, fatty, etc. RENAL C., found in the urine. 2. A stiff bandage or dressing made of crinoline or like material impregnated with plaster of paris or other hardening material, used to immobilize a part in cases of fracture or dislocation, and various orthopedic conditions.

castration (kas-trā′-shun): The removal of testes in the male or ovaries in the female.—castrated, adj.; castrate, n., v.t. C. COMPLEX, fear of losing one's genital organs; usually in children and arising from a sense of guilt over oedipal feelings. See **Oedipus.**

catabasis (ka-tab′-a-sis): The stage during which a disease declines in severity.

catabolism, katabolism (ka-tab′-ō-lizm): The series of chemical reactions in the living body in which complex substances, taken in as food, are broken down into simpler ones accompanied by the release of energy. This energy is needed for anabolism and the other activities of the body.—catabolic, adj.

catalepsy (kat′-a-lep-si): A conscious but trance-like state in which the muscles are rigid so that the subject remains in a fixed position over an indefinite period of time.—cataleptic, adj.

catalysis (ka-tal′-i-sis): A change in the rate at which a chemical action proceeds, produced by an agent which is not itself affected by the reaction. May be positive or negative.—catalytic, adj.

catalyst (kat′-a-list): An agent which produces catalysis (q.v.). It does not undergo any change during the process. Syn., catalyzer, enzyme, ferment.

catamenia (kat-a-mēn′-i-a): Menstruation.—catamenial, adj.

cataphasia (kat-a-fā′-zi-a): A disorder of speech characterized by the constant repetition of certain words or phrases.

cataplasia (kat-a-plā′-zi-a): Atrophy or degeneration of tissues in which they revert to an earlier, or embryonic state.

cataplasm (kat′-a-plazm): A poultice (q.v.).

cataplexy (kat′-a-plek-si): A condition of sudden powerlessness due to muscular rigidity caused by intense emotional upheaval such as fear or shock, or hypnotic suggestion. The patient remains conscious; recovery is usually complete.—cataplectic, adj.

cataract (kat′-a-rakt): An opacity of the crystalline lens or its capsule, or both. It may be congenital, senile, traumatic, or due to diabetes mellitus. HARD C., contains a hard nucleus, tends to be dark in color and occurs in older people. SOFT C., one without a hard nucleus, occurs at any age, but particularly in the young. Cataract usually develops slowly and when mature is called 'ripe.'

catarrh (ka-tar′): An old term for inflammation of mucous membrane with a constant flow of mucus; applied especially to the upper respiratory tract.—catarrhal, adj.

catatonia (kat-a-tō′-ni-a): A type of behavior that may occur in schizophrenia; the patient may assume certain odd postures for indefinite periods, have muscular spasms, refuse to speak, become negative, stuporous or indifferent to the environment.

catchment area: A term used to describe the geographic area from which a mental health facility draws its clientele.

catecholamine (kat-e-kōl-am′-in): Any one of a group of compounds that have the power to cause physiological changes resembling those caused by the action of the sympathetic nerves. Includes dopamine, norepinephrine and epinephrine.

catgut (kat′-gut): A form of ligature and suture of varying thickness, strength and absorbability, prepared from sheep's intestines. After sterilization it is hermetically sealed in glass tubes in sizes 00000 to 8. The 'plain' variety is usually absorbed in 5 to 10 days. 'Chromicized' C. and 'iodized' C. will hold for 20 to 40 days.

catharsis (ka-thar′-sis): 1. A cleansing or purging, said particularly of the intestine. 2. A method used in freudian psychiatry; the analyst urges the patient to talk freely about things that come to mind during a train of thought and thus purge his mind of the memories of painful or unpleasant experiences that may be causing his psychological disturbance. Syn., abreaction (q.v.).

cathartic (ka-thar′-tik): 1. Producing catharsis (q.v.). 2. An agent that promotes evacuation of the intestine. Cathartics are classed as laxatives or purgatives, according to the type and degree of evacuation they produce.

catheter (kath′-e-ter): A hollow, flexible tube of varying length, bore and shape, used for distending a hollow tube or passage or for injecting or withdrawing fluid from a body cavity. Catheters are made of soft and hard rubber, gum elastic, glass, rubberized silk, silver, other metals and plastic materials. FOLEY C., a commonly used type of indwelling C. held in place by an attached inflated thin-walled balloon. INDWELLING OR INLYING C., one which is fastened in place for continuous drainage of the urinary bladder. NASAL C., one used for introducing food into the stomach or for administering oxygen via the nose. TRACHEAL C., one used for suctioning the trachea, particularly after surgery.

catheterization (kath-e-ter-ĭ-zā′-shun): Insertion of a catheter into a body channel or cavity, most usually into the urinary bladder. CARDIAC C., the insertion of a fine, polyethylene or radiopaque nylon tubing via the median basilic vein at the elbow, into the heart to (1) record pressures; (2) introduce an opaque substance prior to x-ray; (3) withdraw samples of blood.—catheterize, v.t.

cathexis (ka-thek′-sis): In psychiatry, the fixing of one's psychic energy on some particular person, thing or concept.

cathode (kath′-ōd): The negatively charged pole of an electrode or electrolytic cell.

cation (kat′-ī-on): A positively charged ion.

catoptrophobia (kat-op-trō-fō′-bi-a): Morbid fear of mirrors or of breaking them.

cat scratch fever: A minor local inflammatory lesion with redness, swelling, slight ulceration or papule formation at the site of a scratch wound; chills, malaise, rash, and fever of an undulating type may develop; probably caused by a virus. Regional lymph nodes may become involved and eventually suppurate. Symptoms usually disappear in 2 to 3 weeks. Apparently worldwide, not seasonal and shows no preference for age or sex.

cauda (kaw′-da): Any tail or tail-like appendage. C. EQUINA, the lower end of the spinal cord; it is a bundle of the roots of all the spinal nerves below the first lumbar. —caudal, caudate, adj.

caudal block: See **epidural.**

caul: A part or all of the amnion which sometimes covers or envelopes the head of the fetus at birth. 'Angel's veil.' In olden days thought to be a good omen.

causalgia (kaw-sal′ji-a): Excruciating burning neuralgic pain, resulting from physical trauma to a cutaneous nerve.

caustic (kaw′-stik): Corrosive or destructive to living tissue, or agents that produce this effect. Used therapeutically to destroy overgrowths of granulation tissue, warts, polypi. Carbolic acid, carbon dioxide snow, and silver nitrate are most commonly employed.

cauterize (kaw′-ter-īz): 1. To apply a cautery. 2. To destroy tissue by heat, chemical action, or electricity.—cauterization, n.

cautery (kaw′-ter-i): A caustic agent such as a chemical or a hot iron used to destroy living tissue. ACTUAL C., a hot iron used to apply direct heat. CHEMICAL C., a chemical substance used to burn or sear tissue. ELEC-

TRIC C., a platinum wire maintained at red heat by an electric current. PAQUELIN'S C., a form of C. in which the hollow platinum point is kept at the required heat by a current of benzene which is constantly pumped into it.—cauterization, n.; cauterize, v.t.

caval infusion (kā′-val in-fū′-shun): A method of treatment in acute renal failure with anuria. A radiopaque nylon cardiac catheter is passed via the femoral vein to lie near the opening of the renal veins or at the entrance to the right atrium. A constant flow of hypertonic fluid is thus possible.

cavamesenteric shunt (kā-va-mes-en-ter′-ik): The upper end of the inferior vena cava is anastomosed to the superior mesenteric vein; used in children when the portal vein is blocked. See **shunt.**

cavernous (kav′-er-nus): Containing hollow spaces. C. SINUS, a channel for venous blood, on either side of the sphenoid bone; it drains blood from the lips, nose and orbits. C. BODY, one of the two erectile columns in the dorsum of the penis and in the clitoris.

cavitation (kav-i-tā′-shun): The formation of a cavity as in pulmonary tuberculosis.

cavity (kav′-i-ti): 1. A hollow; an enclosed area within the body. ABDOMINAL C., that area below the diaphragm and above the pelvis; the abdomen. BUCCAL C., the mouth. CEREBRAL C., the ventricles of the brain. CRANIAL C., the brain box formed by the bones of the cranium. MEDULLARY C., the hollow center of a long bone, containing yellow bone marrow or medulla. NASAL C., that in the nose, separated into right and left halves by the nasal septum. ORAL C., the buccal cavity. PELVIC C., that formed by the pelvic bones, more particularly the part below the iliopectineal line and containing primarily the rectum and reproductive organs. PERITONEAL C., a potential space between the parietal and visceral layers of the peritoneum. Similarly, the PLEURAL C. is the potential space between the pulmonary and parietal pleurae which, in health, are in contact in all phases of respiration. SYNOVIAL C., the potential space in a synovial joint. UTERINE C., that of the uterus, in the form of a small triangle, the base extending between the orifices of the uterine tubes. VENTRAL C., the body C., in front of the spinal column; encloses the mouth, throat, thorax, abdomen and pelvis; it is differentiated from the DORSAL C. which is the space enclosed by the vertebrae

cavus

and the bones of the cranium. 2. In dentistry, a hollow formed in a tooth as a result of decay of the organic matter following decalcification of the inorganic outer part of the tooth; syn., caries.

cavus (kā'-vus): An exaggerated curve of the longitudinal arch of the foot. Clubfoot.

CBC: Abbreviation for complete blood count.

cc: Abbreviation for cubic centimeter.

CCU: Abbreviation for coronary care unit (*q.v.*).

cecectomy (sē-sek'-to-mi): Operation for removal of the cecum.

cecitis (sē-sī'-tis): Inflammation of the cecum.

cecocolostomy (sē-kō-kō-los'-to-mi): The creation of an anastomosis between the cecum and the colon.

cecoileostomy (sē-kō-il-ē-os'-to-mi): A surgically created anastomosis between the cecum and the ileum.

cecorectostomy (sē-kō-rek-tos'-to-mi): A surgically created anastomosis between the cecum and the rectum.

cecosigmoidostomy (sē-kō-sig-moid-os'-to-mi): A surgically created anastomosis between the cecum and the sigmoid flexure of the colon.

cecostomy (sē-kos'-to-mi): A surgically established fistula between the cecum and the anterior abdominal wall.

cecotomy (sē-kot'-ō-mi): The operation of making an incision into the cecum.

cecum (sē'-kum): The blind, pouchlike

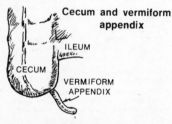

Cecum and vermiform appendix

ILEUM
CECUM
VERMIFORM APPENDIX

commencement of the colon in the right iliac fossa; it is separated from the ileum by the ileocecal valve. The vermiform appendix is attached to it.—cecal, adj.

-cele: Denotes: (1) tumor; (2) hernia.

celiac (sē'-li-ak): Relating to the abdominal cavity. Applied to arteries, veins, nerves and a plexus. C. DISEASE, a condition of wasting, occurring in early childhood, with malabsorption of fats and starch indiges-

tion, thought to be due to intolerance to gluten in wheat flour. The clinical picture is one of misery, distended abdomen, bulky stools with a marked excess of fat.

celiectomy (sē-li-ek'-to-mi): The removal by surgery of any abdominal organ.

celiocentesis (sē-li-ō-sen-tē'-sis): Surgical puncture of the abdomen.

celiocolpotomy (sē-li-ō-kol-pot'-o-mi): Surgical incision into the vagina by way of the abdomen.

celiohysterectomy (sē-li-ō-his-ter-ek'-to-mi): Surgical removal of the uterus via an abdominal incision.

celioscopy (sē-li-os'-ko-pi): Syn., laparoscopy, peritoneoscopy (*q.v.*).

celiotomy (sē-li-ot'-o-mi): Surgical incision into the abdomen.

cell: A histological term for a minute mass of protoplasm containing a nucleus; the physiological and structural unit of all living things. Some cells, *e.g.,* the erythrocytes, are non-nucleated; and others, *e.g.,* the leukocytes, may be multinucleated. —cellular, adj.

cellophane (sel'-ō-fān): A derivative of cellulose, made into a thin, transparent, highly impermeable sheet or tube; used in face masks and as a protective covering for wound and surgical dressings.

cellulitis (sel-ū-lī'-tis): A diffuse inflammation of connective tissue, especially the loose subcutaneous tissue. When it involves the pelvic tissues in the female it is called 'parametritis.' When it occurs in the floor of the mouth it is called 'Ludwig's angina.'

cellulose (sel'-ū-lōs): A carbohydrate forming the outer walls of plant and vegetable cells. A polysaccharide which cannot be digested by man but supplies roughage for stimulation of peristalsis.

censor (sen'-sor): Term employed by Freud to define the resistance which prevents repressed material from readily reentering the conscious mind from the subconscious (unconscious) mind.

centesis (sen-tē'-sis): A puncture of a body cavity with a trocar, needle, or aspirator. Often used as a word ending with a combining form that indicates the part of the body involved, *e.g.,* abdominocentesis.

centigrade (sen'-ti-grād): Having one hundred divisions or degrees. Usually applied to the thermometric scale in which the freezing point of water is fixed at 0 and the boiling point at 100.

centiliter (sen'-ti-lē-ter): 1/100 of a liter. Approximately 10 cc.

centimeter (sen′-ti-me-ter): In metric linear measurement, 1/100 of a meter. 0.3937 of an inch. Abbreviated cm.

central nervous system: That part of the nervous system consisting of the brain and spinal cord. Abbreviated CNS.

centrifugal (sen-trif′-ū-gal): Efferent. Having a tendency to move away or outward from a center or from the cerebral cortex.

centrifuge (sen′-tri-fūj): An apparatus that rotates, thereby increasing the force of gravity so that substances of different densities are separated; usually used to separate particulate material from a suspending liquid.—centrifuge, v.t.

centripetal (sen-trip′-et-al): Afferent. Having a tendency to move toward a center or toward the cerebral cortex.

centrosome (sen′-tro-som): A minute spot in the cytoplasm of animal cells supposed to be concerned with division of the nucleus.

cephal-, cephalic-, cephalo-: Denotes the head.

cephalalgia (sef-al-al′-ji-a): Pain in the head; headache.

cephalhematoma (sef-al-hem-a-to′-ma): A collection of blood in the subperiostal tissues of the scalp.

cephalhydrocele (sef-al-hi′-dro-sel): A serous cyst under the scalp.

-cephalic, -cephalism, -cephaly: Denotes: (1) the head; (2) headed or having such a head.

cephalic (sef-al′-ik): Pertaining to the head; near the head. C. VERSION, an obstetric maneuver to change the fetal lie to a head presentation to facilitate delivery.

cephalocele (sef′-a-lo-sel): Hernia of the brain; protrusion of part of the brain through the skull.

cephalocentesis (sef-a-lo-sen-te′-sis): Surgical puncture of the head; usually refers to the insertion of a trocar or cannula into the brain to drain off the fluid of a hydrocephalus or of an abscess.

cephalodynia (sef-a-lo-din′-i-a): Pain in the head; headache.

cephalohematoma (sef-a-lo-he-ma-to′-ma): Cephalhematoma (q.v.).

cephalometry (sef-a-lom′-e-tri): Measurement of the living human head.

cephalopelvic (sef′a-lo-pel′-vik): Pertaining to the size of the head of the fetus in utero in relation to the size of the mother's bony pelvis.

cephalotomy (sef-a-lot′-o-mi): The operation of cutting the head of the fetus in order to assist in its delivery.

cerate (se′-rat): A preparation for external use; has a wax or fat base; consistency is between that of an ointment and a plaster; does not melt at ordinary temperatures.

cerebellum (ser-e-bel′-um): That part of the brain which lies behind and below the cerebrum. Its chief functions are the coordination of fine voluntary movements and the control of posture.—cerebellar, adj.

cerebral (ser′-e-bral): Pertaining to or affecting the cerebrum. C. ACCIDENT or CEREBROVASCULAR ACCIDENT, apoplexy (q.v.) caused by embolism, hemorrhage, or thrombosis in the brain; abbreviated CVA. C. CORTEX, that part of the brain that is responsible for higher mental activities during consciousness. C. HEMORRHAGE, hemorrhage into the cerebrum from a ruptured artery; may result from hypertension or arteriosclerosis. C. HERNIA, a hernia in which some of the brain substance protrudes through an opening in one of the bones of the skull as may occur after surgery or injury. C. LOCALIZATION, the specification of a certain area in the brain that controls a particular function such as speech, vision, etc. C. MENINGITIS, inflammation of the meninges of the brain. See **meningitis.** C. PALSY, an impairment in the development of the nervous system due to birth injury of cerebral motor nerves; covers a large group of disabilities the most common of which is lack of muscular control; symptoms appear in infancy or early childhood.

cerebralgia (ser-e-bral′-ji-a): Headache.

cerebration (ser-e-bra′shun): Mental activity.

cerebritis (ser-e-bri′tis): Inflammation of the cerebrum.

cerebromalacia (ser-e-bro-ma-la′shi-a): Softening of the substance of the cerebrum.

cerebromeningitis (ser-e-bro-men-in-ji′tis): Inflammation of the brain and its meninges.

cerebrosclerosis (ser-e-bro-skler-o′-sis): Hardening of the substance of the cerebrum.

cerebroside (ser′-e-bro-sid): A chemical substance found in body tissues, particularly brain and nerve tissue.

cerebrospinal (ser′-e-bro-spi′-nal): Pertaining to the brain and spinal cord. C. FEVER, an epidemic form of meningitis (q.v.). C. FLUID, the clear fluid filling the ventricles of the brain and central canal of the spinal cord. Also found beneath the cranial and

spinal meninges in the pia-arachnoid space.
See **meningitis**. C. NERVE, one that runs
to or from the brain or spinal cord, *i.e.,* a
central nervous system nerve. C. SYSTEM,
consists of the brain, spinal cord and the
nerves emanating from or running to them.
cerebrovascular (ser -e-brō-vas′-kū-lar):
Pertaining to the blood vessels of the brain,
especially to pathological changes in these
vessels. C. ACCIDENT, the rupture of a
blood vessel within or near the brain: cerebral hemorrhage; a stroke; abbrev. CVA.
cerebrum (ser′-e-brum, se-rē′-brum): The
largest and uppermost part of the brain; it
does not include the cerebellum, pons and
medulla. The longitudinal fissure divides it
into two hemispheres, each containing a lateral ventricle. The internal substance is
white, the outer convoluted cortex is
gray.—cerebral, adj.
certifiable (ser-ti-fī′-a-b′l): Term used in reference to: (1) infectious or industrial diseases which, by law, are reportable to health
authorities; (2) a person who behaves in
such a way that he is considered to have a
psychosis severe enough to require his
placement in a psychiatric institution.
cerumen (se-roo′-men): Earwax. The soft,
yellowish-brown, wax-like secretion of the
ceruminous glands in the external auditory
canal.—ceruminous, ceruminal, adj.
cervical (ser′-vi-kal): Pertaining to: (1) the
neck; (2) the cervix (neck) of an organ.
C. ADENITIS, inflammation of the lymph
nodes of the neck. C. CANAL, the lumen of
the cervix uteri which leads from the body
of the uterus to the vagina. C. NERVES, the
first eight pairs of spinal nerves. C. RIB, a
supernumerary rib which sometimes occurs
on the 7th vertebra; may present no problems or it may press on the brachial plexus.
C. VERTEBRAE, the first (upper) seven
bones of the spinal column.
cervicectomy (ser-vi-sek′-to-mi): Amputation of cervix uteri.
cervicitis (ser-vi-sī′-tis): Inflammation of
the cervix uteri.
cerviocolpitis (ser-vi-kō-kol-pī′-tis): Inflammation of the cervix uteri and the
vagina.
cervicodynia (ser-vi-kō-din′-i-a): A cramp
or pain in the neck.
cervicovaginitis (ser-vi-kō-vaj-i-nī′-tis): Inflammation of the cervix uteri and the
vagina.
cervicovesical (ser-vi-kō-ves′-i-kal): Pertaining to both the cervix uteri and the urinary bladder.

cervix (ser′-viks): A neck or constricted part
of an organ. C. UTERI, the neck of the
uterus.—cervical, adj.
cesarean section (se-sa′-ri-an): Delivery of
a fetus via an incision through the abdominal and uterine walls. So called because
Caesar was supposed to have been born that
way. Also caesarean.
cestode (ses′-tōd): Tapeworm. See **Taenia**.—cestoid, adj.
cestodiasis (ses-tō-dī′-a-sis): Infestation
with cestodes (*q.v.*).
cf.: Abbreviation for compare.
CFT: Abbreviation for complement-fixation
test. See **complement**.
chafing (chāf′-ing): Irritation of the skin due
to two skin surfaces rubbing together or to
irritants.
chalasia (ka-lā′-zi-a): The relaxation of a
body opening, particularly one that is normally guarded by a sphincter muscle. May
be a cause of regurgitation or vomiting by
infants when there is no other sign of distress.
chalazion (ka-lā′-zi-on): A cyst on the edge
of the eyelid from retained secretion of the
meibomian glands. Similar to a stye, but
painless. May disappear or may need to be
surgically evacuated.—chalazia, pl.
chalicosis (kal-i-kō′-sis): A lung disease
caused by inhalation of stone dust. Found
chiefly among stonecutters. Pneumoconiosis (*q.v.*).
chamber: In anatomy, an enclosed space or
cavity, *e.g.,* the C′S. of the heart, or the anterior and posterior C′S. of the eye.
chancre (shang′-ker): The primary lesion of
syphilis, formed at the site of infection 2 to
3 weeks after infection; usually on lips, genitals or fingers. Consists of an ordinary
round or oval red spot that may go unnoticed as it is usually painless; may develop
into a papule, ulcer or erosion that is highly
infectious. Associated with swelling of local
lymph glands.
chancroid (shang′-kroid): A type of non-
syphilitic veneral infection, prevalent in
warmer climates; associated with uncleanliness; transmitted by sexual contact. Also
called 'soft sore.' Causes painful, multiple,
ragged ulcers on the penis or vulva that
have a purulent exudate and are often associated with bubo (*q.v.*) formation.
change of life: The menopause (*q.v.*).
character (kar′-ak-ter): The sum total of the
known and predictable mental characteristics of an individual, particularly his conduct. C. CHANGE, denotes change in the

form of conduct, to one foreign to the patient's natural disposition, *e.g.*, indecent behavior in a hitherto respectable person. Common in the psychoses.

characteristic (kar-ak-ter-is′-tik): 1. A specific, distinguishing attribute or trait. 2. A structural or functional feature of an organism.

charcoal (char′-kōl): The residue after burning organic substances at a high temperature in an enclosed vessel. Used in medicine for its adsorptive and deodorant properties.

Charcot's joint (shar′-kōs): Complete disorganization of a joint associated with syringomyelia or advanced cases of tabes dorsalis (locomotor ataxia). Condition is painless. C. TRIAD, late manifestations of disseminated sclerosis—nystagmus, intention tremor and staccato speech. [Jean Martin Charcot, French neurologist and clinician. 1825-1893.]

charlatan (shar′-la-tan): One who pretends to have knowledge or skills which he does not possess; a quack.

charley horse: Soreness, stiffness and pain in a muscle or tendon following injury or excessive athletic activity. Term usually restricted to the quadriceps muscle. Slang.

chart: An individual record kept for each hospital patient. Common usage refers to a collection of forms for recording various types of information, *e.g.*, laboratory and x-ray examination reports; patient's temperature, pulse, and respirations; nurses' notes including their observations of the patient's condition, food intake, etc. The chart becomes part of the hospital's permanent records.

cheil-, cheilo-: Denotes the lip.

cheilectomy (kī-lek′-to-mi): Surgical excision of part of the lip.

cheilitis (kī-lī′-tis): Inflammation of the lip.

cheilophagia (kī-lō-fā′-ji-a): Lip-biting.

cheiloplasty (kī′-lō-plas-ti): Any plastic operation on the lip.

cheilorrhaphy (kī-lor′-a-fi): Suturing of a cut or lacerated lip, or repair of a harelip.

cheiloschisis (kī-lōs′-ki-sis): Harelip.

cheilosis (kī-lō′-sis): A condition of the lips, especially at the angles of the mouth, usually resulting from riboflavin deficiency. Pallor of the mucosa is followed by reddening, scaling, maceration and fissuring.

cheir-, cheiro-: Denotes relationship to the hand.

cheiragra (kī-rag′-ra): Pain in the hand.

cheirarthritis (kī-rar-thrī′-tis): Inflammation of the joints of the fingers and hands.

cheiromegaly (kī-rō-meg′-a-li): Abnormal enlargement of the hands.

cheiropompholyx (kī-rō-pom′-fo-liks): Symmetrical eczematous eruption of the skin of the hands (especially fingers) characterized by the formation of tiny vesicles and associated with itching or burning. On the feet the condition is called 'podopompholyx.'

cheirospasm (kī′-rō-spazm): Writer's cramp.

chelating agents (kē-lā′-ting): Soluble organic compounds that can fix certain metallic ions into their molecular structure. When given in cases of poisoning, the new complex so formed is excreted in the urine.

cheloid: See **keloid.**

chemo-: Denotes relationship to: (1) chemistry; (2) a chemical.

chemoceptor (kē′-mō-sep-tor): Chemoreceptor (*q.v.*).

chemopallidectomy (kē-mō-pal-i-dek′-to-mi): The destruction of a predetermined section of globus pallidus by the injection of chemicals. The operation is performed for the relief of parkinsonism and other similar conditions that are marked by muscle rigidity.

chemoprophylaxis (kē-mō-prō-fi-lak′-sis): The prevention of a specific disease (or recurrent attack) by administration of chemical drugs.—chemoprophylactic, adj.

chemoreceptor (kē-mō-rē-sep′-tor): 1. A chemical linkage in a living cell having an affinity for, and capable of combining with, certain other chemical substances. 2. A sensory end organ capable of reacting to a chemical stimulus.

chemosis (kē-mō′-sis): An edema or swelling of the bulbar conjunctiva.—chemotic, adj.

chemosuppressive (kē-mō-sup-pres′-iv): Syn., chemoprophylactic. See **chemoprophylaxis.**

chemosurgery (kē-mō-sur′-jer-i): The destruction of diseased or unwanted tissue by the application of chemical agents.

chemotaxis (kē-mō-tak′-sis), **chemotaxy:** Response of organisms to chemical stimuli, attraction towards a chemical being positive C.; repulsion is negative C.—chemotactic, adj.

chemothalamectomy (kē-mō-thal-a-mek′-to-mi): Destruction of part of the thalamus by the injection of a chemical; similar to chemopallidectomy (*q.v.*). Done for the relief of tremor.

chemotherapy (kē-mō-ther′-a-pi): Use of a

specific chemical agent to arrest the progress of, or eradicate, disease in the body without causing irreversible injury to healthy tissue, *e.g.*, employment of sulpha drugs in lobar pneumonia, of arsenic in syphilis, of nitrogen mustard in Hodgkin's disease. Chemotherapeutic agents are administered mainly by oral, intramuscular and intravenous routes, and are distributed usually by the bloodstream.

chest: The thorax (*q.v.*).

chestmobile: A vehicle outfitted as a clinic which travels from place to place for the purpose of making chest x-rays of the general population.

Cheyne-Stokes respiration: See **respiration.**

chiasm (kī'-azm): An X-shaped crossing or decussation. OPTIC C. or CHIASMA OPTICUM, the meeting of the optic nerves; where the fibers from the medial or nasal half of each retina cross the middle line on the ventral surface of the brain to join the optic tract of the opposite side. Also chiasma.

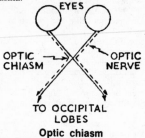

Optic chiasm

chickenpox: A mild, specific disease of childhood, caused by a virus. Successive crops of vesicles appear first on the trunk; they scab and heal without causing scars. Syn., varicella.

chigger (chig'-er): A minute larval mite that burrows into the skin of warm-blooded animals. In man its bite produces a wheal (*q.v.*) which itches intensely. Not the same as jigger.

chilblain (chil'-blān): Congestion and swelling attended with severe itching and burning sensation in reaction to damp, cold weather; fingers, toes and ears are affected particularly. Erythema pernio.

childbearing: Pregnancy and the delivery of a child. C. PERIOD, the years of a woman's life during which she can normally bear children.

childbed: The state of a woman being in labor or bringing forth a child. C. FEVER, puerperal fever (*q.v.*).

childbirth: Term applied to the normal termination of pregnancy with the birth of an infant.

childhood: The period of life between infancy and puberty. C. SCHIZOPHRENIA, that which occurs before puberty; characterized by autism (*q.v.*) and immaturity.

chill: A sudden sensation of cold, accompanied by shivering, often followed by rise in body temperature. Sometimes the initial symptom of an acute infection such as pneumonia: a characteristic symptom of malaria.

chimney sweep's cancer: Scrotal epithelioma (*q.v.*).

chionablepsia (kī-ō-na-blep'-si-a): Snow-blindness.

chirology (kī-rol'-ō-ji): A method of communicating with or between deaf-mutes through hand signals. Dactylology.

chiropodist (kī-rop'-o-dist): One qualified in chiropody (*q.v.*).

chiropody (kī-rop'-o-di): The treatment of corns, callosities, bunions and toenail conditions. Podiatry.

chiropractic (kī-rō-prak'-tik): A system of treatment based on the theory that disease is caused by impingement on the spinal nerves and that relief or cure can be effected through manual manipulation of the spinal column.

chiropractor: One who practices chiropractic (*q.v.*).

chloasma (klō-az'-ma): Painless yellowish to dark brown patches on the skin. Sometimes occur during menopause or pregnancy. Called also 'liver spots.'

chlorate (klō'rāt): Any salt of chloric acid.

chloremia (klō-rē'-mi-a): 1. Decrease in the hemoglobin and red cells; chlorosis (*q.v.*). 2. The presence of more than the normal amount of chlorides in the blood.

chloride (klō'-rīd): A salt of hydrochloric acid; a compound composed of two substances one of which is chlorine that carries a negative charge of electricity.

chloride of lime: See **chlorinated.**

chloriduria (klōr-i-dū'-ri-a): More than the normal amount of chlorides in the urine.

chlorinated (klōr'-in-ā-ted): Said of a substance to which chlorine has been added, *e.g.*, water. C. LIME, a substance made by passing chlorine over hydrated lime; formerly much used as a disinfectant, fumigant and deodorant; also called chloride of lime.

chlorination (klōr-in-ā'-shun): The procedure of adding chlorine to a substance to
disinfect it, *e.g.*, water, sewage.

chlorine (klō'-rēn): A yellowish-green gaseous element with an irritating, suffocating
odor. Represented by the symbol Cl.

chloro-: Denotes a green color.

chloroform (klōr'-ō-form): A clear, colorless, volatile, heavy liquid with a sweetish
taste, once much used as a general anesthetic.

chloroma (klō-rō'-ma): A condition in
which multiple malignant greenish-yellow
growths develop, especially on the periosteum of the facial and cranial bones and the
vertebrae. Observed most frequently in children and young adults.

chlorophenothane (klō-rō-fen'-ō-thān):
dichloro-diphenyl-trichloro-ethane; DDT.
See **dicophane, DDT.**

chlorophyll (klōr'-ō-fil): The coloring matter of green plants; essential for photosynthesis (*q.v.*). Now prepared synthetically for
use in medicine and as a deodorant.

chlorosis (klō'-rō-sis): An old name for simple iron deficiency occurring especially in
young women.

chloruresis (klōr-ūr-ē'-sis): Excretion of
chlorides in the urine.

choana (kō'-a-na): Funnel-shaped opening.
The posterior nasal orifices or nares
(*q.v.*).—choanae, pl.; choanal, adj.

choked disk: Swelling and protrusion of the
optic disk (*q.v.*); occurs in several disease
conditions including brain tumor.

chol-, chole-, cholo-: Denotes bile, gall.

cholagogue (kōl'-a-gog): A drug that causes
an increased flow of bile into the intestine.

cholangiogram (kōl-an'-ji-ō-gram): X-ray
film demonstrating the gallbladder and bile
ducts.

cholangiography (kōl-an-ji-og'-ra-fi): Radiographic examination of hepatic, cystic,
and bile ducts. Can be performed: (1) after
oral or intravenous administration of radiopaque substance; (2) at operation to detect
any further stones in the ducts; (3) after
operation by way of a T-tube in the common bile duct; (4) by means of an injection
via the skin on the anterior abdominal wall
and the liver.—cholangiographic, adj.; cho-
liangiograph, n.; choliangiographically,
adv.

cholangiohepatitis (kōl-an-ji-ō-hep-a-tī'-
tis): Inflammation of the liver and bile
ducts.

cholangitis (kōl-an-jī'-tis): Inflammation of
a bile duct.

cholecyst (kōl'-ē-sist): The gallbladder.—
cholecystic, adj.

cholecystagogue (kōl-ē-sis'-ta-gog): An
agent that stimulates activity of the gallbladder and promotes the flow of bile from
it.

cholecystangiogram (kōl-ē-sist-an'-ji-ō-
gram): Film demonstrating gallbladder,
cystic and common bile ducts after administration of opaque medium.

cholecystectomy (kōl-ē-sis-tek'-to-mi):
Surgical removal of the gallbladder.

cholecystenterostomy (kōl-ē-sist-en-ter-
os'-to-mi): Literally, the establishment of an
artificial opening (anastomosis) between the
gallbladder and the small intestine. Specific
terminology more frequently used.

cholecystitis (kōl-ē-sis-tī'-tis): Inflammation of the gallbladder.

cholecystocolostomy (kōl-ē-sis-tō-kō-los'-
to-mi): The surgical establishment of an
anastomosis between the gallbladder and
some portion of the colon.

cholecystoduodenostomy (kōl-ē-sis -tō-
du-ō-dēn-os'-to-mi): The establishment of
an anastomosis between the gallbladder and
the duodenum. Usually necessary in cases
of stricture of common bile duct, which
may be congenital or due to previous inflammation or operation.

cholecystogastrostomy (kōl-ē-sis-tō-gas-
tros'-to-mi): The establishment of an anastomosis between the gallbladder and the
stomach; a palliative operation when the
common bile duct is obstructed by an ir-
removable growth.

cholecystogram (kōl-ē-sis'-tō-gram): An x-
ray picture of the gallbladder obtained by
cholecystography (*q.v.*).

cholecystography (kōl-ē-sis-tog'-ra-fi):
Radiographic examination of the gallbladder after it has been rendered opaque by the
ingestion or intravenous injection of an
opaque medium.—cholecystographic, adj.;
cholecystographically, adv.; cholecysto-
graph, n.

cholecystojejunostomy (kōl-ē-sis-tō-jē-
jūn-os'-to-mi): An anastomosis between the
gallbladder and the jejunum. Performed for
obstructive jaundice due to growth in the
head of the pancreas.

cholecystokinin (kōl-ē-sis-tō-kī'-nin): A
hormone that induces contraction of the
gallbladder. Secreted by the upper intestinal
mucosa.

cholecystolithiasis (kōl-ē-sis-tō-lith-ī'-a-
sis): The presence of stone or stones in the
gallbladder.

cholecystolithotomy (kōl-ē-sis-tō-li-thot'-o-mi): The surgical removal of stones from the gallbladder.

cholecystopathy (kōl-ē-sis-top'-a-thi): Any pathology of the gallbladder.

cholecystostomy (kōl-ē-sis-tos'-to-mi): A surgically established fistula between the gallbladder and the abdominal surface; used to provide drainage in empyema of gallbladder or after removal of stones.

cholecystotomy (kōl-ē-sis-tot'-o-mi): Incision into the gallbladder.

choledochal (kōl-ē-dok'-al): Pertaining to or affecting the common bile duct.

choledochoduodenostomy (kō-led-ō-kō-dū-ō-den-os'-to-mi): Surgical anastomosis between the common bile duct and the duodenum.

choledocholithiasis (kō-led-ō-kō-li-thī'-a-sis): The presence of a stone or stones in the common bile duct.

choledocholithotomy (kō-led-ō-kō-li-thot'-om-i): Surgical removal of a stone from the common bile duct.

choledochostomy (ko-led-ō-kos'-to-mi): Drainage of the common bile duct through the abdominal wall, usually after exploration for a stone.

choledochotomy (ko-led-ō-kot'-o-mi): Incision into the common bile duct.

cholelith (kōl'-ē-lith): A gallstone.

cholelithiasis (kōl-ē-li-thī'-a-sis): The presence of stones in the gallbladder or bile ducts.

cholelithotomy (kōl-ē-li-thot'-o-mi): Operation for the removal of gallstones.

cholemesis (kō-lem'-e-sis): Vomiting of bile.

cholemia (kō-lēm'-i-a): The presence of bile in the blood.—cholemic, adj.

cholepoiesis (kō-lē-poi-ē'-sis): The formation of bile in the liver.

cholera (kol'-e-ra): An acute epidemic disease, caused by *Vibrio comma*, occurring in the East. The main symptoms are the evacuation of copious 'rice-water' stools accompanied by agonizing cramp and severe collapse. Spread mainly by contaminated water, overcrowding and insanitary conditions. Mortality very high.

choleric temperament (kol'-er-ik): One of the four classical types of temperament (*q.v.*); hasty and prone to emotional outbursts.

cholerrhagia (kol-er-rā'-ji-a): Excessive flow of bile.

cholestasis (kōl-ē-stā'-sis): Diminution or arrest of the flow of bile.—cholestatic, adj.

cholesteatoma (kō-lē-stē-a-tō'-ma): A benign encysted tumor containing cholesterol. Mainly occurs in the middle ear.—cholesteatomatous, adj.

cholesteremia (kō-les-ter-ē'-mi-a): Excess cholesterol in the blood. Also cholesterolemia.

cholesterol (kō-les'-ter-ol): A crystalline substance of a fatty nature found in the brain, nerves, liver, blood and bile. It is not easily soluble and may crystallize in the gallbladder and along arterial walls. When irradiated it forms vitamin D.

cholesterolemia (kō-les-ter-ol-ē'-mi-a): Cholesteremia (*q.v.*).

cholesteroluria (kō-les-ter-ol-ū'-ri-a): Cholesterol in the excreted urine.

cholesterosis (kō-les-ter-ō'-sis): Abnormal deposition of cholesterol, as in the gallbladder.

choline (kō'-lēn): A chemical found in animal tissues as a constituent of lecithin and acetylcholine. Thought to be part of the vitamin B complex, and is known to be a growth factor. Appears to be necessary for fat transportation in the body. Useful in preventing fat deposition in the liver in cirrhosis. Richest sources are dairy products.

cholinergic (kō-lin-er'-jik): Applied to parasympathetic nerves which liberate acetylcholine at their terminations when a nerve impulse passes. See **adrenergic.**

cholinesterase (kō-lin-es'-ter-ās): An enzyme, which hydrolyzes acetylcholine into choline and acetic acid, at nerve endings. Present in all body tissues.

choluria (kō-lū'-ri-a): The presence of bile in the urine.—choluric, adj.

chondr-, chondri-, chondro-: Denotes cartilage.

chondral (kon'-dral): Cartilaginous; relating to cartilage.

chondritis (kon-drī'-tis): Inflammation of cartilage.

chondroblast (kon'-drō-blast): The embryonic cell which produces cartilage.

chondrocostal (kon-drō-kos'-tal): Pertaining to the costal cartilages and ribs.

chondrocyte (kon'-drō-sīt): A cartilage cell.

chondrodynia (kon-drō-din'-i-a): Pain in a cartilage.

chondrolysis (kon-drol'-i-sis): Dissolution of cartilage.—chondrolytic, adj.

chondroma (kon-drō'-ma): A benign tumor of cartilage. Tends to recur after removal. It causes no pain.

chondromalacia (kon-drō-mal-ā'-shi-a): Softening of cartilage.

chondroplasty (kon′-drō-plas-ti): Plastic surgery on cartilage.

chondrosarcoma (kon-drō-sar-kō′-ma): A rapidly growing malignant neoplasm of cartilage occurring most frequently near the ends of long bones.—chondrosarcomatous, adj.; chondrosarcomata, pl.

chondroseptum (kon-drō-sep′-tum): The part of the nasal septum that is composed of cartilage.

chondrosis (kon-drō′-sis): The formation of cartilage.

chondrosternal (kon′-drō-ster′-nal): Pertaining to the rib cartilages and sternum.

chord (kord): Cord.

chorda (kor′-da): A collection of fibers forming a cord; a tendon. CHORDAE TENDINEAE, fine white glistening cords stretching between the valves and the ventricular walls of the heart. When the muscles contract, the chordae are tightened, thus preventing the cusps of the atrioventricular valves from being swept back ìnto the atria. C. TYMPANI, a branch of the facial nerve which passes through the tympanic cavity and joins the lingual branch of the trigeminal nerve.—chordal, chordate, adj.; chordae, pl.

chordee (kor-dē′): Painful erection of the penis, usually due to urethritis; common in gonorrhea. Also may be due to congenital hypospadias.

chorditis (kor-dī′-tis): Inflammation of a cord; usually refers to the spermatic or vocal cords.

chordotomy (kor-dot′-o-mi): Surgical division of any cord, particularly the anterolateral nerve pathways in the spinal cord, to give relief from intractable pain. Temporary relief, as for severe burns or shingles, may be obtained by direct electric chordotomy under local anesthesia. Also cordotomy.

chorea (kō-rē′-a): A nervous disorder associated with rheumatic fever and characterized by ceaseless, rapid, irregular and spasmodic movements that are beyond the patient's control. Even voluntary movements are rendered jerky and ungainly. The childhood type is also called 'rheumatic chorea' or 'St. Vitus's dance'; the adult form is part of a cerebral degenerative process called 'Huntington's chorea.'—choreal, choreatic, choreic, adj.

choreiform (kō-rē′-i-form): Resembling chorea (q.v.).

choreoathetosis (kō-rē-ō-ath-e-tō′-sis): A nervous condition characterized by both choreic and athetoid movements. See **athetosis.**—choreoathetoid, adj.

choreomania (kō-rē-ō-mā′-ni-a): Dancing mania; term often used to describe a type of mania seen in the Middle Ages.

choreophrasia (kō-rē-ō-frā′-zi-a): The constant repetition of senseless words or phrases.

chorion (kō′-ri-on): The outer membrane forming the embryonic sac.—chorial, chorionic, adj.

chorionepithelioma (kō-ri-on-ep-i-thē-li-ō-ma): A highly malignant tumor arising from chorionic cells, usually those of the uterus but also those of other female generative organs and the testes; may follow hydatidiform mole (q.v.), abortion, or even normal pregnancy; quickly metastasizes, especially to the lungs. Syn., Choriocarcinoma. Also chorioepithelioma.

chorionic villi (kō-ri-on′-ik vil′-lī): Projections from the chorion (q.v.) from which the fetal part of the placenta is formed. Through the C. V. diffusion of gases, nutrient, and waste products occurs from the maternal to the fetal blood and vice versa.

chorioretinitis (kō-ri-ō-ret-i-nī′-tis): Inflammation of the choroid and retina.

choroid (kō′-roid): The middle pigmented, vascular coat of the posterior five-sixths of the eyeball, continuous with the iris in front. It lies between the sclera externally and the retina internally, and prevents the passage of light rays.—choroidal, adj.

choroiditis (kō-roid-ī′-tis): Inflammation of the choroid. TAY'S C., degenerative change affecting the retina around the macula lutea; believed to be caused by an atheromatous condition of the arteries; seen in older people. [Warren Tay, English physician. 1843-1927.]

choroidocyclitis (kō-roi-dō-sik-lī′-tis): Inflammation of the choroid and ciliary body.

choroidoretinitis: Syn., chorioretinitis (q.v.).

Christian Science: A religion founded by Mary Baker Eddy in 1866; it teaches that cause and effect are mental and that sin, illness, and death may be overcome through the practice of spiritual healing that is based on a full understanding of the principles of healing as taught by Jesus.

Christmas disease: Allied to hemophilia (q.v.). Caused by a hereditary deficiency of clotting factor IX (plasma thromboplastin component). Named for the patient in whom it was first described.

chrom-, chromat-, chromato-, chromo-, -chromia, -chromio: Denotes: (1) color; (2) pigment.

chromatelopsia (krō-mat-e-lop'-si-a): Imperfect perception of colors; color blindness.

chromatic (krō-mat'-ik): Pertaining to: (1) color; (2) chromatin (q.v.).

chromatin (krō'-ma-tin): That part of the cell nucleus which stains most readily; thought to be the physical basis of heredity.

chromatodermatosis (krō-ma-tō-der-ma-tō'-sis): Any disease of the skin accompanied by discoloration. Also chromodermatosis.

chromatopsia (krō-ma-top'-si-a): A visual defect in which objects that are normally seen as colorless are seen as having color. Also chromopsia.

chromatosis (krō-ma-to'-sis): Abnormal pigmentation of the skin, as in Addison's disease (q.v.).

chromaturia (krō-ma-tū'-ri-a): The excretion of urine of an abnormal color.

chromium (krō'-mi-um): A hard, grayish metallic element.

chromocytometer (krō-mō-sī-tom'-e-ter): An instrument for measuring color, particularly one which measures the hemoglobin in red blood cells.

chromosome (krō'-mo-sōm): Any one of the microscopic, dark-staining, thread-like bodies which develop from the nuclear material of the cell and which split longitudinally during cell division, one half going into the nucleus of each daughter cell. They carry the hereditary factors (genes), the number being constant for each species; they are also responsible for the determination of sex.—chromosomal, adj.

chronic (kron'-ik): Lingering, lasting; opposed to acute.—chronically, adv.; chronicity, n.

chronognosis (kron-og-nō'-sis): Sensitivity to the passage of time.

chronological age (kron-ō-loj'-i-kal): Age from birth; one's calendar age.

chrysotherapy (kris-ō-ther'-a-pi): Treatment with compounds of gold.

chthonophagia (thon-ō-fā'-ji-a): The habit of eating dirt. Syn., geophagia. Also chthonophagy.

Chvostek's sign (shvos'-teks): Excessive twitching of the face on tapping the facial nerve. A sign of tetany. [Franz Chvostek, Austrian surgeon. 1835-1884.]

chyle (kīl): Digested fats which, as an alkaline milky fluid, pass from the small intestine via the lymphatics to the blood stream.—chylous, adj.

chylosis (kī-lō'-sis): The conversion of food into chyle in the intestine and its absorption by the tissues.

chyluria (kī-lū'-ri-a): Chyle in the urine giving it a milky appearance. Can occur in some nematode infestations, when either a fistulous communication is established between a lymphatic vessel and the urinary tract, or the distension of the urinary lymphatics causes them to rupture.—chyluric, adj.

chymase (kī'-mās): An enzyme found in the gastric juice; it acts to hasten the action of pancreatic juice.

chyme (kīm): Partially digested food which as an acid, creamy-yellow, thick fluid, passes from the stomach to the duodenum. Its acidity controls the pylorus so that c. is ejected at frequent intervals.—chymous, adj.

chymotrypsin (kī-mō-trip'-sin): Proteolytic enzyme of the pancreatic secretion. Also prepared synthetically.

cicatrix (sik'-a-triks): A scar; formed from connective tissue. See keloid.—cicatricial, adj.; cicatrization, n; cicatrize, v.i., v.t.

cilia (sil'-i-a): 1. The eyelashes. 2. Microscopic hair-like projections from certain epithelial cells. Membranes containing such cells are known as ciliated membranes, for example, those lining the trachea and fallopian tubes.—cilium, sing.; ciliary, ciliated, cilial, adj.

ciliary (sil'-i-a-ri): Hair-like. C. APPARATUS, the nerves, muscles, and other structures of the eye that are concerned with adjusting the lens of the eye for vision at varying distances. C. BODY, a specialized structure in the eye connecting the anterior part of the choroid to the circumference of the iris; it is composed of the ciliary muscles and processes. C. MUSCLES, fine hair-like muscle fibers arranged in a circular manner to form a grayish-white ring immediately behind the corneoscleral junction. C. PROCESSES, about 70 in number, are projections on the under surface of the choroid which are attached to the C. muscles.

cillosis (sil-lō'-sis): Spasmodic twitching of the muscles of the eyelid.

Cimex (sī'-meks): A genus of insects of the family Cimicidae. C. LECTULARIUS, the common bedbug, parasitic to man; bloodsucking. See bedbug.

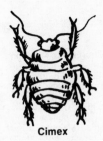

Cimex

cinchonism (sin'-kon-izm): Poisoning from cinchona or one of its alkaloids; quininism (*q.v.*).

cinclisis (sin'-kli-sis): Rapidly repeated movements, particularly winking or breathing.

cineangiocardiography (sin-ē-an-ji-ō-kar-di-og'-ra-fi): Motion picture of the passage of contrast medium through the heart and blood vessels.

cineangiography (sin-ē-an-ji-og'-ra-fī): Motion picture angiography (*q.v.*).

cineradiography (sin-ē-rā-di-og'-ra-fi): Moving picture radiography, *e.g.*, showing joints or heart in action.

cionectomy (sī-ō-nek'-to-mi): Excision of part or all of the vulva.

cionitis (sī-ō-nī'-tis): Inflammation of the vulva.

circadian rhythm (ser-kā-dē'-an): Rhythm within a periodicity of 24 hours, especially in relation to biologic variations.

circinate (ser'-si-nāt): In the form of a circle or segment of a circle, *e.g.*, the skin eruptions of late syphilis, ringworm, etc.

circle of Willis: An anastomosis of arteries at the base of the brain, formed by the union of the branches of the internal carotids with the branches of the basilar artery. [Thomas Willis, physician to James II. 1621-1675.]

CircOlectric bed (ser-kō-lek'-trik): A hospital bed that permits vertical turning of the patient, rather than lateral. An electric motor turns the entire bed frame which is suspended between two hoop-like supports; can be operated by patient or nurse and permits many different positions.

circulation (ser-kū-lā'-shun): Passage in a circle.—circulatory, adj.; circulate, v.i. and v.t. C. OF BILE, the passage of bile from the liver cells where it is formed, via the gallbladder and bile ducts to the small intestine, where its constituents are partly reabsorbed into the blood and thus return to the liver. C. OF CEREBROSPINAL FLUID, takes place from the ventricles of the brain to the cisterna magna, from whence the fluid bathes the surface of the brain, and cord, including its central canal. It is absorbed into the blood in the cerebral venous sinuses. COLLATERAL C., that established through anastomotic communicating channels, when there is interference with main blood supply. CORONARY C., that of blood through the heart walls. EXTRACORPOREAL C., blood is taken from the body, directed through a machine ('heart-lung,' 'artificial kidney') and returned to the general C. FETAL C., that of blood through the fetus, umbilical cord and placenta. LYMPH C., that of lymph collected from the tissue spaces, which passes via capillaries, vessels, glands and ducts to be poured back into the blood stream. PORTAL C., that of venous blood (collected from the intestines, pancreas, spleen and stomach) to the liver before return to the heart. PULMONARY C., deoxygenated blood leaves the right ventricle, flows through the lungs where it becomes oxygenated and returns to the left atrium of the heart. SYSTEMIC C., oxygenated blood leaves the left ventricle and after flowing throughout the body, returns deoxygenated to the right atrium.

circum-: Denotes around, surrounding, on all sides.

circumanal (ser-kum-ā'-nal): Surrounding the anus.

circumcision (ser-kum-sizh'-un): Excision of the prepuce or foreskin.

circumcorneal (ser-kum-kor'-nē-al): Around the cornea.

circumduction (ser-kum-duk'-shun): 1. The circular movement of an organ or part around a central axis; *e.g.*, the eye or a limb. 2. The action of swinging a limb, such as the arm, in such a manner that it describes a cone-shaped figure, the apex of the cone being formed by the joint at the proximal end, while the complete circle is formed by the free distal end of the limb.

circumflex (ser'-kum-fleks): Winding round, designating particularly an artery or nerve that has a winding course. C. NERVE, that supplying the deltoid muscle.

circumocular (ser-kum-ok'-ū-lar): Surrounding the eye.

circumoral (ser-kum-ō'-ral): Surrounding the mouth. C. PALLOR, a pale appearance of the skin around the mouth, in contrast to the flushed cheeks. A characteristic of scarlet fever.—circumorally, adv.

circumscribed (ser'-kum-scrībd): Limited; confined to a limited area.

circumvallate (ser-kum-val'-lāt): Surrounded by a raised ring as the lingual papillae. See **papilla.**

cirrhosis (sir-ō'-sis): Hardening of an organ. Applied almost exclusively to degenerative changes in the liver with resulting fibrosis. Associated developments may include ascites (*q.v.*), obstruction of the circulation through the portal vein with hematemesis (*q.v.*), jaundice and enlargement of the spleen.—cirrhotic, adj.

cirsectomy (ser-sek'-to-mi): The surgical excision of part of a varicose vein.

cirsenchysis (ser-sen'-ki-sis): Treatment of a varicose vein by injecting into it a solution that causes sclerosis.

cirsoid (ser'-soid): Resembling a tortuous, dilated vein (varix, *q.v.*). C. ANEURYSM, a tangled mass of pulsating blood vessels, usually seen as a subcutaneous tumor on the scalp.

cissa (sis'-a): Pica (*q.v.*).

cisterna (sis-ter'-na): Any closed space serving as a reservoir for a body fluid. C. CHYLI, the dilated part at the beginning of the thoracic duct which receives lymph from several lymph-collecting vessels. C. MAGNA, a subarachnoid space in the cleft between the medulla oblongata and the cerebellum.—cisternal, adj.

cisternal puncture: See **puncture.**

cisvestitism (sis-ves'-ti-tizm): Dressing appropriately for one's sex but not for one's position, *e.g.,* a civilian dressing in a uniform of one of the armed services.

citric acid (sit'-rik): Occurs widely in fruits, especially in lemons and limes. Prevents scurvy; also has a diuretic action.

citrin (sit'-rin): [Syn., vitamin P.]. Thought to enhance the action of vitamin C in the prevention of scurvy in human beings. Capillary fragility is associated with lack of this substance. It is found in rose hips, citrus fruits and black currants.

citta (sit'-a), **cittosis** (sit-tō'-sis): Pica (*q.v.*).

clairvoyance (klar-voi'-ans): The act or power of knowing about events without the use of the senses. Extrasensory perception; insight; divination.

clap: A slang term for gonorrhea.

Clark's rule: A formula for calculating the correct dose of medicine for a child:

$$\frac{\text{weight of child in lbs.}}{150} \times \text{adult dose} = \text{child's dose}$$

claudication (klaw-di-kā'-shun): Limping because there is interference with the blood supply to the legs. The cause may be spasm or disease of the vessels themselves. In 'intermittent claudication' patient experiences severe pain in the calves when he is walking; after a short rest he is able to continue.

claustrophilia (klaws-trō-fil'-i-a): Morbid fear of open spaces; desire to remain behind locked doors and windows.

claustrophobia (klaws-trō-fō'-bi-a): Morbid fear of enclosed places, or of being locked in.—claustrophobic, adj.

clavicle (klav'-i-k'l): The collarbone. It articulates with the sternum at one end and the acromion process of the scapula at the other.—clavicular, adj.

clavus (klā'-vus): A corn or horny area on the skin. C. HYSTERICUS, a pain described as feeling like having a nail driven into one's head.

clawfoot (klaw'-foot): Deformity in which the longitudinal arch of the foot is increased in height, and associated with clawing of the toes. It may be acquired or congenital in origin. Syn., pes cavus.

clawhand: The hand is clawed and radially deviated, due to paralysis of the flexor carpi ulnaris, ulnar half of the flexor digitorum longus, and the small muscles of the hand. Occurs in leprosy, syringomyelia, and in lesions of the ulnar nerve.

clean: Uncontaminated; free of microorganisms. Frequently used to refer to objects that have had no contact with patients in isolation units, or to instruments, etc., that have been sterilized and kept free from contact with microorganisms.

cleft: A long, narrow fissure, particularly one that develops in the embryo. C. PALATE, congenital failure of fusion between the right and left palatal processes; if complete, it extends through both hard and soft palates thus forming a single cavity for the nose and mouth; often associated with harelip (*q.v.*). C. LIP, harelip.

cleid-, cleido-: Denotes the clavicle.

cleptomania (klep-tō-mā'-ni-a): Kleptomania (*q.v.*).

climacteric (klī-mak'-te-rik): The menopause or 'change of life.' The end of the period of possible sexual reproduction, as evidenced by the cessation of the menstrual periods. Other bodily and mental changes may occur.

climatotherapy (klī-ma-tō-ther′-a-pi): The treatment of disease by exposure to a climate different from the one in which the patient normally lives.

climax (klī-maks): 1. The period of greatest intensity of a disease; the crisis of a disease. 2. The sexual orgasm.

clinic (klin′-ik): 1. A center for examination, study and treatment of outpatients. 2. Medical instruction, with the examination of patients, before a group of medical students; usually conducted at the bedside.

clinical (klin′-i-k′l): 1. Pertaining to a clinic. 2. Practical observation and treatment of sick persons as opposed to theoretical study. C. DIAGNOSIS, D. that is based on physical signs of disease, physical examination, and the patient's history; does not include laboratory tests.

clinician (kli-nish′-an): A physician who is engaged in clinical practice rather than research.

Clinitest: A method of testing urine for sugar; used particularly by patients at home. Kit consists of reagent tablets, dropper, test tube, and color chart.

clithrophobia (klith-rō-fō′-bi-a): Claustrophobia (*q.v.*).

clitoridectomy (klit-or-i-dek′-to-mi): Surgical removal of the clitoris; female circumcision.

clitoriditis (klit-or-id-ī′-tis): Inflammation of the clitoris. Also clitoritis.

clitoris (klit′-or-is): A small, erectile, highly erotogenic organ situated just below the mons veneris at the junction anteriorally of the labia minora; the homologue of the penis in the male.—clitoral, clitoridean, adj.

cloaca (klō-ā′-ka): 1. The common opening of the intestinal and urogenital tract in fishes and birds and reptiles. 2. In osteomyelitis, the opening through the involucrum which discharges pus.—cloacal, adj.

clonus (klō′-nus): A series of intermittent muscular contractions and relaxations. Opp. tonus (*q.v.*).—clonic, adj.; clonicity, n.

Clostridium (klos-trid′-i-um): A bacterial genus. Large gram-positive anaerobic bacilli found as commensals of the gut of animals and man, and as saprophytes in the soil. Endospores are produced which are widely distributed. Many species are pathogenic for man because of the exotoxins produced—*e.g., C. tetani* (tetanus); *C. botulinum* (botulism); *C. welchii* (gas gangrene).

Mechanism of clot formation

Injury to blood vessel causes
↓
Blood platelets to disintegrate and release
↓
Thromboplastin which is converted into
↓
Prothrombin which unites with calcium to form
↓
Thrombin which causes
↓
Fibrinogen in the blood to be converted into
↓
Fibrin which unites with the cellular elements in the blood to form a
↓
Clot

clot: 1. A semisolid mass. Usually refers to blood; fibrin forms a network that holds the formed elements in the blood in a mass. 2. To form into a clot, or coagulate.

clotting time: The time it takes for shed blood to clot. This is determined by test and differs from bleeding time in that it involves only the ability of the blood to clot, whereas B.T. also involves the ability of the small capillaries to constrict.

clubbed fingers: Seen in chronic heart and lung disease. See **clubbing.**

clubbing: Refers to the bulbous enlargement of the ends of the phalanges due to proliferation of the soft tissues without the same degree of change in the bones.

clubfoot: A congenital malformation in which the foot is twisted out of shape or position; may be either unilateral or bilateral. See **talipes.**

clubhand: A congenital deformity analogous to clubfoot; type most commonly seen is the result of defective development of the radius.

clumping: See **agglutination.**

cluttering (klut′-ter-ing): Confused speech which is rapid and indistinct with syllables and letters being dropped.

Clutton's joints: Symmetrical swelling of joints, usually painless, the knees often being involved. Associated with congenital syphilis. [Henry Hugh Clutton, English surgeon. 1850-1909.]

clysis (klī′-sis): 1. The cleansing or washing out of a cavity. 2. Term used when administering fluids by other than the oral route: subcutaneously (hypodermoclysis); intravenously (venoclysis); rectally (proctoclysis).

cm: Abbreviation for centimeter.

CNS: Abbreviation for central nervous system.

CO: Carbon monoxide. See **carbon.**

CO₂: Carbon dioxide. See **carbon.**

coagulant (kō-ag′-ū-lant): 1. An agent that causes or speeds clotting of the blood. 2. Having the effect of increasing the tendency of the blood to clot.

coagulase (kō-ag′-ū-lās): A clotting enzyme, *e.g.,* thrombin, rennin. Produced by some bacteria (*e.g., Staph. aureus*), which clot plasma. Used to type bacteria into C. negative and positive.

coagulate (kō-ag′-ū-lat): 1. To change from a fluid to a solid jelly-like mass, or to clot. 2. To cause a clot or curdle.—coagulation, n.

coagulation time: See **clotting time.**

coagulum (kō-ag′-ū-lum): Any coagulated mass. Scab.

coalesce (kō-a-les′): To grow together; to unite into a mass. Often used to describe the development of a skin eruption, when discrete areas of affected skin coalesce to form sheets of a similar appearance, *e.g.,* psoriasis, pityriasis rubra pilaris.—coalescence, n.; coalescent, adj.

coal tar: Thick black substance obtained from coal by distillation. Used in a variety of pharmaceutical preparations.

coarctation (kō-ark-tā′-shun): Contraction, stricture, narrowing; applied to a vessel or canal.

coating: A covering. C. OF PILLS, a covering to conceal an unpleasant taste. ENTERIC C., covering for a medicament which prevents its being absorbed from the stomach; the coating dissolves in the intestine only.

cobalt (kō′-bawlt): A mineral element considered nutritionally essential in minute traces. Thought to be linked with iron and copper in prevention of anemia. Co⁵⁸, used as tracer in study of Co metabolism. Co⁶⁰,

now superseding radium in radiotherapy (Co BOMB).

cocainism (kō′-kān-izm): Mental and physical degeneracy caused by a morbid craving for, and excessive use of cocaine.

coccidioidomycosis (kok-sid-i-oi-dō-mī-kō′-sis): An acute infection caused by inhalation of the spores of a fungus. Initial symptoms resemble those of tuberculosis—cough, fever, sweats. Later, cutaneous nodules may develop. Also called desert fever, valley fever, San Joaquin Valley fever.

coccobacillus (kok-ō-ba-sil′-us): A short, thick, somewhat ovoid bacterial cell.

coccus (kok′-us): A spherical, or nearly spherical bacterium. Often classified according to the way it arranges itself, as can be seen under the microscope: diplococcus, when it occurs in pairs; streptococcus, when it occurs in chains; staphylococcus, when it occurs in bunches resembling bunches of grapes.—cocci, pl.; coccal, coccoid, adj.

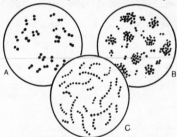

Cocci. A, diplococci
B, staphylococci. C, streptococci

-coccus: Denotes berry-shaped. Used primarily in forming generic names of microorganisms.

coccyalgia (kok-sē-al′-ji-a): Coccydynia (*q.v.*).

coccydynia (kok-sē-din′-i-a): Pain in the region of the coccyx.

coccygectomy (kok-sē-jek′-to-mi): Surgical removal of the coccyx.

coccygodynia (kok-sē-go-din′-i-a): Syn., coccydynia (*q.v.*).

coccyx (kok′-siks): The last bone of the vertebral column. It is triangular in shape and curved slightly forward. It is composed of four rudimentary vertebrae, cartilaginous at birth, ossification being completed at about the 30th year.—coccygeal, adj.

cochlea (kok′-lē-a): A spiral canal resembling the interior of a snail shell, in the anterior part of the bony labyrinth of the inner ear. Contains the organ of Corti, the essential organ of hearing.—cochlear, adj.

cocoa (kō'-kō): The seeds of *Theobroma cacao.* The powder is made into a nourishing pleasant beverage. Contains theobromine and caffeine. C. BUTTER, obtained from the roasted seeds; is used in suppositories, ointments and as an emollient.

cod liver oil: The oil extracted from the liver of fresh codfish. Contains vitamins A and D and on that account is used as a dietary supplement in cases of mild deficiency. Also used as a preventive of rickets in children. Now often replaced by purer forms or concentrates of vitamins A and D.

coelom (sē'-lom): A cavity in the embryo; eventually it divides into the pericardial, pleural and peritoneal cavities.

coenzyme (kō-en'-zīm): An enzyme activator, *e.g.,* bile which facilitates the action of lipase in the digestion of fats.

cognition (kog-nish'-un): Awareness of objects or thoughts; one of the three aspects of mind, the others being affection (feeling or emotion), and conation (willing or desiring). They work as a whole but any one of the three may dominate any mental process.

cognitive (kog'-ni-tiv): Related to or involving perception, including the elements of comprehension, judgment, memory, and reasoning.

cohabitation (kō-hab-i-tā'-shun): The living together of a man and woman as man and wife; they may or may not be legally married.

coitus (kō'-i-tus): The act of sexual intercourse; copulation.

cold: 1. Opp. of heat. 2. A catarrhal inflammation of the upper respiratory tract; may be caused by infection or allergy.

cold sleep: Hypothermia (*q.v.*).

cold sore: A small vesicle or blister that appears, usually around or within the mouth, during a cold or a disease attended by fever. Often multiple. See **herpes.** Also fever blister.

colectomy (kō-lek'-to-mi): Excision of part or the whole of the colon.

coleitis (kōl-ē-ī'-tis): Vaginitis.

coleoptosis (kōl-ē-op-tō'-sis): Prolapse of the vaginal wall.

coleotomy (kōl-ē-ot'-ō-mi): Colpotomy (*q.v.*).

colibacillus (kō-li-ba-sil'-us): The colon bacillus; found in the intestine of man and many animals. *Escherichia coli.*

colic (kol'-ik): Severe pain resulting from

periodic spasm in an abdominal or tubular organ. BILIARY C., spasm of smooth muscle in a bile duct caused by a gallstone. INTESTINAL C., abnormal peristaltic movement of an irritated gut. PAINTER'S (LEAD) C., spasm of intestine and constriction of mesenteric vessels. RENAL C., spasm of ureter due to a stone. UTERINE C., dysmenorrhea (*q.v.*).—colicky, adj.

coliform (kō'-li-form): A word used to describe any bacterium of fecal origin which is morphologically similar to *Esch. coli.*

colitis (kō-lī'-tis): Inflammation of the colon; acute or chronic. ACUTE C., occurs suddenly as result of infection or irritation; accompanied by pain and diarrhea. AMEBIC C., caused by an ameba. MUCOUS C., often seen in neurotic individuals; accompanied by colic, diarrhea and passage of mucus in stools. ULCERATIVE C., an inflammatory and ulcerative condition of the colon of unknown cause. Characteristically it affects young and early middle-aged adults, producing periodic bouts of diarrheal stools containing mucus and blood, and it may vary in severity from a mild form with little constitutional upset to a severe, dangerous and prostrating illness.

collagen (kol'-a-jen): An albuminoid substance arranged in bundles. It is the main constituent of white fibrous tissue and the organic substance of bone. The 'collagen diseases' are characterized by an inflammatory lesion of unknown origin affecting C. and small blood vessels. They include dermatomyositis, lupus erythematosus, polyarteritis (periarteritis) nodosa, and scleroderma; frequently fatal.—collagenic, collagenous, adj.

collapse: 1. Extreme physical or nervous prostration. 2. The 'falling in' of a hollow organ or vessel, *e.g.,* collapse of lung from change of air pressure inside or outside the organ. C. THERAPY, artificial pneumothorax (*q.v.*), induced to collapse and immobilize a lung. Also collapsotherapy.

collarbone: The clavicle (*q.v.*).

collateral (ko-lat'-er-al): Accessory, secondary. C. CIRCULATION, established by blood flowing in vessels alternative to the direct, main one.

Colles' fracture: See **fracture.**

colliquative (ko-lik'-wa-tiv): 1. Profuse; excessive. 2. Characterized by excessive fluid discharge.

collodion (ko-lō'-di-on): An inflammable viscous solution of pyroxylin, ether and alcohol. It forms a flexible film on the skin

colloid

and is used mainly as a protective dressing. FLEXIBLE C., collodion mixed with camphor and castor oil.

colloid (kol'-oid): A glue-like noncrystalline substance; diffusible but not soluble in water; unable to pass through an animal membrane. Some drugs can be prepared in their colloidal form. C. GOITER, abnormal enlargement of the thyroid gland, due to the accumulation in it of viscid, iodine-containing colloid.

colloidal gold test (kol-oid'-al): One of the laboratory tests of cerebrospinal fluid with special application in the diagnosis of neurosyphilis, although positive results may also be obtained in meningitis, multiple sclerosis, poliomyelitis, encephalitis, and other serious diseases of the nervous system. Normal spinal fluid does not precipitate colloidal gold, whereas abnormal fluid does. The degree of precipitation is shown by corresponding color changes and the colors are reported as numbers from 1 to 5. Ten dilutions are commonly tested. General paralysis of the insane (GPI) gives a pattern of numbers such as 5 5 5 5 4 4 3 2 1 0, tabes dorsalis such as 0 0 1 2 3 4 4 3 2 1.

coloboma (kol-ō-bō'-ma): A congenital fissure or gap in the eyeball or one of its parts, *e.g.,* C. iridis.—colobomata, pl.

colocecostomy (kō-lō-sē-kos'-tō-mi): Cecocolostomy (*q.v.*).

colocentesis (kō-lō-sen-tē'-sis): Surgical puncture of the colon, usually to relieve distention.

coloclysis (kō-lok'-li-sis): Irrigation of the colon.

colocystoplasty (kōl-ō-sis'-tō-plas-ti): Operation to increase the capacity of the urinary bladder by using part of the colon. —colocystoplastic, adj.

colon (kō'-lon): The large bowel extending from the cecum to the rectum. In its various parts it has appropriate names—ascending C., transverse C., descending C., sigmoid C. IRRITABLE C., one in which there is a tendency to hyperperistalsis, colic, and sometimes diarrhea.—colonic, adj.

colonorrhagia (kō-lon-o-rā'-ji-a): Hemorrhage from the colon.

colonorrhea (kō-lon-o-rē'-a): Discharge of mucus from the colon.

colonoscope (kō-lon'-o-skōp): An instrument for examining the lower part of the colon.—colonoscopy, n.

colony (kol'-on-i): A mass of bacteria, growing on a culture, which is the result of multiplication of one or more organisms. A colony may contain many millions of individual organisms and become macroscopic (*q.v.*); its physical features are often characteristic of the species.

color blindness: Achromatopsia. See **blindness**.

color index: A term used to indicate the relative amount of hemoglobin in red blood cells of a patient. It is the ratio of the percentage of hemoglobin (100 percent = 14.6 G of hemoglobin per 100 ml) to the percentage of red blood cells (100 percent = 5 million per cu mm). The normal index ranges from 0.85 to 1.1.

colorrhaphy (kō-lor'-a-fi): Suture of the colon.

colostomy (kō-los'-to-mi): A surgically established fistula between the colon and the surface of the abdomen; this acts as an artificial anus and may be temporary or permanent.

colostrum (kō-los'-trum): The relatively clear fluid secreted in the breasts during the first few days after parturition, before the formation of true milk is established. It is rich in lactalbumin and acts as a laxative.

colotomy (kō-lot'-o-mi): Incision into the colon.

colp-, colpo-: Denotes vagina.

colpalgia (kol-pal'-ji-a): Pain in the vagina.

colpatresia (kol-pa-trē'-zi-a): Atresia or closing up of the vagina.

colpectomy (kol-pek'-to-mi): Surgical excision of the vagina, or part of it.

colpitis (kol-pī'-tis): Inflammation of the vagina.

colpocele (kol'-pō-sēl): A hernia into the vagina.

colpohysterectomy (kol-pō-his-ter-ek'-to-mi): Surgical removal of the uterus through the vagina.

colpoperineoplasty (kol-pō-per-i-nē'-ō-plas-ti): Plastic repair of the vagina and perineum.

colpoperineorrhaphy (kol-pō-per-in-ē-or'-a-fi): The surgical repair of an injured vagina and deficient perineum.

colpoptosis (kol-pō-tō'-sis): Prolapse of the vagina.

colporrhaphy (kol-por'-a-fi): Surgical repair of the vagina. ANTERIOR C. for repair of cystocele (*q.v.*) and POSTERIOR C. for repair of a rectocele (*q.v.*).

colposcope (kol'-pō-skōp): An endoscope for viewing the vagina. Biopsy can be taken. —colposcopic, adj.; colposcopically, adv.; colposcopy, n.

colpostenosis (kol-pō-ste-nō'-sis): Constriction or narrowing of the vaginal canal.

colpotomy (kol-pot'-ō-mi): Incision of the

vaginal wall. POSTERIOR C., performed to drain an abscess in the pouch of Douglas through the vagina.

columella (kol-u-mel'-a): A column. Describes the nasal septum and the modiolus (*q.v.*).

column (kol'-um): In anatomy, a structure of the body resembling a column or pillar, *e.g.,* the spinal column.

coma (kō'-ma): Complete loss of consciousness from which the patient cannot be wakened. Seen in poisonings, alcoholism, disease, or injury.

comatose (kōm'-a-tōs): In a state of coma.

combat fatigue: A state of physical and emotional fatigue experienced by soldiers in military combat. Also called combat neurosis and battle neurosis.

comedo (kom'-ē-dō): Blackhead. A worm-like cast formed of sebum which occupies the outlet of a sebaceous gland in the skin. Comedones have a black color because of oxidation; a feature of acne vulgaris. Syn., blackhead.—comedones, pl.

commensal (ko-men'-sal): One of two organisms living in a state of commensalism (*q.v.*). Some commensals are potentially pathogenic.

commensalism (ko-men'-sal-izm): The harmonious living together of two organisms, one of which obtains food, protection or other benefit from the other without either damaging or benefitting the other.

comminuted (kom'-i-nūt-ed): Broken or shattered into a number of small pieces; term often used to denote a shattering fracture of a bone.

commissure (kom'-mi-shur): 1. The point or line of union between two parts, *e.g.,* the angle or corner of the eyelids or lips. 2. A band of nerve fibers that cross from one side of the brain or spinal cord to the other.

commissurotomy (kom-is-shur-ot'-o-mi): Surgical division of a fibrous band or ring. Usually refers to that surrounding the mitral orifice; relieves mitral stenosis.

commitment (ko-mit'-ment): The legal placing of a mentally ill person in an institution that is devoted to the care of such persons.

common cold: See **cold.**

communicable (kom-ūn'-ik-a-b'l): Transmissible directly or indirectly from one person to another.

community mental health center: A facility or network of facilities in a community or neighborhood for the treatment and prevention of mental disorders. The stress is on prevention, but facilities for inpatients, outpatients, and hospital and clinic patients are often included in such a center.

compact (kom-pakt', kom'-pakt): Dense or solid in structure. C. BONE, the hard outer layer of bones, especially the long bones.

compatibility (kom-pat-i-bil'-i-ti): Suitability; congruity. The power of a substance to mix with another without unfavorable results, *e.g.,* two medicines, blood plasma and cells. See **blood groups.**—compatible, adj.

compensation (kom-pen-sā'-shun): 1. A psychic mechanism employed by a person to cover up a weakness by exaggerating a more socially acceptable quality. 2. The state of counterbalancing or making up for a structural or functional defect or deficiency through overgrowth of another organ or increased function of unimpaired parts of the same organ. CARDIAC C., a condition in which adequate circulation is maintained in patients with cardiac disease.

complaint (kom-plānt'): A lay term used to describe a disease, ailment, or group of symptoms.

complement (kom'-ple-ment): A normal constituent of plasma which is of great importance in immunity mechanisms, as it combines with antigen-antibody complex (complement fixation), and this leads to the completion of reactions such as bacteriolysis and the killing of bacteria. Complement is thermolabile and nonspecific and believed to consist of four fractions. C. FIXATION TEST, measures the amount of C. fixed by any given antigen-antibody complex.

complemental (kom-ple-men'-tal): Complementary C. AIR, see **air.**

complementary (kom-ple-men'-ta-ri): Supplying a deficiency.

complement fixation test: See **complement.**

complex (kom'-pleks): A freudian term for a series of emotionally charged ideas, repressed because they conflict with ideas acceptable to the individual, *e.g.,* OEDIPUS C., a syndrome attributed to suppressed sexual desire of a son for his mother; ELECTRA C., of daughter for father. INFERIORITY C., an abnormal feeling of being inferior which causes an individual to behave either timidly or in an assertive, aggressive manner; may stem from organic inferiority, low social status or from an emotional disturbance resulting from not being able to attain one's personal goals. SUPERIORITY C., (1) an exaggerated feeling of being superior; (2) intense striving for superiority as a compensation for supposed inferiority.

complication (kom-pli-kā'-shun): In medicine, a concurrent condition or disease, or an accident or second disease arising in the course of a primary disease and which adds to its severity.

compos mentis (kom´-pos men´-tis): Of sound mind.

compound (kom´-pownd): A substance composed of two or more elements, chemically combined in a definite proportion to form a new substance with new properties. C. FRACTURE, see **fracture.**

comprehension (kom-prē-hen´-shun): Mental grasp of meaning and relationships.

compress (kom´-pres): A pad or folded piece of cloth applied firmly to a part to cover a wound, exert pressure or control hemorrhage, or to relieve pain, swelling or inflammation. May be dry or wet, hot or cold.

compression (kom-presh´-un): The state of being compressed. The act of pressing or squeezing together. CEREBRAL C., arises from any space-occupying, intracranial lesion. DIGITAL C., the pressure is applied by the fingers, usually to an artery to stop bleeding. C. BANDAGE, see **bandage.**

compromise (kom´-pro-mīz): A mental mechanism whereby a conflict (q.v.) is evaded by disguising the repressed wish to make it acceptable in consciousness.

compulsion (kom-pul´-shun): An irresistible urge to engage in some act that the individual knows is irrational, or against his best judgment or his usual standards of behavior. The term is also descriptive of thoughts, fears, and use of words over which the individual has no control.

compulsive (kom-pul´-siv): 1. Having the power of compulsion (q.v.). 2. Pertaining to acts performed under compulsion. C. PERSONALITY, one characterized by an irresistible impulse to perform, under compulsion, acts that have to do with such qualities as orderliness or cleanliness.

conation (kō-nā´-shun): Willing or desiring. The conscious tendency to action. One of the three aspects of mind, the others being cognition (awareness, understanding) and affection (feeling or emotion.)

concatenation (kon-kat´-e-nā-shun): A series of events or objects occurring in sequence or together.

concave (kon-kāv´): Having a somewhat depressed or hollowed out surface like the inner surface of a bowl. Opp. to convex.

concavity (kon-kav´-i-ti): A hollowed out space or depression on the surface of an organ or structure.

conceive (kon-sēv´): 1. To become pregnant. 2. To form a conception of.

concentrate (kon´-sen-trāt): 1. To bring together at a common point. 2. To increase the strength of a substance by condensing it, usually through evaporation of part of its liquid content. 3. A pharmaceutical preparation that has been strengthened by evaporation of some of its nonactive liquid content.

concept (kon´-sept): A mental image resulting from abstracting and recombining certain qualities or characteristics of a number of ideas and forming them into a generalization, or C., e.g., the individual's C. of honor, love, a rose, a house, etc.

conception (kon-sep´-shun): 1. The act of becoming pregnant by the impregnation of an ovum by a spermatozoon. 2. An abstract mental idea of anything.—conceptive, adj.

conceptus (kon-sep´-tus): That which is conceived; a fetus; an embryo.

concha (kong´-ka): In anatomy, a part or structure that resembles a shell in shape, e.g., the hollow part of the external ear or the turbinate bone in the nose.

concoction (kon-kok´-shun): A mixture of two or more substances such as foods or drugs.

concomitant (kon-kom´-i-tant): Occurring at the same time or together.

concrescence (kon-kres´-ens): A growing together or union of parts that are normally separate.

concretion (kon-krē´-shun): A deposit of hard material in the tissues or in a natural cavity of the body; a calculus.

concurrent (kon-kur´-ent): Occurring at the same time or acting together. C. DISINFECTION, the immediate disinfection of infectious discharges from the body of an infected person or of materials that have been contaminated by such discharges or by the patient.

concussion (kon-kush´-un): A condition resulting from a violent jar, blow, or shock. CEREBRAL C., characterized by loss of consciousness, pallor, coldness and usually an increase in the pulse rate. There may be incontinence of urine and feces.

condensation (con-den-sā´-shun): The process of becoming thicker or more dense or compact, or of being concentrated into a smaller volume, e.g., the changing of a gas to a liquid.

conditioning: A process whereby a person learns to modify or adapt his behavior when certain stimuli are applied. OPERANT C., C.

that is the result of rewarding (or punishing) an individual when he responds to a certain stimulus in a particular manner.

condom (kon'-dom): A rubber sheath used by the male as a contraceptive or as protection against venereal infection.

conduction (kon-duk'-shun): The transmission of heat, light, or sound waves through suitable media; also the passage of electrical currents and nerve impulses through body tissues.—conductivity, n.

conductor (kon-duk'-tor): A substance or medium which transmits heat, light, sound, electric current, etc. POOR, GOOD, or NON-CONDUCTOR, designates degree of conductivity.

condyle (kon'-dīl): A rounded, knuckle-like projection at the articular end of a bone.—condylar, adj.

condyloid (kon'-di-loid): Resembling a condyle.

condyloma (kon-di-lō'-ma): Papilloma. Condylomata acuminata are acuminate (pointed) dry warts found under prepuce (male), on the vulva and vestibule (female), or on the skin of the perianal region. They are not necessarily venereal. Condylomata lata are the highly infectious, moist, warty excrescences found in moist areas of the body as a manifestation of late secondary syphilis (vulva, anus, axilla, etc.).—condylomatous, adj.; condylomata, pl.

cone: A solid figure that has a circular base and tapers to a point. In anatomy, usually refers to one of the cone-like bodies found along with the rods in one of the layers of neurons in the retina; together the rods and cones are the receptors for light stimuli.

confabulation (kon-fab-ū-lā'-shun): A symptom common in confusional states when there is impairment of memory for recent events. The gaps in the patient's memory are filled in with fabrications of his own invention. Occurs in senile and toxic confusional states, cerebral trauma and Korsakoff's syndrome (q.v.).

confection (kon-fek'-shun): In pharmacology, a preparation in which drugs are mixed with honey, syrup, or sugar.

confinement (kon-fīn'-ment): Giving birth to a child; lying-in.

conflict (kon'-flikt): In psychiatry, a painful state of consciousness caused by the simultaneous presence of two incompatible contrasting impulses, desires, or tendencies which are of equal or comparable intensity. When the conflict becomes intolerable, repression (q.v.) of one of the wishes may occur. Mental conflict and repression are the basic causes of many neuroses, especially hysteria.

confluent (kon'-floo-ent): Becoming merged; flowing together. In medicine, a uniting as of neighboring pustules, e.g., C. SMALLPOX, a variety in which the pustules coalesce.—confluence, n.

confusion (kon-fū'-zhun): Term used to describe a mental state which is out of touch with reality and associated with clouding of consciousness and impairment of the patient's ability to think, perceive and respond; often accompanied by disorientation as to time, place, and person. May be present following epileptic fits, in cerebral arteriosclerosis, trauma or severe toxemia.

congener (kon'-jen-er): One of two or more substances or things that are allied or akin. In anatomy, term is applied to muscles that have a common action or function. See **synergism.**

congenital (kon-jen'-it-al): Referring to mental or physical conditions that are present at birth, regardless of cause; they are acquired during development in the uterus. To be differentiated from conditions that are hereditary (q.v.). C. DISLOCATION OF THE HIP is due to faulty formation of the acetabulum. C. HEART DISEASE, developmental anomalies of the heart, resulting postnatally in imperfect oxygenation of the blood, manifested by cyanosis and breathlessness. Later there is clubbing of the fingers. See **clubbing, blue baby.** C. SYPHILIS is acquired by the fetus from the mother just after the fourth month of intrauterine life.

congestion (kon-jest'-yun): Hyperemia; abnormal accumulation of blood in a part or an organ. ACTIVE C. is due to increased flow of blood to the part or to dilatation of the vessels. HYPOSTATIC C. occurs in the lowest part of an organ or part; due to gravity and impaired circulation. PASSIVE C. results from slowing down of venous return as in the lower limbs or the lungs.—congest, v.i., v.t.; congestive, adj.

congestive heart failure: A chronic inability of the heart to maintain an adequate output of blood from one or both ventricles resulting in manifest congestion and overdistension of certain veins and organs with blood, and in an inadequate blood supply to the body tissues.

conglutinate (kon-gloo'-ti-nāt): To adhere or stick together as if by a glutinous substance.—conglutination, n.; conglutinant, adj.

Congo red: A coal tar dye which is injected into the blood stream in a test for free acid in the gastric contents or for the presence of amyloid disease.

coniasis (ko-nī′-a-sis): The presence of dust-like particles in the gallbladder or bile ducts.

coniosis (kō-ni-ō′-sis): A pulmonary disease caused by the inhalation of dust. See **pneumoconiosis.**

conization (kon-i-zā′-shun): Removal of a cone-shaped part of the cervix by the knife or cautery.

conjugate (kon′-jū-gāt): 1. Coupled or joined together, especially in pairs. 2. In obstetrics, a measurement of the bony pelvis. DIAGONAL C., the measurement from the lower border of the symphysis pubis to the sacral promontory. OBSTETRICAL C., the available space for the fetal head, *i.e.,* the distance from the sacral promontory to the posterior surface of the top of the symphysis pubis. TRUE C., the distance from the sacral promontory to the summit of the symphysis pubis.

conjunctiva (kon-jungk-tī′-va): The delicate transparent membrane that lines the inner surface of the eyelids and reflects over the exposed anterior surface of the eyeball. —conjunctival, adj.

conjunctivitis (kon-jungk-ti-vī′-tis): Inflammation of the conjunctiva. INCLUSION C. or INCLUSION BLENNORRHEA, caused by a virus; may be transmitted to the infant from the mother's genital tract during birth.

connective tissue: The binding and supportive tissues of the body, the principal varieties of which are (1) areolar, (2) fibrous and (3) elastic. Adipose and lymphoid tissue, bone and cartilage belong to the same group of bodily structures.

consanguinity (kon-san-gwin′-i-ti): Blood relationship.—consanguineous, adj.

conscious (kon′-shus): 1. Being aware; capable of voluntary perception in response to stimuli and of having subjective experiences. 2. Refers to all mental phenomena of which one is aware. 3. Being awake and in full possession of one's mental faculties.

consciousness (kon′-shus-nes): 1. Being conscious (*q.v.*). 2. Awareness of one's psychic experiences and perceptions that result from sensory stimuli. 3. The total of one's perceptions, ideas, sensations and emotions that one is aware of at any given time. 4. In psychoanalysis, that part of

one's psychic or mental life of which one is aware and that is accessible to others through verbal report or by inference from one's behavior.

conservative (kon-serv′-a-tiv): Descriptive of a treatment aimed at preserving health or restoring diseased or injured parts to normal, as opposed to radical or heroic treatment measures.

consolidation (kon-sol-i-dā′-shun): Becoming solid, as, for instance, the state of the lung due to exudation and organization in pneumonia.

constipation (kon-sti-pā′-shun): An implied chronic condition of infrequent and often difficult evacuation of feces due to insufficient food or fluid intake, or to sluggish or disordered action of the bowel musculature or nerve supply, or to habitual failure to empty the rectum. Acute constipation signifies obstruction or paralysis of the gut; of sudden onset.

constitution (kon-sti-tū′-shun): The makeup of the body as a whole.—constitutional, adj.

constitutional type: Bodily makeup. See **Kretschmer's personality types.**

consultation (kon-sul-tā′-shun): A discussion by two or more physicians concerning the specific aspects of a pathological condition in a particular patient.

consumption (kon-sump′-shun): 1. The act of consuming or using up. 2. A wasting of body tissues; in this sense, the term was formerly much used for pulmonary tuberculosis (which 'consumed' the body).—consumptive, adj.

contact (kon′-takt): 1. Direct or indirect exposure to infection. 2. A person who has been so exposed. C. DERMATITIS, a type of eczema due to irritants, friction, sensitivity. C. LENS, of glass or plastic, worn under the eyelids in direct contact with conjunctiva (in place of spectacles) for therapeutic or cosmetic purposes.

contactant (kon-tak′-tant): A substance that may come into contact with the skin; often refers to an allergen (*q.v.*) or other substance that may cause contact dermatitis.

contagion (kon-tā′-jun): 1. Communication of disease from person to person. 2. A contagious disease. 3. The living organism by which a disease is transferred from person to person.—contagious, adj.; contagiousness, n.

contagious (kon-tā′-jus): 1. Capable of transmission from one person to another, by direct or indirect contact. 2. Highly communicable, referring to a disease that is easily transmitted from one person to another.

contaminant (kon-tam′-i-nant): A substance or object that contaminates (*q.v.*).

contaminate (kon-tam′-i-nāt): 1. To soil or infect with extraneous matter, particularly pathogenic bacteria. 2. To render unfit for human use by pollution with unhealthful or disease-producing elements, *e.g.,* pollution of drinking water.—contamination, n.

continence (kon′-ti-nens): 1. Self-restraint; refusal to yield to an impulse or desire, *e.g.,* voluntary refrainment from sexual intercourse. 2. The ability to retain a bodily discharge until the conditions are proper for evacuation, *e.g.,* urine or feces.

continent (kon′-ti-nent): In medicine, the state of being able to control such normal bodily functions as defecation or urination until conditions are proper for carrying them out.

contra-: Denotes against, opposed.

contraception (kon-tra-sep′-shun): The voluntary and artificial prevention of conception or impregnation.

contraceptive (kon-tra-sep′-tiv): An agent used to prevent conception, *e.g.,* condom, spermaticidal vaginal cream, soft diaphragm to cover the mouth of the uterus, intrauterine contraceptive device (IUD), pills that are taken orally.—contraception, n.

contract (kon-trakt′, kon′-trakt): 1. Draw together; shorten; decrease in size. 2. Acquire by contagion or infection.

contractile (kon-trak′-til): Possessing the ability to shorten—usually when stimulated.—contractility, n., special property of muscle tissue.

contraction (kon-trak′-shun): Shortening, especially applied to muscle fibers.

contracture (kon-trak′-chur): Permanent shortening of muscle or scar tissue, producing deformity. DUPUYTREN′S C., painless, chronic flexion of the digits, especially the third and fourth, toward the palm: etiology uncertain. [Guillaume Dupuytren, French surgeon. 1777-1835.] See **Volkmann.**

contraindication (kon-tra-in-di-kā′-shun): A sign, symptom, or condition suggesting that a certain line of treatment (usually used for that disease) should be discontinued or avoided.

contralateral (kon-tra-lat′-er-al): Pertaining to, located on, or occurring in or on the opposite side.—contralaterally, adv.

contrast medium: A substance that is radiopaque (*q.v.*).

contrecoup (kon′-tr-koo): Injury or damage at a point opposite the impact, resulting from transmitted force. More likely to occur in an organ or part containing fluid, as the skull.

contusion (kon-tū′-zhun): A bruise; slight bleeding into tissues while the skin remains unbroken.—contuse, v.t.

convalescence (kon-va-les′-ens): The period of recovery following an illness, operation, or accident.—convalescent, adj. and n.

convalescent serum: Blood serum of a patient recently recovered from a specific disease which is sometimes given by injection to another person to prevent the occurrence of the disease.

convection (kon-vek′-shun): Transfer of heat from the hotter to the colder part; the heated substance (air or fluid), being less dense, tends to rise. The colder portion, flowing in to be heated, rises in its turn, thus c. currents are set in motion.

conversion (kon-ver′-zhun): 1. An unconscious defense mechanism in which psychological conflict is manifested as a physical symptom. 2. Correction of the position of a fetus, or part of it, during labor.

convex (kon-veks′): Having an evenly rounded external surface that bulges outward. Opp. to concave (*q.v.*).

convolutions (kon-vō-loo′-shunz): Folds, twists or coils as found in the intestine, renal tubules and surface of brain.—convoluted, adj.

convulsant (kon-vul′-sant): An agent that causes convulsions.

convulsion (kon-vul′-shun): Violent involuntary contraction of voluntary muscles resulting from abnormal cerebral stimulation from many causes. Occurs with or without loss of consciousness. CLONIC C., alternating contraction and relaxation of muscle groups. TONIC C., sustained rigidity.—convulsive, adj. Also fit, seizure.

convulsive (kon-vul′-siv): Related to, producing, or characterized by convulsions. C. DISORDER, any condition characterized by convulsions, particularly the various types of epilepsy. C. THERAPY, one of the physical methods of treatment for mental disorders, notably depressive states, mania, stupor; before introduction of electroshock therapy, drugs were widely used to produce the convulsions that are basic to this kind of therapy. Also known as electroplexy, electrotherapy, electroconvulsive therapy. See **insulin shock.**

Cooley's anemia: Thalassemia (*q.v.*). [Thomas Benton Cooley, American pediatrician. 1871-1945.]

Coombs' test: DIRECT C. TEST, used in early diagnosis of erythroblastosis fetalis and in crossmatching blood for high-risk recipients. INDIRECT C. TEST, used to detect various minor blood type factors, including the Rh factor.

coordination (kō-war-din-ā′-shun): Moving or functioning in harmony. MUSCULAR C., the harmonious action of muscles, permitting free, smooth and efficient movements under perfect control.

co-ossify (kō-os′-i-fī): To grow or become joined together by ossification (*q.v.*).

cootie (koo′-ti): The body louse (slang).

copiopia (kōp-i-ō′-pi-a): Eyestrain; asthenopia (*q.v.*).

copper: Present in traces in all animal tissues. Copper salts have little use in medicine except the sulphate. This is used occasionally as an astringent lotion, and in phosphorus poisoning. Copper sulphate is also used in Benedict's and Fehling's solutions for testing urine for glucose.

copr-, copra-, copro-: Denotes feces, dung, filth.

copracrasia (kop-ra-krā′-si-a): Lack or loss of ability to control the discharge of feces.

copremesis (kop-rem′-e-sis): The vomiting of material containing feces.

coprolalia (kop-rō-lā′-li-a): The use of filthy speech, especially of words relating to feces; occurs as a symptom in mentally disordered persons, most commonly in those suffering from cerebral deterioration or trauma affecting the frontal lobes of the brain.

coprolith (kop′-rō-lith): A stony concretion or hard mass of fecal material in the intestine.

coprophagy (kop-rof′-a-ji): The eating of dung or feces; in man, a symptom of severe neurosis.

coprophilia (kop-rō-fil′-i-a): An abnormal interest in filth, especially feces.

coproporhyrin (kop-rō-por′-fir-in): Naturally occurring porphyrin in the feces; formed by bilirubin. Also found in the urine of patients with coproporphyrinuria, a metabolic disorder.

coprostasis (kop-ros′-ta-sis): Fecal impaction in the intestine. Also coprostasia.

coprozoic (kop-rō-zō′-ik): Found in or living in feces.

copulation (kop-u-lā′-shun): Sexual intercourse.

cor (kor): The muscular organ that keeps the blood circulating in the body; the heart. COR PULMONALE, pulmonary heart disease, following disease of the lung (emphysema, silicosis, etc.) which strains the right ventricle.

coracoid (kor′-a-koid): 1. Beak-shaped. 2. Denoting a process of the scapula.

cord: A long, rounded, flexible, thread-like structure. SPERMATIC C., that which suspends the testes in the scrotum. SPINAL C., a cord-like structure which lies in the spinal column, reaching from the foramen magnum to the first or second lumbar vertebra. It is a direct continuation of the medulla oblongata and is about 18 in. long in the adult. UMBILICAL C., the navel-string, attaching the fetus to the placenta; gives passage to the umbilical vein and arteries; it is about two feet long and ½ inch in diameter. VOCAL CORDS, membranous bands in the larynx, the vibrations of which are responsible for the production of voice.

cordate (kor′-dāt): Heart-shaped.

cordial (kord′-yal): 1. An invigorating preparation used for its stimulating effect on the heart and circulation. 2. An alcoholic preparation with a pleasant taste, used for its stimulating effect on the digestion.

cordotomy (kor-dot′-om-i): See **chordotomy.**

core: Central portion, usually applied to the mass of necrotic material in the center of a boil.

corediastasis (kō-rē-dī-as′-ta-sis): Dilatation of the pupil or a state of dilatation of the pupil of the eye.

corium (kō′-ri-um): The internal layer of the skin lying immediately beneath the epidermis, composed of a dense bed of connective tissue with many blood vessels. The dermis; true skin; cutis.

corn: A cone-shaped overgrowth and hardening of epidermis, with the point of the cone in the deeper layers, as on a toe; produced by friction or pressure. HARD C. usually occurs over a toe joint. SOFT C. occurs between the toes. Lay term for clavus.

cornea (kor′-nē-a): The outwardly convex transparent membrane forming part of the anterior outer coat of the eye. It covers the iris and the pupil and admits light. It occupies about one-sixth of the circumference of the eyeball and merges backwards into the sclera.—corneal, adj.

corneal graft (kor′-nē-al): The replacement of opaque corneal tissue with healthy, transparent human cornea from a donor. Corneal transplant; keratoplasty.

corneoplasty (kor′-nē-ō-plas-ti): Syn., keratoplasty. See **corneal graft.**

corneoscleral (kor′-nē-o-sklē′-ral): Pertaining to the cornea and sclera, as the circular junction of these structures.

corneum (kor′-nē-um): The horny outer layer of the skin; the stratum corneum.

cornu (kor′-nū): Any horn-shaped structure.—cornual, adj.; cornua, pl.

corona (kor-ō′-na): A crown; any structure resembling a crown. C. DENTIS, the crown of a tooth.—coronal, adj.

coronal suture (kor-ō′-nal sū′-chur): The tranverse line of union between the frontal and parietal bones in the skull.

coronary (kor′-o-nar-i): Crown-like; encircling in the manner of a crown; said of a blood vessel or nerve that encircles a part or organ. C. ARTERIES, those supplying the heart, the first pair to be given off by the aorta as it leaves the left ventricle. Spasm or narrowing of these vessels produces angina pectoris. C. OCCLUSION, stoppage of flow through the coronary arteries by an obstruction. C. SINUS, the channel receiving most cardiac veins and opening into the right atrium. C. THROMBOSIS, occlusion of a coronary vessel by a clot of blood.

coronary care unit: A specially equipped and staffed area in a hospital that provides concentrated, specialized care for the treatment of patients who have suffered a coronary (*q.v.*) thrombosis.

coroner (kor′-o-ner): A public official whose main duty is to hold inquests, in the presence of a jury, in cases of sudden, violent, or unexplained deaths.

coronoid (kor′-o-noid): Crown-like, *e.g.,* C. process of ulna and mandible.

corporeal (kor-po-rē′-al): Pertaining to the physical, material body; not spiritual.

corpse (korps): A dead body. Cadaver.

corpulence (kor′-pū-lens): Obesity; fatness. —corpulent, n. Also corpulency.

corpus (kor′-pus): 1. A discrete mass of material, *e.g.,* specialized tissue. 2. The body of an animal or man, especially a dead body. 3. The main part of an organ or structure. C. CALLOSUM, a band of white nerve fibers passing beneath the longitudinal fissure and connecting the two cerebral hemispheres. C. LUTEUM, the yellow body formed in the ovary after rupture of a graafian follicle; it secretes progesterone and persists and en-

larges if pregnancy supervenes. The false C.L. is formed in the nonpregnant state and persists for approximately one month, when it is reabsorbed. The true C.L. occurs in pregnancy, persists for 6 months, and has almost disappeared by the end of the 9th month. C. STRIATUM, a stalk-like arrangement of gray and white matter at the base of the brain, thought to have a steadying effect on voluntary movement, but no power of initiation of same.—corpora, pl.

corpuscle (kor′-pus′l): A microscopic mass of protoplasm. There are many varieties but the term generally refers to the red and white blood cells. See **erythrocytes** and **leucocytes.**—corpuscular, adj.

corrective (ko-rek′-tiv): 1. Changes, counteracts or modifies something harmful. 2. A drug that modifies the action of another drug.

Corrigan's pulse: See **pulse.**

corrosion (ko-rō′-zhun): The slow wearing away or destruction of a part or tissue.

corrosive (ko-rō′-siv): 1. A caustic; a substance that weakens or destroys the surface or substance of a tissue or other material. 2. Having the power to weaken or destroy the surface or substance of tissue or other material.

cortex (kor′-teks): 1. The outer bark or covering of a plant. 2. The outer layer of an organ beneath its capsule or membrane.— cortices, pl.; cortical, adj.

Corti: ORGAN OF C., the elongated spiral structure lying on the basilar membrane of the cochlea and containing the hair cells where the fibers of the auditory nerve begin; the actual receptor for hearing. [Alfonso Corti, Italian anatomist. 1822-1888.]

corticifugal (kor-ti-sif′-ū-gal): Moving or conducting away from the cortex; said particularly of nerve fibers. Also corticofugal.

corticoid (kor′-ti-koid): A name for the several groups of steroid substances produced by the adrenal cortex and for synthetic compounds with similar actions. Examples of the three main groups are: hydrocortisone, cortisone, prednisolone and prednisone in the first, deoxycortone acetate (DCA or DOCA) in the second, and the sex hormones in the third.

corticospinal (kor-ti-kō-spī′-nal): Pertaining to the cortex of the brain and the spinal cord.

corticosteroids (kor-ti-kō-stěr′-oids): Steroid substances produced in the adrenal cortex, some of which are hormones; corticoids.

corticosterone (kor-ti-kō-stēr′-ōn): A secretion of the adrenal cortex; influences carbohydrate metabolism.

corticotropin (kor-ti-kō-trō′-pin): The hormone of the anterior pituitary gland which specifically stimulates the adrenal cortex to produce corticoids. Available commercially as a purified extract of animal anterior pituitary glands (ACTH). Only active by injection. Also corticotrophin.

cortisone (kor′-ti-sōn): One of the principal hormones of the adrenal gland. Converted into cortisol before use by the body. It has powerful anti-inflammatory properties, and is used in ophthalmic conditions, rheumatoid arthritis, pemphigus and Addison's disease. Side-effects, such as salt and water retention, may limit therapy, and newer derivatives are now preferred for some conditions.

Corynebacterium (kor-ī′-nē-bak-tēr′-i-um): A bacterial genus: gram-positive, rod-shaped bacteria, averaging 3 microns in length, showing irregular staining in segments (metachromatic granules). Many strains are parasitic; some are pathogenic, *e.g., C. diphtheriae,* which produces a powerful exotoxin.

coryza (kō-rī′-za): An acute upper respiratory infection of short duration, due to a filterable virus; highly contagious; attacks produce only temporary immunity.

cosmetic (koz-met′-ic): 1. Relating to that which is done to improve the appearance or prevent disfigurement. 2. A preparation used to improve the appearance.

cost-, costi-, costo-: Denotes rib(s).

costa (kos′-ta): A rib.—costae, pl.; costal, adj.

costectomy (kos-tek′-to-mi): Surgical removal of one or more ribs.

costicartilage (kos-ti-kar′-ti-lij): The cartilage of a rib.

costive (kos′-tiv): 1. Pertaining to or producing constipation. 2. An agent that slows intestinal motility.

costoclavicular (kos-tō-kla-vik′-ūl-ar): Pertaining to the ribs and the clavicle. C. SYNDROME, syn. for cervical rib syndrome. See **cervical.**

costotomy (kos-tot′-o-mi): Excision of all or part of a rib.

cot: FINGER C., a rubber or plastic covering for the finger; used when examining a body passage as the rectum or vagina, or as a protective covering over a bandage. Also finger stall.

cotyledon (kot-il-ē′-don): One of the subdivisions of the uterine surface of the placenta.

cotyloid (kot′-i-loid): Cup-shaped; pertaining to the acetabular cavity.

cough (kawf): A sudden forcible noisy expulsion of air from the lungs in an effort to expel mucus or other extraneous matter from the air passages.

counter-: Denotes: (1) contrary, opposite, adverse; (2) complementary, corresponding, alternate.

counterextension (kown-ter-eks-ten′-shun): Traction upon the proximal extremity of a fractured limb opposing the pull of the extension apparatus on the distal extremity.

counterirritant (kown-ter-ir′-it-ant): An agent, which, when applied to the skin, produces an inflammatory reaction (hyperemia) relieving congestion in underlying organs.—counterirritation, n.

counterstain: A second stain of a different color applied to a smear to make the organisms that are to be viewed microscopically more distinct.

Cowper's glands (kow′-perz): Bulbourethral glands. Two in number, lying lateral to the membranous urethra, below the prostate gland, and deep to the perineal membrane. They open via short ducts into the anterior (penile) urethra. [William Cowper, English surgeon. 1666-1709.]

cowpox: Vaccinia. Virus disease of cows. Lymph is used in vaccination of humans against smallpox (variola).

coxa (kok′-sa): The hip joint.—coxae, pl. C. VALGA, an increase in the normal angle between neck and shaft of femur. C. VARA, a decrease in the normal angle between the neck and shaft of the femur.

coxalgia (kok-sal′-ji-a): Literally, pain in the hip joint. Often used as syn. for hip joint disease.

coxitis (kok-sī′-tis): Inflammation of the hip joint.

coxodynia (kok-sō-din′-i-a): Coxalgia (*q.v.*).

coxotuberculosis (kok-sō-tū-ber-cū-lō′-sis): Tuberculosis of the hip joint.

Coxsackie viruses: First isolated at Coxsackie, N.Y. A heterogeneous group of related but serologically distinct viruses that apparently are related to the poliomyelitis virus and which in man produce a disease that resembles poliomyelitis but without paralysis. Divided into two main groups, A and B. Said to produce such conditions as aseptic meningitis, herpangina, epidemic pleurodynia, encephalitis, and an influenza-like fever.

crab louse (krab lows): Pediculus pubis (*q.v.*).

cradle: A frame, usually of wood or wire, used to keep the bed clothes from contact with an injured or fractured limb; also used when dry heat is being applied to an extremity. C. CAP, an accumulation of grayish-yellow crust-like material on the crown of the scalp of an infant with eczema or one who is not shampooed regularly.

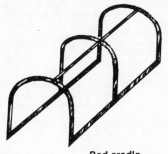

Bed cradle

cramp: Spasmodic, involuntary, painful contraction of a muscle or group of muscles. Occurs in tetany, food poisoning and cholera. In gynecology, a colloquial term for dysmenorrhea. HEAT C., muscular spasm attended by weak pulse, dilated pupils and prostration, seen in those who work in intense heat and who lose much salt and water through perspiration, *e.g.,* stokers, miners. WRITER'S C., an occupational disease characterized by spasmodic contraction of muscles of fingers, hand and forearm; a similar condition occurs in others whose occupations involve use of fine muscles.

crani-, cranio-: Denotes skull.

cranial (krā'-ni-al): Pertaining to the cranium (*q.v.*). C. DECOMPRESSION, reduction of excessive pressure on the brain by means of surgery. C. FOSSA, any one of the three shallow depressions on the upper surface of the base of the skull. C. NERVE, any one of the twelve pairs of nerves given off by the brain rather than the spinal cord; they are named and numbered in the following order: 1, olfactory; 2, optic; 3, oculomotor; 4, trochlear; 5, trigeminal; 6, abducent; 7, facial; 8, acoustic; 9, glos-

sopharyngeal; 10, vagus; 11, accessory; 12, hypoglossal.

craniectomy (krā-ni-ek'-to-mi): Surgical removal of a portion of skull.

craniocele (krā'-ni-ō-sēl): Protrusion of part of the cranial contents through a defect in the bones of the cranium.

craniofacial (krā-ni-ō-fāsh'-al): Pertaining to the cranium and the face.

craniofenestria (krā-ni-ō-fen-es'-tri-a): A condition in which there is defective development of the bones of the cranium; in some areas no bone whatever is formed.

craniometry (krā-ni-om'-e-tri): The science that deals with the measurement of skulls.

cranioplasty (krā'-ni-ō-plas-ti): Operative repair of a skull defect.—cranioplastic, adj.

craniosacral (krā-ni-ō-sā'-kral): Pertaining to the skull and sacrum. Applied to the parasympathetic nervous system.

craniostenosis (krā-ni-ō-stē-nō'-sis): Premature fusion of the cranial sutures with consequent cessation of growth, resulting in deformity and a small skull.

craniotabes (krā-ni-ō-tā'-bēz): A softening and wasting of the cranial bones and widening of the sutures and fontanels occurring in infancy, due to lack of normal mineralization of the bones. Can occur in syphilis, rickets and marasmus.—craniotabetic, adj.

craniotome (krā'-ni-ō-tōm): An instrument used in performing craniotomy (*q.v.*); it is operated by a high-speed drill powered by compressed air.

craniotomy (krā-ni-ot'-o-mi): A surgical opening of the skull in order to remove a growth, relieve pressure, evacuate blood clot, arrest hemorrhage, or to reduce the size of the head of an unborn dead infant to facilitate its delivery. See **leukotomy.**

cranium (krā'-ni-um): The part of the skull enclosing the brain. It is composed of eight bones: the occipital, two parietals, frontal, two temporals, sphenoid and ethmoid.—cranial, adj.

creatine (krē'-a-tin): A protein derivative found in muscle. The serum C. is raised in hyperthyroidism, values above 0.6 mg per 100 ml of blood being suggestive.

creatine test: See **creatine.**

creatinine (krē-at'-in-in): A waste product of protein (endogenous) metabolism found in muscle, blood and urine. Probably derived from creatine of muscle.

creatinuria (krē-at-in-ū'-ri-a): Increased or abnormal amounts of creatinine in the urine. Occurs in metabolic disorders and conditions in which muscle is rapidly broken down, *e.g.,* acute fevers, starvation.—creatinuric, adj.

Credé's method (kre-dāz'): 1. A method of delivering the placenta by gently rubbing the fundus uteri until it contracts, and then, by squeezing the fundus, expressing the placenta into the vagina from whence it is expelled. 2. The placing of one drop of 1 or 2 percent silver nitrate in each eye of a newborn child to prevent ophthalmia neonatorum (*q.v.*). [Karl Sigmund Franz Credé, German obstetrician. 1819-1892.]

cremation (krē-mā'-shun): The burning or incineration of the body of a deceased person.

crenate (krē'-nāt): Scalloped, indented or notched. In physiology, descriptive of the indented edges of red blood cells that have shrunken from exposure to air or to a hypertonic solution. Also crenated.

crenation (kre-nā'-shun): The process of becoming crenate (*q.v.*).

creosote (krē'-ō-sōt): Colorless to yellowish oily liquid obtained from wood tar; used in expectorants.

crepitant (krep'-i-tant): Pertaining to, having, or producing a crackling sound.

crepitation (krep-i-tā'-shun): 1. Grating of bone ends in fracture. Also crepitus. 2. Crackling sound heard via stethoscope in lung infections. 3. Crackling sound elicited by pressure on emphysematous tissue.

cresol (krē'-sol): Colorless to brownish aromatic liquid obtained from wood tar; disinfectant. Lysol is a proprietary name for a compound solution of C.

crest: A projection or ridge, especially at the border of a bone.

cretin (krē'-tin): A person affected with cretinism (*q.v.*).

cretinism (krē'tin-ism): A condition originating in fetal life or early infancy; due to congenital thyroid deficiency; characterized by stunted mental and physical development, dwarfism, large head, thick legs, pug nose, dry skin, scanty hair, swollen eyelids, short neck, protruding abdomen, clumsy uncoordinated gait.—cretin, n.; cretinistic, cretinoid, cretinous, adj.

crib death: Death of an infant who has presented no symptoms of illness; occurs usually during first four or five months of life; sometimes thought to result from a sudden overwhelming infection.

cribriform (krib'-ri-form): Perforated, like a sieve. C. PLATE, that portion of ethmoid bone that forms the roof of the nasal cavity; has many perforations for the passage of fibers of the olfactory nerve.

cricoid (krī'-koid): Ring-shaped. Applied to the cartilage forming the inferior posterior part of larynx.

crisis (krī'-sis): 1. The turning point of a disease—as the point of defervescence in fever. 2. Muscular spasm in tabes dorsalis referred to as visceral crisis (gastric, vesical, rectal, etc.). See **Dietl's crisis.** CHOLINERGIC C., respiratory failure resulting from overtreatment with anticholinesterase drugs. MYASTHENIC C., sudden deterioration with weakness of respiratory muscles due to an increase in severity of myasthenia. OCULOGYRIC C., see **oculogyric.** THYROTOXIC C., sudden return of symptoms of thyrotoxicosis, due to shock, injury or thyroidectomy.

crisis intervention: A term used to describe a brief type of treatment in which a psychotherapist or a team intervenes in a situation in order to assist the family and the patient to secure help in solving an immediate problem; may include medications, referral to a community agency, changing the patient's environment, etc.

crista galli (kris'-ta gal'-lī): Superior triangular portion of ethmoid bone. Likened to a cock's comb.

Crohn's disease: Syn., regional ileitis (*q.v.*). [Burrill Bernard Crohn, American gastroenterologist. 1884- .]

cross-eye: Convergent strabismus (*q.v.*). A squint in which one or both eyes turn inward toward the nose.—cross-eyed, adj.

cross infection: A second infection superimposed upon another infectious disease from which the patient is suffering.

crossmatching: A test for determining the compatibility of bloods before transfusion. See **blood types, blood crossmatching.**

cross section: A cut or slice made through an object at right angles to the long axis.

crotch (krotch): The angle formed by the parting of two leg-like parts or branches. In anatomy, the angle formed by the inner side of the thigh and the trunk.

croup (kroop): A condition resulting from acute spasmodic laryngitis, occurring in infants and children, most often at night; characterized by harsh, brassy cough, crowing inspirations, dyspnea, and with or without membrane formation. Croupy breathing in a child is often called 'stridulous,' meaning noisy or harsh-sounding. Narrowing of the airway gives rise to the typical attack with crowing inspiration; may result from edema, allergy, inflammation of the larynx, spasm. C. KETTLE, a kettle for producing steam or medicated vapor which is either directed into a C. tent or allowed to escape into the air to humidify it; used in croup and bronchial conditions. C. TENT, a covering for the head and shoulders into which a stream of steam or medicated vapor is directed; used to relieve croup and some other respiratory conditions.

crown: The highest or topmost part of anything. In anatomy, the topmost part of an organ or structure, *e.g.,* the top of the head.

crucial (kroo′-shal): 1. Cross-shaped. 2. Severe; essential, as being decisive.

cruciate (kroo′-shi-āt): Shaped like a cross.

crural (kroor′-al): 1. Pertaining to the leg. 2. Leg-like.

crus (kroos): 1. The leg from the knee to the foot. 2. A term applied to various parts of the body which resemble a leg or root.— crural, adj.; crura, pl.

crush injury: An injury in which the physical force caused by crushing, pressure, or by blast is transmitted to the soft tissues, bones or viscera. See **crush syndrome.**

crush syndrome: Traumatic uremia. A condition resulting from damage to the renal tubules because their blood supply has been interfered with. Following an extensive trauma to muscle, there is a period of delay before the effects of renal damage manifest themselves. There is an increase of nonprotein nitrogen of the blood, with oliguria, proteinuria and urinary excretion of myohemoglobin. Loss of blood plasma to damaged area is marked. Symptoms include thirst, nausea, somnolence, hypertension, features of severe shock, pulmonary edema, and cardiac involvement.

crust: A hardened covering formed on a lesion on the surface of the skin from the accumulation of dried serum and other debris. A scab.

crutch: A staff to support and aid the disabled in walking; it is long enough to reach from the armpit to the ground, has a concave crosspiece to fit the armpit and a crossbar for the hand. C. PALSY, paralysis of extensor muscles of wrist, fingers and thumb from repeated pressure of a crutch upon the radial nerve in the axilla.

cryalgesia (krī-al-jē′-zi-a): Pain resulting from the application of cold.

cryanesthesia (krī-an-es-thē′-zi-a): Loss of sensation or perception for cold.

cry-, cryo-: Denotes cold, freezing.

crym-, crymo-: Denotes cold, frost.

crymodynia (krī-mō-din′-i-a): Rheumatic pain brought on by damp or cold weather.

crymotherapy (krī-mō-ther′-a-pi): Cryotherapy (*q.v.*).

cryobiology (krī-ō-bī-ol′-o-ji): The branch of biology that deals with the effects of low temperatures, or freezing, on living tissues.

cryocautery (krī-ō-kaw′-ter-i): The destruction of living tissue by the application of extreme cold, *e.g.,* carbon dioxide snow.

cryogenic (krī-ō-jen′-ik): 1. Pertaining to or causing low temperatures. 2. Describing any means or apparatus involved in the production of low temperatures.

cryopexy (krī-ō-pek′-si): Surgical fixation with freezing, as replacement of a detached retina.

cryoprobe (krī′-ō-prōb): An instrument used for freezing tissue. Can be used for biopsy; causes little tissue damage and seeding of malignant cells. Also used in surgical treatment of conditions in various areas of the body, *e.g.,* brain, eye, prostate gland; the cells die and then may be removed surgically or by the body's own waste removal system.

cryosurgery (krī-ō-sur′-jer-i): The destruction of tissue by the application of extreme cold, *e.g.,* the destruction of an area in the thalamus for treatment of parkinsonism, or the treatment with cold of malignant tumors of the skin. Also chryosurgery, crymosurgery.

cryothalamectomy (krī-ō-thal-a-mek′-to-mi): The destruction of part of the thalamus by cold, done to relieve the tremor and rigidity of Parkinson's disease and other hyperkinetic conditions.

cryotherapy (krī-ō-ther′-a-pi): Therapeutic use of cold, either local or general.

crypt (kript): In anatomy, a small sac, follicle or tube-like depression opening on a free surface of an organ or of the body.

crypt-, crypto-: Denotes: (1) hidden, covered, invisible; (2) latent.

Cryptococcus (krip-tō-kok′-us): A genus of fungi. C. NEOFORMANS is pathogenic to man. It has a marked predilection for the central nervous system causing subacute or chronic disease. It may also affect the skin, lungs, liver, spleen or joints.

cryptogenic (krip′-tō-jen′-ik): Of unknown or obscure cause.

cryptomenorrhea (krip′-tō-men-o-rē-a): Retention of the menses, due to a congenital obstruction such as an imperforate hymen or atresia of the vagina. Syn., hematocolpos.

cryptorchism (krip-tor′-kizm): A developmental defect whereby the testes do not descend into the scrotum; they are retained within the abdomen or inguinal canal.— cryptorchid, cryptorchis, n.

crystallin (kris'-ta-lin): A globulin; principal constituent of the lens of the eye.

crystalline (kris'-ta-līn): Like a crystal; transparent. Applied to various structures. C. LENS, a biconvex body, oval in shape, which is suspended just behind the pupil and the iris of the eye, and separates the aqueous from the vitreous humor. It is slightly less convex on its anterior surface and it refracts the light rays so that they focus directly on the retina.

crystalluria (kris-tal-lū'ri-a): Excretion of crystals in the urine.—crystalluric, adj.

CSF: Abbreviation for cerebrospinal fluid.

cubic centimeter (kū-bik sen'-ti-mē-ter): 1. A mass of material that, in cube form, measures 1 centimeter on each side. Abbreviated cu cm or cc. 2. In liquid capacity it is equal to one one-thousandth of a liter or 0.27 fluidrams; called milliliter and abbreviated ml.

cubitus (kū'-bi-tus): 1. The forearm. 2. The bend between the arm and the forearm. —cubital, adj.

cuboid (kū'-boid): Shaped like a cube; one of the tarsal bones.

cu cm: Abbreviation for cubic centimeter.

cuirass (kwir-as'): 1. A covering, bandage or cast for the chest. 2. A mechanical apparatus fitted to the chest for artificial respiration.

cul-de-sac (kul'-de-sak): A blind pouch or a cavity closed at one end. C. OF DOUGLAS, see **Douglas' pouch.**

culdoscope (kul'-dō-skōp): An endoscope used via the vaginal route.

culdoscopy (kul-dos'-kō-pi): Passage of a culdoscope through the posterior vaginal fornix, behind the uterus to enter the peritoneal cavity, for viewing same.—culdoscopic, adj.; culdoscopically, adv. A form of peritoneoscopy, laparoscopy.

-cule: Denotes small.

Culex (kū'-leks): A genus of mosquitoes that act as vectors of certain diseases. *C. fatigans* or *quinquefasciatus* is the most common vector of *Wuchereria bancrofti*, a species of filaria found in warm regions throughout the world.

Culicidae (kū-lis'-i-de): The Diptera family of insects which includes the mosquitoes.

culicide (kū'-li-sīd): An agent that destroys gnats and mosquitoes.—culicidal, adj.

Cullen's sign: A discoloration of the skin about the umbilicus; may be indicative of a ruptured extrauterine pregnancy; also sometimes seen in acute pancreatitis.

culture (kul'-chur): 1. The development of microorganisms on artificial media under ideal conditions for growth. 2. A growth of microorganisms on a culture medium. 3. The act of cultivating microorganisms on an artificial medium.

cu mm: Abbreviation for cubic millimeter.

cumulative action (kū'-mū-lā-tiv): If the dose of a slowly excreted drug is repeated too frequently, an increasing action is obtained. This can be dangerous as, if the drug accumulates in the system, toxic symptoms may occur, sometimes quite suddenly. Long acting barbiturates, thyroid extract, strychnine, mercurial salts and digitalis are examples of drugs with a cumulative action.

cuneiform (kū-nē'-i-form): 1. Wedge-shaped. 2. Any one of the three small wedge-shaped bones of the tarsus, or the pyramidal bone of the wrist.

cunnus (kun'-us): The female genitalia; the vulva.

cupping (kup'ing): A method of counter-irritation. A small, bell-shaped glass (in which the air is expanded by heating, or exhausted by compression of an attached rubber bulb) is applied to the skin, resultant suction producing hyperemia—dry C. When the skin is scarified before application of the cup it is termed 'wet C.'

curative (kūr'-a-tiv): Having a tendency to heal or cure; related to or useful in curing of diseases.

cure (kūr): 1. To heal or restore to health. 2. A restoration to health. 3. A system or special course of treatment. 4. A medicine or agent used in treating a disease.

curet, curette (kū-ret'): 1. A spoon-shaped instrument or metal loop for scraping the walls of a cavity or other surface (curetting) to remove growths or other abnormal or diseased tissue. 2. To remove growths or other abnormal tissue from a surface such as bone or from the walls of a cavity, as the uterus, by scraping with a spoon-shaped instrument.

curettage (kū-re-tazh'): The scraping of unhealthy or exuberant tissue from a cavity or from a surface such as bone. This may be treatment or may be done to establish a diagnosis.

curettings (kū-ret'-ingz): The material obtained by scraping or curetting and usually sent for examination in the pathology department.

curie (kū'-rē): A unit of radioactivity. [Marie Curie, Polish-born French chemist; discoverer, with Pierre Curie, of radium. 1867-1934.]

curietherapy (kū-rē-ther′-a-pi): Radium therapy.

curvature of the spine: An abnormal curve in the spinal column; may be to the front (lordosis), to the back (kyphosis) or to the side (scoliosis).

Cushing's disease: A rare disorder, mainly of females, characterized principally by virilism, obesity of trunk and face, hyperglycemia, glycosuria, and hypertension. Due to intrinsic and excessive hormone stimulation of the adrenal cortex by tumor or by hyperplasia of the anterior pituitary gland.

Cushing's syndrome: A disorder clinically similar to Cushing's disease, but commoner, in which excessive hormonal activity of the adrenal cortex is due to intrinsic hyperplasia, or to tumor, of the adrenal cortex *per se.* Symptoms include edema; fatness of face, neck and trunk; abnormal distribution of hair; atrophy of genital organs; impotence; amenorrhea, decalcification of bones; elevated blood pressure. [Harvey Williams Cushing, American surgeon. 1869-1939.]

cusp (kusp): A projecting point such as the edge of a tooth or a leaflet of one of the heart valves. The tricuspid valve has three cusps, the mitral valve has two.

cut-, cuti-: Denotes skin, cuticle.

cutaneous (kū-tā′nē-us): Relating to the skin. C. URETEROSTOMY, the ureters are transplanted so that they open on to the skin of the abdominal wall.

cutdown (kut′-down): Cutting into a vein in order to insert a needle or cannula for the administration of intravenous fluids or medication.

cuticle (kū′-ti-k'l): The epidermis (*q.v.*); dead epidermis, as that which surrounds a nail.—cuticular, adj.

cutis (kū′-tis): The corium or deeper layer of the skin; derma; true skin. C. ANSERINA, erection of the papillae of the skin due to contraction of the arrectores pilorum; produced by fear, cold, excitement or other stimulus. Often called gooseflesh or goose pimples.

CVA: Abbreviation for cerebrovascular accident; a stroke. See **cerebrovascular.**

cyanemia (sī-a-nē′-mi-a): Bluishness of the blood, as in cyanosis; due to insufficient oxygen.

cyanide (sī′-a-nīd): Any compound containing cyanogen with the CN radical; all are deadly poisons.

cyanocobalamin (sī-an-ō-kō-bal′-a-min):

Also called vitamin B_{12}. Apparently identical with the antianemic factor in liver. Specific in pernicious anemia; also useful in other macrocytic anemias, herpes zoster, sprue, polyneuritis and megaloblastic anemia of infants. Especially useful in patients who cannot tolerate liver. Given by intramuscular injection. See **vitamin B_{12}.**

cyanoderma (sī-a-nō-der′-ma): A bluish discoloration of the skin.

cyanosis (sī-a-nō′-sis): A bluish tinge manifested by hypoxic tissue, observed most frequently under the nails, lips and skin. It is always due to lack of oxygen, and the causes of this are legion.—cyanosed, cyanotic, adj. CENTRAL C., blueness seen on warm surfaces such as the oral mucosa and tongue. Increases with exertion.

cybernetics (sī-ber-net′-iks): The comparative study of electronic communication systems which combines the disciplines of neurophysiology, mathematics, and electrical engineering; it is concerned with the processes of information flow through which the brain controls the body and through which computers control machines. It supports the hypothesis that the functioning of the human brain is similar to that of electronic control devices.

cyclamate: A sugar substitute; noncaloric. Sucaryl is a trade name.

cyclarthrodial (sik-lar-thrō′-di-al): Pertaining or referring to a cyclarthrosis (*q.v.*).

cyclarthrosis (sik-lar-thrō′-sis): A pivot joint; one which allows for rotation.

cycle (sī-k'l): A regular series of movements or events; a sequence which recurs. CARDIAC C., the series of movements through which the heart passes in performing one heart beat which corresponds to one pulse beat and takes about one second. See **diastole** and **systole.** MENSTRUAL C., the periodically recurring series of changes in breasts, ovaries and uterus culminating in menstruation.—cyclic, cyclical, adj.

cyclical (sīk′-lik-al): Pertaining to or occurring in a cycle or cycles. C. SYNDROME, term used currently for premenstrual symptom complex, to emphasize that these symptoms are due to normal physiological interaction between several endocrine glands under the cyclical control of the hypothalamus and pituitary. C. VOMITING, periodic attacks of vomiting, associated with ketosis: no demonstrable pathological cause; occurs in nervous persons, children in particular.

cyclitis (sī-klī′-tis): Inflammation of the ciliary body of the eye, often coexistent with inflammation of the iris. See **iridocyclitis**.

cyclodialysis (sī-klō-dī-al′-i-sis): Surgical establishment of communication between the anterior chamber of the eye and the suprachoroidal space to relieve intraocular pressure in glaucoma.

cyclodiathermy (sī-klō-dī′-a-ther-mi): Destruction by diathermy of a portion of the ciliary body; done in cases of glaucoma.

cycloid (sī′-kloid): In psychiatry, descriptive of a type of personality characterized by alternating periods of well-being and happiness with mild depression.

cycloplegia (sī-klō-plē′-ji-a): Paralysis of the ciliary muscle of the eye.—cycloplegic, adj.

cycloplegic (sī-klō-plē′-jik): 1. Pertaining to cycloplegia. 2. A drug or agent that causes paralysis of the ciliary muscle.

cyclothymia (sī-klō-thim′-i-a): A temperament characterized by a tendency to alternate between moods of elation and depression. Manic-depressive psychosis.

cyclotomy (sī-klot′-o-mi): A drainage operation for the relief of glaucoma, consisting of an incision through the ciliary body.

cyesis (sī-ē′-sis): Pregnancy. PSEUDOCYESIS, signs and symptoms simulating those of early pregnancy occurring in a childless person with an overwhelming desire to have a child.

cylindroma (sil-in-drō′-ma): A tumor containing elongated twisted cords of hyaline material, found in malignancy of salivary glands, basal cell carcinomas and endotheliomas.

cyllosis (sil-ō′-sis): Clubfoot.

cynanthropy (sī-nan′-thrō-pi): A delusion or mania in which the patient believes himself to be a dog and imitates one by barking and growling.

cynophobia (sī-nō-fō′-bi-a): A morbid or unreasonable fear of dogs.

cynorexia (sī-nō-rek′-si-a): Morbidly excessive hunger or appetite.

cypridophobia (sip-ri-dō-fō′-bi-a): 1. A morbid fear of contracting a venereal disease. 2. Morbid fear of sexual intercourse.

cyst (sist): A sac with a membranous wall, enclosing fluid or semisolid matter. ADVENTITIOUS C., one formed about a foreign body or exudate. BRANCHIAL C., one in the neck region arising from anomalous development of the embryonal branchial cleft(s). CHOCOLATE C., an endometrial c. containing altered blood. The ovaries are the most usual site. DERMOID C., congenital in ori-

gin, usually in the ovary, containing elements of hair, nails, skin, teeth, etc. HYDATID C. is the envelope in which *Taenia echinococcus* (tapeworm) produces its larvae—usually in the human liver. MEIBOMIAN C., see **chalazion**. OVARIAN C., ovarian new growth. Most are cystic, but some such as the fibroma are solid. To be differentiated from a cystic ovary (*q.v.*). O. C. is enucleated from the ovary which is conserved. PAPILLARY C., an ovarian C. in which there are nipple-like (papillary) outgrowths from the wall. May be benign or malignant. PILONIDAL C., see **pilonidal**. RETENTION C., caused by blocking of a duct, as a ranula (*q.v.*). SEBACEOUS C., retention C. of a sebaceous gland (wen). THYROGLOSSAL C., a cystic distension of thyroglossal duct near the hyoid bone, in the neck region.

cyst-, cysti-, cysto-: Denotes a fluid-containing sac, as the gallbladder, urinary bladder.

-cyst: Denotes a bladder.

cystadenoma (sist-ad-en-ō′-ma): An innocent cystic new growth of glandular tissue. Liable to occur in the female breast.

cystalgia (sis-tal′-ji-a): Pain in a bladder, especially the urinary bladder.

cystathioninuria (sis-ta-thī-ō-nin-ū′-ri-a): Excessive excretion of thionine, an intermediate product in conversion of methionine (*q.v.*) to cysteine; an inherited condition. Associated with mental subnormality.

cystectomy (sis-tek′-to-mi): 1. Usually refers to the removal of part or the whole of the urinary bladder. This may involve transplantation of one or both ureters, cutaneously or into the bowel. 2. Excision of a cyst.

cysteine (sis′-tē-in): An amino acid that is produced during the digestion or hydrolysis of proteins.

cystic (sis′-tik): 1. Pertaining to the urinary bladder or the gallbladder. 2. Pertaining to or resembling a cyst. C. DEGENERATION, degeneration with formation of cysts. C. DISEASE OF THE BREAST, the formation in the female breast of cysts that contain straw-colored fluid; usually occurs at menopause. C. DISEASE OF THE LUNG; FIBROSIS OF THE PANCREAS, names given to a condition that affects about one child in 2500; due to a recessive gene mutation. The key to survival is control of pulmonary infection. Prognosis is poor beyond adolescence. Involves the endocrine glands, particularly the pancreas, and the exocrine glands, particularly those that secrete mucus; viscous mucus blocks the small tubular structures of various organs, there is a high level of electrolytes in the sweat, pancreatic functioning is deficient, and there are signs of chronic pulmonary disease. Symptoms include dyspnea, productive cough, bulky greasy malodorous stools, cramps in the abdomen, diarrhea, voracious appetite, impaired growth, malnutrition. See **mucoviscidosis.** C. DUCT, tube connecting the gallbladder to the hepatic and common bile ducts; conveys bile to and from the gallbladder.

cysticercosis (sis-ti-ser-kō′-sis): Infection of man with Cysticercus (*q.v.*).

Cysticercus (sis-ti-ser′-kus): The larval form of various tapeworms. After ingestion, the ova do not develop beyond this form in man. Symptoms include loss of weight, nervousness, muscular pains; in severe cases the brain may be invaded and convulsions or paralysis occur.

cystine (sis′-tin): A sulphur-containing amino acid, produced by the breaking down of proteins during the digestive process.

cystinosis (sis-tin-ō′-sis): Metabolic disorder in which crystalline cystine is deposited in the body, especially in the kidneys. Cystine and other amino acids are excreted in the urine. Renal insufficiency, renal rickets or dwarfism may result. Fanconi syndrome. See **amino-aciduria.**

cystinuria (sis-tin-ū′-ri-a): Metabolic disorder in which cystine appears in the urine; often associated with liver disease or jaundice. A cause of renal stones.—cystinuric, adj.

cystitis (sis-tī′-tis): Inflammation of a bladder, particularly the urinary bladder; exciting cause usually bacterial. The condition may be acute or chronic, primary or secondary to stones, etc. More frequent in females as the urethra is short.

cystitomy (sis-tit′-o-mi): Incision into: (1) the urinary bladder; (2) the gallbladder; (3) the capsule of the crystalline lens of the eye.

cystocele (sis′-tō-sēl): Prolapse of the posterior wall of the urinary bladder into the anterior vaginal wall. See **colporrhaphy.**

cystodynia (sis-tō-din′-i-a): Pain in the urinary bladder.

cystogram (sis′-tō-gram): An x-ray film demonstrating the urinary bladder. MICTURATING C., taken during the act of passing urine.

cystography (sis-tog′-ra-fi): Radiography of

the urinary bladder after it has been rendered radiopaque.—cystographic, adj.; cystographically, adv.

cystoid (sis′-toid): 1. Like a bladder; like a cyst. 2. A tumor that resembles a cyst; it contains fluid or pulpy matter but has no capsule.

cystolith (sis′-tō-lith): A stone in the urinary bladder.

cystolithiasis (sis-tō-lith-ī′-as-is): The presence of a stone or stones in the urinary bladder.

cystolithotomy (sis-tō-li-thot′-o-mi): The removal of stones from the urinary bladder following surgical incision into the bladder. Also cystolithectomy.

cystoma (sis-tō′-ma): A tumor containing cysts, especially one in or near an ovary.

cystometer (sis-tom′-e-ter): An instrument used to measure the pressure within the urinary bladder in relation to its capacity; used in studying the neuromuscular mechanism of the bladder.

cystometrogram (sis-tō-met′-rō-gram): A graphic record, made with a cystometer (*q.v.*), of the changes in pressure within the urinary bladder under various conditions; used in the study of certain disorders of bladder function.

cystoplasty (sis′-tō-plas-ti): Surgical repair of the bladder.—cystoplastic, adj.

cystoplegia (sis-tō-plē′-ji-a): Paralysis of the urinary bladder.

cystorrhagia (sis-tō-rā′-ji-a): Hemorrhage from the urinary bladder.

cystorrhaphy (sis-tor′-a-fi): Suturing of the urinary bladder.

cystorrhea (sis-tō-rē′-a): Mucous discharge from the urinary bladder.

cystoscope (sis′-tō-skōp): An endoscope (*q.v.*) for examining the urinary tract.—cystoscopy, n.; cystoscopic, adj.; cystoscopically, adv.

cystostomy (sis-tos′-to-mi): The operation whereby a fistulous opening is made into the bladder via the abdominal wall.

cystotomy (sis-tot′-o-mi): 1. Incision into the urinary bladder or gallbladder; may be done to remove calculi or a tumor. PERINEAL C., one in which the opening into the urinary bladder is made through the perineum. SUPRAPUBIC C., one in which the opening into the urinary bladder is made just above the symphysis pubis. 2. Incision into the capsule of the crystalline lens.

cystourethritis (sis-tō-ū-rē-thrī′-tis): Inflammation of the urinary bladder and urethra.

cystourethrogram (sis-tō-ū-rē′-thrō-gram): An x-ray film demonstrating the urinary bladder and the urethra.

cystourethrography (sis-tō-ū-rē-throg′-ra-fi): Radiographic examination of the urinary bladder and the urethra after they have been rendered radiopaque.—cystourethrographic, adj.; cystourethrographically, adv.

cystourethropexy (sis-tō-ūr-ēth′-rō-pek-si): Forward fixation of the bladder and upper urethra in an attempt to combat incontinence of urine.

cyt-, cyto-: Denotes: (1) cell(s); (2) cytoplasm.

cytochrome (sī′-tō-krōm): Pigment occurring in almost all types of plant and animal cells.

cytocide (sī′-tō-sīd): An agent that destroys cells.

cytodiagnosis (sī-tō-dī-ag-nō′-sis): Diagnosis by microscopic study of cells. EXFOLIATIVE C., diagnosis by the examination of cells from the external or internal surfaces of the body. See **cytology.**

cytogenetics (sī-tō-je-net′-iks): That branch of biology concerned with the origin, development, structure, functions, etc. of cells, particularly of the chromosomes and genes.—cytogenesis, n.

cytology (sī-tol′-ō-ji): Subdivision of biology, consisting of the microscopic study of the body cells. EXFOLIATIVE C., microscopic study of cells from the surface of an organ or lesion after suitable staining.

cytolysin (sī-tol′-i-sin): A substance or antibody that is capable of causing cells to dissolve. When a C. acts upon a specific type of cell, it is named accordingly, *e.g.,* hemolysin.

cytolysis (sī-tol′-i-sis): The degeneration, destruction, disintegration or dissolution of cells.—cytolytic, adj.

cytoma (sī-tō′-ma): A tumor consisting almost entirely of neoplastic cells, *e.g.,* sarcoma (*q.v.*).

cytomegalic inclusion disease: A disease of the newborn especially; due to infection with a cytomegalovirus (*q.v.*) which often occurs before birth; characterized by enlarged spleen and liver, small head, diarrhea, hematemesis, hematuria, cerebral hemorrhage, anemia, mental and motor retardation. Diagnostic cells that contain large acidophil intranuclear inclusions are found in the ducts or acini of the salivary glands, also sometimes in other organs, *e.g.,* liver, kidney. Congenital form is the most severe; formerly thought to be rare in adults but it has recently been reported to occur in adults as an illness resembling infectious mononucleosis.

cytomegalovirus (sī-tō-meg-a-lō-vī′-rus): One of a group of several viruses that infect monkeys and rodents as well as man; belongs to the same group as the virus of herpes simplex. Affects primarily the newborn but studies show that by age 35 most adults have been infected with it. The carrier rate is high. See **cytomegalic inclusion disease.**

cytometer (sī-tom′-e-ter): A standardized device for measuring and counting cells, especially blood cells.

cytopathic (sī-tō-path′-ik): Pertaining to pathologic changes in cells.

cytoplasm (sī′-tō-plazm): The living material (protoplasm) of the cell other than that of the nucleus.

cytostasis (sī-tos′-ta-sis): Arrest or hindrance of cell development.—cytostatic, adj.

cytotoxic (sī-tō-tok′sik): Any substance that is toxic to cells. Applied to the group of drugs used for the treatment of carcinomas and reticuloses.

cytotoxin (sī-tō-tok′sin): A toxin or antibody that is destructive to specific cells of certain organs, or which inhibits their functioning. See **antibodies, cytotoxic.**

cytozoic (sī-tō-zō′-ik): Living on or within cells; parasitic.

cyturia (sī-tū′-ri-a): An abnormal number of cells, of any kind, in the urine.

D

D: Abbreviation for: (1) diopter (*q.v.*); (2) dexter, meaning right, *e.g.,* OD, *oculus dexter* (right eye).

dacry-, dacryo-: Denotes: (1) lacrimal; (2) tears.

dacryagogatresia (dak-ri-a-gog-a-trē′-zi-a): Obstruction of a lacrimal duct.

dacryagogue (dak′-ri-a-gog): An agent that promotes the flow of tears.

dacryoadenitis (dak-ri-ō-ad-en-ī′-tis): Inflammation of a lacrimal gland. It is a rare condition which may be acute or chronic. Also dacryadenitis.

dacryocyst (dak′-ri-ō-sist): Old term for the tear sac (lacrimal sac). The word is still used in its compound forms.

dacryocystectomy (dak-ri-ō-sis-tek′-to-mi): Excision of any part of the lacrimal sac.

dacryocystitis (dak-ri-ō-sis-tī′-tis): Inflammation of the tear sac, which usually results in abscess formation and obliteration of the tear duct, giving rise to epiphora (*q.v.*).

dacryocystography (dak-ri-ō-sis-tog′-ra-fi): Radiographic examination of the tear drainage apparatus after it has been rendered radiopaque.—dacryocystographic, adj.; dacryocystogram, n.

dacryocystorhinostomy (dak′-ri-ō-sis′-to-rīn-os′-to-mi): An operation to establish drainage from the lacrimal sac into the nose when there is obstruction of the nasolacrimal duct.

dacryolith (dak′-ri-ō-lith): A concretion in the lacrimal passages.

dactyl (dak′-til): A digit; finger or toe.—dactylar, dactylate, adj.

dactylion (dak-til′-i-on): Syndactyly (*q.v.*).

dactylitis (dak-til-ī′-tis): Inflammation of finger or toe. The digit becomes swollen due to periostitis. Met with in congenital syphilis, tuberculosis, sarcoid, etc.

dactylogram (dak-til′-ō-gram): A fingerprint.

dactylography (dak-ti-log′-ra-fi): The scientific study of fingerprints.

dactylology (dak-til-ol′-o-ji): The finger sign method of communication with deaf and dumb people.

dactylomegaly (dak-ti-lō-meg′-a-li): Enlargement of one or more of the fingers or toes.

daltonism (dawl′-ton-izm): 1. Color blindness, named after John Dalton, English chemist and physicist [1766–1844], who was afflicted with it. 2. Red-green color blindness.

D and C: Abbreviation for dilatation of the cervix and curettage (*q.v.*) of the uterus.

dander: In medicine, minute scales of skin, hair, fur, or feathers of animals which may cause allergic reactions in persons sensitive to them.

dandruff (dand′-ruf): The common scaly condition of the scalp or the material shed from it. Also scurf.

dandy fever: Dengue (*q.v.*).

dartos (dar′-tos): A thin layer of smooth muscle tissue that makes up part of the superficial fascia of the scrotum; it envelops the testes. Cold causes it to contract, thus bringing the testes closer to the abdomen for warmth; warmth causes it to relax, thus the testes are kept at a fairly even temperature. Also tunica dartos.

db: Abbreviation for decibel, decibels.

DDT: An insecticide widely used against lice, flies, mosquitoes and many other insects. Toxic to humans. See **dicophane.**

deaf-mute (def′-mūt): A person who lacks both the sense of hearing and the ability to speak.

deafness: Lack, loss, or impairment of the sense of hearing; may be acute or chronic; congenital or acquired. AVIATOR'S D. is an occupational disease of aviators. BOILER-MAKER'S or OCCUPATIONAL D. occurs in individuals who work in extremely noisy places. CONDUCTION D. results from interference with the conduction of sound waves within the ear. NERVE D. results from damage to the auditory nerve. PSYCHIC D. occurs when the patient hears sounds but does not comprehend them. TONE D., inability to distinguish musical sounds.

deamination (dē-am-in-ā′-shun): 1. The removal of an amino from an organic compound. 2. A process occurring in the liver whereby amino acids are broken down and urea formed. Also deaminization.

death: The permanent cessation or end of life. D. CERTIFICATE, a document that the physician is required to file after the death of a patient; it contains vital information about the person and the cause of death. D. INSTINCT, an unconscious tendency toward self-destruction. D. RATE, the ratio of deaths over a certain period of time in a certain area. D. RATTLE, sound sometimes heard in dying patients; caused by the loss of the cough reflex and the breathing of air through mucus that has collected in the trachea. D. STRUGGLE, AGONY, THROE, a final twitching or convulsion sometimes seen in a dying person.

debilitating (dē-bil′-i-tāt-ing): Weakening.

debility (dē-bil′-i-ti): A state of weakness, feebleness or infirmity.—debilitate, n.

débridement (dā-brēd′-mon): In surgery, thorough cleansing of a wound with removal of all foreign matter and devitalized, injured or infected tissue.—debride, v.t.

decalcification (dē-kal-si-fik-ā′-shun): Removal of calcium or calcium salts, as from teeth in dental caries, bone in disorders of metabolism.

decant (dē-kant′): To pour off a liquid without disturbing the sediment or precipitate in it.

decapitation (de-cap-i-tā′-shun): The removal of the head as from the body, or from a part of the body as from a bone.—decapitate, v.t.

decapsulation (dē-kap-sū-lā′-shun): Surgical removal of a capsule, as of the kidney.

decerebrate (dē-ser′-e-brāte): 1. To remove the cerebrum. 2. Without cerebral function; a state of deep unconsciousness. D. POSTURE, a condition of the unconscious patient in which all four limbs are spastic and which indicates severe damage to the cerebrum.

deci-: Denotes one-tenth (in the metric system).

decibel (des′-i-bel): A standard unit that has been adopted for measuring the amount of sound perceptible to the normal ear.

decidua (dē-sid′-ū-a): The endometrial lining of the uterus thickened and altered for the reception of the fertilized ovum. It is shed when pregnancy terminates. D. BASALIS, that part which lies under the embedded ovum and forms the maternal part of the placenta. D. CAPSULARIS, that part that lies over the developing ovum. D. VERA, the decidua lining the rest of the uterus; also called the D. parietalis.—decidual, adj.

deciduoma malignum (dē-sid-ū-ō′-ma malig′-num): Chorionepithelioma (q.v.); a tumor which forms at the site of the placenta during or following pregnancy.

deciduous (dē-sid′-ū-us): Not permanent; said of something that is shed, or that falls off or out, at maturity. Term often applied to the teeth of the first dentition (baby teeth).

decoction (dē-kok′-shun): In pharmacology, a medicinal substance prepared by boiling.

decompensation (dē-kom-pen-sā′-shun): A failure of compensation, particularly in heart disease; inability of the heart to maintain adequate circulation.

decompression (dē-kom-presh′-un): Removal of pressure or a compressing force. ABDOMINAL D., currently being used in pregnancy and labor. Apparatus applied to anterior abdominal wall. Improves blood supply and results in shorter and less painful labor. Of value in pre-eclamptic toxemia. D. OF BRAIN is achieved by trephining the skull. D. OF BLADDER is achieved in cases of chronic urinary retention by continuous or intermittent drainage via catheter inserted into the urethra. D. CHAMBER is used when returning deep-sea divers to the surface. See **caisson disease.**

decongestion (dē-kon-jest′-yun): Relief of congestion (q.v.).—decongestive, adj.

decontamination (dē-kon-tam-in-ā′-shun): The process of destroying, removing, or neutralizing harmful agents, e.g., war gas or radioactive materials, from persons, objects, or an area.

decortication (dē-kort-ik-ā′-shun): Surgical removal of cortex or outer covering of an organ such as the brain, kidney, or lung. D. OF LUNG is carried out when thickening of the visceral pleura prevents re-expansion of lung as may occur in chronic empyema. The visceral pleura is peeled off the lung, which is then re-expanded by positive pressure through an anesthetic apparatus.

decubitus (de-kū′-bi-tus): The recumbent position; lying down. D. ULCER, an ulceration or pressure sore, usually occurring in a patient long confined to bed, arising from continual pressure of the flesh over a bony prominence or from friction, obesity, emaciation, impaired circulation to the part, paralysis, old age, lowered vitality, lack of cleanliness, failure to keep the bed dry, smooth and free of irritating particles. The usual sites are the buttock, hip, shoulder, heel, elbow. The first warning is redness of the area, which becomes hot and tender, later smarting. Discoloration ensues and is followed by breaking of the skin, thus producing an open sore which may or may not become infected and which sloughs before healing takes place by granulation. Skin grafting may be necessary. See **pres-**

sure areas.—decubiti, pl.; decubital, adj.

decussation (de-kus-ā′-shun): Intersection; crossing of nerve fibers in the form of an X at a point beyond their origin, as in the optic and pyramidal tracts. Chiasm.—decussate, adj. and v.

defecation (de-fe-kā′-shun): Discharge of fecal matter from the rectum; evacuation of the bowels.—defecate, v.t.

defense mechanism: In psychiatry, a process used unconsciously in order to gain relief from anxiety or emotional distress.

deferens (def′-er-ens): Vas deferens (*q.v.*).

defervescence (def-er-ves′-ens): The time during which a fever is declining. If the body temperature falls rapidly it is spoken of as 'crisis'; if it falls slowly the term 'lysis' is used.

defibrillation (de-fib-ri-lā′-shun): The arrest of fibrillation of the cardiac muscle (atrial or ventricular), and restoration of normal cycle.—defibrillate, v.

defibrillator (de-fib′-ri-lā′-tor): 1. Any agent (*e.g.*, an electric shock) that arrests ventricular fibrillation and restores normal rhythm. 2. A machine that administers the electric shock used for defibrillation.

defibrinated (de-fī′-brin-āt-ed): Rendered free from fibrin (*q.v.*). A necessary process in the preparation of serum (*q.v.*).—defibrinate, v.

deficiency disease: Disease resulting from dietary deficiency of any substance essential for good health, especially the vitamins.

deformity (de-for′mi-ti): Congenital or acquired malformation, disfigurement or distortion of the body or a part of it when the deviation from normal is apparent.

degeneration (de-jen-er-ā′-shun): Deterioration in quality or function. Regression from more specialized to less specialized type of tissue. AFFERENT D., degeneration spreading up sensory nerves. AMYLOID D., a wax-like change in tissues. CASEOUS D., cheese-like tissue resulting from atrophy in a tuberculoma or gumma. COLLOID D., mucoid degeneration of tumors. FATTY D., droplets of fat found in atrophic tissue, as in the myocardium. HYALINE D., affects connective tissue, especially of blood vessels, in which the tissue takes on a homogeneous or formless appearance. SENILE D. is the clinical picture of old age in which the acuity of thought and performance is blunted. SUBACUTE COMBINED D. of the spinal cord, heralded by paresthesia (*q.v.*), is a complication of untreated pernicious anemia.—degenerative, adj.; degenerate, v.

degenerative disease: One in which loss of efficiency or function of an organ, structure, or tissue is gradual and progressive and usually nonreversible, *e.g.*, arteriosclerosis.

deglutition (deg-loo-tish′-un): The process of swallowing, partly voluntary, partly involuntary.

dehiscence (de-his′-ens): The process of splitting or bursting open, as of a wound. —dehisce, v.t.; dehiscent, adj.

dehydrant (de-hī′-drant): An agent that reduces the amount of water in the body by dehydration (*q.v.*).

dehydration (de-hī′drā-shun): Loss or removal of fluid. In the body this condition arises when the fluid intake fails to replace fluid loss. This is liable to occur when there is bleeding, diarrhea, excessive exudation from a raw area, excessive sweating, polyuria or vomiting, and usually upsets the body's electrolyte balance. If suitable fluid replacement cannot be achieved orally, then parenteral administration must be instituted.—dehydrate, v.t.

déjà vu phenomenon (dā-zha voo′ fe-nom′-e-non): Intense feeling of familiarity as if everything had happened before. Occurs in epilepsy involving the temporal lobes of the brain and in certain epileptic dream states.

dejection (de-jek′-shun): 1. Mental depression. 2. Defecation (*q.v.*).

delactation (de-lak-tā′-shun): 1. Weaning. 2. Cessation of the secretion of milk.

deleterious (del-e-te′-ri-us): Hurtful, injurious, destructive, noxious, pernicious.

Delhi boil: See **oriental sore.**

delinquency (de-lin′-kwen-si): Unacceptable, antisocial or criminal behavior. Used especially with reference to children or adolescents.

deliquescent (del-i-kwes′-ent): Capable of absorbing moisture, thus becoming fluid.

delirium (de-lir′-i-um): Abnormal mental condition characterized by disorientation, confusion, excitement and restlessness; often accompanied by hallucinations and delusions. May be present in various forms of mental disease but more frequently seen in patients with high fever, toxic conditions or injury. D. TREMENS, a violent form of delirium resulting from excessive and prolonged use of alcohol; is represented by a picture of confusion, terror, restlessness, hallucinations, tremor.—delirious, adj.

delivery: Expulsion or extraction of a child from the uterus. The process of being born.

CESAREAN D., D. through an incision in the mother's abdominal wall. FORCEPS D., D. achieved with instruments. PRECIPITATE D., occurs with great suddenness, lack of preparation, or without the presence of a physician.

deltoid (del'-toid): Triangular. D. MUSCLE, base lies over shoulder region, apex inserted into midshaft of humerus.

delusion (dē-lū'-zhun): A false belief that cannot be altered by argument or reasoning. Found as a psychotic symptom in several types of insanity, notably schizophrenia, paraphrenia, paranoia, senile psychoses, mania and depressive states including involutional melancholia. D. OF GRANDEUR, an exaggerated idea of one's status or importance. D. OF PERSECUTION, the idea that one is being willfully persecuted by a particular person or group of persons.

demarcation (dē-mar-kā'-shun): 1. A separation or distinction. 2. An outlining of the junction of diseased and healthy tissue; often used to refer to the line formed at the edge of a gangrenous area.

dementia (dē-men'-shi-a): 1. Madness. 2. An irreversible deterioration of mentality characterized by a marked decline in an individual's intellectual level. D. PARALYTICA, general paralysis of the insane. See **general**. D. PRAECOX, premature schizophrenia (q.v.). PRESENILE D., Alzheimer's disease (q.v.).

demi-: Denotes half; one-half.

demise (dē-mīs'): Death.

demography (dem-og'-ra-fi): Social science. The study of mankind or of human populations, especially their geographic distributions and physical environments, and including vital statistics.

demoniac (dē-mō'ni-ak): 1. Frenzied. 2. A lunatic.

demulcent (dē-mul'-sent): 1. Soothing; softening. 2. A slippery mucilaginous fluid that allays and soothes inflammation, especially of the mucous membranes.

demyelinate (dē-mī'-e-lin-āt): To remove or destroy the myelin sheath of a nerve or nerves.

denatured (dē-nā'churd): 1. Having its natural characteristics modified so as to make it unfit for human consumption, *e.g.*, alcohol. 2. Adulterated.

dendrite or **dendron** (den'-drīt; den'-dron): One of the branched filaments which are given off from the body of a nerve cell. That part of a neuron which transmits an impulse to the nerve cell.—dendritic, adj.

dendritic ulcer: Linear corneal ulcer that sends out tree-like branches. Caused by herpes simplex.

denervation (dē-ner-vā'-shun): The act of depriving an area of its nerve supply. Usually refers to incision, excision or blocking of a nerve.

dengue (den'gā): A disease that occurs epidemically and sporadically in the Middle East, Egypt, Iran, the West Indies and the South Pacific. The causative agent is a virus conveyed by a mosquito. Characterized by rheumatic pains, fever and a skin eruption. Sometimes called 'break-bone fever.'

Denis Browne splint: An apparatus for the correction of congenital clubfoot in young children. Consists of a flexible horizontal bar attached to a pair of metal footplates that have a device that permits them to rotate. The plates are strapped to the child's feet; later in the treatment shoes may be attached to the plates. [Denis Browne, British surgeon. 1892– .]

dens: 1. A tooth.—dentes, pl. 2. The odontoid (q.v.) process of the atlas (q.v.).

dental (den'-tal): Pertaining to the teeth.

dentalgia (den-tal'-ji-a): Toothache.

dentate (den'-tāt): Having teeth or pointed, teeth-like projections.

dentifrice (den'-ti-fris): A powder, paste or liquid for cleansing the teeth.

dentin(e) (den'-tēn): The hard material, similar to bone, that makes up the chief substance of the teeth. It encloses the pulp cavity, is covered with enamel on the crown and cementum on the root of a tooth.

dentition (den-tish'-un): 1. The process of teething. 2. The character and arrangement of an individual's teeth. PRIMARY D., eruption of the deciduous, 'milk' or temporary teeth. SECONDARY D., eruption of the 'adult' or permanent teeth.

denture (den'-chur): A set of teeth. Term usually designates an artificial replacement of one, several or all of the natural teeth.

deodorant (dē-ō'-dor-ant): Any substance that destroys or masks an (unpleasant) odor.—deodorize, v.t.

deossification (dē-os-i-fi-kā'-shun): Removal or reduction in the amount of mineral content of a bone or bones.

deoxidation (dē-ok-si-dā'-shun): The removal of all or part of the oxygen from a compound.—deoxidate, v.t.

deoxycortone (dē-ok-si-kor'-tōn): Desoxycorticosterone (q.v.).

deoxygenate (dē-ok'si-jen-āt): To deprive an organism of oxygen. To remove all or part of the oxygen from a compound. —deoxygenation, n.

deoxyribonucleic acid (dē-ok-si-rī-bō-nūk'-lē-ik): A nucleic acid present in the nuclei of animal and vegetable cells, especially the genes. In conjunction with deoxyribonucleoprotein, it makes up the autoreproducing component of chromosomes and of many viruses; together these substances are the fundamental components of living tissue. Abbreviated DNA. Formerly spelled desoxyribonucleic.

depersonalization (dē-per-sun-al-ī-zā'-shun): A subjective feeling of having lost one's personality, sometimes that one no longer exists. Occurs in schizophrenia and more rarely in depressive states.

depigmentation (dē-pig-men-tā'-shun): Partial or complete loss of pigment.

depilate (dep'-i-lāt): To remove hair from. —depilatory, adj., n.; depilation, n.

depilatories (dē-pil'-a-tor-ēz): Substances usually made in pastes (*e.g.*, barium sulphide) which remove excess hair only temporarily; they do not act on the papillae, consequently the hair grows again. See **epilation.**

deplete (dē-plēt'): 1. To empty or deprive of a principal substance. 2. To reduce the strength of a person or substance.

depletion (dē-plē'-shun): 1. Withdrawal or removal of fluid, especially blood. 2. An exhausted state, often refers to results of loss of blood.

deposit (dē-poz'-it): 1. Sediment; dregs; a precipitate. 2. Morbid particles of matter that have collected in a body tissue or cavity.

depravation (dep-ra-vā'-shun): 1. Deterioration or degeneration. 2. Perversion.

depraved (dē-prāvd'): 1. Deteriorated. 2. Abnormal; perverted.

depressant (dē-pres'-ant): An agent that reduces or slows the functional activity of an organ or system of the body.

depression (dē-presh'-un): 1. A hollow place or indentation, *e.g.*, a fossa in a bone. 2. Diminution of power or activity. 3. A low condition, either mental or physical. In psychiatry, emotional disorder. Of two distinct types, neurotic and psychotic. The neurotic type, REACTIVE D., occurs as a reaction to stress; when the situation causing the stress is removed, the depression disappears. The psychotic type, ENDOGENOUS D., arises spontaneously in the mind. The symptoms are almost the same in both conditions, and vary from mild to fatal and

are: insomnia, headaches, exhaustion, anorexia, irritability, emotionalism or loss of affect, loss of interest, impaired concentration, feelings that life is not worth living and suicidal thoughts. INVOLUTIONAL D., that occurring at the climacteric.

depressor (dē-pres'-or): Anything that depresses a bodily activity or function. Applies to muscles, drugs, nerves, as well as instruments. TONGUE D., a spatula-like blade, usually of wood, used to hold the tongue down during examination of mouth and throat.

deprivation (dep-ri-vā'-shun): The loss, absence, removal or withholding of parts, powers, or things that are needed. D. SYNDROME, usually the result of parental rejection of offspring; including malnutrition, dwarfism, pot-belly, gluttonous appetite, superficial attachment to any adult.

derangement (dē-rānj'-ment): 1. Mental disorder; insanity. 2. A disturbance in the normal order or arrangement of a part or an organ.

derealization (dē-rē-a-lī-zā'-shun): Feelings of unreality, such as occur to normal people during dreams. D. is a symptom often found in schizophrenia and depressive states.

dereistic (dē-rē-is'-tik): Thinking not adapted to reality. Autistic thinking.

derivative (dē-riv'-a-tiv): A chemical substance that is not original or fundamental, but which is derived from another substance.

derm-, derma-, dermat-, dermato-, dermo-: Denotes the skin.

-derm: Denotes: (1) the skin, integument; (2) a covering.

derma: The skin; specifically, the corium (*q.v.*).—dermic, dermal, adj.

dermabrasion (der-ma-brā'-zhun): A surgical procedure for the removal of acne scars or nevi. Wire brushes, sandpaper or other abrasives are used.

Dermacentor (der-ma-sen'-tor): A genus of ticks. D. ANDERSONI, the vector of the western type of Rocky Mountain spotted fever. D. VARIABILIS, the dog tick, vector of the eastern type of Rocky Mountain spotted fever.

dermatalgia (der-ma-tal'-ji-a): Localized pain in the skin with no lesion at the site of the pain; sometimes due to a nervous disorder. Syn., dermatodynia, dermalgia.

dermatitis (der-ma-tī'-tis): Inflammation of the skin, acute or chronic. (By custom limited to an eczematous condition.) There are many types all of which present with one or more of the following symptoms at some stage: itching, redness, blisters, crusting, scaling, oozing, fissuring, thickening, hardening, or increase in pigment. ACTINIC D., caused by sunlight; not a sunburn. CONTACT D., caused by touching a substance to which the individual is sensitive, e.g., a chemical, cosmetic, or such plants as poison ivy, oak, or sumac. Syn., ivy poisoning; atopic D. D. DYSMENORRHOEICA, occurs during the menstrual period, usually on the face. EXFOLIATIVE D. is characterized by pink to deep red skin, intense itching, branny desquamation. EXFOLIATIVE D. OF INFANCY, a type of pemphigus; starts with a red patch or blister. D. HERPETIFORMIS, an intensely itchy skin eruption of unknown cause, most commonly characterized by vesicles, bullae and pustules on urticarial plaques, which remit and relapse. When occurring in pregnancy it is known as 'hydros gravidarum.' D. HIEMALIS, a recurrent eczema occurring in cold weather; winter itch. OCCUPATIONAL or INDUSTRIAL D. occurs as a result of handling some sensitizing agent while at work. D. MEDICAMENTOSA, eruption due to drugs taken internally. SECONDARY EXFOLIATIVE D., may arise during treatment with certain drugs, e.g., arsenic, mercury, gold, etc. SENSITIZATION D. may be due to contact with, or ingestion of, foods to which the person is sensitive. D. SEBORRHEICA, occurs in areas where oil glands abound, e.g., face, scalp, pubic area, around the anus; characterized by yellowish-gray oily scales. TRAUMATIC D., due to exposure to irritating substances or physical agents. VARICOSE D., usually in the lower part of the leg, due to varicosities of the smaller veins. WEEPING D., an oozing D. that results from scratching to relieve itching. X-RAY D., due to exposure to x-rays.

dermato-autoplasty (der-ma-tō-aw′-tō-plas-ti): The grafting of skin taken from some part of the patient's own body.

dermatoglyphics (der-ma-tō-glif′-iks): The skin patterns or surface markings, especially those found on the palms of the hands and soles of the feet.

dermatoheteroplasty (der-ma-tō-het′-er-ō-plas-ti): The grafting of skin taken from the body of another.

dermatologist (der-ma-tol′-o-jist): One who studies skin diseases and is skilled in their treatment. A skin specialist.

dermatology (der-ma-tol′-o-ji): The science which deals with the skin, its structure, functions, diseases and their treat-

ment.—dermatological, adj.; dermatologically, adv.

dermatolysis (der-ma-tol′-i-sis): Abnormal looseness of the skin, usually congenital; causing the skin and subcutaneous tissues to hang in folds.

dermatome (der′-ma-tōm): An instrument for cutting slices of skin of varying thickness, usually for grafting.

dermatomycosis (der-ma-tō-mī-kō′-sis): Fungal infection of the skin.—dermatomycotic, adj.

dermatomyositis (der-ma-tō-mī-o-sī′-tis): An acute, non-suppurative inflammation of the skin and muscles that presents with edema and muscle weakness; abrupt or sudden in onset. May result in the atrophic changes of scleroderma. See **collagen.**

dermatoneurosis (der-ma-tō-nū-rō′-sis): An inflammation of the skin that is due to some nerve abnormality or is a symptom of some form of neurosis.

dermatophylaxis (der-ma-tō-fī-lax′-is): Protection of the skin against infection.

dermatophyte (der′-ma-tō-fīt): One of a group of fungi that invade the superficial skin.

dermatophytosis (der-ma-tō-fī-tō′-sis): An eruption caused by one of the dermatophytes (q.v.). Most commonly seen on the feet (athlete's foot). Characterized by itching, small vesicles, fissures and scaling. See **tinea pedis.**

dermatoplasty (der′-ma-tō-plas-ti): Plastic repair of the skin; skin grafting.

dermatorrhagia (der-ma-tō-rā′-ji-a): Hemorrhage into or from the skin.

dermatosis (der-ma-tō′-sis): Generic term for skin disease.—dermatoses, pl.

dermatoxerasia (der-ma-tō-ze-rā′-si-a): Roughening or drying of the skin. Syn., xeroderma (q.v.).

dermis (der′-mis): The true skin; the cutis vera; the layer below the epidermis.

dermitis (der-mī′-tis): Dermatitis (q.v.).

dermographia (der-mō-graf′-i-a): A condition in which wheals occur on the skin after a blunt instrument or fingernail has been lightly drawn over it. Seen in vasomotor instability and urticaria. Also dermatographia.

dermoid (der′-moid): Pertaining to or resembling skin. D. CYST, a congenital tumor filled with fluid or sebaceous matter; of dermal origin. See **cyst.**

dermotropic (der-mō-trop′-ik): Having an affinity for the skin.

Descemet's membrane: The fine, elastic

membrane that lines the posterior surface of the cornea.

desensitization (dē-sen-si-tī-zā'-shun): The neutralization or lessening of acquired hypersensitiveness to some agent acting on the skin or internally. Used in asthma and for treatment of people who have become allergic to drugs such as penicillin and streptomycin. The process usually consists of giving small, repeated doses of the protein to which the person is sensitive.—desensitize, v.t.

desexualize (dē-seks'-ū-a-līz): To castrate (q.v.).

desiccant (des'-i-kant): Promoting dryness of a substance by absorbing or expelling water from it, or an agent that does this.

desiccate (des'-i-kāt): To dry up thoroughly.—desiccation, n.

desmodynia (des-mō-din'-i-a): Pain in a ligament.

desoxycorticosterone (des-ok-sē-kor-ti-kos'-ter-ōn): One of the steroid substances produced in the adrenal cortex, chiefly concerned with the metabolism of salt and water. Also deoxycortone.

desoxyribonucleic: Deoxyribonucleic (q.v.).

desquamation (des-kwa-mā'-shun): Shedding or flaking off; usually refers to the peeling off of loose scales from skin or mucous membrane. Commonly seen after diseases attended by a rash, e.g., scarlet fever, measles.—desquamate, v.t., v.i.

dest: Abbreviation for distilled.

detelectasis (de-tel-ek'-ta-sis): Collapse of an organ due to loss of normal inflation.

detergent (dē-ter'-jent): A purifying or cleansing agent.

deterioration (dē-tēr-i-ō-rā'-shun): The state of being worse or becoming worse.

determinism (dē-term'-min-izm): In psychiatry, the postulate that all emotional and mental life is determined by pre-existing conditions or forces and never by chance or choice by the individual.

detoxication (dē-tok-si-kā'-shun): The process of removing the poisonous property of a substance.—detoxicant, adj., n.; detoxicate, v

detrition (dē-trish'-un): A wearing off or away by friction, rubbing, or use.

detritus (dē-trī'-tus): Matter produced by detrition; waste matter from disintegration.

detrusor (dē-troo'-ser): The muscle of the urinary bladder.

detumescence (dē-tū-mes'-ens): Diminution or subsidence of swelling.

deviant (dē'-vi-ant): 1. Varying from an accepted normal standard. 2. Something that differs from what is considered normal, especially a person whose behavior or characteristics vary from what is acceptable in the group to which he belongs.

deviation (dē-vē-ā'-shun): 1. A departure from normal. 2. Failure to conform to normal standards. In optics, strabismus (q.v.).

devitalize (dē-vīt'-a-līz): To destroy or deprive of life, vitality, force, effectiveness. In dentistry, to destroy the pulp and nerve supply of a tooth.

devolution (dev-ō-lū'-shun): Catabolism; degeneration.

dexter (deks'-ter): Related to or situated on the right. In anatomy, on the right-hand side.

dextr-, dextro-: Denotes the right, toward or on the right side.

dextran (deks'-tran): A blood plasma substitute, obtained by the action of a specific bacterium on sugar solutions. Given intravenously in hemorrhage, shock, etc.

dextrimaltose (deks-tri-mal'-tōs): A sugar preparation used in infant formulas; contains maltose and dextrin.

dextrin (deks'-trin): A soluble polysaccharide formed during the hydrolysis of starch.

dextrocardia (deks-trō-kar'-di-a): Transposition of the heart to the right side of the thorax.—dextrocardial, adj.

dextromanual (deks-trō-man'-ū-al): Right-handed.

dextrose (deks'-trōs): 1. Glucose (q.v.); a soluble, readily absorbed and utilized carbohydrate (monosaccharide); may be given by almost any route; widely used by intravenous infusion in dehydration, shock and postoperatively. Also given orally as a readily absorbed sugar in acidosis and other nutritional disturbances. 2. The end product of carbohydrate digestion.

dhobie itch (dō'-bē): Tinea cruris (q.v.); tropical ringworm of the groin, a contact dermatitis found in the laundrymen of India; thought to be caused by laundry-marking fluid.

di-: Denotes two, twice, double.

diabetes (dī-a-bē'-tēz): A disease characterized by polyuria. Used without qualification it means D. MELLITUS. D. INNOCENS, renal glycosuria, where there is unusual permeability of the kidneys to glucose, the concentration in the blood remaining within normal limits. D. INSIPIDUS, a disease (congenital or following injury or infection) of the posterior pituitary gland or its adnexa.

There is dehydration, polydipsia, polyuria. The urine is pale and of *low* specific gravity. D. MELLITUS, a condition in which there is faulty carbohydrate metabolism, mainly due to a lack of insulin. This results in hyperglycemia and glycosuria. Other features are dehydration and polydipsia. The urine is pale, and of *high* specific gravity because of its contained sugar. Other symptoms include loss of weight, lassitude, pruritus, lowered resistance to infection, decreased ability of wounds to heal. Especially serious in the young. In more advanced stages there is coma and ketosis. Maternal latent D.M. is responsible for 80 percent of deformed children. BRONZE D., a type of D. in which the skin is deeply pigmented and the liver and pancreas are also involved. See **hemochromatosis.** STARVATION D., glycosuria following ingestion of glucose, after prolonged fasting; attributed to a reduced ability to form glycogen.

diabetic (dī-ab-et′-ik): 1. Pertaining to diabetes. 2. An individual suffering from diabetes. D. IDENTIFICATION CARD, one carried by diabetics; lists patient's and doctor's names, addresses and telephone numbers, states the kind and amount of insulin the patient is receiving and directions for treatment, should the person become ill when in a public place.

diabetogenic (dī-a-bet-ō-jen′-ik): Causing diabetes.

diacetic acid (dī-a-sē′-tik as′-id): Syn., acetoacetic acid (*q.v.*).

diagnosis (dī-ag-nō′-sis): The act or art of distinguishing one disease from another. CLINICAL D., one made by a study of the presenting symptoms. DIFFERENTIAL D., one arrived at after comparing the symptoms of two or more diseases. LABORATORY D. one arrived at after a study of specimens taken from the patient. TENTATIVE D., one judged by the apparent symptoms and facts pending further study and examination. See **cytodiagnosis.**

diagnostic (dī-ag-nos′-tik): 1. Pertaining to diagnosis. 2. Serving as evidence in diagnosis.—diagnostician, n.

diagnostician (dī-ag-nos-tish′-un): A physician whose chief field of interest and practice is in making diagnoses.

dialysis (dī-al′-i-sis): Separation of substances in solution by taking advantage of their differing diffusibility through a porous membrane as in the artificial kidney. PERITONEAL D., a method of irrigating the peritoneum; urea and other waste products

are exuded into the irrigation fluid and withdrawn from the abdominal cavity. —dialyze, v.t.; dialyses, pl. See **hemodialysis.**

dialyzer (dī′a-līz-er): The apparatus used in performing dialysis, or the membrane in the apparatus.

diapedesis (dī-a-pe-dē′-sis): The passage of blood cells through the unbroken vessel walls into the tissues; usually refers to passage of white cells through capillary walls in response to infection or injury.

diaphoresis (dī-a-fō-rē′-sis): Visible perspiration.

diaphoretic (dī-a-fō-ret′-ik): 1. An agent which induces diaphoresis. 2. Pertaining to diaphoresis.

diaphragm (dī′-a-fram): 1. The dome-shaped muscular partition between the thorax above and the abdomen below. 2. Any partitioning membrane or septum. —diaphragmatic, adj.

diaphragmatocele (dī-a-frag-mat′-ō-sēl): Hernia through the diaphragm.

diaphysis (dī-af′-i-sis): The shaft of a long bone.—diaphyseal, adj.; diaphyses, pl.

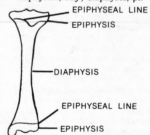

EPIPHYSEAL LINE
EPIPHYSIS
DIAPHYSIS
EPIPHYSEAL LINE
EPIPHYSIS

The tibia—diaphysis and epiphyses

diarrhea (dī-a-rē′-a): Loose and frequent evacuation of the bowels. 'Epidemic diarrhea of the newborn' is a highly contagious infection in maternity hospitals. SUMMER D., acute gastroenteritis of infants occurring in the hot weather chiefly.—diarrheic, diarrheal, adj.

diarthrosis (dī-ar-thrō′-sis): A synovial, freely movable joint, such as the hip joint.—diarthrodial, adj.; diarthroses, pl.

diastase (dī′-a-stās): A specific enzyme in certain plant cells and in the digestive juice; it converts starch into sugar. PANCREATIC D. is excreted in the urine (and saliva) and therefore estimation of urinary D. may be used as a test of pancreatic function.

diastasis (dī-as′-tas-is): 1. A separation of

bones without fracture; dislocation. 2. The separation of the epiphysis from the body of a bone.

diastole (dī-as′-to-li): The relaxation period of the cardiac cycle, as opposed to systole.—diastolic, adj.

diastolic murmur (dī-as-tol′-ik): An abnormal sound heard during diastole; occurs in valvular diseases of the heart.

diathermy (dī′-a-ther-mi): The passage of a high frequency electric current through the tissues whereby heat is produced. When both electrodes are large, the heat is diffused over a wide area according to the electrical resistance of the tissues. In this form it is widely used in the treatment of inflammation, especially when deeply seated (*e.g.*, sinusitis, pelvic cellulitis). When one electrode is very small the heat is concentrated in this area and becomes great enough to destroy tissue. In this form (surgical diathermy) it is used to stop bleeding at operation by coagulation of blood, or to cut through tissue in operation for malignant disease.

diathesis (dī-ath′-e-sis): An inherited predisposition to certain diseases or classes of diseases.

dicephalous (dī-sef′-a-lus): Two-headed.

dichotomy (dī-kot′-ō-mē): A division into two parts, classes, or groups.

dichromatism (dī-krō′-ma-tizm): Color blindness in which either the red-green or the blue-yellow system is lacking, the first type being relatively common and the second being the rarest of all forms of color blindness.

dichromatopsia (dī-krō-ma-top′-si-a): Ability to distinguish only two colors.

Dick test: A small amount of scarlet fever toxin is injected intracutaneously; the appearance of a small area of reddened skin at the site of injection within 24-48 hours indicates susceptibility to scarlet fever. [George F. and Gladys R. H. Dick, Chicago physicians. Both b. 1881.]

dicophane (dī′-ko-fān): Dichloro-diphenyl-trichloroethane (DDT). Well-known insecticide sometimes used against pediculosis capitis and other body parasites as lotion or dusting powder. Also chlorophenothane.

dicrotic (dī-krot′-ik): Pertaining to, or having a double beat, as indicated by a second expansion of the artery during diastole. D. PULSE, a small wave of distension of the blood vessel after the normal beat. D. WAVE, the second rise in the tracing of a dicrotic pulse.

diencephalon (dī-en-sef′-a-lon): That part of the brain lying between the telencephalon and the mesencephalon; contains the thalamus and hypothalamus.

diet: 1. The food normally consumed in the course of living. 2. A prescription of food that is required by a patient or permitted to him. 3. To eat only simple, easily digested food in limited quantities. BALANCED D., one that contains all the elements in the correct quantities needed for growth and repair of body tissues. BLAND D., one that contains no stimulating or irritating foods. DIABETIC D., one adapted to the needs of a diabetic patient; contains weighed amounts of fats, carbohydrates and proteins. KETOGENIC D., one high in fat, low in protein and carbohydrate. LIGHT D., one suitable for a person taking little exercise, *e.g.*, bed patient, convalescent. LOW SODIUM or LOW SALT D., one low in sodium, often used in treatment of edema, hypertension, congestive heart disease. SOFT D., one containing such foods as milk, eggs, custards, mashed potatoes, ice cream or other nonirritating, easily digested foods.—dietary, dietetic, adj.

dietetics (dī-e-tet′-iks): The interpretation and application of the scientific principles of nutrition to feeding in health and disease.

dietitian (dī-e-tish′-un): One who applies the principles of nutrition to the feeding of an individual, or a group of individuals in a heterogeneous setting of economics or health, *e.g.*, in schools, hospitals, institutions, restaurants, hotels, etc.

Dietl's crisis (dēt′-lz kri′-sis): A complication of 'floating kidney' (nephroptosis). Kinking of the ureter is thought to be responsible for the severe colic produced in the lumbar region. The urine is scanty and often blood-stained. [Jósef Dietl, Polish physician. 1804-1878.]

dietotherapy (dī-et-ō-ther′-a-pi): Scientific management of the diet in the treatment of disease.

differential: D. BLOOD COUNT, the estimation of the relative proportions of the different leukocyte cells in the blood. The normal differential count is: polymorphs, 65 to 70 percent; lymphocytes, 20 to 25 percent; monocytes, 5 percent; eosinophils, 0 to 3 percent; basophils, 0 to 0.5 percent. D. DIAGNOSIS, diagnosis based on comparing the symptoms of diseases that have similar manifestations and evaluating the signs and symptoms that are dissimilar.

diffusion (di-fū′-zhun): 1. The process

whereby gases and liquids of different densities intermingle when brought into contact, until the density is equal throughout. 2. Dialysis.

digest (dī-jest'): In physiology, to change food by mechanical and chemical processes, in the mouth, stomach and intestines, so that it can be absorbed by the body.

digestant (dī-jest'-ant): An agent that aids in digestion of food.

digestion (dī-jest'-chun): The mechanical and chemical process by which food is broken down in the gastrointestinal tract and rendered absorbable.—digestible, digestive, adj.; digestibility, n.; digest, v.t., v.i.

digestive (dī-jes'-tiv): Pertaining to digestion. D. TUBE, that part of the digestive system that includes the esophagus, stomach, small and large intestine.

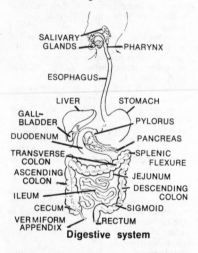

SALIVARY GLANDS
PHARYNX
ESOPHAGUS
LIVER
STOMACH
GALL-BLADDER
PYLORUS
DUODENUM
PANCREAS
TRANSVERSE COLON
SPLENIC FLEXURE
ASCENDING COLON
JEJUNUM
ILEUM
DESCENDING COLON
CECUM
SIGMOID
VERMIFORM APPENDIX
RECTUM

Digestive system

digit (dij'-it): A finger or toe.—digital, adj.

digitalis (dij-i-tal'-is): The leaf of the common foxglove plant which is the source of a large group of drugs used extensively in cardiac conditions to strengthen and slow the heart beat. Especially useful in auricular fibrillation and congestive heart failure. The purple foxglove furnishes the glycosides digitalin and digitoxin while the white foxglove furnishes digoxin. These drugs have a cumulative effect.

digitalism (dij'-i-tal-izm): 1. The effect of digitalis in the body. 2. Symptoms caused by overdosage or poisoning by digitalis.

digitalization (dij-it-al-ī-zā'-shun): Physiological saturation with digitalis, to obtain optimum therapeutic effect.

dilatation (dil-a-tā'-shun): The condition of being stretched or enlarged. May occur physiologically, pathologically, or be induced artificially.—dilate, v.; dilation, n.

dilation (dī-lā'-shun): The act of dilating or stretching.

dilator (dī'-lā-tor): Anything that dilates or stretches an opening or canal or a part of the body, e.g., a muscle, drug, or instrument.

diluent (dil'-ū-ent): A diluting agent.

dilute (dī-lūt'): To make weaker or thinner by the addition of liquid.

dilution (dī-lū'-shun): 1. The state of being diluted. 2. That which has been diluted.

dimple (dim'-p'l): A slight depression in bone or other body tissue.—dimpling, n.

diopter, dioptre (dī-op'-ter): A unit of measurement in refraction. A lens of one diopter has a focal length of 1 meter.

dioxide (di-ok'-sīd): An oxide whose molecules contain two atoms of oxygen to one of another element.

diphtheria (dif-thē'-ri-a): An acute, specific, highly infectious disease caused by the *Corynebacterium diphtheriae* [Klebs-Loeffler bacillus]. Characterized by formation of a grayish, leathery, adherent false membrane growing on a mucous surface, usually that of the upper respiratory tract. Locally there is pain, swelling, and may be suffocation. Systemically, the toxins attack the heart muscle and nerves. Transmitted by direct and indirect contact and carriers. Primarily a disease of childhood; protection obtained through immunization.—diphtheric, diphtheritic, diphtherial, adj.

diphtheroid (dif'-ther-oid): 1. Any bacterium resembling the *Corynebacterium diphtheriae*. 2. A disease that resembles diphtheria but is not caused by the *Corynebacterium diphtheriae*.

Diphyllobothrium latum (dī-fil-ō-both'-rē-um lā'-tum): A genus of broad tapeworms, including the common fish tapeworm. Occurs in man as a result of eating raw or improperly cooked infected fish.

diplegia (dī-plē'-ji-a): Symmetrical paralysis of the same parts on both sides of the body. Cf. **paraplegia.** See **Little's disease.**

diplococcus (dip-lō-kok'-us): A coccal bacterium characteristically occurring in pairs. Diplococcus may be used in a binomial to describe a characteristically paired coccus, *e.g., Diplococcus pneumoniae* = pneumococcus.—diplococcal, adj.

diploë (dip´-lō-e): The cancellous tissue between the outer and inner layers of compact bone, *e.g.,* the flat bones of the skull.

diploneural (dip-lō-nū´-ral): Being supplied with two nerves; said of certain muscles.

diplopia (dip-lō´-pi-a): Double vision.

dipsesis (dip-sē´-sis): Thirst.—dipsetic, adj.

dipsomania (dip-sō-mā´-ni-a): Alcoholism in which uncontrollable drinking occurs in bouts, often with long periods of sobriety between.—dipsomaniac, adj., n.

dipsosis (dip-sō´-sis): Abnormal thirst, or a craving for unusual drinks.

dipsotherapy (dip-sō-ther´-a-pi): Treatment by withholding or limiting the amount of fluid allowed the patient.

direct contact: Refers to the passing of a disease directly from one person to another.

director (di-rek´-tor): A grooved instrument used for guiding the knife in surgical operations.

dirt-eating: Geophagia or chthonophagia (*q.v.*).

dis-: Denotes: (1) to do the opposite of, reverse, deprive of, exclude; (2) absence of, opposite of; (3) not; (4) same as dys-.

disaccharide (dī-sak´-ar-īd): Any one of a class of sugars (carbohydrates) that yields two molecules of monosaccharide on hydrolysis, *e.g.,* lactose, maltose, sucrose.

disarticulation (dis-art-ik-ū-lā´-shun): Amputation or separation at a joint.

disc (disk): Disk (*q.v.*).

discharge (dis-charj´): 1. To liberate or set free. 2. Material that is expelled, evacuated, or flows away from a body cavity or wound, *e.g.,* feces, urine, pus.

dischronation (dis-krōn-nā´-shun): A disturbance in one's consciousness of time.

discission (di-sizh´-un): A cutting or division; specifically the rupturing of the lens capsule to allow absorption in the condition of cataract. Syn., needling.

discography (dis-kog´-ra-fi): X-ray of an intervertebral disc after it has been rendered radiopaque.—discographic, adj.; discographically, adv.; discograph, n.

discrete (dis-krēt´): Separate; not continuous. Often said of lesions that do not blend or join others. Opp. to confluent (*q.v.*).

disease (di-zēz´): Sickness; illness. A departure from a state of health caused by an interruption or modification of any of the vital functions and characterized by a definite train of symptoms.

disequilibrium (dis-ē-kwi-lib´-ri-um): Loss

or lack of balance, physical or mental.

disinfect (dis-in-fekt´): To free a substance or area of pathogenic organisms or to cause them to become inert.

disinfectant (dis-in-fek´-tant): An agent that is used to destroy pathogenic organisms or to cause them to be inert.—disinfectant, adj.

disinfection (dis-in-fek´-shun): A vague term, implying the destruction of all microorganisms, except spores, and can refer to the action of antiseptics as well as disinfectants.

disinfestation (dis-in-fes-tā´-shun): Extermination of such infesting agents as insects, parasites or rodents, especially lice. Delousing.

disintoxication (dis-in-tok-si-kā´-shun): 1. Detoxication (*q.v.*). 2. Treatment to assist an addict to overcome his drug habit.

disk: A circular or rounded flattened organ or structure. Also disc, discus.

diskitis (dis-kī-tis): Inflammation of a disk, particularly an intervertebral disk. Also discitis.

diskography: Discography (*q.v.*).

dislocation (dis-lō-kā´-shun): A displacement of organs or articular surfaces, more especially of a bone at a joint; accompanied by pain and deformity. Syn., luxation.—dislocated, adj.; dislocate, v.t.

dismemberment (dis-mem´-ber-ment): Amputation of an extremity or part of it.

disobliteration (dis-ob-lit-er-ā´-shun): Rebore. Removal of that which blocks a vessel, most often intimal plaques in an artery, when it is called endarterectomy (*q.v.*).

disorder (dis-or´-der): A disturbance or abnormality of physical or mental health or function.

disorientation (dis-or-i-en-tā´-shun): Loss of orientation (*q.v.*).

dispensary (dis-pen´-sa-ri): 1. A place where the indigent sick may receive medicines at little or no cost to them. 2. A pharmacy in a hospital or clinic where medicines are dispensed.

dispense (dis-pens´): To prepare and deliver medicines.

disposition (dis-pō-zish´un): A prevailing tendency, mood, attitude.

dissect (dis-sekt´): 1. To cut apart or separate; applied particularly to tissues of a cadaver for anatomical study. 2. In surgery, to separate a structure by cutting or tearing along the natural lines rather than by making a wide incision.

disseminated (dis-sem′-i-nā-ted): Widely extended, scattered or distributed.

dissociation (dis-sō-shi-ā′-shun): In psychiatry, an abnormal mental process by which the mind achieves non-recognition and isolation of certain unpalatable facts. This involves the actual splitting off from consciousness of all the unpalatable ideas so that the individual is no longer aware of them. D. is commonly observed in such involuntary states as hysteria, schizophrenia, fugue, somnambulism, and dual personality, but is seen in its most exaggerated form in delusional psychosis.

dissolution (dis-sō-lū′-shun): 1. The chemical separation of a compound into its component elements. 2. The liquefaction of a solid substance. 3. Death.

dissolve (di-zolv′): 1. To cause a substance to pass into solution by placing it in a solvent. 2. To melt or liquefy a substance.

dissonance (dis′-sō-nans): A combination of tones that produce harsh or disagreeable sounds.

dist: Abbreviation for distilled or distil.

distal (dis′-tal): Farthest from the head, center, or any point of reference. Located away from the center of the body.—distally, adv.; distad, adj. Cf. **proximal.**

distention (dis-ten′-shun): The state of being enlarged or distended. ABDOMINAL D., occurs after some operations when there is an abnormal accumulation of gas in the intestines.

distil, distill (dis-til′): To change a liquid to vapor by the application of heat, then by cooling change the vapor to a liquid.

distillation (dis-til-ā′-shun): The process of driving off gas or vapor by heating solids or liquids, and then condensing the resulting product(s).—distil, distill, v.t.

distortion (dis-tor′-shun): The state of being twisted out of the natural position or shape. In psychiatry, a mechanism through which material that is offensive to the superego is repressed or disguised so as to be acceptable.

distractibility (dis-trak′-ti-bil-i-ti): Inability to focus the attention on any one subject; susceptibility to distraction.

distress (dis-tres′): Anguish or suffering, physical or mental.

diuresis (dī-ū-rē′-sis): Increased secretion of urine.

diuretic (dī-ū-ret′-ik): 1. Increasing the flow of urine. 2. An agent which increases the flow of urine.

diurnal (dī-er′-nal): 1. Occurring or recur-

ring during the daytime. 2. Recurring every day.

divergence (dī-ver′-jens): A spreading out or drawing apart. In ophthalmology, the abduction of both eyes at the same time.

diversional (dī-ver′-zhen-al): Tending to produce relaxation or diversion. D. THERAPY, a pastime that causes a person to turn his thoughts away from himself and his problems.

diverticulitis (dī-ver-tik′-ū-lī′-tis): Inflammation of a diverticulum (q.v.).

diverticulosis (dī-ver-tik-ū-lō′-sis): A condition in which there are many diverticula, especially in the intestines.

diverticulum (dī-ver-tik′-ū-lum): A circumscribed pouch or sac of variable size protruding from the wall of a tube or hollow organ; occurs chiefly in the intestine, but also in the rest of the alimentary tract and the urinary tract. May be congenital or acquired.—diverticula, pl.

divulse (di-vuls′): To separate or pull apart forcibly.—divulsion, n.

dizziness (diz′-i-nes): A disturbed, unpleasant sense of one's relationship to space in which objects seem to whirl about. Giddiness; vertigo.—dizzy, adj.

DNA: Deoxyribonucleic acid (q.v.).

DOA: Abbreviation for dead on arrival.

dochmiasis (dōk-mī′-a-sis): Ancylostomiasis (q.v.).

Döderlein's bacillus (*Lactobacillus acidophilus*): Gram-positive rod bacterium which produces acid. Occurs in the normal vagina, and the *p*H of the vaginal secretions is largely due to the growth of the organism. Also found in the intestine in large numbers when diet is rich in milk or milk products. The bacillus is nonpathogenic. [Albert Döderlein, German obstetrician and gynecologist. 1860-1941.]

dolor (dō′-lor): Pain.

dominance (dom′-in-ans): 1. In genetics, the ability of one of a pair of genes to suppress the other (recessive) gene. 2. In neurology, the tendency of one side of the brain to be more important than the other in controlling certain functions.

dominant (dom′-in-ant): In genetics, refers to a character possessed by one parent, which in the offspring, masks the corresponding alternative character derived from the other parent. Opp. to recessive. See **Mendel's law.**

donee (dō-nē′): One who receives something from another, as blood in a transfusion.

donor (dō′-nor): One who supplies living tis-

sue or material to be used by another.
UNIVERSAL D., a person who has group O
blood which, in an emergency, can safely be
given to patients with blood of any type.

Donovan bodies: See **Leishman-Donovan.**

dopamine (dōp′-a-mēn): An intermediate
product in the synthesis of norephineph-
rine. It increases cardiac output and renal
blood flow but does not produce peripheral
vasoconstriction.

dorsad (dor′-sad): Toward the back.

dorsal (dor′-sal): Pertaining to the back, or
the posterior part of an organ. Opp. to ventral.

dorsalgia (dor-sal′-ji-a): Pain in the back.

dorsalis pedis (dor-sā′-lis pē′-dis): The
main artery on the upper side of the foot.

dorsiduct (dor′-si-dukt): To draw toward
the dorsum or the back.

dorsiflexion (dor-si-flek′-shun): Bending
backwards, as of the hand or foot. In the
case of the great toe—upwards. See **Babinski's reflex.**

dorsocentral (dor-sō-sen′-tral): At the back
and in the center.

dorsolumbar (dor-sō-lum′-bar): Referring
to the back in the region of the lower
thoracic and upper lumbar vertebrae.

dorsonasal (dor-sō-nā′-sal): Referring to
the bridge of the nose.

dorsum (dor′-sum): The back or the surface
that corresponds to the back.—dorsa, pl.

dosage (dō′-sij): 1. The determination of
the proper amount of a medicinal agent to
be given. 2. The giving of prescribed
amounts of a medicinal agent.

dose (dōs): A quantity of any therapeutic
agent to be given at any one time, as an
amount of medicine or a quantity of radiation. BOOSTER D., one given some time after a primary immunization to maintain
protection of the individual. DIVIDED D.,
one given in fractional amounts at specific
intervals. LETHAL D., one likely to cause
death. MAINTENANCE D., one given in pro-
tracted illness to keep the patient under an
influence achieved by an initial dose of a
drug. MAXIMUM D., the largest amount
that can be given with safety. MINIMUM D.,
the smallest one that will produce the
desired effect.

dossier (dōs′-ē-ā): The file that contains the
case history of a patient.

dotage (dō′-tij): Senility; feeblemindedness
in the aged.

dotard (dō′-tard): A person who is feebleminded from old age.

double blind: Descriptive of an experiment
in which neither the experimenter nor the
subject knows what is being used, e.g., an
experiment in which the effect of a certain
drug is being tested.

douche (doosh): A stream of water, gas or
vapor directed against the body externally
or into a body cavity.

Douglas' pouch: A cul-de-sac of the pelvic
cavity in the female, which lies between the
posterior surface of the uterus and the anterior surface of the rectum. [James
Douglas, anatomist and 'man-midwife.'
1675-1742.]

Down's syndrome: See **mongolism.**

dracontiasis (drā-kon-tī′-a-sis): Infestation
with the guinea worm (q.v.).

draft, draught (draft): 1. A current of air
circulating in a limited space. 2. A large
dose of liquid medicine to be taken at a
single swallow.

dragée (dra-zhā′): A large sugar-coated capsule or pill.

drain (drān): 1. To draw off by degrees an
accumulation of such material as pus,
lymph, or secretion. 2. A device or substance that provides a channel or means of
exit for the discharge from a wound or
cavity.

drainage (drān′-ij): The withdrawal or flow
of fluid from a wound or cavity. POSTURAL
D., that achieved by putting the patient in
a position in which gravity aids the process.
D. TUBE, one inserted into a body cavity to
facilitate escape of fluids.

dram, drachm: Sixty grains by weight; 60
minims by fluid measurement, or 1 teaspoonful.

drape (drāp): A sheet or other material used
to cover parts of the body that do not need
to be exposed for examination or carrying
out a procedure.—drape, v.t.

drastic (dras′-tik): Term applied to a treatment or medication that has a powerful or
thorough effect.

draw sheet: A narrow sheet placed crosswise of the bed to protect the lower sheet.
It can be removed when soiled by pulling
to the side.

dressing (dres′-ing): 1. Any material or
substance applied to a wound or lesion to
cover it, to prevent infection, to aid in healing, or to absorb drainage. 2. The application of any one of various materials to
protect or cover a wound or lesion.

dribble (drib′l): 1. To drool. 2. To fall in
drops, as urine from the bladder.

Drinker respirator: An alternate pressure
machine for administering artificial respi-

ration; often also called an iron lung.

drip: 1. To instill a medication drop by drop, as eye drops. 2. The slow continuous administration of a solution into a body cavity. INTRAVENOUS D. (IV), continuous drop-by-drop instillation of a solution into a vein; nutrients or drugs may be added to the sol. MURPHY D., continuous drop-by-drop instillation of fluid into the rectum. POSTNASAL D., dripping of irritating material from the posterior nares into the pharynx.

drive: 1. An urgent, instinctive need that causes one to press for its satisfaction, *e.g.,* the sex drive. 2. A powerful concern or interest that motivates one to consistent and continual effort.

drool: 1. To let saliva or other liquid run from the mouth. 2. To flow from the mouth, as saliva.

drop foot: An abnormal downward position of the foot due to paralysis of the flexors of the foot. Often due to pressure of bedclothes on the foot or to pressure from poorly fitting casts or splints. Also footdrop.

droplet (drop'-let): A very small drop. D. INFECTION, one transmitted by small droplets expelled when talking, sneezing or coughing.

dropsy (drop'-si): A popular term used to describe an abnormal accumulation of fluid in cellular tissue or a cavity. See **anasarca, ascites, hydrocephalus, hydrops, hydrothorax.**—dropsical, adj.

drop wrist: Flaccid paralysis of the wrist, usually due to injury to a nerve caused by fracture or trauma.

drug: A substance used in the diagnosis, prevention, or treatment of disease; often of vegetable or chemical origin. A medicine. D. ABUSE, misuse of a drug by a person whose pathological craving for it seems unrelated to his physical dependence on it. D. ADDICTION, see **addiction.** D. DEPENDENCE, state arising from repeated use of a drug over a period of time, and thus includes both drug abuse and drug addiction. Dependence on alcohol, the hallucinogens, opiates, narcotics, analgesics, tranquilizers, marihuana are forms of D. dependence. D. RESISTANCE, the ability of certain bacteria to develop the power to resist the bacteriostatic action of certain drugs.

drug-fast: A term used to describe resistance of bacteria to the bacteriostatic action of drugs.

drum: In anatomy, the ear drum or tympanic membrane.

DTP: Abbreviation for diphtheria and tetanus toxoids combined with pertussis vaccine, used for active immunization of normal infants and children.

DT's: Abbreviation for delirium tremens. See **delirium.**

Ducrey's bacillus (*Haemophilus ducreyi*) (dū-krāz'): Small gram-negative rod. The causative organism of soft chancre (chancroid), a venereal disease. [Augosto Ducrey, Italian dermatologist. 1860-1940.]

duct (dukt): A passage or tube, especially one for the passage of secretions or excretions.—ductal, adj.

ductless (dukt'-les): Having no duct, as the ductless glands. See **endocrine gland.**

ductus arteriosus (duk'-tus ar-tē-ri-ō'-sus): A blood vessel connecting the left pulmonary artery to the aorta, to bypass the lungs, in the fetal circulation. It normally closes at birth. PATENT D. A. is a form of congenital heart defect wherein this 'shunt' remains open.

ductus venosus (duk'-tus vē-nō'-sus): A blood vessel in the fetus; it connects the umbilical vein to the inferior vena cava, thus the venous blood bypasses the liver. It ceases to function at birth but remains in the liver as a ligament.

dull: 1. Lacking mental alertness. 2. Not sharp. 3. Not resonant, said of sounds heard on examination by percussion.

dumb (dum): Unable to speak.

dummy: Term sometimes used synonymously with placebo (*q.v.*).

'dumping syndrome': The name given to the symptoms which often follow a partial gastrectomy—bilious vomiting, nausea, sweating, palpitation, and a feeling of faintness and weakness after meals.

duodenitis (dū-od-e-nī'-tis): Inflammation of the duodenum.

duodenocholangeitis (dū-ō-dē-nō-kōl-an-jē-ī'-tis): Inflammation of the duodenum and the common bile duct.

duodenocholecystostomy (dū-ō-dē-nō-kō-lē-sis-tos'-tō-mi): Surgical creation of a passage between the gallbladder and the duodenum.

duodenojejunostomy (dū-ō-dē-nō-je-joo-nos'-to-mi): Surgical formation of a communication between the duodenum and the jejunum.

duodenostomy (dū-od-e-nos'-to-mi): Surgical creation of an opening into the duodenum with the establishment of a fistula between it and another cavity or the outside.

duodenum (dū-ō-dē′-num): The fixed, curved, first portion of the small intestine, connecting the stomach above to the jejunum below.—duodenal, adj.

dupp (dup): A syllable used to describe the second sound heard at the apex of the heart in auscultation. It is higher pitched and shorter than the first sound, lupp.

dura mater (dū′-ra mā′-ter): The outermost, fibrous, and toughest of the three meninges which surround the brain and spinal cord.—dural, adj.

dwarf (dwarf): An abnormally short or undersized person. Condition is found in achondroplasia, hypothyroidism (cretinism), congenital heart disease, etc.—dwarfism, n.

dyad (dī′-ad): A pair.—dyadic, adj.

dynamic (dī-nam′-ik): Pertinent to or having energy or force. D. PSYCHOLOGY, a psychological theory that stresses the element of energy in mental processes.

dynamometer (dī-na-mom′-et-er): An apparatus that measures the strength of a muscular contraction. SQUEEZE D., a D. that measures the strength of the grip.

dys-: Denotes painful, difficult, abnormal, diseased, impaired, faulty, poorly.

dysacousia (dis-a-koo′-zi-a): An impairment of hearing in which certain ordinary sounds produce pain or discomfort.

dysaphia (dis-ā′-fi-a): Impairment in the sense of touch (pressure).

dysarthria (dis-ar′-thri-a): 1. Difficulty in articulating words, due to a cerebellar disorder. Stammering. 2. Difficulty in articulating the joints; dysarthrosis.

dysarthrosis (dis-ar-thrō′-sis): Any joint condition limiting movement.

dysbasia (dis-bā′-zi-a): Difficulty in walking, particularly when it is due to a nervous system lesion.

dyschesia (dis-kē′-zi-a): Constipation with accumulation of feces in the rectum and difficult or painful defecation. Also dyschezia.

dyschondroplasia (dis-kon-drō-plā′-zi-a): A disease affecting the growth of long bones, metacarpals and phalanges; the cartilage develops regularly but ossifies very slowly thus arresting the growth of the long bones while the head and trunk develop normally. This produces a condition of stocky dwarfism.

dyschromatopsia (dis-krō-ma-top′-si-a): Disorder or impairment of color vision.

dyscoria (dis-kō′-rē-a): Abnormal shape, form or reaction of the pupil.

dyscrasia (dis-krā′-zi-a): A morbid general state resulting from the presence of toxic materials in the blood; an old term used to describe abnormality of the humors (q.v.) of the body. See **humoralism.** BLOOD D., usually refers to a diseased condition in which the abnormality of the blood cells is more or less permanent in character.

dysdipsia (dis-dip′-si-a): Difficulty in drinking.

dysentery (dis′-en-ter-i): Covers a variety of disorders that may be epidemic or endemic and that are characterized by inflammation and sometimes ulceration of the intestines accompanied by evacuation of stools containing blood and mucus and attended by colic and tenesmus. Causative agent is usually a bacterium, protozoon or parasitic worm that is spread chiefly through contaminated food or water. AMEBIC D. is caused by the *Entamoeba histolytica;* BACILLARY D. by a bacillus of the genus *Shigella.* See **amebiasis.**—dysenteric, adj.

dysesthesia (dis-es-thē′-zi-a): Impairment of touch sensation.

dysfunction (dis-fungk′-shun): Abnormal functioning of any organ or part.

dysgammaglobulinemia (dis-gam-ma-glob-ū-li-nē′-mi-a): Imperfect production or abnormality of the gamma globulins in the blood serum; often associated with poor resistance to infection.

dysgenesis (dis-jen′-e-sis): Malformation during embryonic development.—dysgenetic, adj.

dysgerminoma (dis-jer-mi-nō′-ma): A solid ovarian or testicular tumor of low grade malignancy. It is not hormone-secreting, as it is developed from cells which date back to the undifferentiated state of gonadal development, *i.e.,* before the cells have either male or female attributes.

dysgeusia (dis-gū′-si-a): Impairment in the sense of taste or perversion of taste; those affected say that all foods have a vile taste.

dysgraphia (dis-graf′-i-a): 1. Impairment of the power to write; often a result of a brain lesion. 2. Writer's cramp.

dyshidrosis (dis-hid-rō′-sis): 1. Any abnormality in the production of sweat. 2. A vesicular skin eruption, thought to be caused by a blockage of the sweat glands at their orifices; pompholyx (q.v.).

dyskinesia (dis-kī-nē′-zi-a): Impairment of voluntary movement.—dyskinetic, adj.

dyslalia (dis-lā′-li-a): Difficulty in talking due to defect of speech organs.—dyslalic, adj.

dyslexia (dis-leks′-i-a): Impairment of the ability to read understandingly; the child usually has difficulty with groups of letters, but the intelligence is unimpaired. Often associated with mirror-writing.—dyslexic, adj.

dysmaturity (dis-ma-tūr′-it-i): Signs and symptoms of growth retardation. 'Small for dates.'

dysmenorrhea (dis-men-ō-rē′-a): Painful or difficult menstruation.

dysmnesia (dis-nē′-si-a): Impairment of memory.

dysmorphogenic (dis-mor-fō-jen′-ik): Now preferred to teratogenic (see **teratogen**) when applied to drugs taken during pregnancy.

dysopia (dis-ō′-pi-a): 1. Painful or defective vision. 2. Any serious pathology of the eye or its accessory organs.

dysorexia (dis-o-rek′-si-a): An abnormal or unnatural appetite.

dysosteogenesis (dis-os-tē-ō-jen′-e-sis): Defective bone formation. Also dysostosis.

dyspareunia (dis-pa-rū′-ni-a): Painful or difficult coitus in women.

dyspepsia (dis-pep′-si-a): Disturbed digestion, characterized by heartburn, gas, nausea and a sense of over-fullness; indigestion. May be due to morbid condition of some part of the digestive system or to the psychic effects of emotional tension, anxiety, fits of temper, etc.

dysphagia (dis-fā′-ji-a): Painful or difficult swallowing.—dysphagic, adj.

dysphasia (dis-fā′-zi-a): Loss or impairment of power to use or understand language due to injury or damage to the brain.—dysphasic, adj.

dysphonia (dis-fō′-ni-a): Unnatural sound of the voice, as hoarseness, or difficulty in speaking; due to organic, functional, or psychic causes.

dysplasia (dis-plāz′-i-a): Abnormal development of organs, tissues or cells.—dysplastic, adj.

dyspnea (disp-nē′-a): Difficult or labored breathing.—dyspneic, adj.

dysrhythmia (dis-rith′-mi-a): Disordered or abnormal rhythm. CEREBRAL D., disturbance or irregularity of brain waves as recorded by electroencephalography.

dystaxia (dis-tak′-si-a): Difficulty in controlling voluntary movements.—dystaxic, adj.

dystocia (dis-tō′-si-a): Difficult or slow labor or delivery.

dystonia (dis-tō′-ni-a): Disordered or defective muscle tone.

dystopia (dis-tō′-pi-a): Displacement or malposition of an organ.—dystopic, adj.

dystrophia adiposogenitalis (dis-tro′-fi-a ad-i-pō-sō-jen-i-tāl′-is): See **Fröhlich's syndrome.**

dystrophy (dis′-trō-fi): Defective nutrition.—dystrophic, adj. MUSCULAR D., genetically determined primary degenerative myopathy.

dysuria (dis-ū′-ri-a): Difficult or painful urination.

E

Eagle test: A precipitation test for syphilis.
ear: The organ of hearing. EXTERNAL E., consists of the semicircular flap on the side of the head called the auricle or pinna and the external auditory meatus or canal that extends to the middle ear from which it is separated by the tympanum or ear drum. MIDDLE E., consists of an air-containing cavity, bounded laterally by the tympanum; anteriorly it communicates with the eustachian tube and thus with the throat. Stretched across this cavity are three tiny

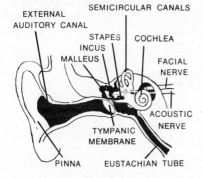

The ear

bones, the malleus, incus and stapes; these bones are in contact with the tympanic membrane and with one of the openings into the inner ear; their function is to transmit sound waves from the tympanum to the inner ear. INTERNAL or INNER E., the deepest part of the ear; consists of a bony labyrinth in which a similar membranous labyrinth is suspended in a fluid called perilymph. It is divided into the vestibule, cochlea and three semicircular canals and contains a fluid called endolymph. Its walls hold the endings of the nerve of hearing. E. DRUM, the membrane that separates the external from the middle ear; also called tympanic membrane, tympanum. E. LOBE, the lower, usually fleshy part of the pinna. E. PLUG, a small device of wax, rubber, or plastic worn in the external auditory canal to keep out noise, water when swimming, etc.
earwax: Cerumen (*q.v.*).

Eaton agent: Isolated in 1944 from secretions of patients with non-bacterial pneumonia and in 1962 identified as a member of PPLO group of organisms. Causes an acute pneumonitis that sometimes progresses to bronchitis or pneumonia, *e.g.,* primary atypical pneumonia, Eaton agent pneumonia. See **PPLO.**
Eberth's bacillus: *Salmonella typhosa,* the causative agent of typhoid fever. [Karl J. Eberth, German physician. 1835-1926.]
ebonation (ē-bō-nā′-shun̯): Removal of bone fragments from a wound after an injury.
ebriety (ē-brī′-e-ti): Drunkenness. Also inebriety, ebrietas.
ebullition (eb-ū-lish′-un): The state or process of boiling; effervescence.
eburnation (ē-bur-nā′-shun): A disease condition in which bone becomes dense and hard like ivory.
ecbolic (ek-bol′-ik): Any agent that stimulates contraction of the gravid uterus and hastens expulsion of its contents.
ecchondroma (ek-kon-drō′-ma): A benign tumor composed of cartilage that protrudes from the surface of the bone in which it arises. Also ecchondrosis.
ecchymoma (ek-i-mō′-ma): A slight hematoma or swelling due to a bruise and resulting from subcutaneous extravasation of blood.
ecchymosis (ek-i-mō′-sis): An extravasation of blood under the skin; marked by purple discoloration gradually changing to brown, green, yellow. Syn., bruise.—ecchymoses, pl.; ecchymosed, ecchymotic, adj.
ecdemic (ek-dem′-ik): Neither epidemic nor endemic. A disease that is carried to an area from without.
ECG: Abbreviation for electrocardiogram. Also EKG.
Echinococcus (ek-ī′-nō-kok′-us): A genus of tapeworms, the adults infesting a primary host, *e.g.,* a dog. In man (secondary host) the encysted larvae cause 'hydatid disease.'
echoencephalography (ek-ō-en-sef-a-log′-ra-fi): The passing of penetrating sound waves (ultrasound) across the head; useful in detecting abscess, blood clot, injury, or tumor within the brain.

echolalia (ek-ō-lā′-li-a): Pathologic, meaningless repetition of words or phrases heard. Occurs most commonly in schizophrenia and dementia; sometimes in toxic delirious states. A characteristic of all infants' speech.—echolalic, adj.

echophony (ek-of′-o-ni): The echo of a vocal sound heard during auscultation of the chest.

echopraxia (ek-ō-prak′-si-a): Pathologic, involuntary repetition of acts one has seen performed by others; often performed without any expression or emotion.—echopractic, adj.

ECHO viruses: Enteric Cytopathic Human Orphan. Given this name because these viruses were originally found in the stools of diseaseless children. They have caused non-bacterial meningitis, enteritis, and various infections with and without fever and/or rash.

eclampsia (ek-lamp′-si-a): 1. A severe manifestation of toxemia of pregnancy, often accompanied by convulsions and sometimes coma; associated with hypertension, edema or proteinuria. May also occur during the puerperium. 2. A sudden convulsive attack.—eclamptic, adj.

ecmnesia (ek-nē′-zi-a): Impaired memory for recent events with normal memory of remote ones. Common in old age and in early cerebral deterioration.

ecology (ē-kol′-o-ji): The science that deals with the interactions of organisms with their environments and with each other.

écraseur (ā-kra-zer′): An instrument with a wire loop that can be tightened around the pedicle of a new growth so as to sever it.

ecstasy (ek′-sta-sē): A state of exaltation, exhilaration or delight; a trance.—ecstatic, adj.

ecstrophy (ek′-strō-fī): Exstrophy (*q.v.*).

ECT Abbreviation for electroconvulsive therapy. See **electrotherapy.**

ect-, ecto-: Denotes: (1) external, outside; (2) out of place.

ectasia (ek-tā′-si-a): An overstretching or dilatation of a tubular organ or vessel. See **bronchiectasis.**

-ectasia, -ectasis: Denotes dilatation, stretching.

ecthyma (ek-thī′-ma): An eruption of impetigo contagiosa on the thighs and legs, most often seen in children and characterized by large flat pustules with hardened bases and thick brownish crusts that heal with pigmented scars. A similar condition occurs in syphilis.

ectocardia (ek-tō-kar′-di-a): A congenital condition in which the heart is misplaced, either within or without the thoracic cavity.

ectoderm (ek′-tō-derm): The external primitive germ layer of the embryo. From it are developed the skin structures, the nervous system, organs of special sense, mucous membrane of the mouth and anus, pineal gland and part of the pituitary and adrenal glands.—ectodermal, adj.

ectodermosis (ek-tō-der′-mō-sis): Any disease or disorder due to congenital maldevelopment of an organ or tissue derived from the ectoderm, *e.g.*, skin, eyeball, retina, nervous system.

ectogenous (ek-toj′-e-nus): 1. Introduced from or originating outside of the body. 2. Capable of developing apart from the host; said of bacteria, particularly the pathogens.—ectogenic, adj.

-ectomy: Denotes a cutting out; surgical removal.

ectoparasite (ek-tō-par′-a-sīt): A parasite that lives on the exterior surface of its host. —ectoparasitic, adj.

ectopia (ek-tō′-pi-a): Malposition of an organ or structure, usually congenital. E. VESICAE, an abnormally placed urinary bladder which protrudes through or opens on to the abdominal wall.—ectopic, adj.

ectopic (ek-top′-ik): Situated outside of the normal position, said of an organ or part; may be congenital or acquired. E. PREGNANCY, extrauterine pregnancy; the fertilized ovum fails to reach the uterus but becomes implanted elsewhere; in most cases the site is the fallopian tube but sometimes it is the peritoneal cavity. At about the 6th week of pregnancy, the tube ruptures causing a surgical emergency. This is a serious condition and may be accompanied by severe pain, shock and intra-abdominal hemorrhage. Prognosis is good if diagnosis and treatment are early, poor if treatment is omitted or unduly delayed.

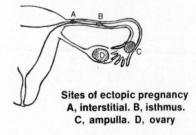

**Sites of ectopic pregnancy
A, interstitial. B, isthmus.
C, ampulla. D, ovary**

ectoplasm (ek'-tō-plazm): The outer layer of protoplasm of a cell.

ectozoa (ek-tō-zō'-a): Animal parasites living on the outside of the body of the host.—ectozoon, sing.

ectrodactylia (ek-trō-dak-til'-i-a): Congenital absence of one or more fingers or toes or parts of them.

ectromelia (ek-trō-mē'-li-a): Congenital absence of one or more of the long limb bones. Also, congenital absence of one or more of the limbs. See **amelia.**

ectropion (ek-trō'-pi-on): An abnormal turning out of a part, as of an eyelid.

eczema (ek'-ze-ma): An all-inclusive term used to describe a non-catagious condition of the skin; may be acute or chronic. Characterized by redness; inflammation; swelling; itching; formation of vesicles, papules, or pustules that discharge and later become scaly and crusted. Cause is unknown but the condition is usually associated with allergies, drug sensitivity, fungus infection, nutritional deficiency, uncleanliness. IN-FANTILE E., an allergic E. of infants from about two months to two years, often limited to forehead and cheeks; very irritating; due to an allergy to foods, baby oil or powder, etc.—eczematous, eczematoid, adj.

edema (e-dē'-ma): Dropsy. The accumulation of abnormally large amounts of fluid in the intercellular tissue spaces. AN-GIONEUROTIC E., localized, acute, transitory edematous areas appear in the skin due to allergy to a protein; may also be of neurotic origin. CARDIAC E., due to failure of the blood to reach the kidney for filtration; most marked in the extremities. HEPATIC E., that caused by osmotic pressure changes in the blood. NUTRITIONAL E. occurs in starvation or prolonged malnutrition; results from protein deprivation. PULMO-NARY E., a form of waterlogging of the lungs resulting from left ventricular failure or mitral stenosis. RENAL E., results from disturbed kidney function in nephritis. SUBCUTANEOUS E., that which is demonstrable by the 'pits' produced when pressure is applied with a finger. Generalized edema is called **anasarca.**—edematous, adj.

edentulous (e-den'-tū-lus): Without teeth.

Edmonton vaccine: A live-virus vaccine against measles; may be given with gamma globulin (*q.v.*) to minimize the febrile response that often occurs about a week after administration.

EEG: Abbreviation for electroencephalogram.

effector (e-fek'-tor): A motor or secretory nerve ending in a muscle, gland or organ. Opp. to receptor.

efferent (ef'-er-ent): Carrying, conveying, or conducting away from a center. Opp. to afferent. E. NERVE, one that conveys impulses away from the central nervous system to a part of the body such as a muscle or gland.

effervescent (ef-er-ves'-ent): Bubbling, foaming; giving off gas bubbles.

effleurage (ef-loo-razh'): A long, deep or superficial stroking movement used in massage.

efflorescent (ef-lō-res'-ent): Descriptive of a crystalline substance that has become dry and powdery due to loss of water content.

effort syndrome: A form of anxiety neurosis, manifesting itself in a variety of cardiac symptoms including precordial pain, for which there is no pathological explanation.

effusion (e-fū'-zhun): Extravasation or escape of fluid into a tissue or cavity; may be serous, bloody, or purulent. HEMOR-RHAGIC E., occurs when a blood vessel ruptures. PLEURAL E., presence of fluid in the space between the lungs and pleura. PUL-MONARY E., the presence of fluid in the air sacs and interstitial tissue of the lung.

egesta (e-jes'-ta): Excreta.

ego (e'-gō): 1. Self-esteem. 2. In psychology, refers to the unconscious self, the 'I,' that part of personality that deals with reality and is influenced by social forces. It modifies behavior by unconscious compromise between the primitive instinctual urges (the id), internalized parental and social prohibitions (the superego), and reality.

egocentric (e-gō-sen'-trik): Self-centered in the extreme.

egomania (e-gō-mā'-ni-a): Morbid preoccupation with self.

egotistic (e-gō-tis'-tik): Conceited; vain.

Ehrlich's theory of immunity: Postulated that tissue cells receive molecules of antigen by means of receptors. Under certain conditions these receptors are over-produced and released into the body fluids. The free receptor groups become the antibodies and are capable of combining specifically with antigen molecules. E.'S '606,' Salvarsan, discovered in 1909 as a result of the 606th experiment. [Paul Ehrlich, German bacteriologist. 1854-1915.]

eiweissmilch (ī'-vīs-milkh): A preparation for infant feeding; consists of milk with added casein and calcium oxide and a reduced amount of lactose. Used in nutritional disturbances.

ejaculation (ē-jak-ū-lā′-shun): A sudden emission or expulsion, as of semen.

ejaculatory ducts (ē-jak′-ū-la-tor-i dukts): Two fine tubes, one on either side, commencing at the union of the seminal vesicle with the vas deferens, and terminating at their union with the prostatic urethra.

EKG: Abbreviation for electrocardiogram. Also ECG.

Elastoplast: Trademark for a type of elastic bandage made of cotton cloth without rubber; has porous, adhesive, non-fray edges.

elation (ē-lā′-shun): Joyfulness; excitement that is marked by increased physical and mental activity. It becomes pathological when not consistent with the patient's circumstances.

elbow: The joint between the arm and forearm. E. JERK, involuntary bending of the elbow when the triceps muscle is struck suddenly. MINER'S E., inflammation and enlargement of the bursa over the tip of the elbow caused by leaning on the elbow while digging. When seen in students it is called STUDENT'S E. TENNIS E., radiohumeral bursitis; inflammation of the epicondyle of the humerus; occurs in those who engage in certain sports including tennis; due to repeated sudden, jerky, vigorous movement of the extended forearm.

elective (ē-lek′-tiv): Term applied to procedures, usually surgical, that may be advantageous to the patient but not necessary to save his life; either the physician or the patient may make the choice.

Electra complex (e-lek′-tra kom′-plex): Term derived from Greek mythology. Refers to excessive fondness of a daughter for her father. The female counterpart of the Oedipus complex (*q.v.*).

electrocardiogram (ē-lek-trō-kar′-di-ō-gram): A graphic record of the electric current produced by the contraction of the heart muscle; obtained with the electrocardiograph (*q.v.*). Abbreviated EKG.

electrocardiograph (ē-lek-trō-kar′-di-ō-graf): An instrument containing a string galvanometer through which passes the electrical current produced by the heart's contraction. A permanent record (electrocardiogram) of these oscillations is made on a moving drum of graph paper.
—electrocardiographic, adj.; electrocardiographically, adv.

electrocautery (ē-lek-trō-kaw′-ter-i): A platinum wire that is heated by electricity and used for cauterizing tissue. See **cautery.**

electrocoagulation (ē-lek-trō-kō-ag-ū-lā′-shun): A technique of surgical diathermy. Coagulation of bleeding points, or hardening of tumors or diseased tissue by the application of electricity.

electroconvulsive shock therapy (ē-lek-trō-kon-vul′-siv): See **electroshock therapy.**

electrocorticography (ē-lek-trō-kor-ti-kog′-ra-fi): An electroencephalogram in which the electrodes are attached directly to the cortex of the brain.—electrocorticographic, adj.; electrocorticographically, adv.

electrode (ē-lek′-trōd): In electrotherapy, a conductor in the form of a pad or plate whereby electricity enters or leaves the body.

electrodesiccation (ē-lek-trō-des-i-kā′-shun): A technique of surgical diathermy in which a high-frequency current is applied to tissue with a needle electrode; there is drying and subsequent removal of the tissue.

electrodiagnosis (ē-lek-trō-dī-ag-nō′-sis): The use of graphic recordings of electrical irritability of tissues in diagnosis.—electrodiagnostic, adj.

electroencephalogram (ē-lek-trō-en-sef′-a-lō-gram): A graphic record made with the electroencephalograph (*q.v.*).

electroencephalograph (ē-lek-trō-en-sef′-a-lō-graf): An instrument for obtaining a recording of the electric currents developed in the brain by means of electrodes that may be attached to the scalp or the surface of the brain, or placed within the substance of the brain. The record is an electroencephalogram (EEG). Useful in studying some forms of mental disorder and brain functions.—electroencephalographic, adj.; electroencephalographically, adv.

electrohemostasis (ē-lek-trō-hē-mos′-ta-sis): The arrest of hemorrhage by the use of electrocautery.

electrolysis (ē-lek-trol′-i-sis): 1. Chemical decomposition of a substance by passing an electric current through it. 2. Destruction and permanent removal of hairs (epilation), moles, spider nevi, etc. by means of electricity.

electrolyte (ē-lek′-trō-līt): A liquid or solution of a substance that is capable of conducting electricity and is decomposed by it. The chemical change that takes place as the current passes through the substance is called 'electrolysis.' E. BALANCE, a normal state in which there is correct balance between the positive and negative ions in the body fluids, tissues and blood.—electrolytic, adj.

electromyography (ē-lek-trō-mī-og′-ra-fĭ): Graphic recording of electrical currents generated when a muscle contracts as a result of the application of an electric stimulus. EMG.—electromyogram, n.; electromyographical, adj.; electromyographically, adv.

electron (ē-lek′-tron): The unit of negative electricity that, revolving around a nucleus of positive electricity, constitutes the atom. Thought to be the ultimate constituent of all matter. E. MICROSCOPE, a modern M. that differs from the ordinary M. in several ways; in particular, instead of using ordinary light it utilizes electron beams that have a much shorter wave length than ordinary visible light and this allows for much greater magnification.

electronarcosis (ē-lek-trō-nar-kō′-sis): Narcosis or unconsciousness produced by passing an electric current through the brain. Used in treating certain mental disorders.

electronic (ē-lek-tron′-ik): Relating to or carrying electrons (q.v.), or referring to devices that operate on the principles of electronics (q.v.).

electronics (ē-lek-tron′-iks): A special branch of physics that deals with the behavior of electrons in gases or vacuums, and with the operation and functioning of electronic devices.

electrophoresis (ē-lek-trō-fō-rē′-sis): Migration of colloidal particles in solution to the positive or negative pole when an electric current is passed through it.

electroplexy (ē-lek′-trō-plek-si): Electric shock; may be intentional as in electroshock therapy or accidental by lightning or electrocution.

electropyrexia (ē-lek-trō-pī-rek′-si-a): High body temperature produced by a special electrical apparatus. Used in fever therapy.

electroradiology (ē-lek-trō-rā-di-ol′-ō-ji): The branch of medicine that deals with the use of electricity and x-ray in the treatment of disease.

electroretinogram (ē-lek-trō-ret′-i-nō-gram): Graphic record of electrical currents generated in the active retina after stimulation by light. Abbreviated ERG.

electroshock (ē-lek′-trō-shok): Shock produced by applying an electric current to the brain. E. THERAPY, the treatment of mental disorders by the induction of coma through the use of an electric current.

electrosurgery (ē-lek-trō-ser′-jer-i): The use of electricity in surgery, e.g., the electric knife, electric needle, or hot electric wire.

electrotherapy (ē-lek-trō-ther′-a-pi): Treatment of disease by means of electricity, e.g., diathermy, electroshock therapy. Also electrotherapeutics.

element (el′-e-ment): One of the constituents of a compound. The elements are the primary substances which in pure form, or combined into compounds, constitute all matter. In chemistry, an E. is a simple substance made up of like atoms and which cannot be broken down or decomposed by chemical means.—elementary, adj.

elephantiasis (el-e-fan-tī′-a-sis): A chronic disease, usually of the tropics, caused by an obstruction in the lymphatics. Often due to filaria (q.v.) but in non-tropical areas may occur as a result of syphilis or recurrent streptococcal infections. Characterized by thickening and hardening of the skin and subcutaneous tissues and hypertrophy of the affected areas; legs and external genitalia most often affected. Also Barbados leg, pachydermia.—elephantoid, elephantiasic, adj.

elimination (ē-lim-i-nā′-shun): The removal of wastes from the body.

elixir (ē-liks′-er): A clear, sweetened, flavored, often alcoholic, solution containing a drug.

elliptocytosis (ē-lip-tō-sī-tō′-sis): A rare hereditary type of anemia in which the red blood cells are oval in shape.

emaciation (e-mā-shi-ā′-shun): Excessive leanness, or wasting of body tissue.—emaciate, v.t.

emanation (em-a-nā′-shun): 1. Exhalation. 2. That which is given off, such as the gaseous disintegration products of radioactive substances.

emasculation (e-mas-kū-lā′-shun): Castration.

embalm (em-balm′): To treat a dead body with preservatives to prevent its decay.

embolectomy (em-bō-lek′-to-mi): Surgical removal of an embolus.

embolic (em-bol′-ik): Pertaining to an embolism or an embolus.

embolism (em′-bō-lizm): The sudden obstruction of a blood vessel by a solid body brought to the site by the blood current. See **embolus.**

embolus (em′bō-lus): A body such as a clot

or an air bubble transported in the circulation until it causes obstruction by blocking a blood vessel. Besides clots and air bubbles, emboli may consist of masses of bacteria, parasites, tissue fragments, or fat globules. —emboli, pl.

embryo (em′-brē-ō): The early stage in the development of any organism, particularly one that is produced by the fertilization of an egg. In human anatomy the term is applied to the developing ovum in the first two months or until it shows human characteristics, after which it is called a fetus. —embryonal, embryonic, adj.

embryology (em-brē-ol′-o-ji): Study of the development of an organism from fertilization to extrauterine life.—embryological, adj.; embryologically, adv.

embryoma (em-brē-ō′-ma): Teratoma (*q.v.*).

embryopathy (em-brē-op′-a-thi): A disease or abnormal condition resulting from interference with the development of the embryo or fetus. More serious if it occurs during the first three months. Includes the 'rubella syndrome,' anomalies that occur in the fetus as a result of the mother's having had German measles early in pregnancy.

embryotomy (em-brē-ot′-o-mi): Mutilation of the fetus to facilitate removal from uterus when natural birth is impossible.

emesis (em′-e-sis): Vomiting.

-emesis: Denotes vomiting.

emetic (ē-met′-ik): 1. Causing vomiting. 2. Any agent used to produce vomiting.

-emia: Denotes: (1) blood; (2) a condition of the blood.

eminence (em′-i-nens): A prominence or projection, especially on the surface of a bone.

emission (ē-mish′-un): An ejaculation or sending forth, specifically an involuntary ejaculation of semen.

emmenagogue (ē-men′-a-gog): An agent or measure used to regulate or induce menstruation.

emmenia (ē-mē′-ni-a): The menses (*q.v.*).

emmetropia (em-e-trō′-pi-a): Normal or perfect vision.—emmetropic, adj.

emollient (ē-mol′-i-ent): An agent that softens and soothes skin or mucous membrane.

emotion (ē-mō′-shun): A strong feeling such as fear, anger, grief, joy, or love, or an aroused mental state recognized in ourselves by certain bodily changes, and in others by certain characteristic behavior. Aroused usually by ideas or concepts.

emotional (ē-mō′-shun-al): Characteristic of or caused by emotion. E. BIAS, tendency of E. attitude to affect logical judgment. E. STATE, effect of emotions on normal mood, *e.g.*, agitation.

empathy (em′-pa-thi): The ability to perceive and share the feelings of another through insightful awareness of that person's feelings and emotions and what they mean. To be distinguished from sympathy.

emphysema (em-fi-sē′-ma): Gaseous distension of the tissues. PULMONARY E., alveolar distension: (1) generalized—often accompanies chronic bronchitis; (2) localized —either distal to partial obstruction of a bronchus or bronchiole (obstructive E.) or in alveoli adjacent to a segment of collapsed lung (compensatory E.). SURGICAL E., air in the subcutaneous tissue planes following trauma by surgery or injury.—emphysematous, adj.

empirical (em-pir′-i-kal): Based on observation and experience and not on scientific reasoning.—empiricism, n.

emprosthotonos (em-pros-thot′-o-nos): A tetanic spasm in which the body becomes tense and the feet and head are brought forward; when face downward, the body is incurving with only the forehead and feet touching the bed. The position is opposite to that seen in opisthotonos (*q.v.*).

empyema (em-pī-ē′-ma): A collection of pus in a cavity, hollow organ or space; when unspecified refers to pus in the pleural cavity.—empyemic, adj.

emulsion (ē-mul′-shun): A fluid containing fat or oil particles in a state of fine subdivision and suspension, so that a smooth, milky white fluid results.

enamel (en-am′-el): The hard external covering of the crown of a tooth.

enanthem (en-an′-them), **enanthema** (en-an-thē′-ma): An eruption on a mucous surface, *e.g.*, strawberry tongue in scarlet fever or Koplik's spots in measles.—enanthematous, adj.

enarthrosis (en-ar-thrō′-sis): A ball and socket joint such as the hip joint.

encanthis (en-can′-this): A small neoplasm or excrescence at the inner canthus of the eye.

encapsulation (en-kap-sū-lā′-shun): Enclosure within a capsule.

encephal-, encephala-, encephalo-: Denotes the brain.

encephalalgia (en-sef-a-lal′-ji-a): Pain in the head.

encephalitis (en-sef-a-lī′-tis): Inflammation of the brain; may be a specific disease or occur as a sequel of another disease. Characterized by headache, malaise, fever, slowed mental and motor responses and stuporous sleep. E. EQUINE, once thought to be a disease of horses, but now known to be transmitted to man by vectors such as mosquitoes. E. LETHARGICA, a sporadic and occasionally epidemic form of virus infection. Profound cerebral damage with cranial nerve palsies, stupor and delirium can occur. Reversal of sleep rhythm common. May be followed by alteration of personality or Parkinson's disease (q.v.).

encephalocele (en-sef′-a-lō-sēl): Hernia of the brain with protrusion of the brain substance through an opening in the skull. Often associated with hydrocephalus when the protrusion occurs at a suture line.

encephalogram (en-sef′-a-lō-gram): An x-ray picture of the contents of the skull. See **pneumoencephalogram.**

encephalography (en-sef-a-log′-ra-fi): Roentgenology of the skull contents, particularly of the brain. See **pneumoencephalography.**

encephaloma (en-sef-a-lō′-ma): A tumor within the brain.—encephalomata, pl.

encephalomalacia (en-sef-a-lō-mal-ā′-shi-a): Softening of the brain.

encephalomeningitis (en-sef-a-lō-men-in-jī′-tis): Inflammation of the brain and its meninges.

encephalomeningocele (en-sef-a-lō-me-nin′-jō-sel): Protrusion of cerebral membranes and brain substance through a defect in the bones of the skull.

encephalomyelitis (en-sef-a-lō-mī-e-lī′-tis): Inflammation of the brain and spinal cord.

encephalomyelopathy (en-sef-a-lō-mī-e-lop′-a-thi): Disease affecting both brain and spinal cord.—encephalomyelopathic, adj.

encephalon (en-sef′-a-lon): The brain.

encephalopathy (en-sef-a-lop′-a-thi): Any disease or dysfunction of the brain.—encephalopathic, adj.

encephalorrhagia (en-sef-a-lō-rā′-ji-a): Hemorrhage from the brain or within it.

encephalosclerosis (en-sef-a-lō-skler-ō′-sis): Hardening of the brain.

enchondroma (en-kon-drō′-ma): A benign cartilaginous tumor occurring in a part where cartilage is not normally found or within a bone near the epiphyseal line.—enchondromata, pl.; enchondromatous, adj.

encopresis (en-kō-prē′-sis): Involuntary passage of feces not due to disease or organic defect.—encopretic, adj.; n.

encysted (en-sis′-ted): Enclosed in a cyst or sac or surrounded by a membrane.

end-, endo-: Denotes within, inside.

Endamoeba: See **Entamoeba.**

endarterectomy (end-ar-ter-ek′-to-mi): Surgical removal of atheromatous plaques or of the thickened atheromatous tunica intima of an artery.

endarteritis (end-ar-ter-ī′-tis): Inflammation of the tunica intima or lining coat of an artery. E. OBLITERANS, a form of E. in which the lumina of smaller vessels become obliterated.

endaural (end-awr′-al): Pertaining to the inner portion of the external auditory canal.

end bulb: A term used to describe certain sensory nerve endings in some areas of the skin or mucous membrane.

endemic (en-dēm′-ik): Peculiar to a certain area; said of diseases that are habitually present within a given locality.

endemiology (en-dēm-i-ol′-o-ji): The special study of endemic diseases.

endermic (en-der′-mik): Acting by absorption through the skin; an agent that acts by absorption through the skin.

endocarditis (en-dō-kar-dī′-tis): Inflammation of the inner lining of the heart and/or the covering of the valves of the heart; most commonly due to rheumatic fever. ACUTE E., the nonbacterial E. often due to rheumatic fever. ACUTE BACTERIAL E., caused by pyogenic organisms, usually streptococcus, pneumococcus, meningococcus, gonococcus; rapidly progressive; often fatal. SUBACUTE BACTERIAL E., usually due to *Streptococcus viridans;* gradual onset; usually confined to the valves; seen most often in young adults. VALVULAR E., affects one or more of the heart valves.

endocardium (en-dō-kar′-di-um): The thin serous membrane lining the chambers of the heart and covering the surfaces of the heart valves. It is continuous with the lining of the vessels entering and leaving the heart.

endocervicitis (en-dō-ser-vi-sī′-tis): Inflammation of the mucous membrane lining the cervix of the uterus.

endocervix (en-dō-ser′-vix): The lining of the cervix of the uterus.—endocervical, adj.

endocrine (en′-dō-krēn): Secreting within; term applied to the ductless glands of the body whose function is to secrete substances that pass directly from the gland into the blood or lymph and which affect the functioning of another organ(s) or part. Opp. to exocrine.—endocrinal, adj. E. GLANDS include pineal, pituitary, thyroid, parathyroid, thymus, adrenals, ovaries, testes, pancreas. E. THERAPY, treatment with endocrine preparations. E. SECRETIONS, those produced by endocrine glands; they have important influence on metabolic processes. E. SYSTEM, all of the glands that deliver their secretions directly into the bloodstream.

endocrinology (en-dō-krin-ol'-o-ji): The study of the ductless glands and their internal secretions.

endocrinopathy (en-dō-krin-op'-ath-i): Abnormality or disease of one or more of the endocrine glands, or abnormality of their secretions.

endoderm (en'-dō-derm): The inner layer of cells that forms during the early development of the embryo.—endodermal, adj.

endogenous (en-doj'-e-nus): Originating within a structure, organ, or organism, as contrasted with exogenous.

endolymph (en'-dō-limf): The fluid contained in the membranous labyrinth of the internal ear.

endolysin (en-dol'-i-sin): An intracellular, leukocytic substance that destroys engulfed bacteria.

endometrioma (en-dō-mē-tri-ō'-ma): A tumor containing shreds of misplaced endometrium; found most frequently in the ovary. Adenomyoma (*q.v.*). See **cyst** (chocolate).—endometriomata, pl.

endometriosis (en-dō-mē-tri-ō'-sis): The presence of endometrium in abnormal sites. See **cyst** (chocolate).

endometritis (en-dō-mē-trī'-tis): Inflammation of the endometrium.

endometrium (en-dō-mē'tri-um): The lining mucosa of the uterus.—endometrial, adj.

endomorph (en'-dō-morf): An individual whose body build differs from the normal in that the digestive viscera are large, there are accumulations of fat about the abdomen, the trunk and thighs are large and the extremities are tapering.—endomorphic, adj.

endomyocarditis (en-dō-mī-ō-kar-dī'-tis): Inflammation of both the inner lining and muscular portions of the heart.

endomysium (en-dō-mis'-i-um): The delicate connective tissue sheath that surrounds individual muscle fibers within a fasciculus and serves to support blood vessels and nerves that branch between the fibers.

endoneurium (en-dō-nū'-ri-um): The delicate, inner connective tissue surrounding the nerve fibers.

endoparasite (en'-dō-par'-a-sīt): Any parasite living within its host.—endoparasitic, adj.

endophlebitis (en-dō-flē-bī'-tis): Inflammation of the internal lining of a vein.

endophthalmitis (en-dof-thal-mī'-tis): Inflammation of any of the internal structures of the eye. May occur as a complication of such infections as pneumonia or measles or as a result of a perforating injury.

endoplasm (en'-dō-plazm): The central more fluid portion of a unicellular organism, as distinguished from the ectoplasm (*q.v.*).

end organ: An encapsulated structure containing the terminal part of a sensory nerve fibril in muscle tissue, skin, mucous membrane or a gland.

endoscope (en'-dō-skōp): A tubular, lighted instrument for visualization of body cavities or organs.—endoscopic, adj.; endoscopy, n.

endospore (en'-dō-spōr): A bacterial spore that has a purely vegetative function. It is formed by the loss of water and probable rearrangement of the protein of the cell, so that metabolism is minimal and resistance to environmental conditions, especially high temperature, desiccation and antibacterial drugs, high. The only genera which include pathogenic species that form spores are *Bacillus* and *Clostridium*.

endosteitis (en-dos-tē-ī'-tis): Inflammation of the endosteum (*q.v.*).

endosteoma (en-dos-tē-ō'-ma): A tumor in the medullary canal of a bone.

endosteum (en-dos'-tē-um): The thin vascular connective tissue lining the medullary canal of a long bone.

endothelioid (en-do-thē'-li-oid): Resembling endothelium.

endothelioma (en-dō-thē-li-ō'-ma): A tumor derived from the epithelial cells that make up the lining of blood or lymph vessels or serous cavities; may be benign or malignant.

endothelium (en-dō-thē'-li-um): The lining membrane of serous cavities, heart, blood and lymph vessels.—endothelial, adj.

endotoxin (en-dō-tok'sin): A toxic product of bacteria which is associated with the structure of the cell, and can only be obtained by destruction of the cell.—endotoxic, adj. Opp. to exotoxin.

endotracheal (en-dō-trā'kē-al): Within the trachea.

endotracheitis (en-dō-trā-kē-ī'-tis): Inflammation of the mucosa of the trachea.

endotrachelitis (en-dō-trā-kel-ī′-tis): Inflammation of the membrane lining the uterine cervix.

enema (en′-e-ma): The injection of a liquid into the rectum, to be returned or retained. It can be further designated according to the function of the fluid: to promote evacuation of feces; to provide nutrients or medicinal substances; to introduce opaque material in x-ray examination of the lower intestinal tract.

energy (en′-er-ji): The capacity to do work; manifested in various forms such as motion, light, heat.

enervation (en-er-vā′-shun): 1. General weakness; loss of strength; lack of vigor or nervous energy. 2. Removal of a nerve or part of one.

engagement (en-gāj′-ment): In obstetrics, the entrance of the presenting part of the fetus into the superior pelvic strait. The beginning of the descent through the pelvic canal. Usually occurs about the fourth week before delivery and often accompanied by a sensation called 'lightening.'

engorged (en-gorjd′): Distended or swollen with blood or other fluid; term is applied to a tissue, an organ or a vessel.—engorgement, n.

engram (en′-gram): An enduring mark or trace. In psychology, a lasting impression made by an experience.

enophthalmos (en-of-thal′-mos): Abnormal retraction of an eyeball within its orbit.

enostosis (en-os-tō′-sis): A bony growth within the medullary canal of a bone. See **exostosis**.

ensiform (en′-si-form): Sword-shaped. Term applied to the process at the lower end of the breast bone. Syn., xiphoid.

entamebiasis (en-ta-me-bī′-a-sis): Infestation with a species of the Entamoeba; amebic dysentery.

Entamoeba (en-ta-mē′-ba): A genus of protozoon parasites, some species of which affect man. E. COLI, nonpathogenic, infests the human intestinal tract. E. GINGIVALIS, infests the mouth about the gums and found in tartar on teeth. E. HYSTOLYTICA, pathogenic; causes amebic dysentery (*q.v.*).

enter-, entero-: Denotes intestine.

enteral (en′-ter-al): Within the gastrointestinal tract, as distinguished from parenteral.

enteralgia (en-ter-al′-ji-a): Abdominal pain; cramps; colic.

enterectasis (en-ter-ek′-ta-sis): Distention or dilatation of the small intestine.

enterectomy (en-ter-ek′-to-mi): Surgical removal of part of the small intestine.

enteric (en-ter′-ik): Pertaining to the intestine. E. COATED, a pill or other medicine that is coated with a substance that will not dissolve until it reaches the intestine. E. FEVER, includes typhoid and paratyphoid fever (*q.v.*).

enteritis (en-ter-ī′-tis): Inflammation of the intestine, the small intestine in particular.

enteroanastomosis (en′-ter-ō-a-nas-tō-mō′-sis): The surgical union of two parts of the intestine; term usually refers to the small intestine.

enterobiasis (en-ter-ō-bī′-a-sis): Infestation with worms of the genus *Enterobius vermicularis* (*q.v.*).

Enterobius vermicularis (en-ter-ō′-bi-us ver-mik-ū-lar′-is): A nematode which infests the small and large intestine. Threadworm; pinworm; seatworm. Found more often in children than adults. Presence in the rectum causes intense itching. Transmitted in the ova of the worm which is found in feces of infected persons. Prevalent among those whose environmental and personal hygiene are poor. Distribution is worldwide.

enterocele (en′-ter-ō-sēl): 1. Hernia of the intestine. 2. Prolapse of the intestine; can be into the upper part of the vagina.

enterocentesis (en-ter-ō-sen-tē′-sis): Surgical puncture of the intestine to withdraw gas or fluid.

enterocholecystostomy (en-ter-ō-kō-le-sis-tos′-to-mi): Surgical creation of an opening from the gallbladder into the small intestine.

enteroclysis (en-ter-ok′-li-sis): The introduction of nutrient or medicinal fluid into the bowel; a high enema. Syn., proctoclysis.

enterococcus (en-ter-ō-kok′-us): A grampositive encapsulated streptococcus that occurs in short chains and is relatively resistant to heat. It is found in the human intestine; sometimes is the causative organism in infections of the urinary tract, ear, and wounds and, more rarely, in endocarditis.

enterocolitis (en-ter-ō-kō-lī′-tis): Inflammation of the mucous membrane lining of the small intestine and colon.

enterocolostomy (en-ter-ō-kō-los′-to-mi): The surgical creation of an artificial opening between the small intestine and colon.

enteroenterostomy (en-ter-ō-en-ter-os′-to-mi): The surgical anastomosis of two parts of the intestine that do not normally adjoin each other.

enterogenous (en-ter-oj′-en-us): Originating within the intestine.

enterokinase (en-ter-ō-kī′-nās): An enzyme in intestinal juice. It converts inactive trypsinogen into active trypsin.

enterolith (en′-ter-ō-lith): An intestinal concretion.

enterolithiasis (en-ter-ō-lith-ī′-a-sis): The presence of calculi or concretions in the intestine.

enterolysis (en-ter-ol′-i-sis): The surgical freeing of the intestine from adhesions.

enteron (en′-te-ron): The gut, the small intestine in particular.

enteropexy (en′-ter-ō-pek-si): The surgical fixation of a part of the intestine to the abdominal wall.

enteroplasty (en′-ter-ō-plas-ti): Any plastic surgery on the bowel, but particularly that employed for enlarging the caliber of the bowel.

enteroplegia (en-ter-ō-plē′-ji-a): Paralysis of the intestine.

enteroptosis (en-ter-op-tō′-sis): Descent or downward displacement of the intestines, usually associated with the downward displacement of other abdominal organs. Also called enteropsia, abdominal ptosis, visceroptosis.—enteroptotic, adj.

enterorrhagia (en-ter-ō-rā′-ji-a): Hemorrhage in or from the intestine.

enteroscope (en′-ter-ō-skōp): An endoscope (q.v.) for examining the intestine.

enterostasis (en-ter-ō-stā′-sis): Intestinal stasis; cessation or delay of the passage of intestinal contents.

enterostenosis (en-ter-ō-ste-nō′-sis): A stricture or narrowing of a portion of the intestine.

enterostomy (en-ter-os′-to-mi): The surgical establishment of an artificial opening into the intestine through the abdominal wall.

enterotomy (en-ter-ot′-o-mi): An incision into the intestine, the small intestine in particular.

enterotoxin (en-ter-ō-tok′-sin): A toxin produced in the intestine by a certain species of bacteria and which produces symptoms associated with food poisoning.

enterovirus (en′-ter-ō-vī′-rus): One of a group of human viruses including the three polioviruses, Coxsackie virus and the ECHO group of viruses. Enter the body through the alimentary tract and tend to invade the central nervous system.

enterozoon (en-ter-ō-zō′on): Any animal parasite that infests or inhabits the intestines.—enterozoa, pl.

enthesis (en′-the-sis): The use of an inorganic material in the repair of a defect or deformity.

entoderm (en′-tō-derm): The innermost of the three primary layers of the embryo from which is derived the epithelial lining of the whole of the digestive tube except part of the mouth, pharynx, and rectum; the lining cells of the glands that empty into the digestive tube; the epithelium lining the respiratory tract and the auditory canal and part of the genitourinary tract; and part of the thyroid, thymus and parathyroid glands.—entodermal, adj.

entrails (en′-trāls): Intestines.

entropion (en-trō′-pē-on): The turning inward of a margin or edge, particularly the inversion of an eyelid so that the lashes are in contact with the globe of the eye.

enucleation (ē-nū-klē-ā′-shun): The removal of an organ or tumor in its entirety, as of an eyeball from its socket.—enucleate, v.t.

enuresis (en-ū-rē′-sis): Involuntary urination, especially bedwetting, when it is not due to any organic disease of the urinary organs.

environment (en-vī′-ron-ment): External surroundings. The total of all the conditions and forces that surround and act upon an organism or any of its parts.

enzyme (en′-zīm): A complex organic compound, frequently a protein, produced by living cells, capable of accelerating or producing some chemical change without itself being changed. Syn., catalyst (q.v.).—enzymic, enzymatic, adj.

enzymology (en′-zī-mol′-ō-ji): The science dealing with the structure and function of enzymes.—enzymological, adj.; enzymologically, adv.

eosin (ē′-ō-sin): A red staining agent used in histology and laboratory diagnostic procedures.

eosinopenia (ē-ō-sin-ō-pē′-ni-a): An abnormally small number of eosinophils in the blood.

eosinophil(e) (ē-ō-sin′-ō-fil): 1. Cell having an affinity for eosin. 2. A type of white blood cell (eosinophil polymorphonuclear).

eosinophilia (ē-ō-sin-ō-fil′-i-a): Increased eosinophils in the blood.

ep-, epi-: Denotes upon, above, over.

ependyma (ep-en′-di-ma): The membrane lining the ventricles of the brain and the central canal of the spinal cord.—ependymal, adj.

ependymoma (ep-en-di-mō′-ma): Neoplasm arising in the lining of the cerebral ventricles or central canal of the spinal cord. Occurs in all age groups.

ephebiatrics (e-fē-bi-at′-riks): That branch of medicine that deals with the diseases of adolescents as compared with pediatrics and geriatrics.

ephebiatrist (e-fē-bī′-a-trist): A physician who specializes in the diseases of adolescents.

ephelis (e-fēl′-is): A freckle.—ephelides, pl.

ephemeral (ē-fem′-er-al): Fleeting; transient.

epicanthus (ep-i-kan′-thus): The congenital occurrence of a fold of skin that may obscure the inner canthus and caruncle of the eye. Characteristic of the Mongolian.—epicanthal, adj.

epicardium (ep-i-kar′-di-um): The visceral or inner layer of the pericardium that immediately invests the heart.—epicardial, adj.

epicondyle (ep-i-kon′-dīl): A bony projection situated above a condyle (*q.v.*).

epicranium (ep-i-krān′-i-um): The scalp; that is, the muscle, skin, etc., that form the covering of the cranium.

epicritic (ep-i-krit′-ik): Term applied to a set of nerve fibers in the skin and oral mucosa that enable one to discriminate fine variations in the sensations of touch, temperature, or pain, and to localize these sensations. The opposite of protopathic (*q.v.*).

epidemic (ep-i-dem′-ik): 1. Simultaneously affecting many people in an area. Cf. **endemic.** 2. The occurrence in a community or region of a group of illnesses of a similar nature, in excess of normal expectancy, and derived from a common source.

epidemiology (ep-i-dē-mi-ol′-o-ji): The scientific study of the incidence, distribution and control of disease in a population, especially epidemic and endemic diseases.—epidemiological, adj.; epidemiologically, adv.

epidermis (ep-i-der′-mis): The external, nonvascular layer of the skin; composed of several individual layers; the cuticle. Also known as the 'scarf' skin.—epidermal, adj.

epidermitis (ep-i-der-mī′-tis): Inflammation of the epidermis or external layers of the skin.

epidermoid (ep-i-der′-moid): 1. Resembling epidermis or epidermal cells. 2. A tumor made up of aberrant epidermal cells.

epidermomycosis (ep-i-der-mō-mī-kō′-sis): Dermatitis caused by a fungus.

Epidermophyton (ep-i-der-mof′-i-ton): A genus of fungi that affects the skin and nails. E. FLOCCOSUM, the causative agent of several types of ringworm including ringworm of the scalp and athlete's foot.

epidermophytosis (ep-i-der-mō-fī-tō′-sis): Infection with fungi of the genus Epidermophyton.

epididymectomy (ep-i-did-i-mek′-to-mi): Surgical removal of the epididymis.

epididymis (ep-i-did′-i-mis): A small oblong body attached to the posterior surface of the testis. Consists of the first, convoluted portion of the excretory duct of the testis; conveys the spermatozoa from the testis to the vas deferens.

epididymitis (ep-i-did-i-mī′-tis): Inflammation of the epididymis (*q.v.*).

epididymo-orchitis (ep-i-did-i-mō-or-kī′-tis): Inflammation of the epididymis and the testis.

epidural (ep-i-dūr′-al): Upon or external to the dura. E. BLOCK, injection of local anesthetic, usually in the lumbar or caudal region prior to rectal examination and surgery, a forceps delivery or cesarean section. Currently used for crush injuries to the chest; the analgesia can be maintained for a week or more.

epigastrium (ep-i-gas′-tri-um): The abdominal region lying directly over the stomach; the 'pit' of the stomach.—epigastric, adj.

epiglottis (ep-i-glot′-is): The thin leaf-shaped flap of cartilage behind the tongue which, during the act of swallowing, covers the opening leading into the larynx.

epiglottitis (ep-i-glot-tī′-tis): Inflammation of the epiglottis. Also epiglottiditis.

epilation (ep-il-ā′-shun): Extraction or destruction of hair roots, *e.g.*, by coagulation necrosis, electrolysis, or forceps.—epilate, v.t.

epilatory (ē-pil′-a-tor-i): An agent that produces epilation.

epilepsy (ep′-i-lep-si): A recurrent paroxysmal disorder of cerebral function characterized always by variable clouding of consciousness, often associated with localized or generalized convulsions, and due to an abnormal discharge of nerve impulses in the brain. E. can be classified on causation; (1) symptomatic (known), *e.g.,* cerebral tumor, trauma and vascular abnormality; (2) idiopathic (unknown). Or on clinical features; (1) grand mal—loss of consciousness with generalized convulsions; (2) petit mal—clouding of consciousness with no generalized convulsions; (3) jacksonian—convulsions beginning in one muscle group and either remaining localized or else spreading in an orderly march to involve wider muscle groups, and which may then involve loss of consciousness. See **akinetic.** —epileptic, adj.

epileptic (ep-i-lep′-tik): 1. A person affected with epilepsy. 2. Pertaining to epilepsy. E. AURA, premonitory subjective phenomena (tingling in the hand or visual or auditory sensations) that precede an attack of grand mal. E. CRY, the croak or shout heard from the epileptic person as he falls unconscious.

epileptiform (ep-i-lep′-ti-form): 1. Resembling epilepsy. 2. Descriptive of a convulsion that resembles the convulsions of epilepsy; accompanied by loss of consciousness.

epileptogenic (ep-i-lep-tō-jen′-ik): Causing epilepsy or an epileptic seizure.

epiloia (ep-i-loi′-a): An inherited abnormality of brain tissue resulting in a syndrome consisting of mental deficiency, hypertrophic sclerosis of the brain, nodules on the floor of the third ventricle, sometimes growths in the kidneys and spleen. Also known as 'tuberous sclerosis.' May be associated with epilepsy.

epimenorrhagia (ep-i-men-ō-rā′-ji-a): Too frequent and too excessive menstruation.

epimenorrhea (ep-i-men-ō-rē′-a): Reduction in the length of the menstrual cycle resulting in too frequent menstruation.

epimysium (ep-i-miz′-i-um): The external connective tissue sheath of a muscle.

epinephrectomy (ep-i-ne-frek′-to-mi): Adrenalectomy (q.v.).

epinephrine (ep-i-nef′-rin): The chief hormone of the normal adrenal medulla; is also produced synthetically. A powerful vasopressor substance. Contracts arterioles of skin, mucous membrane and viscera; dilates arterioles of skeletal muscles and brain; increases strength and rate of heart beat; increases heart output, blood pressure, blood sugar and metabolism; speeds blood clotting; relaxes bronchial muscles. Used therapeutically to control local bleeding as in epistaxis, and to relieve anaphylaxis, allergic conditions, asthmatic attacks, heart and circulatory failure. Adrenaline.

epineurium (ep-i-nū′-ri-um): The connective tissue covering of a nerve trunk.

epiphora (ē-pif′-o-ra): Pathological overflow of tears onto the cheek. May be due to excessive secretion or obstruction of the lacrimal passages.

epiphysial, epiphyseal (ep-i-fiz′-i-al): Referring to or related to an epiphysis (q.v.). E. FRACTURE, the separation of the epiphysis from a long bone; results from injury. E. LINE, the line of junction between the epiphysis and diaphysis of a long bone; it is where growth in length of the bone occurs.

epiphysiolysis (ep-i-fiz-i-ol′-i-sis): Abnormal separation of an epiphysis from the shaft of a bone.

epiphysis (ē-pif′-i-sis): The growing part of a bone, especially a long bone. Separated from the end of the main shaft by a plate of cartilage which disappears and becomes part of the bone due to ossification when growth ceases. SLIPPED E., displacement of an E., especially the upper femoral.—epiphyses, pl.; epiphysial, adj.

epiphysitis (ē-pif-i-sī′-tis): Inflammation of an epiphysis.

epiplocele (ē-pip′-lō-sēl): A hernia that contains omentum.

epiploic (ep-i-plō′-ik): Related to or referring to the epiploon (q.v.).

epiplomphalocele (ep-i-plom-fal′-o-sēl): An umbilical hernia containing omentum.

epiploon (ē-pip′-lō-on): The great omentum (q.v.).—epiploic, adj.

episclera (ep-i-sklē′-ra): Loose connective tissue between the sclera and conjunctiva.—episcleral, adj.

episcleritis (ep-i-sklē-rī′-tis): Inflammation of the episclera.

episiorrhaphy (ē-piz-i-or′-ra-fi): The surgical repair of a vulva or of an episiotomy after childbirth.

episiotomy (ē-piz-i-ot′-o-mi): A perineal incision made during the birth of a child when the vaginal orifice does not stretch enough and laceration of the perineum seems imminent.

epispadias (ep-i-spā′-di-as): A congenital malformation in which the opening of the urethra is on the upper side of the penis.

epispastic (ep-i-spas′-tik): A blistering agent.

epistaxis (ep-i-stak′-sis): Bleeding from the nose.—epistaxes, pl.

epistropheus (ep-i-strō′-fē-us): The second cervical vertebra; the axis.

epithelialization (ep-i-thē-li-al-ī-zā′-shun): The growth of epithelium over a raw area;

the final stage of healing. Also epitheliza-tion.

epithelioma (ep-i-thēl-i-ō′-ma): A ma-lignant growth arising in epithelial tissue, usually the skin; a squamous cell carci-noma.

epithelium (ep-i-thē′-li-um): The surface layer of cells covering cutaneous, mucous and serous surfaces. It is classified accord-ing to the arrangement and shape of the cells it contains.—epithelial, adj.

epizoon (ep-i-zō-on): An animal parasite liv-ing on the outside of the host's body. —epizoa, pl.

epulis (ep-ū′-lis): A tumor growing on or from the gums.

equilibrium (ē-kwi-lib′-ri-um): 1. A state of balance between forces or processes. 2. The normal, oriented state of the body in respect to its position in space, maintained through the labyrinthine sense. ACID-BASE E., the state of the body when the acids and bases in body fluids are present in their normal ratio. NITROGENOUS E., the condition of the body when the amount of nitrogen ex-creted is in the normal ratio to that taken in.

equinia (ē-kwin′-i-a): A mild form of glan-ders (*q.v.*) in man; contracted from horses with glanders.

equinovarus (ē-kwī-nō-va′-rus): The most common form of clubfoot; the sole turns inward and the heel does not touch the ground when walking.

erasion (ē-rā′-zhun): Surgical removal of tis-sue by scraping. E. OF A JOINT, arthrec-tomy (*q.v.*).

Erb's palsy: Paralysis of a group of muscles of the shoulder and arm, due to injury to the brachial plexus or lower cervical nerve roots. [Wilhelm H. Erb, German neurolo-gist. 1840-1921.]

erectile (ē-rek′-tīl): Upright; capable of be-ing elevated. E. TISSUE, highly vascular tis-sue, which, under stimulus, becomes rigid and erect from hyperemia.

erection (ē-rek′-shun): The condition achieved when erectile tissue is made rigid or elevated due to hyperemia. The enlarged, rigid penis of the male (or clitoris of the female) under stimulus of sexual excitement is said to be in a state of erection.

erector (ē-rek′-tor): A muscle that achieves erection of or raises a part.

erepsin (ē-rep′-sin): A proteolytic enzyme in succus entericus (*q.v.*).

erethism (er′-e-thizm): Heightened respon-siveness of the nervous system.

ERG: Abbreviation for electroretinogram (*q.v.*).

ergasiomania (er-gās-i-ō-mā′-ni-a): 1. An abnormal desire to keep oneself continually working. 2. An intense desire to perform surgical operations. Also ergomania.

ergometry (er-gom′-et-ri): Measurement of work done by muscles.—ergometric, adj.

ergonomics (er-gō-nom′-iks): The applica-tion of various biological disciplines in rela-tion to man and his working environ-ment.

ergosterol (er-gos′-ter-ol): A provitamin present in the subcutaneous fat of man; also found in plants and foodstuffs. On irradia-tion with sunlight or ultraviolet light it is converted into vitamin D_2 which has antira-chitic properties.

ergot (er′-got): A fungus that is parasitic on rye. It is the source of several valuable al-kaloids used in medicine; causes contrac-tion of muscular coat of the arteries, raises blood pressure and contracts uterine mus-cle. Widely used in control of postpartum hemorrhage.

ergotism (er′-got-izm): Chronic poisoning due to excessive or wrong use of ergot as a medicine or from eating food made from rye or wheat that was infected with the fun-gus; marked by muscle spasms, cerebrospi-nal symptoms and dry gangrene. Has been called St. Anthony's fire (*q.v.*).

erode (ē-rōd′): To diminish or destroy gradually; to wear away.

erogenous (ē-roj′-e-nus): Erotogenic (*q.v.*).

erosion (ē-rō′-zhun): The wearing away of a tissue or a surface; often due to ulceration.

erotic (ē-rot′-ik): Pertaining to sexual pas-sion or interest; lustful.

erotica (ē-rot′-i-ka): Artistic or literary work that has an erotic theme or quality.

eroticism (ē-rot′-i-sizm), **erotism:** Exces-sive sexual desire or interest.

erotogenic (ē-rot-ō-jen′-ik): Descriptive of body areas or skin that respond to stimula-tion by giving rise to sexual stimulation, *e.g.*, the oral, anal and genital areas. Also erogenous.

erotomania (ē-rot-ō-mā′-ni-a): Morbid preoccupation with erotic activites or im-aginings.

erotophobia (ē-rot-ō-fō′-bi-a): Morbid fear of sexual love or aversion to its physical expression.

erratic (e-rat′-ik): 1. Wandering; said of pain or other symptoms. 2. Queer, eccen-tric.

eructation (ē-ruk-tā′-shun): Noisy, oral expulsion of gas from the stomach. The act of belching.

eruption (ē-rup′-shun): 1. The act of becoming visible or breaking out. 2. The appearance of a rash or visible lesion on the skin due to disease; characterized by redness, prominence, or both.—erupt, v.i.

erysipelas (er-i-sip′-e-las): An acute inflammatory contagious disease of the skin and subcutaneous tissues, caused by a hemolytic streptococcus. The inflammation begins around a wound, often too small to be noticeable. The characteristic rash is painful, red with small blebs, and is raised at the edge, often spreading over the nose and cheeks in a butterfly pattern. Disease is accompanied by fever and other severe constitutional symptoms. Syn., St. Anthony's fire.

erysipeloid (er-i-sip′-e-loid): A specific infective dermatitis resembling erysipelas, occurring primarily in persons who handle fish or meat. Usually confined to the hands but may become generalized and septicemic.

erythema (er-i-the′-ma): Reddening of the skin.—erythematous, adj. E. INDURATUM is Bazin's disease (*q.v.*). E. MULTIFORME is a form of toxic or allergic skin eruption that breaks out suddenly and lasts for days; the lesions are in the form of violet-pink papules or plaques and suggest urticarial wheals. Severe form called Stevens-Johnson syndrome (*q.v.*). E. NODOSUM is an eruption of painful red nodules on the front of the legs. It occurs in young women and is generally accompanied by rheumatic pains. May be a symptom of many diseases including tuberculosis, acute rheumatism, gonococcal septicemia; also caused by certain drugs or food poisoning. E. PERNIO, chilblain (*q.v.*).

erythr-, erythro-: Denotes erythrocyte.

erythrasma (er-i-thraz′-ma): A chronic skin infection, now thought to be caused by a bacterium; characterized by a reddish-brown eruption that occurs in the axilla, groin, inner surface of the thigh, and the pubic area; the patches desquamate but cause little or no discomfort.

erythredema (er-ith-rē-dē′-ma): A disease of infancy characterized by bluish-red swollen extremities, tachycardia, photophobia; cause unknown. Nervous irritability is extreme, leading to anorexia and disordered digestion, followed by multiple arthritis and muscular weakness. Syn., pink disease, Swift's disease, infantile acrodynia, dermatopolyneuritis.

erythremia (er-i-thrē′-mi-a): An increase in the blood corpuscles, especially the red ones. See **erythrocythemia**.

erythroblast (ē-rith′-rō-blast): A nucleated red blood cell found in the red bone marrow and from which the erythrocytes are derived.—erythroblastic, adj.

erythroblastosis (ē-rith-rō-blas-tō′-sis): Presence of erythroblasts in the circulating blood. E. FETALIS or NEONATORUM is a pathological condition in the fetus or the newborn; occurs when the mother's blood is Rh negative, causing the development of antibodies against the fetus whose blood is Rh positive. Red blood cell destruction occurs with anemia, jaundice, an excess of erythroblasts in the blood, enlarged liver and spleen and often generalized edema. Immunization of women at risk with gamma globulin containing a high titre of anti-D is being tried with success.

erythrocyanosis (ē-rith-rō-sī-a-nō′-sis): A condition characterized by swollen, bluish-red areas of discoloration on the skin that burn and itch. E. FRIGIDA, a vasoplastic disease in which there is hypertrophy of the arteriolar muscular coat; marked by bluish-red discoloration of the legs, especially of young women when exposed to cold.

erythrocyte (ē-rith′rō-sīt): A non-nucleated red cell of the circulating blood; a red blood corpuscle.—erythrocytic, adj.

erythrocyte sedimentation rate: The rate at which red blood cells settle to the bottom of a glass tube. The rate is increased in infections and conditions in which cell destruction occurs. Useful in diagnosing and following such illnesses as rheumatic fever, arthritis and myocardial infarction. Abbreviated ESR.

erythrocythemia (ē-rith-rō-sī-the′-mi-a): Overproduction of red blood cells. 1. This may be a physiological response to the need for greater oxygenation of the tissues (congenital heart disease) and is referred to as erythrocytosis or secondary polycythemia. 2. The idiopathic condition is polycythemia vera; see **polycythemia**.—erythrocythemic, adj.

erythrocytolysis (ē-rith-rō-sī-tol′-i-sis): Destruction or dissolution of red blood cells with escape of hemoglobin into the plasma.

erythrocytometer (ē-rith-rō-sī-tom′-e-ter): An instrument for measuring or counting red blood cells.

erythrocytopenia (ē-rith-rō-sī-tō-pē′-ni-a): Deficiency in the number of red blood cells. —erythrocytopenic, adj.

erythrocytosis (ē-rith-rō-sī-tō′-sis): An increase in the red cells in the blood resulting from a known cause; secondary polycythemia. Cf. **polycythemia vera.**

erythroderma (ē-rith′-rō-der-ma): Excessive redness of the skin. Also erythrodermia.

erythrodermatitis (ē-rith-rō-der-ma-tī′-tis): Reddening and inflammation of the skin.

erythrogenic (ē-rith-rō-jen′-ik): 1. Producing or causing a rash. 2. Producing red blood cells.

erythropenia (ē-rith-rō-pē′-ni-a): Deficiency in the number of red cells in the blood.

erythropoiesis (ē-rith-rō-poi-ē′-sis): The production of red blood cells. See **hemopoiesis.**]

eschar (es′-kar): A slough, as results from a burn, application of caustics, diathermy, etc. See **slough.**

escharotic (es-ka-rot′-ik): 1. Any agent capable of producing an eschar. 2. Corrosive; caustic.

Escherichia (esh-er-ik′-i-a): A genus of bacteria. Motile, gram-negative rod bacteria which are very widely distributed in nature, especially in the intestinal tract of vertebrates. Some strains are pathogenic to man, causing enteritis, peritonitis, pyelitis, cystitis and wound infections. The type species is *Esch. coli.*

eschrolalia (es-krō-lā′-li-a): Coprolalia (*q.v.*).

Esmarch's bandage: A rubber roller bandage used to procure a bloodless operative field in the limbs. [Johann Friedrich August von Esmarch, German military surgeon. 1823-1908.]

esophagalgia (ē-sof-a-gal′-ji-a): Pain in the esophagus.

esophageal (ē-sof-a-jē′-al): Belonging or pertaining to the esophagus. E. DIVERTICULUM, a circumscribed pouch-like protrusion from the wall of the esophagus. See **diverticulum.** E. HIATUS, the opening in the diaphragm through which the esophagus passes before it joins the stomach. E. VARICES, varices in the esophageal wall; see **varix.**

esophagectasia (ē-sof-a-jek-tā′-si-a): Dilatation of the esophagus.

esophagectomy (ē-sof-a-jek′-to-mi): Excision of a portion or the whole of the esophagus.

esophagism (ē-sof′-a-jizm): Spasmodic stricture of the esophagus, due to contraction of the circular muscle fibers.

esophagocele (ē-sof′-a-gō-sēl): Hernia, diverticulum, or distention of the esophagus.

esophagoduodenostomy (ē-sof-a-gō-dū-ō-dē-nos′-to-mi): The creation of a surgical anastomosis between the esophagus and the duodenum.

esophagogastrostomy (ē-sof-a-gō-gas-tros′-to-mi): The creation of an artificial communication between esophagus and stomach.

esophagoplasty (ē-sof′-a-gō-plas-ti): A plastic operation for the repair of damage to the esophagus.

esophagoscope (ē-sof′-a-gō-skōp): An endoscope (*q.v.*) fitted with a light and lenses; used for examining the esophagus.

esophagospasm (ē-sof′-a-gō-spazm): Spasm of the muscles of the esophagus.

esophagostenosis (ē-sof-a-gō-ste-nō′-sis): Constriction or stricture of the esophagus.

esophagostomy (ē-sof-a-gos′-to-mi): A surgically created fistula between the esophagus and the exterior; used temporarily for feeding after excision of some part of the throat, usually for cancer.

esophagotomy (ē-sof-a-got′-o-mi): An incision into the esophagus.

esophagus (ē-sof′-a-gus): A musculomembranous tube, about 10 inches long, that extends from the pharynx through the diaphragm to join the cardiac end of the stomach. Serves as a passageway for food.

ESP: Abbreviation for extrasensory perception (*q.v.*).

espundia (es-pun′-di-a): South American mucocutaneous leishmaniasis (*q.v.*). Causes ulceration of the legs with later involvement of the nose and throat.

ESR: Erythrocyte sedimentation rate (*q.v.*).

essence (es′-sens): 1. That which is the real nature of a thing and so causes it to have its particular qualities. 2. A solution of a volatile oil in alcohol.

essential (ē-sen′-shal): Of great importance; indispensable. In medicine the term is often used to describe conditions of unknown origin, *e.g.,* essential hypertension.

EST: Electroshock therapy (*q.v.*).

ester (es′-ter): Any organic compound formed by the combination of an acid and an alcohol with the elimination of water.

esterification (es-ter-i-fi-kā′-shun): The reaction between an alcohol and an acid to form an ester.

esthesia (es-thē′-zi-a): The capacity for feeling, sensation, or perception, as opposed to anesthesia.

esthesio-: Denotes: (1) sensation, feeling; (2) perception.

esthetic (es-thet′-ik): 1. Pertaining to sensation or feeling. 2. Pertaining to beauty.

estival (es′-ti-val): Pertaining to summer or occurring during the summer months.

estradiol (es-tra-dī′-ol): A steroid hormone, produced by the ovarian follicles; stimulates follicle growth, proliferation of the endometrium, and uterine contractions. Also influences the pituitary gland, stimulating production of gonadotropic hormones.

estrogen (es′-trō-jen): The collective name for the female sex hormones, secreted within the ovary. Applied to the ovarian follicular hormone estradiol and its excretion derivative estrone, and to synthetic compounds of similar activity.—estrogenic, adj.

estrogenic (est-rō-jen′-ik): Having the action of the female sex hormones. See **estrogen.** E. HORMONES, the substances secreted within the ovary that stimulate activity of the female sex organs; those produced in animals (mare) may be used in medicine when the normal supply is lacking or deficient. The active ingredient of the contraceptive pill.

estrus (es′-trus): The sexually receptive state in females. In humans, it occurs during that phase of the menstrual cycle when changes in the lining of the uterus prepare it for receiving the fertilized ovum, should conception occur.

ether (ē′-ther): Inflammable liquid; one of the oldest volatile anesthetics and less toxic than chloroform. Occasionally used orally for its carminative action.

ethics (eth′-iks): A code of moral principles that govern conduct. NURSING E., the code governing the nurse's behavior, especially to her patients, visitors, and colleagues. It implies loyalty to the employing authority and to the profession.—ethical, adj.

ethmoid (eth′-moid): 1. Sievelike; cribriform. 2. The sievelike bone that separates the nasal cavity from the brain; the olfactory nerves pass through perforations in it; contains small cavities called ethmoid sinuses.

ethmoidectomy (eth-moid-ek′-to-mi): Surgical removal of a part of the ethmoid bone, usually that forming the lateral nasal walls.

ethnic (eth′-nik): Pertaining to race or to the races of mankind.

ethnology (eth-nol′-o-ji): The science that treats of the races of mankind.

ethyl (eth′-il): The univalent alcohol radical, present in many compounds, *e.g.,* ethyl alcohol, ethyl ether.

ethyl chloride (eth′-il klō′-rīd): A volatile general anesthetic for short operations, and a local anesthetic by reason of the intense cold produced when applied to the skin.

etiology (ē-ti-ol′-o-ji): The science that deals with causation of diseases.—etiologic, etiological, adj.; etiologically, adv.

eu-: Denotes: (1) well, good; (2) a feeling of well-being.

Eubacteriales (ū-bak-ter-i-ā′-lēz): An order of bacteria important in medicine; includes those that are spheroid or rod-shaped, *e.g.,* the gonococcus and the typhoid bacillus.

eudipsia (ū-dip′-si-a): Normal, ordinary thirst.

eugenics (ū-jen′-iks): The science dealing with those factors which improve successive generations of the human race.—eugenic, adj.

eunuch (ū-nuk): A human male from whom the testes have been removed; a castrated male.

eupepsia (ū-pep′-si-a): Normal digestion.

euphoria (ū-fō′-ri-a): A state of bodily comfort; well-being. In psychology, an exaggerated state of well-being, usually not justified by the circumstances.—euphoric, euphoretic, euphoriant, adj.

eupnea (ūp-nē′-a): Normal respiration.

eurhythmic (ū-rith′-mik): 1. Harmonious development and relationship of the body parts. 2. Descriptive of a pulse beat that is regular.

eurhythmics (ū-rith′-miks): Harmonious body movements performed to music.

eustachian (ū-stā′-ki-an): A canal, partly bony, partly cartilaginous, measuring 1 to 2 in. in length, connecting the pharynx with the tympanic cavity. It allows air to pass into the middle ear, so that the air pressure is kept even on both sides of the eardrum. E. CATHETER, an instrument used for dilating the eustachian tube when it becomes blocked. E. VALVE, the valve guarding the entrance of the inferior vena cava into the right atrium of the heart. [Bartolommeo Eustachius, Italian anatomist. 1520-1574.]

euthanasia (ū-tha-nā′-zi-a): 1. A painless death. 2. The painless killing of a person suffering from an incurable disease.

euthyroid (ū-thī′-roid): Denoting a state in which the thyroid function is normal.

eutocia (ū-tō′-si-a): A natural and normal labor without any complications.

evacuant (ē-vak′-ū-ant): An agent which

causes an evacuation, particularly of the bowel. E. ENEMA, fluid injected into the rectum, to be returned, as distinct from retained.

evacuation (ē-vak-ū-ā'-shun): The act of emptying a cavity; generally refers to the discharge of fecal matter from the rectum.

evagination (ē-vaj-i-nā'-shun): An outpouching or protrusion of a layer or a part of an organ or of a tissue.

evanescent (ev-a-nes'-ent): Fleeting, unstable, unfixed, vanishing.

evaporate (ē-vap'-o-rāt): To convert from the liquid or solid state to the gaseous state. —evaporation, n.

evaporating lotion: One which, applied as a compress, absorbs heat in order to evaporate, and so cools the skin.

eventration (ē-ven-trā'-shun): 1. Protrusion of some of the contents of the abdomen through the abdominal wall. 2. Surgical removal of the contents of the abdominal cavity.

eversion (ē-ver'-zhun): A turning inside out or back upon itself, as the eversion of an eyelid to expose the conjuctival sac.

evisceration (ē-vis-e-rā'-shun): Removal of the internal organs; disembowelment.

evolution (ev-ō-lū'-shun): 1. The process of continual, gradual and orderly growth and development or advance. 2. The theory that living things have developed to their present state by a series of changes that raised them from lower to higher orders of biological species.

evulsion (ē-vul'-shun): Forcible tearing away of a structure.

Ewald's test meal: Employed in test for gastric secretion or function. Consists of two unbuttered slices of bread and 300 cc of water given in the morning on an empty stomach and later withdrawn at stated intervals to be examined for acidity.

Ewing's tumor: Sarcoma involving shaft of long bone before twentieth year. Current view holds that it is a secondary bone deposit from a malignant neuroblastoma of the adrenal gland. [James Ewing, American pathologist. 1866-1943.]

ex-, exo-: Denotes out, outside, outside of, away from, lacking. Opp. to end-, endo-. Variants are e-, ef-.

exacerbation (eks-as-er-bā'-shun): Increased severity as of symptoms, or a flareup of symptoms that have subsided.

examination (eks-am-i-nā'-shun): The procedure of inspecting a patient to determine his physical condition and to aid in diagnosing his ailment. PHYSICAL E., examining the physical state of a person by inspection, palpation, percussion and auscultation.

exania (ek-sā'-ni-a): Prolapse of the rectum.

exanthema (ek-san-thēm'-a): 1. A skin eruption. 2. Any eruptive disease such as measles.—exanthemata, pl.; exanthematous, adj.

exchange transfusion: See **transfusion.**

excision (ek-sizh'-un): Removal of a part by cutting.—excise, v.t.

excitability (ek-sīt-a-bil'-i-ti): 1. The state of readiness of cells or an organism to respond to stimuli. 2. A state of being easily irritated.

excitation (ek-sī-tā'-shun): The act of stimulating an organ or tissue.

excoriation (eks-kō-ri-ā'-shun): Loss or removal of skin such as that produced by scratching, scraping, burns or chemicals. Abrasion (*q.v.*).—excoriate, v.t.

excrement (eks'-kre-ment): Waste matter cast off by body; usually refers to feces.

excrescence (eks-kres'-ens): Any abnormal protuberance or growth of the tissues; usually refers to surface outgrowths.

excreta (eks-krē'-ta): The waste matter which is normally discharged from the body, particularly urine and feces.

excrete (eks-krēt'): To separate and throw off from the body as waste matter.

excretion (eks-krē'-shun): The elimination of waste material from the body, and also the matter so discharged.—excretory, adj.; excrete, n.; v.t.

excretory (eks'-kre-tor-i): Pertaining to excretion. E. SYSTEM, term used to describe groups of organs that eliminate waste products from the body; urinary, digestive, respiratory systems, and the skin.

excruciating (eks-krū'-shi-āt-ing): 1. Agonizing or torturing, as pain. 2. Causing severe suffering.

exenteration (eks-en-te-rā'-shun): Evisceration. Removal of the viscera. PELVIC E., the removal of pelvic organs, a radical operation for malignant growths.

exercise (ek'-ser-sīz): Physical exertion engaged in for the purpose of improving one's health, correcting a deformity or developing a particular athletic skill. ACTIVE E., voluntary muscular activity performed by one's own efforts. PASSIVE E., massage, manipulation or movement of the body or parts of it, performed by another person, a machine or other outside force without any effort on the part of the patient.

exfoliation (eks-fō-li-ā'-shun): The scaling off of tissues in layers.—exfoliative, adj.

exhalation (eks-ha-lā'-shun): In physiology, the forcing of air out of the lungs.

exhale (eks-hāl'): To breathe out; to force or let air out of the lungs.

exhaustion (eg-zaws'-chun): 1. Extreme weariness or fatigue. 2. Inability to respond to stimuli. 3. The using up of a supply of anything. HEAT E., a condition caused by excessive heat, either from exposure to the sun or from working in hot places; characterized by prostration, subnormal temperatures, weakness, dehydration, and collapse.

exhibitionism (eks-i-bish'-un-izm): Any kind of 'showing off'; extravagant behavior to attract attention including such perverted behavior as indecent exposure.—exhibitionist, n.

exitus (ek'-si-tus): Fatal termination of a disease; death.

exocrine (ek'-sō-krēn): Term applied to glands that deliver their secretions to an epithelial surface either directly or through a duct, or to the secretions such glands produce. Opp. to endocrine (q.v.).—exocrinal, adj.

exodontics (eks-sō-don'-tiks): That branch of dentistry that deals with the extraction of teeth.

exogenous (ek-soj'-en-us): Of external origin.

exomphalos (ek-som'-fa-los): A congenital condition due to failure of the abdominal wall to develop properly; the abdominal viscera herniate through a gap in the umbilical region. Umbilical hernia.

exophthalmos (ek-sof-thal'-mos): Abnormal protrusion of the eyeballs; most frequently occurs in hyperthyroidism. See **goiter**.—exophthalmic, adj.

exostosis (ek-sos-tō'-sis): A bony outgrowth from the surface of a bone or tooth, forming a tumor.

exotoxin (ek-sō-tok'-sin): A toxic product of living bacteria that is passed into the environment of the cell, becomes diffused and attacks specific tissues. The organisms causing diphtheria and typhoid fever produce exotoxins. Opp. to endotoxin.—exotoxic, adj.

exotropia (ek-sō-trō'-pi-a): Outward deviation of the visual axis of one eye. Also divergent strabismus, divergent squint, 'walleye.'

expansiveness (eks-pan'-siv-nes): In psychiatry, behavior marked by euphoria, talkativeness, and an exaggerated sense of one's own importance.

expectorant (eks-pek'-to-rant): An agent that promotes or increases the expectoration of mucus or other exudate from the lungs, bronchi and trachea.

expectoration (eks-pek-tō-rā'-shun): 1. The elimination of secretion from the respiratory tract by coughing and spitting. 2. Sputum (q.v.).—expectorate, v.t.

expel (eks-pel'): To force out.

expiration (ek-spi-rā'-shun): 1. The act of breathing out air from the lungs. 2. Death. —expire, v.t., v.i.; expiratory, adj.

expire (ek-spīr'): 1. To exhale or breathe out. 2. To die.

explant (eks-plant'): To transfer tissue from the body to another medium for growth, or the material so transferred.

exploration (eks-plor-ā'-shun): The act of exploring for diagnostic purposes, particularly in the surgical field.—exploratory, adj.

expression (eks-presh'-un): 1. Expulsion by force, squeezing, or pressing out, as the placenta from the uterus, milk from the breasts, etc. 2. Facial disclosure of feelings, mood, etc.

expulsion (eks-pul'-shun): The act of forcing out, as feces from the rectum or urine from the bladder.—expel, v.t.

exsanguination (eks-sang-wi-nā'-shun): The process of rendering bloodless.

exstrophy (ek'-strō-fi): The congenital turning inside out or eversion of a hollow organ such as the bladder.

ext. Abbreviation for extract.

extension (eks-ten'-shun): 1. Traction upon a fractured or dislocated limb. 2. The act of straightening a flexed limb or part.

extensor (eks-ten'-sor): A muscle which on contraction extends or straightens a part. Opp. to flexor.

exterior (eks-tēr'-i-or): The outside or outer part, or situated on or near the outside.

extern(e) (eks'-tern): A medical student or graduate who does not live in the hospital but is on the staff and assists with the medical and surgical care of patients.

external: Of two parts, the one farther from the center of the body; on the outside or surface of the body. Opp. to internal. E. EAR, see **ear**. E. HEMORRHAGE, that in which blood escapes to the outside of the body; opp. to internal hemorrhage. E. MALLEOLUS, the prominence on the lateral side of the ankle formed by the rounded eminence on the lateral side of the fibula.

exteroceptor (eks-ter-ō-sep'-tor): A sensory

nerve terminal located in the skin or mucous membrane and that receives such external stimuli as heat, cold, pain, touch, taste, and smell.

extirpation (ek-stir-pā′-shun): Complete removal or destruction of a part.

extra-: Denotes outside, beyond.

extra-articular (eks-tra-ar-tik′-ū-lar): Outside a joint.

extracapsular (eks-tra-kap′-sū-lar): Outside a capsule.

extracardial (eks-tra-kar′-di-al): Outside the heart.

extracellular (eks-tra-sel′-ū-lar): Occurring outside a cell or cells.

extracorporeal (eks-tra-kor-pō-rē′-al): Occurring outside of the body. See **circulation.**

extracorpuscular (eks-tra-kor-pus′-kū-lar): Outside of the corpuscles (*q.v.*).

extract (eks′-trakt): A preparation obtained by evaporating a solution of a drug.

extraction (eks-trak′-shun): 1. The preparation of an extract. 2. The act or process of drawing or pulling out. E. OF LENS, surgical removal of the lens of the eye. EXTRACAPSULAR E., the capsule is ruptured prior to delivery of the lens. INTRACAPSULAR E., the lens is removed within its capsule.

extradural (eks-tra-dū′-ral): External to the dura mater.

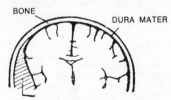

BONE

DURA MATER

Extradural hematoma

extragenital (eks-tra-jen′-i-tal): Not related to, originating in, or occurring on the genital organs. Occurring in areas apart from the genital organs. E. CHANCRE, the primary lesion of syphilis, occurring on the lip, breast, finger, etc.

extrahepatic (eks-tra-hep-at′-ik): Outside the liver.

extramural (eks-tra-mū′-ral): Outside the wall of a vessel or organ.—extramurally, adv.

extraneous (eks-trā′-nē-us): 1. Originating, existing, or coming from outside of the organism. 2. Unessential; not vital.

extraocular (eks-tra-ok′-ū-lar): Outside of the eye.

extraperitoneal (eks-tra-per-i-tō-nē′-al): Outside of the peritoneal cavity.—extraperitoneally, adv.

extrapleural (eks-tra-ploo′-ral): Outside the pleura, *i.e.,* between the parietal pleura and the chest wall. See **plombage.**

extrapyramidal (eks-tra-pi-ram′-i-dal): Outside of or independent of the pyramidal tracts. See **pyramidal.**

extrasensory perception (eks-tra-sen′-so-ri per-sep′-shun): Thought transference. Term pertains to capacities or forms of perception that are not dependent upon the five senses or explainable in relation to the senses. Abbreviated ESP.

extrasystole (eks-tra-sis′-to-li): A premature beat that is independent of the regular pulse rhythm; the beat follows closely the preceding beat and is followed by a long pause before the next beat.

extrathoracic (eks-tra-thō-ras′-ik): Outside the thoracic cavity.

extrauterine (eks-tra-ū′-ter-in): Outside the uterus. See **ectopic pregnancy.**

extravasation (eks-trav-a-sā′-shun): An escape of blood, lymph or fluid from its normal enclosure into the surrounding tissues.

extravascular (eks-tra-vas′-kū-lar): Outside of a vessel or vessels.

extravenous (eks-tra-vē′-nus): Outside a vein.

extraventricular (eks-tra-ven-trik′-ū-lar): Outside a ventricle; term usually refers to ventricles of the heart.

extraversion (eks-tra-ver′-zhun): Extroversion (*q.v.*).

extravert (eks′-tra-vert): Extrovert (*q.v.*).

extremitas (eks-trem′-i-tas): In anatomy, a term used to designate a distal or terminal part of an organ or structure.

extremity (eks-trem′-i-ti): The terminal end of a thing. In anatomy, term refers to a distal or terminal position and is used to designate such structures as arm, leg, hand, foot.

extrinsic (eks-trin′-sik): Developing or having its origin from without; not internal. E. FACTOR, vitamin B_{12} (cyanocobalamin), which is normally present in the diet and absorbed from the gut; it is essential for normal hemopoiesis.

extro-: Denotes outward, outside. Opp. to intro-.

extroversion (eks-trō-ver′-zhun): Turning outward; turning inside out; exstrophy. In psychology, the direction of one's thoughts

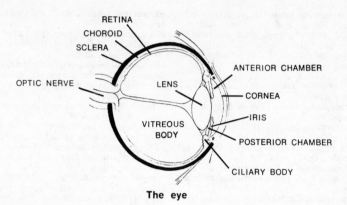

RETINA
CHOROID
SCLERA
OPTIC NERVE
LENS
ANTERIOR CHAMBER
CORNEA
IRIS
VITREOUS BODY
POSTERIOR CHAMBER
CILIARY BODY

The eye

to the external world and the focusing of one's interest on things outside oneself.

extrovert (eks'-tro-vert): Used by Jung to describe one extreme of personality dimension. The person described as E. regulates his behavior in response to other people's attitude to him. He is sociable, a good mixer and interested chiefly in external things and the actions of others.

extrude (eks-trood'): To force or push out of the position normally occupied, or to occupy such a position.—extrusion, n.

extubation (eks-tū-bā'-shun): To remove a tube that has been previously inserted.

exudate (eks'-ū-dāt): The matter which has passed through a vessel wall or membrane by exudation (*q.v.*).

exudation (eks-ū-dā'-shun): The oozing out of serum and cells, mostly leukocytes, through unruptured walls of capillaries or venules.—exudate, n.; exude, v.t., v.i.

exumbilication (eks-um-bil-i-kā'-shun):

Abnormal protrusion of the navel.

eye: The organ of vision, located in the eye socket of the skull.

eyeball: The globe of the eye without any appendages such as the extrinsic muscles.

eyebrow: The line of hairs at the upper edge of the bony orbit that contains the eye.

eyeground: The fundus of the eye as it is visible through the ophthalmoscope (*q.v.*).

eyelash: One of the hairs that project from the edge of the eyelid.

eyelid: One of two folds of skin (upper and lower) that is continuous with the skin of the face, lined with conjunctiva (*q.v.*), and has a row of stiff hairs at the edge. See **meibomian gland, canthus.**

eye-minded (ī-mīnd'-ed): Descriptive of a person who remembers chiefly the impressions made on the eye.

eyestrain: Fatigue of the eye from overuse, poor lighting, or an uncorrected defect in focusing.

F

F: Abbreviation for Fahrenheit (*q.v.*).

fabrication (fab-ri-kā′-shun): The creation of imaginary events or tales and presenting them as true; sometimes indulged in by psychiatric patients whose memory is lacking or deficient.

face: The anterior aspect of the human head, including the chin, mouth, cheeks, nose and forehead. F. LIFTING, plastic surgery for the removal of facial defects. F. PRESENTATION, the position of the fetus when the face presents first during labor and delivery.

facet (fas′-et): A small, smooth, flat surface on a bone.

facial (fā′-shal): Pertaining to the face. F. NERVE, one of the seventh pair of cranial nerves. F. NEURALGIA, neuralgia (*q.v.*) in that part of the face supplied by the trigeminal (fifth cranial) nerve. F. PARALYSIS, paralysis of the muscles supplied by the facial nerve. F. SPASM, muscular spasm on one side of the face or around the eye, irregular and not under conscious control.

-facient: Denotes a person or agent that brings something about or initiates an action.

facies (fā′shi-ēz): An anatomical term used to designate a surface of a body structure or part, the expression on the face, or the face itself. ABDOMINAL F., the expression seen in peritonitis; the skin is livid, the eyes sunken and the lips dry. ADENOID F., openmouthed, vacant expression seen in children with enlarged adenoids. F. HIPPOCRATICA, the drawn, pale, pinched expression indicative of extreme prostration and approaching death. PARKINSON′S F., the masklike appearance seen in persons with Parkinson's disease; saliva may trickle from the corner of the mouth.

facio-: Denotes the face.

facioplegia (fā-shi-ō-plē′-ji-a): Facial paralysis.

factitious (fak-tish′-us): Artificial.

factor (fak′-tor): Something that contributes to the production of a result, *e.g.*, an agent, influence, circumstance, constituent, ingredient. In heredity, a gene (*q.v.*). In nutrition, a desirable or essential element, *e.g.*, a vitamin.

facultative (fak′-ul-tā-tiv): 1. Conditional, optional, voluntary. 2. Able to live and thrive under more than one set of conditions; said of bacteria, *e.g.*, some aerobic bacteria can live and thrive in anaerobic conditions.

faculty (fak′-ul-ti): 1. An inherent normal power, capability, function, or attitude. Used chiefly in reference to the human body or its parts, particularly in reference to mental endowments. 2. The teaching staff of an educational institution.

Fahrenheit (far′-en-hīt): A thermometric scale; the freezing point of water is 32° and its boiling point 212°; the normal body temperature is 98.4°-98.6°. [Gabriel Fahrenheit, German physicist. 1686-1736.]

failure: Inability to perform a normal duty or expected action. HEART F., sudden cessation of the heart's action.

faint: 1. Weak; lacking in strength or courage. 2. A swoon; a state of temporary unconsciousness. Syn., syncope.

Fairbank's splint: Used for treatment of Erb's palsy. Baby's arm is immobilized in abduction and external rotation of the shoulder, flexion of the elbow to 90°, supination of the forearm and extension of the wrist.

falciform (fal′-si-form): Sickle-shaped. F. LIGAMENT, a fold of peritoneum that separates the two main lobes of the liver.

fallopian (fal-lō′-pi-an): F. LIGAMENT, the round ligament of the uterus. F. TUBE, one of the two tubes that open out of the upper part of the uterus. Each measures about 4-5.5 in.; the distal ends are fimbriated and lie near the ovary. The function is to carry the ova from the ovary to the uterus. [Gabriele Fallopius, 16th century Italian anatomist.]

Fallot's tetralogy (fa-lōz′): Tetralogy of Fallot (*q.v.*).

fallout: Radioactive particles that result from a nuclear explosion and descend through the atmosphere.

false: Not true; not genuine. F. PAINS, abdominal pains occurring during pregnancy that are not true labor pains. F. PELVIS, that part of the pelvis above the pelvic brim. F. LABOR, painful contractions of the uterus that resemble those of true labor but without dilatation of the cervix. F. RIBS, the lower five pairs of ribs, so called because they attach to the sternum by means of a cartilage rather than directly.

falx (falks): A sickle-shaped structure. F. CEREBRI, that portion of the dura mater that separates the two cerebral hemispheres.

familial (fa-mil′-i-al): Pertaining to the family, as of a disease affecting several members of the same family, or that occurs in members of the same family in successive generations.

Fanconi syndrome: See **amino-aciduria.** [Guido Fanconi, Swiss pediatrician. 1882– .]

fang: In humans, the root of a tooth.

fantasy (fan′-ta-si): Imagination in which images or chains of images are directed by the desire or pleasure of the thinker, normally accompanied by a feeling of unreality. Occurs pathologically in schizophrenia. Also phantasy.

farad (far′-ad): A unit of electrical capacity.

faradism (far′-a-dizm): Therapeutic application of a rapidly alternating current to stimulate muscles or nerves. Also faradization, faradotherapy.

farinaceous (far-i-nā′-shus): Pertaining to cereal substances, *i.e.,* made of flour or grain. Starchy.

farmer's lung: A form of pneumoconiosis arising from the dust of moldy hay or other moldy vegetable produce. Recognized as an occupational disease.

farsightedness: Hyperopia (*q.v.*).

fascia (fash′-i-a): A connective tissue sheath consisting of fibrous tissue and fat which unites the skin to the underlying tissues. It also surrounds and separates many of the muscles, and, in some cases, holds them together. F. LATA, the strong, tough F. that envelops the muscles of the thigh.—fasciae, pl.; fascial, adj.

fasciculation (fa-sik-ū-lā′-shun): Involuntary contraction or twitching of a group of muscle fibers.

fasciculus (fas-sik′-ū-lus): A little bundle, as of muscle or nerve.—fascicular, adj.; fasciculi, pl.

fasciorrhaphy (fash-i-or′-a-fi): Suturing of torn or cut fascia.

fasciotomy (fash-i-ot′-o-mi): Incision of a fascia.

fascitis (fas-ī′-tis): Inflammation of a fascia.

fast: 1. To abstain from eating. 2. To be resistant to destruction or to staining, said of bacteria.

fastidium (fas-tid′-i-um): Repugnance or aversion to food or to eating. Squeamishness.

fastigium (fas-tij′-i-um): 1. The highest point of a fever; the period of full development of a disease. 2. The highest point in the roof of the fourth ventricle of the brain.

fat: 1. Plump, stout, obese. 2. The oily substance that makes up most of the cell content of adipose tissue. 3. An oil of animal or vegetable origin, either solid or liquid. —fatty, adj. F. SOLUBLE, refers usually to vitamins A, D, E, and K. See **calorific.**

fatal (fā′-tal): Causing death; deadly.

father complex: Electra complex (*q.v.*).

fatigue: Weariness resulting from prolonged or excessive labor or exertion. In physiological experiments on muscle the term is used to denote diminishing reaction to stimuli applied.—fatigability, n.

fatty degeneration: Degeneration (*q.v.*) of tissues which results in appearance of fatty droplets in the cytoplasm: found especially in diseases of liver, kidney and heart.

fauces (faw′-sēz): The opening from the mouth into the pharynx, bounded above by the soft palate, below by the tongue. Pillars of the F., anterior and posterior, lie laterally and enclose the tonsil.—faucial, adj.

favism (fā′-vizm): Hemolytic anemia; thought to be a sensitivity reaction to certain groups of drugs as well as to fava beans (broad beans) or the pollen from the fava bean plant.

favus (fā′-vus): A type of ringworm in which yellow, cup-shaped crusts form around the hair follicles on the scalp; collectively, they resemble a honeycomb in appearance.

FDA: Abbreviation for Food and Drug Administration (*q.v.*).

fear: An unpleasant, strong emotion occurring in response to recognition of danger or a threat; apprehension, dread, alarm. When carried to morbid excess it is called a phobia (*q.v.*).

febri-: Denotes fever.

febricant (feb′-ri-kant): Causing or producing fever. Also fébrifacient, febrific.

febricide (feb′-ri-sīd): An agent that reduces or destroys fever.

febrifuge (feb′-ri-fūj): An agent that decreases fever.

febrile (feb′-ril): Feverish; accompanied by fever. F. ALBUMINURIA, albuminuria that is due to fever.

fecal (fē′-kal): Pertaining to feces. F. IMPACTION, a hard mass of feces that collects in the intestine and is immovable by normal intestinal activity.

fecalith (fē′-ka-lith): A concretion formed in the bowel from fecal matter.

fecaluria (fē-ka-lū′-ri-a): The presence or

evidence of fecal matter in the urine.

feces (fē-sēz): The waste matter excreted from the bowel, consisting of indigestible cellulose, unabsorbed food, intestinal secretions, water, and bacteria.—fecal, adj.

feculent (fek′-ū-lent): Foul. Pertaining to, containing, or of the nature of feces.

fecundation (fē-kun-dā′-shun): Impregnation. Fertilization.

fecundity (fē-kun′-di-ti): Pronounced fertility; the power to reproduce offspring in large numbers.

feeblemindedness (fē-b'l-mīnd′-ed-nes): Lack of mental development or intelligence. Usually divided into the three grades of idiocy, imbecility, and moronity, or slow learner, retarded, and severely retarded.

feedback: In electronics, the return to the input of part of the output constituting information that reports discrepancies between intended and actual operation and leads to self-correction. In psychology, information that is transmitted to a person in order to modify his behavior when it has deviated from its intended course.

feeding: The giving or taking in of food. DEMAND F., feeding an infant when he indicates he is hungry rather than on a set schedule. FORCED F., giving liquid food by nasal tube. TUBE F., introducing food via tube into the stomach, duodenum, or rectum.

feeling: 1. The sense of touch. 2. The awareness of the sensations produced by the special sense organs. 3. An emotion or mental state that is recognized as pleasurable or unpleasurable.

Fehling's solution (fā′-lings): An alkaline, copper solution used to detect presence and amount of sugar. [Hermann von Fehling, German chemist. 1812-1885.]

feldscher (feld′-sher): An old term now used mainly in Russia and other European countries to describe a medical worker who stands between the doctor and the nurse on the professional scale. Several U.S. medical schools have started programs for training such persons who are called in this country 'physician's assistants.'

fellatio (fe-lā′-shi-ō): Insertion of the penis into the mouth of another person, male or female.

felon (fel′-un): A purulent infection involving the end of a finger, usually near the nail.

feminism (fem′-i-nizm): The appearance of female secondary sex characteristics in a male.

feminization (fem-i-nī-zā′-shun): The development of female characteristics in a man, e.g., high-pitched voice, female type of breast.

femoral (fem′-or-al): Pertaining to the femur or to the thigh as a whole. F. CANAL, a conical canal, about 1.25 cm in length, situated in the region between the anterior superior spine of the ilium and the symphysis pubis; it is a frequent site of hernia. F. HERNIA, see **hernia.**

femoropopliteal (fem-or-ō-pop-lit-ē′-al): Usually refers to the femoral and popliteal vessels.

femur (fē′-mur): The thigh bone; the longest and strongest bone in the body.—femoral, adj.; femora, pl.

fenestra (fen-es′-tra): A window-like opening. F. OVALIS, an oval opening between the middle and internal ear. Below it lies the F. ROTUNDA, a round opening.

fenestrated (fen′-es-trāt-ed): Pierced by one or more openings, e.g., the cribriform plate of the ethmoid bone.

fenestration (fen-es-trā′-shun): The surgical creation of an opening or fenestra in the inner ear for the relief of deafness in otosclerosis.

ferment (fer-ment′): 1. To undergo fermentation (q.v.). 2. Any substance that causes other substances to undergo fermentation.

fermentation (fer-men-tā′-shun): The chemical changes brought about by the action of ferments, usually accompanied by liberation of heat and gas. Excellent examples are the making of bread, cheese and wine.

ferric (fer′-ik): Pertaining to trivalent iron, as of its salts and compounds.

ferrous (fer′-rus): Pertaining to divalent iron, as of its salts and compounds.

fertile (fer′-til): Fruitful; not sterile or barren; capable of bearing young.—fertility, n.

fertilization (fer-ti-lī-zā′-shun): The impregnation of an ovum by a spermatozoon. Conception.

fester (fes′-ter): To ulcerate, generate pus, or suppurate superficially.

festination (fes-ti-nā′-shun): An involuntary hastening in gait as seen in paralysis agitans and some other nervous affections.

fetal (fē′-tal): Pertaining to a fetus (q.v.). F. MOVEMENT, movement of the fetus within the uterus and of which the mother may or may not be aware.

fetid (fet′-id): Having an offensive odor; stinking.

fetish (fet′-ish): An inanimate object that is believed to have magical or supernatural power, or that is worshipped or regarded with unreasonable devotion.

fetography (fē-tog′-ra-fi): X-ray of the fetus in utero.

fetology (fē-tol′-o-ji): That branch of medicine that deals with the diagnosis and treatment of conditions of the unborn fetus.

fetometry (fē-tom′-e-tri): Estimation of the size of the fetus in utero, particularly of the size of the head.

fetor (fē′-tor): Offensive odor; stench. F. EX ORE, bad breath; halitosis.

fetus (fē′-tus): An unborn child. In the human the term usually refers to the unborn child from the third month after gestation until birth.—fetal, adj.

fever (fē′-ver): 1. An elevation of body temperature above normal. Syn., pyrexia. 2. Designates some infectious conditions, *e.g.,* PARATYPHOID F., SCARLET F., TYPHOID F., etc. F. BLISTER, see BLISTER. F. THERAPY, the treatment of disease by causing fever in the patient; may be done by drugs, diathermy, or inoculation with an organism like that which causes malaria.

fiber (fī′-ber): A slender, elongated, threadlike structure.—fibrous, adj.

fibr-, fibro-: Denotes: (1) fiber(s); (2) fibrous tissue; (3) fibrin.

fibril (fī′bril): A component filament of a fiber, as of a muscle or nerve. A small fiber. —fibrillar, fibrillary, adj.

fibrillation (fī-bril-ā′-shun): Uncoordinated quivering contraction of muscle; referring usually to atrial (auricular) F. in the myocardium wherein the atria (auricles) beat very rapidly and are not synchronized with the ventricular beat. The result is a total irregularity of the pulse rhythm. VENTRICULAR F., similar to atrial fibrillation and resulting in rapid, wavering and ineffectual contractions of the ventricles.

fibrin (fī′-brin): The matrix on which a blood clot is formed. The substance is formed from soluble fibrinogen of the blood by the catalytic (enzymatic) action of thrombin. —fibrinous, adj.

fibrinogen (fī-brin′-ō-jen): A soluble protein of the blood from which is produced the insoluble protein called fibrin (*q. v.*) essential to blood coagulation.

fibrinogenopenia (fī-brin-ō-jen-ō-pē′-ni-a): Lack of blood plasma fibrinogen. May be congenital or due to liver disease. Fibrinopenia. Hypofibrinogenemia.

fibrinolysin (fi-bri-nol′-i-sin): An enzyme produced by certain bacteria and which causes the destruction of fibrin thereby aiding in the dissolution of blood clots. Thought to dissolve the fibrin that occurs in tissues after minor injuries. Also called streptokinase.

fibrinolysis (fī-bri-nol′-i-sis): The dissolution of fibrin.—fibrinolytic, adj.

fibroadenoma (fī-brō-ad-e-nō′-ma): A benign tumor containing fibrous and glandular tissue.

fibroblast (fī′-brō-blast): A cell which gives rise to connective tissue. Syn., fibrocyte.— fibroblastic, adj.

fibroblastoma (fī-brō-blas-tō′-ma): A tumor arising from the ordinary connective tissue cell or from fibroblasts.

fibrocartilage (fī-brō-kar′-ti-li j): Cartilage containing fibrous tissue.—fibrocartilaginous, adj.

fibrochondritis (fī-brō-kon-drī′-tis): Inflammation of fibrocartilage.

fibrochondroma (fī-brō-kon-drō′-ma): A benign tumor of cartilaginous tissue which contains a considerable amount of fibrous tissue.

fibrocyst (fī′-brō-sist): A fibroma that has undergone cystic degeneration (*q. v.*).—fibrocystic, adj.

fibrocystic (fī-brō-sis′-tik): Pertaining to a fibrocyst. F. DISEASE OF BONE, cysts may be solitary or generalized. The latter condition, when accompanied by decalcification of bone, is due to hyperparathyroidism. F. DISEASE OF THE BREAST, see **mastitis.** F. DISEASE OF PANCREAS, see **mucoviscidosis.**

fibrocyte (fī′-brō-sīt): See **fibroblast.**—fibrocytic, adj.

fibroid (fī′-broid): 1. Being fibrous in nature. 2. A fibromuscular benign tumor, usually found in the uterus.

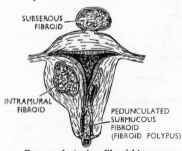

SUBSEROUS FIBROID

INTRAMURAL FIBROID

PEDUNCULATED SUBMUCOUS FIBROID (FIBROID POLYPUS)

Types of uterine fibroid tumor

fibrolymphoangioblastoma (fī-brō-lim-fō-an-ji-ō-blas-tō′-ma): A fibrous tumor of the breast; it is hard and freely movable although somewhat adherent to the skin.

fibroma (fī-brō-ma): A benign tumor composed chiefly of fibrous tissue.—fibromatous, adj.; fibromata, pl.

fibromatosis (fī-brō-ma-tō′-sis): A condition in which several fibromata develop at the same time; they may be quite widely distributed throughout the body.

fibromuscular (fī-brō-mus′-kū-lar): Pertaining to or consisting of fibrous and muscle tissue.

fibromyoma (fī-brō-mī-ō′-ma): A benign tumor consisting of fibrous and muscle tissue.—fibromyomata, pl.; fibromyomatous, adj.

fibroplasia (fī-brō-plā′-zi-a): The formation of fibrous tissue; occurs in the healing of wounds. Usually implies an abnormal increase of fibrous tissue. RETROLENTAL F., see **retrolental**.

fibroplastic (fī-brō-plas′-tik): Giving origin to or producing fibrous tissue.

fibrosarcoma (fī′-brō-sar-kō′-ma): A form of sarcoma. A malignant tumor derived from fibroblastic (fibrocytic) cells.—fibrosarcomata, pl.; fibrosarcomatous, adj.

fibrose (fī′-brōs): 1. The forming of fibrous tissue. 2. Fibrous.

fibrosis (fī-brō′-sis): The formation of fibrous tissue in an organ or part; usually refers to excessive formation as part of a reparative process. It is the cause of adhesions of the peritoneum and other serous tissues. CYSTIC F. OF THE PANCREAS, see **cystic**. F. OF THE LUNGS, the formation of scar tissue in the stroma of the lungs following an infection or inflammation.

fibrositis (fī-brō-sī′-tis): Inflammation of the white fibrous tissue, especially that of some of the muscles. Syn., muscular rheumatism. See **Bornholm disease, lumbago, pleurodynia**.

fibrothorax (fī-brō-thō′-raks): A condition in which the two layers of the pleura adhere to each other. It may result from trauma, tuberculous effusion, or emphysema.

fibrotic (fī-brot′-ik): Characterized by or pertinent to fibrosis.

fibrous (fī′-brus): Consisting of, containing, or like fibers. F. TISSUE, a type of connective tissue that is made up of strong, tough, white fibers; forms tendons, ligaments and fascia.

fibrovascular (fī-brō-vas′-kū-lar): Pertaining to fibrous tissue, which is well supplied with blood vessels.

fibula (fib′-ū-la): One of the longest and thinnest bones of the body; situated on the outer side of the leg and articulating at the upper end with the lateral condyle of the tibia and at the lower end with the lateral surface of the talus (astragalus) and tibia.—fibular, adj.

field (fēld): A limited area; an open space. F. OF HEARING, the space within which sounds are audible. Also called auditory field. F. OF VISION, the area in which objects can be seen by the fixed eye.

filaceous (fi-lā′-shus): Made up of small fibers or filaments.

filament (fil′-a-ment): A delicate fiber or threadlike structure.—filamenta, pl.; filar, adj.

Filaria (fi-lā′-ri-a): A generic term formerly loosely applied to members of the family Filarioidea (*q.v.*); includes several types of nematode worms that infest man.

filaria (fi-lā′-ri-a): A parasitic nematode worm of the family Filarioidea.—filariae, pl.

filariasis (fil-a-rī′-a-sis): Infestation with one of the filariae. See **elephantiasis**.

filaricide (fil-ar′-i-sīd): An agent that destroys filariae.—filaricidal, adj.

Filarioidea (fi-lar-i-oi′-dē-a): A family of parasitic threadlike worms found mainly in the tropics or sub-tropics. Several varieties infest humans; they live in the lymphatics and also invade the connective tissues or mesentery where they may cause obstruction, but the embryos migrate to the bloodstream. Completion of the life cycle is dependent upon passage through a mosquito or other blood-sucking insect.—filarial, adj.

filiform (fil′-i-form): Thread-like. F. PAPILLAE, small projections ending in several minute processes; found on the tongue.

filipuncture (fil′-i-pung-chur): Insertion of wire thread, etc., into an aneurysm to produce coagulation of contained blood.

filter (fil′-ter): 1. To screen out or strain the solids from a substance by passing it through a device that will hold back the solids while letting the liquid pass. 2. Any device that screens or strains out suspended particles. In radiotherapy the term applies to a sheet of metal that lets certain rays pass through while holding others back. F. PAPER, a coarse-grained paper used for filtering solutions. F. PASSING VIRUS, see **virus**.

filterable (fil′-ter-a-b'l): Capable of passing through a filter. F. VIRUS, a pathogenic agent that is so small it passes through the pores of the finest filter available. Also sometimes called filter passing virus.

filtrate (fil'-trāt): That part of a solution that has passed through a filter.

filtration (fil-trā'-shun): The process of straining through a filter. The act of passing fluid through a porous medium. F. UNDER PRESSURE occurs in the kidneys, due to pressure of the blood in the glomeruli.

filum (fi'-lum): Any filamentous or thread-like structure. F. TERMINALE, a strong, fine cord blending with the spinal cord above, and the periosteum of the sacral canal below; the terminal end of the spinal cord.

fimbria (fim'-bri-a): A fringe or frond resembling a frond of a fern, especially one of the frondlike processes at the end of a fallopian tube.—fimbriae, pl.; fimbrial, fimbriated, adj.

finger: A digit of the hand. CLUBBED F., swelling of the terminal phalanx which occurs in many lung and heart diseases. INDEX F., that next to the thumb. WEBBED F., one that is joined to another by a fold of skin. F. COT, see **cot.** F. STALL, a F. cot.

fingerprint: The impression made when the ends of the fingers are inked and then pressed on a piece of paper. Used for identification purposes as no two persons have the same pattern of ridges in the skin at the ends of the fingers.

first aid: The treatment given to a person who is injured or becomes suddenly ill, before the doctor arrives or medical treatment can be obtained.

fish skin disease: Ichthyosis (q.v.).

fission (fish'-un): The action of splitting. In biology, the reproduction of a cell by simple division into two approximately equal parts. In nuclear physics, the splitting of the nucleus of the atom, causing the release of great quantities of energy.

fissure (fish'-ur): A split, cleft or groove;

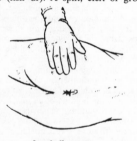

Anal fissure

may be normal or abnormal. ANAL F., a linear ulcer on the margin of the anus.

PALPEBRAL F., the opening between the eyelids. F. OF ROLANDO, see **rolandic.** F. OF SYLVIUS, see **Sylvius.**

fistula (fis'-tū-la): An abnormal communication between two body surfaces or cavities, or between an internal organ and the surface of the body, e.g., gastrocolic F. between the stomach and colon; colostomy, between the colon and the abdominal surface. ABDOMINAL F., one leading from an abdominal viscus to the exterior.—fistular, fistulous, adj.; fistulae, pl.

fistulization (fis-tū-lī-zā'-shun): 1. The surgical creation of a fistula (q.v.). 2. The process of becoming a fistula. Also fistulation.

fit: Convulsion (q.v.). Inappropriate, sudden attack of motor or psychic activity, or both. Typical episode involves patient in involuntary and paroxysmal muscular movements (writhing), associated with loss of consciousness. See **epilepsy.**

fixation (fiks-ā'-shun): 1. The act of fastening something into a fixed position, often by suturing. 2. The condition or state of being fixed in a certain position. 3. In microscopy, a method of treating material to be examined so as to preserve it or to make possible a more thorough examination. 4. In personality development, the arrest of development at a level short of maturity; may result in unnatural behavior, e.g., excessive emotional attachment for a parent. 5. In optics, the direct focusing of one or both eyes so that the image falls on the fovea centralis. COMPLEMENT F., when antigen and homologous antibody unite to form a complex, complement may unite with such a complex, and this is referred to as F.

flaccid (flak'-sid): Soft, flabby, not firm; term is often used to describe muscles that have lost all or part of their tone. Also sometimes used to describe a certain type of personality. See **paralysis.**—flaccidity, n.

flagellate (flaj'-e-lāt): Having flagella. See **flagellum.**

flagellum (fla-jel'-um): A fine, hair-like appendage capable of lashing movement. Characteristic of spermatozoa, certain bacteria and protozoa.—flagella, pl.

flail chest: Unstable thoracic cage due to fracture. See **respiration.**

flank: That part of the trunk of the body that lies between the lowest ribs and the ilia.

flap: A piece of skin or soft tissue that has been surgically detached from the underlying tissue but left attached at some point; used in various plastic operations and to cover the end of bone after amputation of a part.

flatfoot: A congenital or acquired condition in which the arch of the instep is depressed so that the entire sole of the foot touches the ground when one is standing or walking. See **talipes.**

flatulence (flat′-ū-lens): Gastric and intestinal distension with air or gas.—flatulent, adj.

flatus (flā′-tus): Gas or air in the stomach or intestines.

fld: Abbreviation for fluid.

fl dr: Abbreviation for fluid dram, fluidram.

flea (flē): A blood-sucking wingless insect of the order Siphonaptera; it may act as host and transmit such diseases as typhus and plague. Its bite leaves a portal of entry for infection. HUMAN F., Pulex irritans. RAT F., Xenopsylla cheopis, transmitter of plague (*q.v.*).

flesh: The soft tissues of an animal or human body, especially the muscle tissue. GOOSE F., cutis anserina (*q.v.*). PROUD F., the excessive growth of granular tissue in a wound.

flex: Bend.

flexibilitas cerea (flek-si-bil′-i-tas sē′-rē-a): Literally waxy flexibility. A condition of generalized hypertonia of muscles found in catatonic schizophrenia. When fully developed, the patient's limbs retain positions in which they are placed, remaining immobile for hours at a time. Occasionally occurs in hysteria as hysterical rigidity.

flexion (flek′-shun): The act of bending.

Flexner's bacillus (*Shigella flexneri*): A pathogenic gram-negative rod bacterium, which is the most common cause of bacillary dysentery epidemics, and sometimes infantile gastroenteritis. It is found in the feces of cases of dysentery and carriers, from whence it may pollute food and water supplies, or be transferred by contact. [Simon Flexner, American pathologist. 1863-1946.]

flexor (flek′-sor): A muscle which on contraction flexes or bends a part. Opp. to extensor.

flexure (flek′-sher): A bend. HEPATIC F., the bend between the ascending and transverse colon, on the right side near the liver. SPLENIC F., the bend at the junction of the transverse and descending parts of the colon, on the left side near the spleen. SIGMOID F., the S-shaped bend at the lower end

of the descending colon, at its juncture with the rectum below.—flexural, adj.

flight of ideas: Sometimes seen in acute mania when a patient talks continually and repeatedly changes his line of thought.

floating: In anatomy, an organ that is out of, or has become detached from, its normal position in the body. FLOATING KIDNEY, see **nephroptosis.** FLOATING RIBS, a name sometimes given to the 11th and 12th pairs of ribs because they are not attached to the sternum.

floccillation (flok-si-lā′-shun): Carphology (*q.v.*).

flocculation (flok-ū-lā′-shun): The coalescence of colloidal particles in suspension resulting in their aggregation into larger discrete masses which are often visible to the naked eye.

flooding: A popular term to describe excessive bleeding from the uterus.

florid (flor′-id): Flushed; of a bright red color.

fl oz: Abbreviation for fluid ounce, fluidounce.

flu: Abbreviation for **influenza.**

fluctuation (fluk-choo-ā′-shun): A wave-like motion felt on digital examination of an organ or structure containing fluid.—fluctuant, adj.

fluidextract (floo-id-eks′-trakt): A liquid preparation of a plant drug in which 1 cc contains the equivalent of 1 gram of the crude drug. The solvent is usually alcohol.

fluidounce, fluid ounce: In liquid measure, 8 fluidrams (apothecaries' system); 29.57 cc (metric system).

fluidram, fluid dram: A unit of liquid measure (apothecaries' system) equal to 60 minims, 1/8 fluidounce, or approximately 1 teaspoonful. In the metric system it equals 3.7 cc.

fluke (flook): A small, flat, unsegmented trematode worm that may be parasitic to animals and to man, particularly in tropical countries.

fluorescent (floo-o-res′-ent): Having the property of emitting electromagnetic radiation following absorption of radiation from some other source.—fluorescence, n. F. SCREEN, a screen that gives a temporary visualization of a structure when it is interposed between the subject and a source of x-rays.

fluoridation (floo-or-id-ā′-shun): The addition of fluorine salts to water; term usually refers to treatment of the water supply of a community as a public health measure to

fluoride

reduce the incidence of dental caries; the dilution is usually 1:1,000,000. See **fluorine.**

fluoride (floo′-o-rīd): A compound of fluorine and another element; the form of fluorine used as an additive to drinking water to prevent caries.

fluoridize (floo-or′-i-dīz): 1. To add fluoride to the drinking water. 2. To apply a fluoride to the teeth as a preventive measure against the formation of caries.

fluorine (floo′-or-ēn): A non-metallic gaseous element; in the human body it is found chiefly in bones and teeth. When present in natural water supply, it tends to reduce dental decay; in excess it gives a mottled appearance to the teeth. See **fluoridation.**

fluoroscope (floo-or′-o-skōp): A device used in examining the deeper structures of the body. See **fluoroscopy.**

fluoroscopy (floo-or-os′-ko-pi): X-ray examination by means of a fluorescent screen; commonly called 'screening.'

fluorosis (floo-o-rō′-sis): A condition caused by excessive intake of a fluoride substance; characterized by brittleness of bones, discoloration and mottling of the teeth; may occur when the water supply of a community contains an excessive amount of natural fluoride.

flush: A reddening of the skin, especially of the face and neck. 'Hot flush' is a lay term for such reddening when seen in women during menopause.

flutter: A rapid pulsation or vibration; said especially of the heart. ATRIAL F., a type of cardiac arrhythmia in which the atrial contractions may reach 200-400 per minute, but they remain rhythmic and of uniform strength.

flux: 1. An excessive flow of any of the body secretions. 2. Diarrhea. BLOODY F., dysentery.

focal infection: An infection localized more or less in one site from which it spreads to other parts of the body.

focus (fō′-kus): 1. A point at which rays converge; said of light and sound waves. 2. The area of the body where disease or a morbid process is localized.—foci, pl.; focal, adj.

folacin (fōl′-a-sin): Folic acid (*q.v.*).

Foley catheter: See **catheter.**

folic acid: A constituent of the vitamin B complex, found in leafy plants, certain nuts, yeast, liver, kidney. Has antianemic properties and is important in the formation of red blood cells; effective in preventing sprue,

pernicious and other types of anemia.

folie à deux (fŏ′-li a dü′): A situation in which two closely associated persons, usually relatives, have the same delusion.

follicle (fol′-ik′l): 1. A small secreting sac. 2. A simple tubular gland. GRAAFIAN F., minute vesicle in the stroma of the ovary, containing a single ovum. HAIR F., the tubular oil-secreting invagination of epithelium in which the hair grows.—follicular, adj.

follicle-stimulating hormone: A hormone of the anterior pituitary lobe which stimulates the graafian follicles of the ovary, promotes maturation of the follicle and liberation of estrin (*q.v.*). In the male it stimulates the production of spermatozoa through stimulation of the epithelium of the seminiferous tubules.

folliculitis (fŏ-lik-ū-lī′-tis): Inflammation of a follicle (*q.v.*); usually refers to infections around the hair follicles.

fomentation (fō-men-tā′-shun): A hot, wet application used to reduce pain or inflammation. When the skin is intact, strict cleanliness is observed (medical F.); when the skin is broken, aseptic technic is observed (surgical F.). See **stupe.**

fomite (fō′-mīt): Any article that has been in contact with infection and is capable of transmitting same. Also fomes.

fontanel, fontanelle (fon-ta-nel′): A soft spot, particularly in the spaces between certain cranial bones of an unborn or newly born child. The diamond shaped anterior F. (bregma) is at the junction of the frontal and two parietal bones. It ossifies during the second year of life. The triangular posterior F. (lambda) is at the junction of the occipital and two parietal bones. It ossifies within a few weeks of birth.

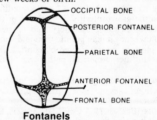

Fontanels

Food and Drug Administration: A federal governmental agency that is charged with the duty of inspecting and passing on the purity and potency of foods and drugs that are offered for sale in the United States.

food poisoning: Vomiting, with or without diarrhea, resulting from eating food contaminated with chemical poison, preformed bacterial toxin, or live bacteria.

foot: That portion of the lower leg that is below the ankle. The sole or bottom is called the plantar surface; the top side is called the dorsal surface. ATHLETE'S F., tinea pedis (*q.v.*). DROP F., or FOOTDROP, inability to dorsiflex the foot as in severe sciatica and nervous conditions affecting lower lumbar regions of the cord; sometimes results from failure to protect feet from pressure of bedclothing. MADURA F., see **mycetoma.** TRENCH F., immersion F., so called because it occurs among soldiers in trenches; also occurs in frostbite and other conditions of exposure when there is local deprivation of blood supply.

footprint: An ink impression of the sole of the foot. Used in maternity hospitals or wards as a means of identification of newborn infants.

foramen (for-ā'-men): A natural hole or opening. Generally used with reference to bones. F. MAGNUM, the opening in the occipital bone through which the spinal cord passes and becomes continuous with the medulla oblongata. OBTURATOR F., found in the anterior portion of the innominate bone. F. OVALE, a fetal cardiac, interatrial communication. Closes at birth.—foramina, pl.

forceps (for'-seps): Surgical instruments with two opposing blades which are used to grasp or compress tissues, swabs, needles and many other surgical appliances. The two blades are controlled by direct pressure on them (tong-like), or by handles (scissorlike). OBSTETRIC F., used to help extract the infant's head from the birth canal.

forearm (fōr'-arm): That part of the arm that is between the elbow and the wrist.

forefinger: The index finger, *i.e.,* the one next to the thumb.

forensic medicine (for-en'-sik med'-i-sin): Medical jurisprudence (*q.v.*).

foreskin (fōr'-skin): The prepuce or skin covering the glans penis.

formaldehyde (for-mal'-de-hīd): A colorless, pungent, irritating gas that has disinfectant and germicidal properties. Used in the gas form and also in solution. See **formalin.**

formalin (for'-ma-lin): Approximately a 40 percent solution of formaldehyde. Used mainly for room disinfection and for fixing and preserving pathological specimens.

formic acid (for'-mik as-id): An organic acid found naturally in ants and other insects as well as in some plants *e.g.,* nettles.

formication (for-mi-kā'-shun): A sensation as of ants running over the skin. Occurs in nerve lesions, particularly in the regenerative phase.

formula (for'-mū-la): 1. A prescription. 2. Recipe for an infant's artificial feeding, or the feeding itself. 3. A simplified statement of a general fact or rule expressed in figures, symbols, or simple language.—formulae, formulas, pl.

formulary (for'-mū-lar-i): A collection of formulas, recipes, prescriptions. NATIONAL F., a book issued periodically by the American Pharmaceutical Association, containing standards for pharmaceuticals that are not included in the U.S. Pharmacopeia.

fornix (for'-niks): An arch; particularly referred to the vagina, *i.e.,* the space between the vaginal wall and the cervix of the uterus.—fornices, pl. CONJUNCTIVAL F., the line of reflection of the conjunctiva from the eyelids onto the eyeball.

fortified (for'-ti-fīd): In nutrition, refers to the addition of substances intended to make food more nutritious.

fossa (fos'-a): In anatomy, a depression, furrow, hollow, or pit.—fossae, pl.

fourchette (foor-shet'): A membranous fold connecting the posterior ends of the labia minora.

fovea (fō'-vē-a): A small depression or fossa, particularly the fovea centralis retinae, the site of most distinct vision.

Fowler's position: The position in which the patient's head or the head of the bed is raised 18-20 inches above the level. The knees are flexed and supported by a pillow. Aids abdominal and pelvic drainage and useful in aiding breathing in respiratory disorders.

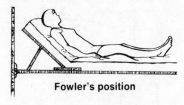

Fowler's position

foxglove (foks'-glov): See **digitalis.**
frac dos: Abbreviation for fractional or divided doses.

fractional sterilization: Sterilizing material by submitting it to temperatures of 60-100° C for three or four successive days to kill the spores that develop in the periods between heatings.

fractional test meal: A method of examining the gastric contents by withdrawing samples at intervals after a standard meal, and subsequently submitting them to chemical analysis.

fracture (frak′-chur): Breach in continuity of a bone. CLOSED (SIMPLE) F., there is no communication with external air. COLLES' F., of the lower end of radius giving typical

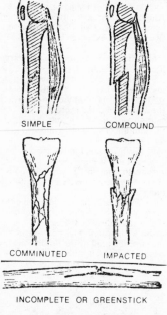

SIMPLE   COMPOUND

COMMINUTED   IMPACTED

INCOMPLETE OR GREENSTICK

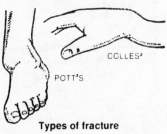

COLLES'

POTT'S

Types of fracture

'dinner fork' deformity. COMMINUTED F., the bone is broken into several pieces. COMPLICATED F., there is injury to surrounding organs and structures. COMPRESSION F., usually of lumbar or dorsal region due to hyperflexion of spine; the anterior vertebral bodies are crushed together. DEPRESSED F., the broken bone presses on an underlying structure, such as brain or lung. IMPACTED F., one end of the broken bone is driven into the other. INCOMPLETE F., the bone is only cracked or fissured—called 'GREENSTICK F.' when it occurs in children. OPEN (COMPOUND) F., there is a wound permitting communication of broken bone end with air. PATHOLOGICAL F., one caused by local disease of bone. POTT'S F., occurs at the lower end of the fibula; often accompanied by dislocation of the tarsal bones and injury to the ligaments. SPONTANEOUS F., one occurring without appreciable violence; may be synonymous with pathological F.

fragilitas (fra-jil′-i-tas): Brittleness. F. CRINIUM, brittleness of the hair. F. OSSIUM, congenital disease characterized by abnormal fragility of bone, multiple fractures and a china-blue discoloration of the sclera. F. SANGUINIS, fragility of the red blood cells. F. UNGUIUM, abnormal brittleness of the nails.

frambesia (fram-bē′-zi-a): Yaws (q.v.).

fraternal twins: Twins that have developed from the fertilization of two ova; need not be of the same sex or identical in appearance.

Fredet-Ramstedt operation: An operation for the correction of congenital pyloric stenosis.

free association: A method in psychoanalytic therapy in which the patient is urged to express verbally whatever ideas and feelings he may have.

freezing: 1. Frostbite. 2. The use of freezing temperatures to produce temporary anesthesia, e.g., spraying the skin with liquid carbon dioxide snow or the use of ice bags. When used for therapeutic purposes, it is called **cryotherapy.**

Freiberg's disease: Osteochondritis of the second metatarsal head. [Albert Henry Freiberg, American orthopedic surgeon. 1868-1940.]

Freijka splint (frā′-ka): Used to correct congenitally dislocated hips. Consists of a pillow stuffed with kapok and held in position between the baby's legs by a special garment made with straps that are placed over the baby's shoulders and pinned securely; it is applied over the regular diaper. The baby's legs are maintained in a position of abduction and flexion.

French chalk: Talc (*q.v.*).

frenetic (fre-net'-ik): Wild, excited, frantic, frenzied.—frenetically, adv.

Frenkel's exercises: Exercises for tabes dorsalis to teach muscle and joint sense in order to restore lost coordination. [Heinrich Frenkel, Swiss neurologist. 1860-1931.]

frenotomy (fre-not'-om-i): Surgical severance of a frenum, particularly for tongue-tie.

frenulum (fren'-ū-lum): A small frenum (*q.v.*). F. LINGUAE, extends from the under surface of the tongue to the floor of the mouth.

frenum (fre'-num): A small fold of membrane that checks or limits the movement of an organ.

frenzy (fren'-ze): Violent, abnormal, compulsive excitement or agitation.

Freud (froid): The originator of psychoanalysis and the psychoanalytical theory of the causation of neuroses. He first described the existence of the unconscious mind, censor, repression, the theory of infantile sexuality, and worked out in detail many mental mechanisms of the unconscious which modify normal, and account for abnormal human behavior. [Sigmund Freud, Austrian psychiatrist. 1856-1939.]

freudian (froid'-ē-an): Pertaining to Freud (*q.v.*) or his doctrines.

friable (frī'-a-b'l): Easily crumbled; readily pulverized.

friction (frik'-shun): Rubbing. F. MURMUR, heard through the stethoscope when two rough or dry surfaces rub together, as in pleurisy and pericarditis.

Friedländer's bacillus: (*Klebsiella pneumoniae*) A large, gram-negative rod bacterium occasionally found in the upper respiratory tract; may cause lobar pneumonia (less than 1 percent of all cases) and other inflammations of the respiratory tract. [Carl Friedländer, German pathologist. 1847-1887.]

Friedman's test: A pregnancy test. The intravenous injection, into a virgin rabbit, twice a day for 2 days, of 4 cc of urine from a pregnant woman will cause ovulation in the rabbit at the end of 2 days. It necessitates sacrifice and postmortem examination of the rabbit. [Maurice H. Friedman, American physician. 1903- .]

Friedreich's ataxia: A progressive familial disease of childhood, in which there develops a sclerosis of the sensory and motor

columns in the spinal cord, with consequent muscular weakness and staggering (ataxia), impairment of speech and lateral curvature of the spine. [Nikolas Friedreich, German neurologist. 1825-1882.]

frigidity (fri-jid'-i-ti): Lack of normal sexual desire or response; usually refers to the female; often a symptom of psychoneurotic disorder.

frigotherapy (frig-ō-ther'-a-pi): The use of low temperatures or of cold in the treatment of disease; cryotherapy.

frog: F. BREATHING, a type of breathing taught to patients with respiratory difficulty to help free them from dependence on mechanical breathing aids such as the iron lung. Air is forced down the throat by the tongue. F. PLASTER, conservative treatment of a congenital dislocation of the hip, whereby the dislocation is reduced by gentle manipulation and both hips are immobilized in plaster of paris, both limbs abducted to 80 degrees. F. TEST, a pregnancy test in which the female African frog, *Xenopus laevis,* is utilized.

Fröhlich's syndrome: A group of symptoms caused by damage to the pituitary gland and hypothalamus, including adiposity, sexual infantilism, excessive somnolence and, occasionally, diabetes insipidus. Also called dystrophia adiposogenitalis. [Alfred Fröhlich, Viennese neurologist. 1871-1953.]

frontal (frun'-tal): 1. Pertaining to the front or anterior aspect of an organ or the body. 2. The bone of the forehead. F. SINUS, a cavity at the inner aspect of each orbital ridge on the F. bone.

frostbite (frost'-bīt): Freezing of the skin and superficial tissues resulting from exposure to extreme cold. The fingers, toes, nose and ears are most frequently affected. The lesion is similar to a burn and may become gangrenous.

frottage (frō-tahzh'): 1. A rubbing movement in massage. 2. A form of sexual perversion in which orgasm is achieved by rubbing against someone.

frozen: F. SECTION, section cut from frozen tissue for histologic examination, *e.g.,* that removed from the body during surgery and examined immediately for possible malignancy. F. SHOULDER, disability of the shoulder joint in which there is limited abduction and rotation of the arm; results from a fibrositis (*q.v.*) of unknown origin; initial pain is followed by stiffness which lasts several months; as the pain subsides exercises are intensified until full recovery is gained.

fructose (fruk'-tōs): A monosaccharide found with glucose in plants. It is the sugar in honey and is a constituent of cane sugar. Syn., levulose.

frustration (frus-trā'-shun): The condition of emotional tension resulting when forces outside oneself block or thwart the performance of acts which, if carried out, would result in satisfaction or gratification of specific needs or desires.

FSH: Abbreviation for follicle-stimulating hormone (*q.v.*).

FTA-ABS test: [Fluorescent treponemal antibody absorption.] A serological test for syphilis.

FTA-IgM test: A serological test to differentiate neonatal syphilis from passive placental transfer of maternal antibodies.

-fugal: Denotes: (1) passing from, driving away; (2) relieving or dispelling.

fugitive (fū'-ji-tiv): Wandering; transient. Descriptive of certain inconstant symptoms.

fugue (fūg): An attempt to escape from reality. A period of loss of memory as to identity but with retention of habits, skills, and mental faculties; sometimes involving flight from familiar surroundings. During the fugue, the patient may appear to act in a purposeful manner, but after recovery he has no memory of what occurred during the state although earlier events are remembered. Occurs in schizophrenia, hysteria; sometimes after an epileptic seizure.

fulgurant (ful'-gū-rant): Suddenly severe and agonizing. A darting, momentary pain.

fulgurate (ful'-gū-rāt): 1. To come and go quickly, like a flash of lightning. 2. To destroy tissue by electricity.—fulguration, n.; fulgurize, v.t.

full term: Mature—when pregnancy has lasted 40 weeks.

fulminating (ful'-mi-nāt-ing): Developing quickly with great severity, characterized by a severe course, and terminating abruptly. Also fulminant.

fumigant (fū'-mi-gant): A substance which emits fumes for fumigation (*q.v.*).

fumigation (fū-mi-gā'-shun): Disinfection by exposure to the fumes of a vaporized disinfectant. Now used primarily for destroying insects and rodents.

fuming (fūm'-ing): Smoking; emitting a vapor, usually unpleasant.

function: The special work performed by an organ or structure in its normal state.

functional: 1. Pertaining to function. 2. Describing a disorder of the function but not the structure of an organ or system. 3. In psychiatry, a disorder of neurotic origin, *i.e.,* psychogenic, without primary organic disease.

fundus (fun'-dus): The basal portion of a hollow structure; the part that is farthest from the opening.—fundi, pl.; fundic, adj.

fungal (fung'-gal): Relating to or caused by a fungus.

fungicide (fun'-ji-sīd): An agent that is lethal to fungi.—fungicidal, adj.

fungiform (fun'-ji-form): Resembling a mushroom in shape.

fungistat (fun'-ji-stat): An agent that inhibits the growth of fungi.—fungistatic, adj.

fungus: A low form of vegetable life including mushrooms, toadstools, molds, and many microscopic organisms capable of producing disease in man.—fungi, pl.; fungoid, fungous, adj. See **actinomycosis, ringworm, tinea pedis.**

funic (fū'-nic): Pertaining to the umbilical cord.

funicle (fū'-ni-k'l): Funiculus (*q.v.*).

funicular (fū-nik'-ū-lar): Pertaining to the spermatic or to the umbilical cord. F. PROCESS, the part of the tunica vaginalis that covers the spermatic cord.

funiculitis (fū-nik'-ū-lī-tis): Inflammation of a funiculus, the spermatic cord in particular.

funiculus (fū-nik'-ū-lus): A cord-like structure.

funnel breast: A congenital deformity in which the breastbone is depressed toward the spine (pectus excavatum). Also funnel chest.

funny bone: Lay term for a place at the back of the elbow that responds with a tingling sensation when struck; it is the place where the ulnar nerve passes over the medial condyle of the humerus.

furor (fū'-ror): Fury, madness, rage.

furuncle (fū'-rung-k'l): An acute, painful, circumscribed inflammatory lesion of the skin and subcutaneous tissue, usually caused by infection of a hair follicle with the *Staphylococcus aureus;* suppuration occurs with the formation of a central core that is eventually discharged. It has but one opening for drainage in contrast to a carbuncle (*q.v.*). A boil.

furunculosis (fū-rung-kū-lō'-sis): The condition of being afflicted with furuncles.

furunculus orientalis (fū-rung'-kū-lus o-ri-en-tā'-lis): Oriental sore (*q.v.*).

fusiform (fū′-zi-form): Resembling a spindle.

fusion (fū′-zhun): In surgery, the induction of bony ankylosis in joints when it is desirable to immobilize them. SPINAL F., the joining of two or more vertebrae to immobilize part of the spinal column; used in cases of abnormality, arthritis or tuberculosis of the spine. BINOCULAR F. The F. of two separate images of an object in the two eyes into one.

G

G, g: Abbreviation for gram(s).

γ: Symbol for the Greek letter gamma (*q.v.*).

gag: 1. A device that is placed between the teeth to keep the mouth open. 2. To prevent one from speaking. 3. To retch or attempt to vomit. GAG REFLEX, the contraction of the constrictor muscle of the pharynx when the back of the pharynx is touched; also pharyngeal reflex.

gait: A manner or style of walking. ATAXIC G., the foot is raised high and then brought down suddenly, the whole foot striking the ground. CEREBELLAR G., reeling, staggering, lurching. SCISSOR G., one in which the legs cross each other in progression. SPASTIC G., stiff, shuffling, the legs being held together. TABETIC G., ataxic G.

galact-, galacto-: Denotes: (1) milk; (2) galactose.

galactagogue (ga-lak′-ta-gog): 1. An agent that induces or increases the flow of milk. 2. Increasing the flow of milk. Also galactogogue.

galactin (ga-lak′-tin): Syn., prolactin (*q.v.*).

galactocele (ga-lak′-tō-sēl): 1. A cyst in the mammary gland containing milk. 2. A hydrocele that contains a milky fluid.

galactorrhea (ga-lak-tō-rē′-a): 1. Excessive flow of milk. 2. Continued flow of milk after a child has been weaned. 3. Spontaneous, excessive flow of milk without there having been a recent pregnancy.

galactose (gal-ak′-tōs): A monosaccharide found with glucose in lactose or milk sugar.

galactosemia (ga-lak-tō-sē′-mi-a): 1. A congenital metabolic disorder, beginning in infancy, in which galactose is present in the blood causing a toxic effect that is particularly damaging to the liver and brain. Symptoms include vomiting, malnutrition, jaundice, poor weight gain. 2. The presence of galactose in the circulating blood.

galactostasis (ga-lak-tos′-ta-sis): Lessening or cessation of milk secretion.

galactosuria (ga-lak-tō-sū′-ri-a): The presence of galactose in the urine.

galacturia (ga-lak-tū′-ri-a): Passing of urine that has a milky appearance.

gall: Bile (*q.v.*).

gallbladder (gawl′-blad-der): A pear-shaped bag on the right underside of the liver. Between meals it concentrates and stores bile; during digestion it releases the bile into the duodenum where it acts on fats. G. SERIES, x-ray examination of the gallbladder for diagnostic purposes.

gallstones (gawl′-stōns): Stones or concretions formed within the gallbladder or bile ducts; they are often multiple and faceted.

galvanic (gal-van′-ik): Pertaining to a direct current of electricity, particularly that produced by a battery.

galvanocauterization (gal-van-ō-kaw-ter-ī-zā′-shun): The use of a wire heated by galvanic current to destroy tissue.

gamete (gam′-ēt): A mature male or female reproductive cell. See **ovum, spermatozoon.**

Gamgee (gam′-jē): A surgical dressing of absorbent cotton enclosed in a fine gauze mesh.

gamma: The third letter in the Greek alphabet; sometimes used in scientific nomenclature to designate the third in a series. G. GLOBULIN, a chemically extracted protein fraction of human plasma, rich in specific antibodies against a variety of viruses, *e.g.*, those of measles and epidemic hepatitis. G. RAYS, electromagnetic radiation given off by certain radioactive substances; of shorter length than x-rays; have great penetrating power; used to destroy tissue.

ganglioma (gang-li-ō′-ma): A tumor or swelling of a lymphatic ganglion (*q.v.*).

ganglion (gang′-li-on): 1. An organized mass of nerve cell bodies outside the brain and spinal cord, forming a subsidiary nerve center that receives and sends out nerve fibers, *e.g.*, the ganglionic masses forming the sympathetic nervous system. 2. A cystic tumor on a tendon or aponeurosis; sometimes on the back of the wrist due to strain such as excessive piano practice. 3. An enlargement on the course of a nerve such as is found on the receptor nerves before they enter the spinal cord. 4. An enlarged lymphatic gland.—ganglia, pl.; ganglionic, adj. GASSERIAN G. is deeply situated within the skull, on the sensory root of the fifth cranial nerve. It is involved in trigeminal neuralgia.

ganglionectomy (gang-li-on-ek′-tom-i): Surgical excision of a ganglion.

gangrene (gang′-grēn): Death of part of the tissues of the body. Usually the result of inadequate blood supply, but occasionally due to direct injury (traumatic G.) or infection (*e.g.,* gas G.). Deficient blood supply may result from pressure on blood vessels (*e.g.,* tourniquets, tight bandages, or swelling of a limb); from obstruction within healthy vessels (*e.g.,* arterial embolism; frostbite, where the capillaries become blocked); from spasm of the vessel wall (*e.g.,* ergot poisoning); or from thrombosis due to disease of the vessel wall (*e.g.,* arteriosclerosis in arteries; phlebitis in veins). DRY G., occurs when the circulation of the blood through an affected part is inadequate; usually starts in the toes; tissues become shrunken and black. GAS G., results from the infection of a dirty, lacerated wound by anaerobic organisms, usually *Clostridium welchii;* the gas that forms spreads through the muscles so that they give a crackling sound when touched; formerly a serious problem in wartime wounds. MOIST G., occurs when venous drainage is inadequate; tissues become swollen with fluid and there is an offensive purulent discharge.—gangrenous, adj.

gargle: 1. The act of washing the throat. 2. A solution used for washing the throat.

gargoylism (gar′-goil-izm): Rare congenital mucopolysaccharide disorder of metabolism with recessive or sex-linked inheritance. Characterized by skeletal abnormalities, dwarfism, coarse fractures, heavy ugly

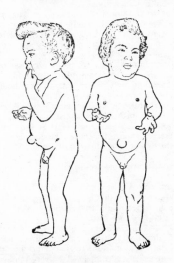

Gargoylism

facies, enlarged liver and spleen, mental subnormality. Hunter-Hurler syndrome.

Gärtner's bacillus: *Salmonella enteritidis.* A motile gram-negative rod bacterium, widely distributed in domestic and wild animals, particularly rodents, and sporadic in man as a cause of food poisoning. [August Gärtner, German bacteriologist. 1848-1934.]

gas: One of the three states of matter. It retains neither shape nor volume when released.—gaseous, adj. LAUGHING G., nitrous oxide (*q.v.*). G. GANGRENE, see **gangrene.** G. POISONING, see **asphyxia, carbon monoxide.**

gasp: 1. To catch one's breath audibly in response to shock or emotion. 2. To breathe with difficulty through the open mouth.

gasserectomy (gas-er-ek′-to-mi): Surgical excision of the gasserian ganglion (*q.v.*).

gasserian ganglion: A large flattened ganglion of the sensory root of the 5th cranial nerve (trigeminal); located in a cleft in the dura mater over the anterior part of the temporal bone; gives off the ophthalmic and maxillary nerves and part of the mandibular nerve.

gaster (gas′-ter): The stomach.

gastr-, gastri-, gastro-: Denotes: (1) the stomach; (2) the ventral area.

gastralgia (gas-tral′-ji-a): Pain in the stomach. Also gasteralgia.

gastratrophia (gas-tra-trō′-fi-a): Atrophy of the stomach.

gastrectasia (gas-trek-tā′-zi-a): Dilatation of the stomach.

gastrectomy (gas-trek′-to-mi): Removal of a part or the whole of the stomach. PARTIAL G. is the commonest operation carried out for peptic ulcer; also subtotal G. TOTAL G. is carried out only for cancer of the stomach.

gastric (gas′-trik): Pertaining to the stomach. G. ANALYSIS, analysis of gastric contents for diagnostic purposes; patient is given a meal and specimens are withdrawn at intervals during digestion in the stomach. G. INFLUENZA, a term used when gastrointestinal symptoms predominate. G. JUICE, secreted by the glands in the mucous lining of the stomach; the two main ingredients are pepsin and hydrochloric acid. G. LAVAGE, a washing out of the stomach. G. SUCTION may be intermittent or continuous to keep stomach empty after abdominal operations. G. ULCER, see **ulcer.**

gastrin (gas′-trin): A hormone secreted by

the gastric mucosa on entry of food, which causes a further flow of gastric juice.

gastritis (gas-trī'-tis): Inflammation of the stomach, especially the mucous membrane lining.

gastroblennorrhea (gas-trō-blen-ō-rē'-a): Excessive secretion of gastric mucus.

gastrocnemius (gas-trok-nē'-mi-us): The large two-headed muscle of the calf.

gastrocolic (gas-trō-kol'-ik): Pertaining to the stomach and the colon. G. REFLEX, sensory stimulus arising on entry of food into stomach, resulting in strong peristaltic waves in the colon.

gastrocolostomy (gas-trō-kō-los'-to-mi): The surgical creation of an artificial opening between the stomach and the colon.

gastroduodenal (gas-trō-dū-ō-dē'-nal): Pertaining to the stomach and duodenum.

gastroduodenostomy (gas-trō-dū-ō-de-nos'-to-mi): A surgical anastomosis between the stomach and the duodenum.

gastrodynia (gas-trō-din'-i-a): Pain in the stomach.

gastroenteritis (gas-trō-en-ter-ī'-tis): Inflammation of mucous membranes of stomach and small intestine; although sometimes the result of dietetic error, the cause is usually a bacterial infection.

gastroenterology (gas-trō-en-ter-ol'-o-ji): Study of the stomach and intestines and their diseases.—gastroenterological, adj. gastroenterologically, adv.

gastroenteropathy (gas-trō-en-ter-op'-a-thi): Any disease of the stomach and intestine.—gastroenteropathic, adj.

gastroenteroptosis (gas-trō-en-ter-op-tō'-sis): Prolapse or downward displacement of the stomach and part of the intestine.

gastroenterostomy (gas-trō-en-ter-os'-to-mi): A surgical anastomosis between the stomach and small intestine.

gastroesophagostomy (gas-trō-ē-sof-a-gos'-to-mi): The surgical formation of an artificial passage from the esophagus into the stomach.

gastrogastrostomy (gas-trō-gas-tros'-to-mi): The surgical removal of part of the stomach and union of the two remaining parts. May be done to relieve a condition known as hourglass stomach.

gastrogavage (gas-trō-ga-vazh'): The introduction of food directly into the stomach via a tube through an opening in the wall of the stomach.

gastrohysterectomy (gas-trō-his-ter-ek'-to-mi): See **abdominohysterectomy**.

gastroileostomy (gas-trō-il-ē-os'-to-mi): The creation of an anastomosis between the stomach and the ileum.

gastrointestinal (gas-trō-in-tes'-ti-nal): Pertaining to the stomach and intestine.

gastrojejunostomy (gas-trō-je-joon-os'-to-mi): A surgical anastomosis between the stomach and the jejunum.

gastrolavage (gas-trō-la-vazh'): Washing out of the stomach.

gastrolith (gas'-trō-lith): A calculus or stone formed in the stomach.

gastromalacia (gas-trō-mal-ā'-shi-a): Abnormal softening of the stomach walls.

gastromegaly (gas-trō-meg'-a-li): Enlargement of the stomach or of the abdomen.

gastropathy (gas-trop'-a-thi): Any disease of the stomach.

gastropexy (gas-trō-peks'-si): Surgical fixation of a displaced stomach to the wall of the abdomen or some other structure.

gastrophrenic (gas-trō-fren'-ik): Pertaining to the stomach and diaphragm.

gastroplasty (gas'-trō-plas-ti): Any plastic operation on the stomach.

gastroplication (gas-trō-pli-kā'-shun): An operation for the cure of dilated stomach by pleating the wall.

gastroptosis (gas-trop-tō'-sis): Downward displacement of the stomach.

gastropylorectomy (gas-trō-pī-lō-rek'-to-mi): Excision of the pyloric end of the stomach. Pylorectomy.

gastrorrhagia (gas-trō-rā'-ji-a): Hemorrhage from the stomach.

gastrorrhea (gas-trō-rē'-a): Excessive secretion of mucus or gastric juice by the stomach.

gastroscope (gas'-trō-skōp): See **endoscope**.—gastroscopic, adj.; gastroscopy, n.

gastrospasm (gas'-trō-spazm): Spasmodic contraction of the walls of the stomach.

gastrostenosis (gas-trō-sten-ō'-sis): A reduction in the size of the stomach.

gastrostomy (gas-tros'-to-mi): A surgically established fistula between the stomach and the exterior abdominal wall; usually for artificial feeding.

gastrotomy (gas-trot'-o-mi): Incision into the stomach.

gastroxynsis (gas-trok-sīn'-sis): Excessive secretion of hydrochloric acid by the stomach; hyperchlorhydria. Also gastroxia.

Gatch bed: See **bed**.

Gaucher's disease (gō'-shāz): A rare familial disorder mainly in Jewish children, characterized by a disordered lipoid metabolism and usually accompanied by very marked enlargement of the spleen. Diagnosis follows sternal marrow puncture and the finding of typical Gaucher cells (distended with lipoid). [Phillippe Charles Ernest Gaucher, French physician. 1854-1918.]

gauze (gawz): A thin open-mesh material used in all surgical procedures and for making surgical and other dressings.

gavage (ga-vazh′): Forced or tube feeding.

GC: Abbreviation for gonococcus.

Gehrig's disease: A popular name for amyolateral sclerosis (see **sclerosis**); so called because it was fatal to an American baseball hero, Lou Gehrig.

Geiger-Müller counter (gī′-ger mil′-er kown′-ter): A device for detecting and registering radioactivity.

gelatin (jel′-a-tin): The protein-containing, glue-like substance obtained by boiling bones, skin and other animal tissues. Used in various ways in pharmaceutical preparations, as a bacteriological culture medium and as a food.—gelatinoid, gelatinous, adj.

gena (jē′-na): The cheek.—genal, adj.

gene (jēn): The factor in the chromosome that is responsible for transmission of hereditary characteristics. Genes are typically in pairs, one of the pair being found in the chromosome received from the father and the other in the corresponding chromosome from the mother.—genetic, adj. DOMINANT G., one that is capable of transmitting its characteristics regardless of whether it is present in the chromosomes of the other parent. RECESSIVE G., one that will transmit its characteristics only if it is present in the chromosomes of both parents.

general: Said of a disease process that affects all or many parts of the body. G. ANESTHETIC, see **anesthetic**. G. PRACTITIONER, a physician who engages in the general practice of medicine as opposed to a specialist; abbreviated GP. G. PARALYSIS OF THE INSANE, involvement of the brain, usually by syphilitic infection, with consequent dementia; onset may be slow or rapid; loss of memory is an early sign along with disintegration of the personality; abbreviated GPI.

generalize: Term is used to describe a disease process that has changed from being primarily local to being general (*q.v.*).

generation (jen-er-ā′-shun): A group of humans, animals or plants that came into being at approximately the same time and are living contemporaneously; in the human a generation is usually considered to represent one-third of a century.

generative (jen′-er-at-iv): Pertaining to reproduction.

generic (je-ner′-ik): 1. Pertaining to a genus (*q.v.*). 2. Distinctive. 3. Not protected by patent or trademark; said of drugs.

genesis (jen′-e-sis): The production, generation or origin of anything.

genetic (je-net′-ik): 1. Relating to origin or reproduction. 2. Inherited or produced by a gene. 3. Relating to the science of genetics.

genetics (je-net′-iks): The study of heredity.

Geneva Convention: An agreement between European nations signed in Geneva, Switzerland in 1864, and later adopted by other nations, specifying that prisoners of war, and the sick, wounded and dead, as well as those caring for them, would be humanely treated.

-genic: Denotes: (1) forming, producing; (2) produced by, formed from; (3) of or relating to a gene; (4) suitable for production or reproduction.

genicular (jen-ik′-ū-lar): Pertaining to the knee.

genital (jen′-it-al): Pertaining to the organs of generation.

genitalia (jen-it-ā′-li-a): The organs of generation.

genito-: Denotes the genital organs.

genitocrural (jen-it-ō-kroo′-ral): Pertaining to the genital area and the leg.

genitourinary (jen-it-ō-ū′-rin-a-ri): Pertaining to the reproductive and urinary systems or to the organs of those systems.

genocide (jen′-ō-sīd): The killing or destruction of an entire group of humans.

genotype (jen′-ō-tīp): 1. The inherent endowment of the individual. 2. A group of organisms in which all members have the same genetic constitution.

genu (jē′-nū): the knee. G. VALGUM, knock knee. G. VARUM, bowleg.—genua, pl.; genicular, adj.

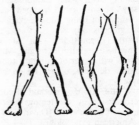

G. valgum   G. varum

genupectoral position (jen-ū-pek′-tor-al): Knee-chest position (*q.v.*).

genus (jē′-nus): A classification ranking between the family (higher) and the species (lower).

geophagia (jē-ō-fā′-ji-a): The habit of eating dirt. Also geophagism, geophagy.

geriatrics (jer-i-at′-riks): The branch of medical science dealing with old age and its diseases.

germ (jurm): 1. A small bit of living substance capable of developing into a new individual. 2. Any microorganism, particularly a pathogenic bacterium. 3. The part of a cereal grain that is separated from the starchy part in the milling process, *e.g.*, wheat germ. 4. A beginning. 5. One of three layers of cells in the embryo from which the organs and structures of the body develop (ectoderm, mesoderm, entoderm).

German measles: See **rubella.**

germicide (jur′-mi-sīd): An agent that kills germs.—Germicidal, adj.

gerontology (jer-on-tol′-oj-i): The scientific study of aging.

gestalt psychology (ges-tawlt′): A school of psychology which teaches that humans respond to meaningful wholes or forms that cannot be broken down into component parts. From the German word *gestalt* meaning appearance or shape. Also called gestalt theory; gestaltism.

gestation (jes-tā′-shun): Pregnancy.—gestational, adj. ECTOPIC G., extrauterine pregnancy, usually in the fallopian tube.

Ghon's focus: Primary lesion of tuberculosis in the lung. [Anton Ghon, Austrian pathologist. 1866-1936.]

GI: Abbreviation for gastrointestinal.

Giardia lamblia: A flagellated beet-shaped organism that attaches itself to the intestinal wall; usually does not cause pathology but may cause giardiasis (*q.v.*). *Lamblia intestinalis.*

giardiasis (ji-ar-dī′-a-sis): Lambliasis (*q.v.*).

gibbosity (gib-bos′-i-ti): A humped back, or the condition of being humpbacked.—gibbus, n.; gibbous, adj.

gigantism (jī′-gan-tizm): An abnormal overgrowth, especially in height. May be associated with anterior pituitary tumor if the tumor develops before fusion of the epiphyses.

Gilliam's operation: A method of correcting retroversion by shortening the round ligaments of the uterus. [David Tod Gilliam, American gynecologist. 1844-1923.]

gingiva (jin-ji′-va): The gum; the vascular tissue surrounding the necks of the teeth.

gingivectomy (jin-ji-vek′-to-mi): Excision of a portion of the gum, usually for pyorrhea.

gingivitis (jin-ji-vī′-tis): Inflammation of the gums.

girdle (ger′-dl): 1. A belt. 2. An encircling structure or part. G. PAIN, a constricting pain round the waist region, occurring in tabetic persons. PELVIC G., comprises the two innominate bones, sacrum, and coccyx. SHOULDER G., comprises the two clavicles and scapulae.

glabrous (glāb′-rus): Smooth, hairless.

gladiolus (glad-i-ō′-lus): The blade-like middle portion of the sternum.

glairy (glā′-ri): Slimy, albuminous; like the white of egg.

gland: An organ, structure or group of cells capable of manufacturing a fluid substance (1) to be eliminated from the body, or (2) to be used in some part of the body other than the place it is made. LYMPHATIC G., (node) does not secrete but is concerned with filtration of the lymph. See **endocrine, exocrine.**—glandular, adj.

glanders (glan′-derz): A contagious, febrile, ulcerative disease communicable from horses, mules and asses to man.

glandular fever: See **infectious mononucleosis.**

glans (glanz): The bulbous termination of the clitoris and penis.

glass arm: Lay term for irritation of the long head of the biceps brachii muscle.

glaucoma (glaw-kō′-ma): A condition of the eye characterized by increased intraocular pressure. In acute stage the pain is severe. May result in hardening of the globe of the eye and blindness.

gleet: A chronic urethral discharge in the male; usually mucoid in character.

glenohumeral (glē-nō-hū′-mer-al): Pertaining to the glenoid cavity of the scapula and the humerus.

glenoid (glē′-noid): Resembling a pit or socket, particularly the cavity on the scapula into which the head of the humerus fits to form the shoulder joint.

glia (glī′-a): Neuroglia (*q.v.*).—glial, adj.

-glia: Denotes neuroglia in which the elements are of a particular kind or size, *e.g.*, microglia.

glioblastoma multiforme (glī-ō-blas-tō′-ma mul′-ti-form): A highly malignant brain tumor.

glioma (glī-ō′-ma): A neoplasm that does not give rise to secondary deposits. Usually malignant. It arises from the neuroglia. One form occurring in the retina is hereditary.—gliomata, pl.

gliomyoma (glī-ō-mī-ō'-ma): A tumor of nerve and muscle tissue.—gliomyomata, pl.

Glisson's capsule: The connective tissue sheath of the blood vessels and bile ducts in the liver. [Francis Glisson, English physician and anatomist. 1579-1677.]

globin (glō'-bin): A protein that combines with hematin to form hemoglobin.

globulin (glob'-ū-lin): A fraction of serum or plasma protein. GAMMA G. contains antibodies against certain bacterial and viral diseases. Prepared from convalescent serum; used in prevention and treatment of measles, poliomyelitis and other infectious diseases.

globulinuria (glob-ū-lin-ū'-ri-a): The presence of globulin in the urine.

globus hystericus (glō'-bus his-ter'-ik-us): Subjective feeling of a lump in the throat; of neurotic origin. Can also include difficulty in swallowing and is due to tension of muscles of deglutition. Occurs in hysteria, anxiety states and depression. Sometimes follows slight trauma to throat, e.g., scratch by foreign body.

glomectomy (glō-mek'-to-mi): The excision of a glomus (q.v.).

glomerulitis (glō-mer-ū-lī'-tis): Inflammation of the glomeruli of the kidney.

glomerulonephritis (glō-mer-ū-lō-nef-rī'-tis): A term used in bilateral, non-suppurative inflammation of the glomeruli of the kidneys.

glomerulosclerosis (glō-mer-ū-lō-skler-ō'-sis): Fibrosis of the glomeruli of the kidney, the result of inflammation. INTERCAPILLARY G. is a common pathological finding in diabetes.—glomerulosclerotic, adj.

glomerulus (glō-mer'-ū-lus): A coil of minute arterial capillaries held together by scanty connective tissue. It invaginates the entrance of a uriniferous tubule in the kidney cortex.—glomerular, adj.; glomeruli, pl.

glomus: In anatomy, a small, encapsulated, globular body containing many arterioles and having a rich nerve supply, especially sensory receptors, e.g., the G. CAROTICUM, situated behind the carotid artery at its bifurcation. G. TUMOR, a neoplasm of unknown cause; consists of a slightly elevated, rounded, firm, nodular mass, occurring chiefly in the skin; generally seen on distal ends of fingers and toes and in the nailbed; treatment is surgical removal.

gloss-, glosso-: Denotes: (1) the tongue; (2) language.

glossa (glos'-a): The tongue.—glossal, adj.

glossectomy (glos-ek'-to-mi): Excision of all or part of the tongue.

glossitis (glos-ī'-tis): Inflammation of the tongue.

glossolalia (glos-ō-lā'-li-a): Unintelligible talk; jargon.

glossopharyngeal (glos-ō-fa-rin'-ji-al): 1. Pertaining to the tongue and pharynx. 2. The ninth pair of cranial nerves.

glossoplegia (glos-ō-plē'-ji-a): Paralysis of the tongue.

glossoptosis (glos-op-tō'-sis): Retraction or downward displacement of the tongue.

glottis (glot'-tis): The part of the larynx that is associated with voice production. RIMA GLOTTIDIS, the opening between the free margins of the vocal cords. See **vocal cords.**—glottic, adj.

gluc-, gluco-: Denotes glucose.

glucagon (gloo'-ka-gon): Hormone produced in alpha cells of pancreatic islets of Langerhans. Causes breakdown of glycogen into glucose, thus preventing blood sugar from falling too low during fasting.

glucase (gloo'-kās): An enzyme from plants and microorganisms that acts as a catalyst in converting starch to glucose.

glucocorticoid (gloo-kō-kor'-ti-koid): Any steroid hormone which promotes gluconeogenesis (i.e., the formation of glucose and glycogen from protein) and which antagonizes the action of insulin. Occurs naturally in the adrenal cortex as cortisone and hydrocortisone; also produced synthetically.

glucogenesis (gloo-kō-jen'-e-sis): The formation in the body of glucose from the breakdown of glycogen.

gluconeogenesis (gloo-kō-nē-ō-jen'-e-sis): Glyconeogenesis (q.v.).

glucose (gloo'-kōs): Dextrose or grape sugar. A common and important monosaccharide, present in most fruits. The chief end product of the digestion of carbohydrates and the form in which they are absorbed from the gastrointestinal tract. A normal constituent of blood and other fluids of the body. Excess over what is needed or utilized by the body is stored in the form of glycogen or in body tissues as fat.

glucose tolerance test: Useful in the diagnosis of diabetes mellitus and other causes of glycosuria. Serial collections of blood are estimated for blood glucose following the oral or intravenous administration of glucose, and urine samples are simultaneously tested for glucose.

glucosuria (gloo-kō-sū′-ri-a): The presence of glucose in the urine.

gluteal (gloo′-tē-al): Pertaining to the buttocks.

gluten (gloo′-ten): A protein constituent of wheat flour. Insoluble in water but an essential component of the elastic 'dough.'

gluteus (gloo′-tē-us): G. MAXIMUS, the largest and most superficial of the three large muscles that form the buttock. G. MEDIUS, the middle of the muscles that form the buttock. G. MINIMUS, the innermost of the muscles that form the buttock.

glyc-, glyco-: Denotes glycogen.

glycemia (glī-sē′-mi-a): The presence of glucose in the blood.

glycerin(e) (glis′-er-in): A clear, syrupy liquid prepared synthetically or obtained as a by-product in soap manufacture. It has a hygroscopic action. Widely used in pharmaceutical preparations as a solvent or vehicle for drugs in syrups, lozenges, suppositories. Useful as an emollient (*q.v.*).

glycerol (glis′-er-ol): Glycerin (*q.v.*).

glycine (glī′-sēn): A nonessential amino acid (*q.v.*).

glycinuria (glī-sin-ū′-ri-a): Excretion of glycine in the urine. Associated with mental subnormality.

glycogen (glī′-kō-jen): Animal starch, the form to which glucose is converted for storage in the body. G. STORAGE DISEASE, an inborn error of metabolism; associated with mental subnormality.

glycogenase (glī-kō′-jen-ās): An enzyme necessary for the conversion of glycogen into glucose.

glycogenesis (glī-kō-jen′-e-sis): The synthesis or formation of glycogen from glucose or other monosaccharides.

glycogenolysis (glī-kō-je-nol′-i-sis): The conversion of glycogen into glucose.

glycogenosis (glī-kō-je-nō′-sis): A chronic metabolic disorder of childhood leading to increased storage of glycogen, particularly in the kidney and liver. Leads to enlargement of liver, glycogen myopathy, hypoglycemia.

glycolysis (glī-kol′-i-sis): The hydrolysis of sugars in the body.—glycolytic, adj.

glyconeogenesis (glī-kō-nē-ō-jen′-e-sis): The formation of sugar from protein or fat when there is lack of available carbohydrate.

glycopenia (glī-kō-pē′-ni-a): A deficiency of sugar in the body tissues.

glycoptyalism (glī-kō-tī-al-izm): Glycosialia (*q.v.*).

glycosemia (glī-kō-sē′-mi-a): Glycemia (*q.v.*).

glycosialia (glī-kō-sī-āl′-i-a): Presence of sugar in the saliva.

glycoside (gli′-kō-sīd): A complex natural substance composed of a sugar with another compound, particularly as found in some plants, *e.g.*, digitalis, strophanthus and others. The non-sugar fragment is sometimes of therapeutic value.

glycosuria (glī-kō-sū′-ri-a): The presence of sugar in the urine.

glycuresis (gli-kū-rē′-sis): The normal appearance of glucose in the urine following a carbohydrate meal.

Gm, gm: Abbreviation for gram. G and g are also used.

gnath-, gnatho-: Denotes the jaw.

gnathalgia (nath-al′-ji-a): Pain in the jaw.

gnathoplasty (nath′-ō-plas-ti): Plastic surgery of the jaw.

gnathoschisis (nath-os′-ki-sis): Congenital cleft in the upper jaw, as occurs in cleft palate.

gnosia (nō′-si-a): The faculty of being able to perceive and recognize objects and persons.

gnotobiotics (nō-tō-bī-ot′-iks): The science of producing and raising germ-free animals such as chickens, guinea pigs, rabbits, monkeys and swine, which are useful in research studies of disease production, immunity, antibody formation, etc., or studies that utilize such animals.

goblet cells: Special secreting cells, shaped like a goblet, found in the mucous membranes.

goiter: An enlargement of the thyroid gland causing a swelling in the front of the neck. ADENOMATOUS G., one in which the gland becomes firm and enlarges more on one side than the other; it may grow slowly and then enlarge greatly during middle age; may become toxic or not. COLLOID G., the gland enlarges and becomes soft due to collection of gelatinous matter in the follicles. ENDEMIC G., occurs in certain areas of the world where the food and water do not contain the normal amount of iodine, but the goiters are usually of the simple type. EXOPHTHALMIC G., gland may or may not enlarge; excess of thyroid hormone is secreted, leading to physical symptoms such as nervousness, loss of weight, profuse sweats, accelerated pulse, psychic disturbances, increased basal metabolism, fine muscle

·tremor, and exophthalmos (*q.v.*). SIMPLE
G., not accompanied by the physical symptoms seen in exophthalmic G.; caused by enlargement of the gland in response to iodine insufficiency in the diet; may disappear spontaneously. TOXIC G., exophthalmic G.

goitrogens (goi'-trō-jens): Agents causing goiter; some occur in plants, others in drugs.

Golgi bodies (gol'-jē): Also **Golgi apparatus.** An anastomosing network of delicate fibrils found in the cytoplasm of nearly all cells. [Camillo Golgi, Italian histologist. 1843-1926.]

gomphosis (gom-fō'-sis): An immovable joint, where a conical eminence fits into a socket, *e.g.,* a tooth, or the styloid process of the temporal bone.

gon-, gono-: Denotes: (1) semen; (2) seed; (3) sexual; (4) reproduction.

gonad (gō'-nad): One of the essential sex glands of the male or female. See **ovary, testis.**—gonadal, adj.

gonadotherapy (gon-ad-ō-ther'-a-pi): Treatment by the use of gonadal hormones or extracts.

gonadotrophic (gon-ad-ō-trō'-fik): Gonadotropic (*q.v.*).

gonadotropic (gon-ad-ō-trō'-pik): Having an affinity for, influencing, or stimulating the gonads; said of the anterior pituitary gland, for example.

gonadotropin (gon-ad-ō-trō'-pin): Any gonad-stimulating hormone. Also gonadotrophin.

gonioscopy (gō-ni-os'-kop-i): Measuring or examining the angle of the anterior chamber of the eye with an instrument called a gonioscope.

goniotomy (gō-ni-ot'-o-mi): Operation for glaucoma. Incision through the anterior chamber angle to the canal of Schlemm.

gonoblennorrhea (gon-ō-blen-ō-rē'-a): Gonorrheal conjunctivitis.

gonococcal complement fixation test: A specific serological test for the diagnosis of gonorrhea.

gonococcus (gon-ō-kok'-us): *Neisseria gonorrhoeae;* a gram-negative, encapsulated diplococcus, usually occurring in pairs; the causative organism of gonorrhea.—gonococci, pl.; gonococcal, adj.

gonorrhea (gon-or-rē'-a): An infectious disease of venereal origin in adults. In children infection is accidental, *e.g.,* gonococcal ophthalmia of the newborn, gonococcal vulvovaginitis of girls before puberty. Chief manifestations of the disease in the male are

a purulent urethritis with dysuria; in the female, urethritis and endocervicitis which may be symptomless. Incubation period is 2 to 5 days.—gonorrheal, adj.

gonorrheal (gon-or-rē'-al): Resulting from gonorrhea. G. ARTHRITIS is a metastatic manifestation of gonorrhea. G. OPHTHALMIA is one form of ophthalmia neonatorum (*q.v.*).

gony-: Denotes the knee.

gonyoncus (gon-ē-ong'-kus): Tumor of the knee.

gooseflesh: Cutis anserina. Roughness of the skin produced by the erection of papillae when the arrectores pilorum muscles attached to the sides of the hair follicles contract under stimulation, usually cold or fear. Also called goose bumps, goose pimples.

gouge (gowj): A chisel with a grooved blade for removing bone.

gout (gowt): A metabolic disorder in which uric acid is retained in the body and sodium urates are deposited around joints and in other places in the body; characterized by redness, swelling, pain, and inflammation of the joints, particularly of the big toe. Frequently said to be due to heavy eating of rich foods and consumption of alcohol, but heredity also seems to be involved. See **tophus, purines, uric acid.**

GP: Abbreviation for general practitioner. See **general.**

GPI: Abbreviation for general paralysis of the insane. See **general.**

gr: Abbreviation for grain.

graafian follicle: See **follicle.**

Graefe's knife (grā'-fes): Finely pointed knife with narrow blade, used for making incision across anterior chamber of eye prior to removal of cataract. [Albrecht von Graefe, German ophthalmologist. 1828-1870.]

graft: A tissue or organ which is transplanted to another part of the same animal (autograft), to another animal of the same species (homograft), or to another animal of a different species (heterograft). Only autografts and homografts are used in man.

grain: The unit of weight in the apothecaries' system; equivalent to about 1/15 of a gram in the metric system. (Sometimes abbreviated gr, but it is advisable to spell it out.)

gram, gramme: The unit of weight in the metric system; equivalent to 15.432 grains in the apothecaries' system. Abbreviated Gm, gm, G, g.

-gram: Denotes: (1) drawing; (2) writing; (3) a record.

Gram's stain: A bacteriological stain for differentiation of microorganisms. Those retaining the stain are gram-positive (+), those unaffected by it are gram-negative (—). [Hans Christian Gram, Danish physician. 1853-1938.]

grand mal (gron mal): Major epilepsy. See **epilepsy.**

granulation (gran-ū-lā′-shun): The outgrowth of new capillaries and connective tissue cells from the surface of an open wound. G. TISSUE, the young, soft tissue so formed.—granulate, v.t., v.i.

granulocyte (gran′-ū-lō-sīt): Any cell containing granules, *e.g.,* a leukocyte with neutrophil, eosinophil, or basophil granules in its protoplasm.

granulocytopenia (gran-ū-lō-sī-tō-pē′-ni-a): Decrease of granulocytes in the blood but not sufficient to warrant the term agranulocytosis (*q.v.*).

granulocytosis (gran-ū-lō-sī-tō′-sis): An abnormally large number of granulocytes in the circulating blood.

granuloma (gran-ū-lō′-ma): A tumor formed of granulation tissue. G. INGUINALE, one of the venereal diseases in which lesions form on the genitalia and in the inguinal regions. See **lymphogranuloma.**—granulomata, pl.; granulomatous, adj.

grape sugar: Dextrose or glucose.

graph (graf): A diagram or curve presenting clinical or experimental data in pictorial form.—graphic, adj.

-graph: Denotes: (1) something written; (2) an instrument used for writing, recording, or transmitting.

graphology (graf-ol′-o-ji): The scientific study of handwriting.

graphospasm (graf′-ō-spazm): Writer's cramp.

-graphy: Denotes: (1) writing; (2) a writing on a particular subject.

grasp reflex: The grasping motion exhibited by the fingers or toes in response to stimulation.

gravel: Minute stones or sandy deposit in the gallbladder or urinary bladder.

Graves' disease: Hyperthyroidism (*q.v.*). [Robert James Graves, Irish physician. 1797-1853.]

gravid (grav′-id): Pregnant.

gravida (grav′-i-da): A pregnant woman. Gravida I designates the first pregnancy, gravida II the second, and so on.

gravidarum (grav-id-ar′-um): Literal translation is 'of the pregnant.' G. STRIAE, the purplish longitudinal marks that occur on the skin of the lower abdomen during the later weeks or months of pregnancy.

gravitational (grav-i-tā′-shun-al): Being attracted by force of gravity. G. ULCER, varicose ulcer (*q.v.*).

gravity (grav′-i-ti): Weight. SPECIFIC G., the weight of a substance compared with that of an equal volume of water.

gray matter: Nervous tissue consisting mostly of the cell bodies of neurons and unmyelinated nerve fibers; of grayish color. Occurs in the cortex of the brain and the central H-shaped portion of the spinal cord.

green sickness: Chlorosis (*q.v.*).

green soap: A soft gelatinous soap; prepared as a tincture in a two to one solution with alcohol, used for cleansing skin before surgery.

greenstick fracture: See **fracture.**

grid: A chart with horizontal and perpendicular lines on which curves may be plotted. WETZEL G., a chart of growth on which weight, height, and other factors of growth and development are plotted; used for evaluating physical fitness of young and adolescent children.

griffado (gri-fa′-dō): A person who is one-eighth Negro; one parent is white and the other is quadroon.

grinders (grīn′-derz): The molars or double teeth.

grinder's asthma: One of the many popular names for silicosis arising from inhalation of metallic dust.

grip: Influenza. Also grippe, la grippe.

gripe (grīp): 1. Colic. 2. A sharp, spasmodic intestinal pain.

gristle: Cartilage (*q.v.*).

grocer's itch: An eczema due to sensitivity to flour, sugar, chocolate, cinnamon, etc.

groin: The junction, or the area of the junction of the thigh with the abdomen.

gross: 1. Large or coarse. 2. Seen as a whole, without fine details. 3. Visible without the use of a microscope.

group psychotherapy: See group therapy, under **therapy, psychotherapy.**

growing pains: Pains in the limbs during youth, thought to be rheumatic in origin.

growth: 1. Normal increase in size of any organism. 2. An abnormal increase in size of cells or of tissues, as in a tumor.

gruel: A cereal that is cooked or diluted with milk or broth; may be used in liquid diets or for tube feedings.

G suit: A pressure suit used by test pilots to prevent blacking out at high speeds of travel in aircraft. Has been used experimentally to control internal bleeding.

gt: Abbreviation for *gutta* meaning drop. Plural, gtt for *guttae.*

GU: Abbreviation for genitourinary.

guillotine (gil′-o-tēn): A surgical instrument for excision of the tonsils.

guilt (gilt): In psychiatry, unconscious G. consists of mental functions that are initiated by unconscious punishment fantasies; suffering that results from gratification, or drive toward gratification, of a repressed wish.

gullet (gul′-let): The tube by which food passes from the mouth to the stomach; includes the pharynx and esophagus.

gum: Gingiva (*q.v.*).

gumboil: An abscess on a gum (gingiva).

gumma (gum′-a): A localized area of soft, gummy, vascular, granulation tissue, such as is seen in the later stages (tertiary) of syphilis; may occur in almost any tissue. Obstruction to the blood supply results in necrosis, and gummata near the surface of the body tend to break down, forming chronic ulcers, *e.g.,* on the nose, lower leg, palate, etc. Probably these ulcers are not infectious.—gummata, gummas, pl.; gummatous, adj.

gustation (gus-tā′-shun): 1. The act of tasting. 2. The sense of taste.

gustatory (gus′-ta-tor-i): Pertaining to the sense of taste.

gut: The intestines.

gutta (gut′-a): A drop. G. PERCHA, a waterproof material, formerly much used for surgical drains, among other purposes; now largely replaced by synthetics.

guttatim (gut-tā′-tim): Drop by drop.

guttur (gut′-ter): The throat.—guttural, adj.

gyn-, gyne-, gynec-, gyneco-, gyno-: Denotes: (1) woman; (2) female reproductive organs.

gynae-: Same as **gyn-**.

gynandrism (jin-an′-drizm): Female hermaphroditism.

gynandromorphism (ji-nan-drō-mor′-fizm): An abnormality in which an individual has both female and male characteristics.

gynatresia (jin-a-trē′-zi-a): The occlusion of part of the female generative tract, particularly the vagina.

gynecography (jin-e-kog′-ra-fi): X-ray visualization of the female generative organs following introduction of air into the peritoneal cavity.—gynecographical, adj.; gynecographically, adv.

gynecologic (jin-e-kō-log′-ik): Affecting or relating to the female reproductive tract.

gynecologist (jin-e-kol′-o-jist): A person who specializes in gynecology (*q.v.*).

gynecology (jin-e-kol′-o-ji): The branch of medical science that deals with disorders of the female genital tract.

gynecomastia (jin-e-kō-mas′-ti-a): Excessive enlargement of the male mammary gland.

gypsum (jip′-sum): Plaster of paris (calcium sulphate).

gyrate (jī′-rāt): 1. To revolve. 2. Twisted into a spiral or ring shape.

gyrectomy (jī-rek′-to-mi): Surgical removal of a gyrus (*q.v.*) of the cortex of the brain.

gyrus (jī-rus): Convolution. Term is used specifically to describe the tortuous elevations on the surface of the cortex of the brain; these elevations are separated from each other by shallow grooves called sulci and deep grooves called fissures.—gyri, pl.

H

H: Abbreviation for (1) hydrogen; (2) hour (h also used for hour).

habit: A constant automatic response in a given situation, acquired by frequent repetition. When applied to thoughts, thinking habits become attitudes. H. SPASM, sudden, rapid, twitching, coordinated movement of muscles of a certain area, habitually repeated; voluntary at first, becoming involuntary.

habituation (ha-bit-ū-ā′-shun): The act or process of becoming accustomed to a stimulus or environment. DRUG H., psychological dependence on a drug after physical need for it is gone; usually there is no tendency to increase the dose and on this basis it is often differentiated from drug addiction.

hacking (hak′-ing): 1. Short, chopping blows; a maneuver used in massage. 2. Short dry, interrupted coughing.

haem (hēm): Heme (*q.v.*).

haem-: See **hem-**.

Haemophilus (hē-mof′-il-us): A genus of bacteria. Small gram-negative rods that show much variation in shape. They are strict parasites, and accessory substances present in the blood are usually necessary for growth. Found in the respiratory tracts of vertebrates and are often associated with acute and chronic disease, *e.g.,* influenza, whooping cough, pinkeye. See **Ducrey's bacillus.**

hahnemannian (hah-ne-man′-i-an): Relating to Hahnemann or to the doctrine of homeopathy which he taught. See **homeopathy.**

hahnemannism (hah′-ne-man-izm): Homeopathy (*q.v.*).

hair: Thread-like filament present on all parts of human skin except the palms, soles, lips, glans penis and that surrounding the terminal phalanges. Also the aggregation of such filaments, especially on the scalp. Consists of a shaft and a bulb-like root. EXCLAMATION-MARK H., the broken off stump found at the periphery of spreading bald patches in alopecia areata; atrophic thinning of the hair shaft gives this characteristic shape—hence its name.

hairball: Trichobezoar (*q.v.*).

halazone (hal′-a-zōn): A white powder containing chlorine, useful in disinfecting drinking water.

half-life: The time required to reduce the radioactivity of a radioactive substance by one-half through radioactive decay.

halfway house: In psychiatry, a special residence for individuals who do not need full-time care in a mental hospital but who are not yet ready to return to independent community living.

halibut liver oil: A very rich source of vitamins A and D. The smaller dose required makes it more acceptable than cod liver oil.

halitosis (hal-i-tō′-sis): Bad breath.

hallucination (hal-ū-si-nā′-shun): A false perception, unique to the individual, occuring without any true sensory stimulus but regarded by him as real. May be auditory, gustatory, olfactory, tactile, visual. A common symptom in severe psychoses (*q.v.*) including schizophrenia, paraphrenia, confusional states. Common in delirium, during toxic states, and following head injuries. May also be induced by drugs, alcohol, or stress.

hallucinogen (hal-ūs′-in-ō-jen): An agent, drug, or specifically, a chemical such as mescaline or LSD, that is capable of producing hallucination. Psychotomimetic.

hallucinosis (hal-ū-si-nō′-sis): A psychosis in which the patient is grossly hallucinated. Usually a subacute delirious state; the predominant symptoms are auditory illusions (*q.v.*) and hallucinations.

hallux (hal′-uks): The great toe. H. RIGIDUS, ankylosis of the metatarsophalangeal articulation caused by osteoarthritis. H. VALGUS, lateral deviation of the great toe, as in a bunion (*q.v.*).—halluces, pl. Syn., hallex, hallus.

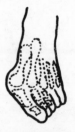

Hallux valgus

halogen (hal'-ō-jen): Any one of the non-metallic elements—bromine, chlorine, fluorine, iodine.

halothane (hal'-ō-thān): A clear, colorless, non-explosive liquid used as an inhalation anesthetic.

hamate (hā'-māt): The medial bone in the second row of wrist bones. Also hamatum.

hammer: The hammer-shaped bone of the middle ear; the malleus. PERCUSSION H., a rubber-headed hammer used to tap various parts of the body to produce sounds for diagnostic purposes. REFLEX H., a rubber-headed hammer for tapping tendons, muscles or nerves to elicit reflexes during physical examination.

hammertoe: A claw-like deformity in which there is a permanent hyperextension of the first phalanx and flexion of the second and third phalanges.

Hammertoe

hamstring: Name given to: (1) the tendons on either side of the popliteal space; (2) the three muscles on the posterior aspect of the thigh; their function is to flex the leg at the knee and to adduct and extend the thigh.

handedness: A tendency to prefer to use one or the other hand in all voluntary motor acts.

handicap: Term applied to a physical or mental defect that interferes with a person's normal activities and achievement.—handicapped, adj.

Hand-Schüller-Christian disease: Inborn error of fat metabolism, associated with mental subnormality. [Alfred Hand, American pediatrician. 1868-1949; Artur Schüller, Austrian neurologist. 1874- ; Henry A. Christian, American internist. 1876-1951.]

hanging drop: A method of preparing microorganisms for microscopic study. A drop of liquid containing the microorganisms is suspended from a cover glass over a depression in a glass slide.

hangnail (hang'-nāl): A narrow strip of skin, partly detached from the nail fold.

hangover: A combination of symptoms that occur, usually the next morning, after overindulgence in alcoholic beverages; includes headache, fatigue, thirst, irritability, gastric discomfort.

Hanot's disease (an'-ōz): Hypertrophic cirrhosis of the liver with jaundice, splenomegaly and fever. [Victor Charles Hanot, French physician. 1844-1896.]

Hansen's disease: Leprosy (q.v.). [Gerhard A. Hansen, Norwegian physician. 1841-1912.]

haploid (hap'-loid): Having half the number of chromsomes normally carried by the particular cell or cells.

hardening: H. OF THE ARTERIES, arteriosclerosis (q.v.).

harelip: A congenital defect in the lip; a fissure extending from the margin of the lip to the nostril; may be single or double, and is often associated with cleft palate.

Harrison Narcotic Act: A Federal law, enacted in 1915, which imposes strict regulations on the purchase, possession, sale or prescription of narcotics such as cocaine, morphine, opium; requires that physicians and hospitals keep accurate records of all narcotics purchased and dispensed. Violations are punishable by heavy fines, imprisonment, or both.

Hartnup disease: A disease believed to be due to an inborn error of protein metabolism. Associated with mental subnormality. Characterized by red scaly rash following exposure to sunlight, cerebellar ataxia, emotional instability, excessive excretion of indican.

hasheesh: Hashish (q.v.).

Hashimoto's disease: A condition in which the thyroid gland is infiltrated with lymphocytes resulting in destruction of the parenchyma and mild hypothyroidism. Occurs in middle-aged females mostly, and is a result of sensitization of patient to her own thyroid protein, thyroglobulin. See **autoimmunization.** [H. Hashimoto, Japanese surgeon. 1881-1934.]

hashish (hash'-ēsh): Cannabis indica (q.v.).

haunch: The hip and buttock.

haustration (haws-trā'-shun): 1. Haustrum (q.v.). 2. The formation of a haustrum.

haustrum (haw'-strum): One of the sacculations in the colon; these sacculations or pouches are caused by the longitudinal bands along the colon that are slightly shorter than the gut itself.—haustra, pl.

haversian canals (ha-ver'-zhan): Spaces containing blood, lymph vessels and nerves; found in the compact tissue of bone. [Clopton Havers, English physician. 1650-1702.]

hay fever: A form of allergic rhinitis in which attacks of catarrh of conjunctiva, nose and throat are precipitated by exposure to a pollen or specific antigen to which the individual is sensitive.

Haygarth's nodes: Swelling of joints sometimes seen in the fingers of patients suffering from arthritis. [John Haygarth, English physician. 1740-1827.]

Hb, hb: Abbreviation for hemoglobin.

HCG: Human chorionic gonadotrophin; obtained from the placenta. Used for cryptorchism (*q.v.*).

headache: Pain in the head. Often accompanied by nausea as in migraine H. Of many types; described both as to location and quality of the pain: frontal, one-sided, top-of-the-head, sharp, dull, pulsating or throbbing, steady, intermittent, depressing. May be gradual or sudden in onset. Causes include worry, lack of sleep, fatigue, hunger, tension, anxiety, high blood pressure, epilepsy, constipation, liver and kidney disorders, indigestion, allergy, eye trouble, sinusitis, fever, onset of a communicable disease, premenstrual tension.

headward acceleration: In aerospace travel, the acceleration of the body forward following the direction of the head; this causes the blood to rush from the head downward in the body.

healing (hē′-ling): The natural process of cure or repair of the tissues.—heal, v.t., v.i. H. BY FIRST INTENTION occurs when the edges of a clean wound are accurately held together; healing occurs with the minimum of scarring and deformity. H. BY SECOND INTENTION occurs when the edges of the wound unite after the formation of granular tissue. H. BY THIRD INTENTION occurs when granular tissue fills the wound cavity followed by the formation of scar tissue.

health: The state of an individual who enjoys physical, mental and social well-being.

heart: The hollow muscular organ that pumps blood through the body; situated behind the sternum, lying obliquely between the two lungs. It weighs 8 to 12 ounces in the female and 10 to 12 ounces in the male. H. ARREST, cardiac arrest (*q.v.*). H. BLOCK, partial or complete inhibition of the speed of conduction of the electrical impulse from the atrium to the ventricle of the heart. The cause may be an organic lesion or a functional disturbance. It its mildest form, it can only be detected electrocardiographically, while in its complete form the ventricles beat at their own slow intrinsic rate uninfluenced by the atria. H. CATHETERIZATION, cardiac catheterization (*q.v.*). H. FAILURE, sudden fatal stoppage of the heart

beat as may occur in coronary thrombosis; when it is the result of failure to maintain adequate circulation in all parts of the body there is congestion of blood in the portal and pulmonary circulations and it is then called congestive heart failure.

heartburn: A scalding or burning sensation felt behind the sternum, usually associated with acid regurgitation.

heart-lung machine: A mechanical pump used in heart surgery; it shunts the blood away from the heart while maintaining the circulation and oxygenation of the blood.

heat exhaustion: Heat syncope. Collapse, with or without loss of consciousness, suffered in conditions of heat and high humidity; results largely from loss of fluid and salt by sweating. If the surrounding air becomes saturated, heat stroke will ensue. Symptoms include pale, cold, clammy skin, rapid pulse, normal or subnormal temperature, dizziness, dyspnea, and abdominal cramps.

heat stroke: A serious condition produced by prolonged exposure to excessive temperatures. Symptoms include hot, dry skin, headache, dizziness, rapid pulse, high fever; in severe cases coma and death may ensue. A complication of electropyrexia (*q.v.*). Cf. **heat exhaustion.**

hebephrenia (hē-be-frē′-ni-a): A type of schizophrenia (*q.v.*) most often seen in adolescents; characterized by silly, uncoordinated, meaningless behavior, giggling, and superficial mannerisms.

Heberden: 1. H'S. disease; angina pectoris. 2. H'S. NODES, small osseous swellings at terminal phalangeal joints occurring in many types of arthritis. [William Heberden, English physician. 1710-1801.]

hedonism (hē′-don-izm): Excessive devotion to pleasure, so that a person's conduct is determined by an unconscious drive to seek pleasure and avoid unpleasant things.

Hegar's sign: Marked softening of the cervix in early pregnancy. [Alfred Hegar, German gynecologist. 1830-1914.]

helcoplasty (hel′-kō-plas-ti): Plastic surgery or repair of tissues damaged by ulcers.

helcosis (hel-kō′-sis): Ulceration; ulcer formation.

heli-, helio-: Denotes: (1) sun, sunlight; (2) solar energy.

heliosensitivity (hē-li-ō-sen-si-tiv′-i-ti): Sensitivity to the sun's rays.

heliosis (hē-li-ō′-sis): Sunstroke.

heliotherapy (hē-li-ō-ther′-a-pi): Treatment by exposure of the body to the sun's rays.

helium (hē′-li-um): A colorless, odorless,

tasteless, inert gas. Sometimes used in medicine as a diluent for other gases.

helix (hē'-liks): 1. The curved fold forming most of the rim of the external ear. 2. A coiled structure. WATSON-CRICK H., a double H. in which each chain contains information specifying the other chain; it represents the manner in which the genetic factors in DNA (deoxyribonucleic acid) reproduce themselves.

Heller's test, Heller's ring test: A test for albumin in the urine. Urine is dropped gently down the side of a test tube containing nitric acid; if an opaque white layer forms at the point of junction of the two liquids, the urine contains albumin.

helminth (hel'-minth): A worm or wormlike parasite, particularly one found in the intestine.

helminthagogue (hel-min'-tha-gog): See **anthelmintic.**

helminthiasis (hel-min-thī'-a-sis): The condition resulting from infestation with worms.

helminthology (hel-min-thol'-o-ji): The study of parasitic worms.

heloma (hē-lō'-ma): Corn, callosity.— helomata, pl.

hem-, hema-, hemat-, hemi-, hemo-: Denotes blood.

hemachromatosis: Hemochromatosis (q.v.).

hemacyte: Hemocyte (q.v.).

hemacytometer (hēm-a-sī-tom'-et-er): An instrument for measuring the number of blood corpuscles.

hemadynamometer: Hemodynamometer (q.v.).

hemafecia (hem-a-fē'-si-a): Blood in the feces.

hemagglutination (hem-a-gloo-tin-ā'-shun): Clumping of red blood cells; may be caused by antibodies or by certain viruses.

hemagglutinin (hem-a-gloo'-ti-nin): A substance that agglutinates (clumps) red blood cells.

hemagogue (hem'-a-gog): An agent that promotes the flow of blood, especially the menstrual flow.

hemangiectasis (hēm-an-ji-ek'-ta-sis): Dilatation of the blood vessels.

hemangioma (hēm-an-ji-ō'-ma): A benign lesion of blood vessels that may occur in any part of the body. When it occurs in the skin it may be called a birthmark, port wine stain or strawberry mark.—hemangiomata, pl.

hemarthrosis (hem-ar-thrō'-sis): The extravasation of blood into a joint or the synovial cavity of a joint.

hematemesis (hem-a-tem'-e-sis): The vomiting of blood.

hematidrosis (hēm-at-ī-drō'-sis): Excretion of sweat containing blood; occurs rarely.

hematin (hem'-a-tin): An iron-containing constituent of hemoglobin. Heme (q.v.).

hematinic (hem-a-tin'-ik): 1. Pertaining to hematin. 2. Any substance required for the production of red blood cells and their constituents. 3. An agent that improves the quality of the blood by increasing the quantity of red blood cells and hemoglobin.

hematoblast (hē-mat-ō-blast): A primitive cell from which a blood cell develops. A blood platelet.

hematocele (hē'-mat-ō-sēl): 1. A swelling filled with blood. 2. An effusion of blood into a body cavity or a sac, particularly into the sac that covers the testes.

hematocolpos: See **cryptomenorrhea.**

hematocrit (hē-mat'-ō-krit): 1. The term commonly used to express the percentage volume of red cells in the blood. 2. The calibrated tube or the procedure used in tests to determine the percentage volume of red cells in the blood.

hematocyst (hē'-mat-ō-sist): 1. A cyst containing blood. 2. Effusion of blood into the urinary bladder.

hematocyte (hē'-mat-ō-sit): A blood corpuscle. Hemocyte.

hematocytometer: Hemacytometer (q.v.).

hematocytopenia (hēm-at-ō-sī-tō-pē'-ni-a): A deficiency or decrease in the cellular content of the blood.

hematocytosis (hēm-at-ō-sī-tō'-sis): An increase in the cellular content of the blood.

hematocyturia (hēm-at-ō-sī-tū'-ri-a): The presence of red blood cells in the urine.

hematogenesis: The production of blood.

hematogenous (hē-ma-toj'-en-us): 1. Concerned with the formation of blood. 2. Carried by the blood stream. 3. Derived from or produced by the blood.

hematoid (hem'-a-toid): Resembling blood.

hematology (hē-ma-tol'-o-ji): The science dealing with the formation, composition, functions and diseases of the blood and the morphology of the blood-forming organs. —hematological, adj.; hematologically, adv.

hematolysis (hē-ma-tol'-i-sis): Destruction of blood cells, and liberation of hemoglobin. —hematolytic, adj.

hematoma (hē-ma-tō'-ma): A localized mass of blood within a tissue or body part;

a swelling filled with blood. SUBDURAL H., one beneath the dura mater of the brain.

hematometra (hē-ma-tō-mē′-tra): An accumulation of blood (or menstrual fluid) in the uterus.

hematomphalocele (hēm-at-om-fal′-ō-sēl): An umbilical hernia that contains blood.

hematopenia (hēm-at-ō-pē′-ni-a): Deficiency of blood.

hematophilia: Hemophilia (q.v.).

hematopoiesis: See **hemopoiesis.**

hematosalpinx (hē-ma-tō-sal′-pinks): An accumulation of blood in a fallopian tube.

hematosepsis (hē-ma-tō-sep′-sis): Septicemia (q.v.).

hematozoa (hē-ma-tō-zō′-a): Animal parasites living in the blood.—hematozoon, sing.

hematuria (hē-ma-tū′-ri-a): The presence of blood in the urine.

heme (hēm): The pigment-carrying nonprotein portion of hemoglobin. Formerly called hematin.

hemeralopia (hem-er-al-ō′-pi-a): Defective vision in a bright light. Term has been incorrectly used for nyctalopia, night blindness (q.v.).

hemi-: Denotes: (1) half of, or one-half; (2) affecting half of an organ or part.

hemiachromatopsia (hem-i-a-krō-ma-top′-si-a): Color blindness in one half the visual field of each eye.

hemianopia (hem-i-an-ō′-pi-a): Defective vision or blindness in one half of the field of vision in one or both eyes.—hemianopic, adj. Also hemianopsia, hemiopia. HOMONYMOUS H., H. that affects the right or left halves of the visual fields of both eyes.

hemianopsia (hem-i-an-op′-si-a): Hemianopia (q.v.).

hemiatrophy (hem-i-at′-ro-fi): Atrophy of one half or one side of the body or of an organ or part. H. FACIALIS, a congenital condition, or a manifestation of scleroderma (q.v.), in which the structures on one side of the face are shrunken.

hemiballismus (hem-i-bal-iz′-mus): Sudden, violent jerking movements on one side of the body, resulting from a brain lesion and occurring on the side of the body opposite to the lesion. Also hemiballism.

hemicardia (hem-i-kar′-di-a): A congenital anomaly in which one lateral half of the heart is lacking.

hemichorea (hem-i-kō-rē′-a): Choreiform movements limited to one side of the body. See **chorea.**

hemicolectomy (hem-i-kō-lek′-to-mi): Removal of approximately half the colon.

hemicorporectomy (hem-i-kor-po-rek′-to-mi): Amputation above the brim of the pelvis, including the lower extremities and all of the tissues and organs of the pelvic area. A radical operation that has been performed in a few cases of inoperable cancer and war injuries in which there is extensive destruction of tissue of and below the pelvis.

hemicrania (hem-i-krā′-ni-a): 1. Unilateral headache, as in migraine 2. Congenital anomaly in which the cerebrum has not developed properly.

hemidiaphoresis (hem-i-dī-a-for-ē′-sis): Profuse sweating on only one side of body.

hemidystrophy (hem-i-dis′-trō-fi): A condition of underdevelopment of one side of the body.

hemigastrectomy (hem-i-gas-trek′-to-mi): Removal of half or part of the stomach.

hemiglossectomy (hem-i-glos-ek′-to-mi): Removal of approximately half the tongue.

hemihypertrophy (hem-i-hī-per′-trō-fi): A congenital anomaly in which one half of the body is overdeveloped; due to faulty division of a zygote in the embryo.

hemilateral (hem-i-lat′-er-al): Pertaining to or affecting one lateral half of the body or of an organ.

hemiparaplegia (hem-i-par-a-plē′-ji-a): Paralysis of one side of the lower half of the body; paralysis of one lower extremity.

hemiparesis (hem-i-par′-e-sis): A slight paralysis or muscular weakness of one half of the body or face.

hemiplegia (hem-i-plē′-ji-a): Paralysis of one side of the body, usually resulting from a cerebrovascular accident on the opposite side.—hemiplegic, adj.

hemisphere (hem′-is-fēr): Half of a sphere or any spherical structure or organ; term commonly applied to either half of the cerebrum or the cerebellum.

hemoagglutination: Hemagglutination (q.v.).

hemoblast (hēm′-ō-blast): An immature blood cell; a blood platelet.

hemochromatosis (hē-mō-krō-ma-tō′-sis): A congenital error in iron metabolism, resulting in brown pigmentation of the skin and cirrhosis of the liver. Syn., 'bronze diabetes.'—hemochromatotic, adj.

hemochromometer (hē-mō-krō-mom′-e-ter): An apparatus for estimating the percentage of hemoglobin in the blood; a colorimeter.

hemocidal (hē-mō-sī′-dal): 1. Destructive to red blood cells. 2. An agent that destroys red blood cells.

hemoclastic (hē-mō-klas′-tik): Pertaining

to or causing destruction of red blood cells.

hemoconcentration (hē-mō-kon-sen-trā'-shun): Relative increase of volume of red blood cells to volume of plasma, usually due to loss of the latter. May occur in such conditions as shock, burns, diabetes mellitus. The degree of concentration is determined by a hematocrit (*q. v.*).

hemocyte (hēm'-ō-sīt): A blood corpuscle.

hemocytolysis (hē-mō-sī-tol'-i-sis): Destruction of blood cells.

hemocytometer: An apparatus for measuring the number of red blood cells in a given quantity of blood.

hemodialysis (hē-mō-dī-al'-i-sis): A process of removing waste products from, and replacing essential constituents in blood by a process of dialysis (*q. v.*). Such a technique is used in the artificial kidney.

hemodynamics (hē-mō-dī-nam'-iks): Study of the movement of blood in the body and of the forces involved.

hemodynamometer (hē-mō-dī-na-mom'-e-ter): An apparatus for measuring blood pressure.

hemoglobin (hē-mō-glō'-bin): The oxygen-carrying coloring matter in the red blood cells. It is composed of an iron-containing substance called heme (*q. v*) combined with globin. Has the reversible function of combining with and releasing oxygen. See **oxy-hemoglobin.**

hemoglobinemia (hē-mō-glō-bin-ē'-mi-a): Free hemoglobin in the blood plasma.—hemoglobinemic, adj.

hemoglobinometer (hē-mō-glō-bin-om'-e-ter): An instrument for estimating the percentage of hemoglobin in the red blood cells.

hemoglobinopathy (hē-mō-glō-bin-op'-a-thi): Abnormality of the hemoglobin.

hemoglobinuria (hē-mō-glō-bin-ū'-ri-a): The presence of free hemoglobin in the urine.

hemoid (hē'-moid): Resembling blood.

hemolith (hēm'-ō-lith): A concretion or stone in the wall of a blood vessel.

hemolysin (hē-mol'-i-sin): An agent that causes disintegration of erythrocytes. See **antibodies.**

hemolysis (hē-mol'-is-is): Disintegration of red blood cells, with liberation of contained hemoglobin. Laking. May be caused by bacterial toxins, snake venom, immune bodies, and hypotonic salt solutions. See **anemia, hemoglobinemia.**—hemolytic, adj.

hemolytic (hē-mō-lit'-ik): Characterized by or referring to hemolysis; causing hemol-

ysis. H. DISEASE OF THE NEWBORN, erythroblastosis fetalis (*q. v.*).

hemometra (hē-mō-mē'-tra): See **hemato-metra.**

hemopericardium (hē-mō-per-i-kar'-di-um): Blood in the pericardial sac.

hemoperitoneum (hē-mō-per-i-to-nē'-um): Blood in the peritoneal cavity.

hemophilia (hē-mō-fil'-i-a): An inherited bleeding disease found only in males and transmitted through carrier females, who are daughters of affected males. Under special genetic circumstances, females with H. may be produced. Patient is subject to prolonged bleeding following even minor injuries.

hemophiliac (hē-mō-fil'-i-ak): 1. Pertaining to hemophilia. 2. A person afflicted with hemophilia.

hemophilic (hē-mō-fil'-ik): 1. Pertaining to hemophilia. 2. Blood-loving; said of microorganisms.

hemophobia (hē-mō-fō'-bi-a): Morbid dread of blood.

hemophthalmia (hē-mof-thal'-mi-a): Bleeding into the eyeball.

hemopneumothorax (hē-mō-nū-mō-thor'-aks): The presence of blood and air in the pleural cavity causing compression of lung tissue.

hemopoiesis (hē-mō-poi-ē'-sis): The formation of blood cells.—hemopoietic, adj. (See diagram, next page.)

hemoproctia (hē-mō-prok'-shi-a): Hemorrhage from the rectum.

hemoptysis (hē-mop'-tis-is): The coughing up of blood or blood-stained sputum.—hemoptyses, pl.

hemorrhage (hem'-or-rij): The escape of copious amounts of blood from a vessel. The terms ARTERIAL H., VENOUS H., and CAPILLARY H. designate the type of vessel from which it escapes. PRIMARY H. occurs at the time of surgery or injury. SECONDARY H. occurs after surgery or injury but after a considerable time has elapsed.—hemorrhagic, adj. ACCIDENTAL ANTEPARTUM H., bleeding from separation of a normally situated placenta after the 28th week of pregnancy. The term placental abruption is now preferred. ANTEPARTUM H., vaginal bleeding after the 28th week of pregnancy and before labor. INTRAPARTUM H., occurs during labor. POSTPARTUM H., excessive bleeding after delivery of child. MASSIVE H., loss of large amount of blood in a short time, often leading to shock. PETECHIAL H., occurs in minute discrete areas beneath the skin.

hemorrhoid (hem'-o-roid): Varicosity of a vein in the rectal area. EXTERNAL H., one outside of the anal sphincter covered with skin. INTERNAL H., one inside the anal sphincter covered with mucous membrane.

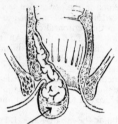

Prolapsed internal hemorrhoid

hemorrhoidal (hem-o-roid'-al): 1. Pertaining to hemorrhoids. 2. Applied to nerves and blood vessels in the anal region.

hemorrhoidectomy (hem-o-roid-ek'-to-mi): Surgical removal of hemorrhoids.

hemosalpinx (hē-mō-sal'-pinks): Hematosalpinx (q.v.).

hemosiderosis (hē-mō-sid-er-ōs'-is): Iron deposits in the tissues.

hemospermia (hē-mō-sper'-mi-a): The discharge of blood-stained semen.

hemostasis (hē-mos'-ta-sis): 1. Arrest of bleeding. 2. Stagnation of blood within its vessel.

hemostat (hē'-mō-stat): 1. An agent that arrests bleeding. 2. An instrument for constricting a blood vessel to stop or control the flow of blood.

hemostatic (hē-mō-stat'-ik): 1. An agent that arrests bleeding. 2. Having the effect of arresting bleeding.

hemothorax (hē-mō-thō'-raks): Blood in the pleural cavity.

hepar (hē'-par): The liver.—hepatic, adj.

heparin (hep'-a-rin): An acid present in several of the body tissues, chiefly the liver. In pharmacy, a preparation made from the livers or lungs of cattle; usually given by intravenous injection to inhibit coagulation of the blood; widely used in prevention and treatment of thrombosis.

hepat-, hepatico-, hepato-: Denotes liver.

hepatalgia (hep-a-tal'-ji-a): Pain in the liver.

hepatectomy (hep-a-tek'-to-mi): Excision of part of the liver.

hepatic (hep-at'-ik): Pertaining to the liver.

hepaticocholedochostomy (hep-at-i-kō-kō-lē-dō-kos'-to-mi): End-to-end union of the severed hepatic and common bile ducts.

hepaticoenteric (hep-at-i-kō-en-ter'-ik): Pertaining to the liver and the intestine.

hepaticoenterostomy (hep-at'-i-kō-en-ter-os'-to-mi): The surgical establishment of an

Hemopoiesis

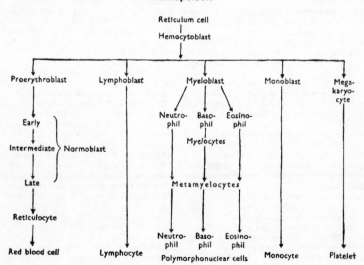

artificial communication between the hepatic duct and the intestine.

hepaticojejunostomy (hep-at′-i-kō-jē-joon-os′-to-mi): Anastomosis of the hepatic duct to a loop of proximal jejunum.

hepatitis (hep-a-tī′-tis): Inflammation of the liver. INFECTIOUS H., a virus (A or IH) infection of the liver; has an incubation period of two to six weeks; causes jaundice after an influenza-like illness; spread by oral-fecal route; may give rise to epidemics in schools or among armed forces. HOMOLOGOUS SERUM H., symptoms are the same as for infectious H., but is caused by a B or SH virus and is spread by contact, blood transfusion or serum therapy, or by improperly sterilized needles or instruments; incubation period is six weeks to six months; can be severe, even fatal; an estimated 2 to 3 percent of the world adult population are carriers of SH virus.

hepatization (hep-a-tī-zā′-shun): Pathological changes in the tissues, which cause them to resemble liver. Occurs in the lungs in pneumonia.

hepatocellular (hep-a-tō-sel′-ū-lar): Pertaining to, or affecting liver cells.

hepatocholangeitis (hep-a-tō-kō-lan-jē-ī′-tis): Inflammation of the liver and the biliary ducts.

hepatocirrhosis (hep-a-tō-si-rō′-sis): Cirrhosis (*q.v.*) of the liver.

hepatocystic (hep-a-tō-sis′-tik): Pertinent to the liver and gallbladder.

hepatogenous (hep-a-toj′-e-nus): Originating in the liver.

hepatolenticular degeneration (hep-a-tō-len-tik′-ū-lar): Descriptive of a group of diseases characterized by degeneration of the liver and the lenticular nucleus (*q.v.*), *e.g.*, Wilson's disease.

hepatolith (hep′-a-tō-lith): A gallstone within the liver.

hepatoma (hep-a-tō′-ma): Primary carcinoma of the liver.

hepatomegaly (hep-a-tō-meg′-al-i): Enlargement of the liver.

hepatorenal syndrome: Term originally used to describe death from hepatic and renal failure after cholecystectomy for prolonged obstructive jaundice. Now used to describe liver and kidney failure from any cause.

hepatorrhea (hep-a-to-rē′-a): Excessive formation or flow of bile from the liver.

hepatorrhexis (hep-a-tō-rek′-sis): Rupture of the liver.

hepatosplenomegaly (hep′-a-tō-splē-nō-meg′-al-i): Enlargement of the liver and the spleen.

hepatotoxic (hep-a-tō-tok′-sik): Having an injurious effect on liver cells.—hepatotoxicity, n.

hept-, hepta-: Denotes (1) seven; (2) division into seven units.

heptadactylia (hep-ta-dak-til′-i-a): The condition of having seven toes or fingers on one hand or foot.

hereditary (he-red′-i-ter-i): Inherited; capable of being inherited.

heredity (he-red′-i-ti): 1. The genetic factor responsible for the persistence of particular characteristics in successive generations. 2. The physical and mental components that are transmitted from parent to offspring at conception.

heredosyphilis (her-e-dō-sif′-i-lis): Syphilis acquired during fetal life.

hermaphrodite (her-maf′-rō-dīt): An individual possessing both ovarian and testicular tissue. Such a person may approximate either to the male or female type, but is usually sterile from imperfect development of the gonads.

hermetic (her-met′-ik): Airtight.—hermetically, adj.

hernia (her′-ni-a): The protrusion of an organ, or part of an organ, through an abnormal aperture in the surrounding structures; commonly the protrusion of an abdominal organ through a gap in the abdominal wall.

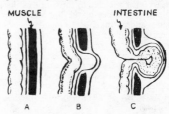

Formation of hernia. A, normal. B, simple hernia. C, strangulation of loop of intestine

Rupture. DIAPHRAGMATIC H., protrusion through the diaphragm, the commonest one involving the stomach at the esophageal opening (HIATUS H.). FEMORAL H., protrusion through the femoral canal, alongside the femoral blood vessels as they pass into the thigh. INGUINAL H., protrusion through the inguinal canal, alongside the spermatic cord in the male. STRAN-

GULATED H., hernia in which the blood supply to the organ involved is impaired, usually due to constriction by surrounding structures. UMBILICAL H., protrusion through the area of the umbilical scar. See **irreducible.**

herniated (her′-ni-ā-ted): 1. Having a hernia. 2. Descriptive of a structure that protrudes like a hernia.

herniation (her-ni-ā′-shun): 1. Formation of a hernia. 2. A hernia.

hernioplasty (her′-ni-ō-plas-ti): An operation for hernia, in which an attempt is made to prevent recurrence, by refashioning the structures to give greater strength.—hernioplastic, adj.

herniorrhaphy (her-ni-or′-a-fi): An operation for hernia, in which the weak area is reinforced by some of the patient's own tissues, or by some other material.

herniotomy (her-ni-ot′-o-mi): An operation to cure hernia by the return of its contents to their normal position, and the removal of the hernial sac.

heroic (he-rō′-ik): Severe or extreme; said of medical or surgical measures taken to save life.

herpangina (her-pan-jī′-na): Minute vesicles and ulcers at the back of the mouth. Short, febrile illness in children caused by a Coxsackie virus.

herpes (her′-pēz): Vesicular eruption due to a virus infection.—herpetic, adj. H. SIMPLEX, characterized by formation of blisters along the border of the lips and external nares and on the mucous membrane of the genitalia. This is the so-called 'fever blister.' H. ZOSTER, a form of herpes characterized by severe pain and eruption of a group of vesicles that follow the course of a nerve, usually on one side of the body only. Also called 'shingles.'

herpetiform (her-pet′-i-form): Resembling herpes.

hesperidin (hes-per′-i-din): Functions as vitamin P (*q.v.*). See **citrin.**

heter-, hetero-: Denotes: (1) different, other than usual; (2) containing several kinds.

heterocellular (het-er-ō-sel′-ū-lar): Made up of different kinds of cells.

heterochromia (het-er-ō-krō′-mi-a): A difference in the color of two anatomical parts that are normally of the same color; *e.g.,* the iris of the eye.

heterogeneous (het-er-ō-jē′-nē-us): Made up of ingredients or constituents that are dissimilar.

heterogenous (het-er-oj′-e-nus): 1. Of un-

like origin. 2. Not originating within the body. Opp. to autogenous (*q.v.*).

heterograft (het′-er-ō-graft): A graft of tissue from an individual of a species other than that of the recipient.

heterolateral (het-er-ō-lat′-er-al): Pertaining to or situated or occurring on the opposite side.

heterologous (het-er-ol′-o-gus): 1. Of different origin; from a different species. 2. Pertaining to or consisting of tissue that is not normal to that part of the body.

heterometropia (het-er-ō-me-trō′-pi-a): A condition in which the degree of refraction is not the same in the two eyes.

heteromorphosis (het-er-ō-mor′-fo-sis): The development of tissue or an organ that is different from the normal type, especially that which occurs in regeneration of tissue or a structure that was destroyed or removed.

heteromorphous (het-er-ō-mor′-fus): Differing in shape or structure from the normal type.

heteroplasia (het-er-ō-plā′-zi-a): The development of tissue in a place where it is not normally found or in a place where another type of tissue is normally found.

heteroplasty (het′-er-ō-plas-ti): Plastic operation using a graft from an individual of another species, or a synthetic material that is not organic.—heteroplastic, adj.

heteropsia (het-er-op′-si-a): Unequal vision in the two eyes.

heterosexual (het-er-ō-seks′-ū-al): Relating to or characterized by heterosexuality (*q.v.*). Opp. to homosexual.

heterosexuality (het-er-ō-seks-ū-al′-i-ti): The characteristic of directing love or sexual attraction toward those of the opposite sex. The expression of the normal sex instinct, as opposed to homosexuality.

heterotopia (het-er-ō-tō′-pi-a): The presence of tissue or an organ in a place where it is not normally located.

heterotropia (het-er-ō-trō′-pi-a): Strabismus (*q.v.*).

hexachlorophene (heks-a-klor′-ō-fēn): An antiseptic used in skin sterilization, and in some bactericidal soaps.

hexose (hek′-sōs): A class of simple sugars, monosaccharides, $C_6 H_{12} O_6$. Examples are glucose, mannose, galactose.

Hg: Symbol for mercury; also sometimes for hemoglobin.

Hgb, hgb: Abbreviation for hemoglobin.

hiatus (hī-ā′-tus): A space or opening. See **hernia.**—hiatal, adj.

Hibb's operation: Operation for spinal fixation, following spinal tuberculosis. [Russell H. Hibbs, American orthopedic surgeon. 1869-1932.]

hibernation (hī-ber-nā'-shun): The winter sleep of some animals. ARTIFICIAL H., lowering of the body temperature of human beings by the external application of cold packs (ice, etc.) in combination with drugs to control shivering. It reduces the oxygen requirements of vital tissues, and is used mainly in the treatment of head injuries and in cardiac surgery. Syn., hypothermia (*q.v.*). See **refrigeration.**

hiccough (hi'-kof): Hiccup (*q.v.*).

hiccup (hik'-up): An involuntary inspiratory spasm of the respiratory organs, ending in a sudden closure of the glottis, with the production of a characteristic sound. Hiccough.

hidrorrhea (hid-rō-rē'-a): Profuse sweating.

hidrosis (hid-rō'-sis): 1. Sweat secretion. 2. Excessive sweating.

hidrotic (hid-rot'-ik): 1. Causing sweating. 2. Any agent that causes sweating; diaphoretic (*q.v.*).

high blood pressure: Blood pressure that is above the normal range. See **blood pressure, hypertension.**

Highmore's antrum: See **antrum.**

hilum (hī'-lum): hilus (*q.v.*).

hilus (hī'-lus): A depression on the surface of an organ where vessels, ducts, etc., enter and leave.—hilar, adj.; hili, pl.

hip: The lateral part of the body on either side between the waist and the thigh.

Hippocrates (hi-pok'-ra-tēz): Famous Greek physician and philosopher (460 to 367 B.C.) who established a school of medicine at Cos, his birthplace. He is often termed the 'Father of Medicine.'

Hippocratic oath: An oath taken by young physicians on entering the profession of medicine; based on an oath required by Hippocrates of his students. It is the ethical guide of physicians. The oath has been adapted for nurses and is often repeated by nursing students at their graduation exercises.

hippuria (hip-pū'-ri-a): An excess of hippuric acid in the urine.

Hirschprung's disease: Megacolon. Congenital hypertrophy and massive enlargement of the colon. The affected part is sometimes removed surgically. [Harold Hirschprung, Danish physician. 1830-1916.]

hirsute (her'-sūt): Being hairy or shaggy.

hirsutism (her'-sūt-izm): Excessive hairi-

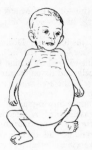

Hirschsprung's disease

ness, especially in women, or the growth of hair in unusual places.

hirudin (hi-roo'-din): A substance secreted by the buccal glands of the leech, which prevents the clotting of blood.

Hirudo (hi-roo'-dō): A genus of leeches including the species sometimes used in medicine.

His (hiss): BUNDLE OF H., a bundle of nerve fibers that arise in the atrioventricular node and extend down the interventricular septum where they divide and pass into the ventricle tissue; they conduct the contraction impulse from the atrioventricular node to the ventricles. [Wilhelm His, German physiologist. 1863-1934.]

hist-, histo-: Denotes tissue.

histaminase (his-tam'-i-nās): An enzyme that is widely distributed in body tissues and that inactivates histamine (*q.v.*).

histamine (his'-ta-mēn): A naturally occurring chemical substance in body tissues which, in small doses, has profound and diverse actions on muscle, blood capillaries, and gastric secretion. Sudden excessive release from the tissues, into the blood, is believed to be the cause of the main symptoms and signs in anaphylaxis (*q.v.*).—histaminic adj.

histidine (his'-ti-dēn): An essential amino acid which is widely distributed and is present in hemoglobin. It is a precursor of histamine.

histiocyte (his'-ti-ō-sīt): A tissue cell; a macrophage.

histioma (his-ti-ō'-ma): Histoma (*q.v.*).

histodiagnosis (his-tō-dī-ag-nō'-sis): Diagnosis that is based on microscopic findings in tissue or cells.

histodialysis (his-tō-dī-al'-i-sis): Disintegration of tissue.

histology

172

histology (his-tol'-o-ji): Microscopic study of tissues.—histological, adj.; histologically, adv.

histolysis (his-tol'-i-sis): Disintegration of organic tissue.—histolytic, adj.

histoma (his-tō'-ma): A benign tumor composed of cells and tissue that are very similar to those of the area where it arises, *e.g.*, a fibroma.

histoplasmosis (his-tō-plas-mō'-sis): A systemic disease caused by infection with the fungus *Histoplasma capsulatum* and involving the reticulo-endothelial system; may produce varying clinical pictures but usually produces fever, emaciation, splenomegaly, anemia, leukopenia and skin lesions.

hives (hīvs): Nettle-rash; urticaria (*q.v.*).

H₂O: Symbol for water.

H₂O₂: Symbol for hydrogen peroxide.

hoarse (hors): Harsh or grating, said of the voice.

hobnail liver: Term is descriptive of the appearance of the liver in one form of cirrhosis; the surface of the liver is covered with small nodules while the body of the organ is shrunken and hard.

Hodgkin's disease: Lymphadenoma. Progressive, painless, fatal disease in the reticulo-endothelial system, shown in generalized enlargement of the lymphatic glands and splenomegaly; of unknown cause. Other features are recurring fever, anemia, and occasionally cutaneous manifestations. Also lymphosarcoma, lymphadenoma, anemia lymphatica, malignant lymphoma, [Thomas Hodgkin, English physician. 1798-1866.]

Hogben test: A test for pregnancy in which a South African toad is injected with a preparation of an early morning specimen of urine. If the subject is pregnant, the toad will lay eggs in 8 to 24 hours. Advantage over the Friedman and Aschheim-Zondek tests is that the toad does not need to be sacrificed and can be used repeatedly. Test is over 99 percent accurate. [Lancelot Hogben, British scientist. 1895- .]

holandric (hōl-an'-drik): Pertaining to characteristics that are transmitted only through the male of the species.

holarthritis (hol-ar-thrī'-tis): Arthritis in all or many of the joints; polyarthritis.

holistic (hō-lis'-tik): Pertaining to a totality or whole; the consideration of man as a complete unit, functioning as a whole.

hollow-back: Lordosis (*q.v.*).

hologynic (hō-lō-jin'-ik): Pertaining to char-

acteristics that are transmitted only through the female.

hom-, homo-: Denotes: (1) alike, similar, one and the same, corresponding in structure or type; (2) from or of the same species.

Homans' sign: Passive dorsiflexion of foot causes pain in calf muscles. Indicative of incipient or established venous thrombosis of leg. [John Homans, American surgeon. 1877- .]

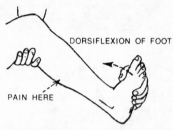
DORSIFLEXION OF FOOT

PAIN HERE

Homans' sign

homeomorphous (hō-mē-ō-morf'-us): Of similar shape and structure.

homeopathy (hōm-ē-op'-a-thi): A method of treating disease by prescribing minute doses of drugs which, in maximum dose, would produce symptoms of the disease. First adopted by Hahnemann.—homeopathic, adj. [Christian Friedrich Samuel Hahnemann, German physician. 1775-1843.]

homeoplasia (hō-mē-ō-plā'-zi-a): The growth of new tissue that is similar to the adjacent tissue.

homeostasis (hō-mē-ō-stā'-sis): 1. The state of relative stability or equilibrium of the internal environment of the body, including the various functions, such measurable conditions as blood pressure, temperature, heart rate, etc., and the chemical composition and reactions of tissues and fluids. 2. The physiological processes by which this status is maintained in the living body.

homicide (hom'-i-sīd): Killing of a man; manslaughter; murder. A murderer.

homocystinuria (hō-mō-sis-tin-ū'-ri-a): Excretion of homocystine (a sulfur-containing amino acid, homologue of cystine) in the urine.

homogeneous (hom-ō-jē'-nē-us): Of the same kind; of the same quality or consistency throughout.

homogenize (ho-moj'-e-niz): To make into the same consistency throughout.

homogenous (ho-moj'-en-us): Having a like nature, *e.g.,* a bone graft from another human being.

homograft (hō'-mō-graft): A tissue or organ which is transplanted from one individual to another of the same species.

homolateral (hō-mō-lat'-er-al): On the same side.—homolaterally, adv.

homologous (hō-mol'-ō-gus): Corresponding in origin and structure, but not necessarily in function.

homonymous (hō-mon'-im-us): In anatomy, being in the same relation or having corresponding halves. See **hemianopia.** In language, having two names or meanings.

homophilic (hō-mō-fil'-ik): Descriptive of an antibody that reacts with, or has affinity for, a specific antigen.

homosexual (hō-mō-seks'-ū-al): 1. Relating to the same sex. 2. An individual who exhibits homosexuality (*q.v.*).

homosexuality (hō-mō-seks-ū-al'-i-ti): 1. Abnormal sexual attraction for or erotic relationship with persons of one's own sex. 2. In psychoanalysis, term is used in relation to the period of development when attraction to the same sex is a normal manifestation. FEMALE H., lesbianism (*q.v.*).

homothermal (hō-mō-ther'-mal): Descriptive of organisms that maintain a constant temperature in spite of changes in the temperature of the environment. Denoting warm-blooded animals.

homotransplantation (hō-mō-trans-plan-tā'-shun): Transfer of tissue or organ to a member of the same species. Syn., homograft.

hookworm: Any one of a number of parasitic nematode worms (including Ancylostoma and Uncinaria) that infest the intestinal tract of man; transmitted by feces. H. DISEASE, a chronic debilitating disease caused by a hookworm; the blood-sucking parasite causes severe anemia. The disease is found mostly in warm areas where disposal of feces is inadequate and people do not wear shoes; the parasite enters the body through the skin, usually of the feet.

HOP: High oxygen pressure.

hordeolum (hor-dē'-ō-lum): Inflammation of one or more of the sebaceous glands of the eyelid; a sty.

hormone (hor'-mōn): A chemical substance manufactured in the body and carried by the blood or lymph to another organ or tissue where it acts as a stimulant or accelerator. Many H.'S are secreted by ductless glands. See **endocrine.**—hormonic, hor-

monal, adj. H. THERAPY, the treatment of certain pathological conditions with hormones, *e.g.,* thyroxine, testosterone.

hormonopoiesis (hor-mō-nō-poi-ē'-sis): The production of hormones.—hormonopoietic, adj. Also hormopoiesis.

hormonoprivia (hor-mōn-ō-priv'-i-a): A pathological condition caused by lack of one or more hormones; may result from surgical removal of all or part of an endocrine gland.

hormonotherapy (hor-mō-nō-ther'-a-pi): Treatment by hormones.

Horner's syndrome: Clinical picture following paralysis of cervical sympathetic nerves, on one side. There is myosis, slight ptosis of the upper eyelid with enophthalmos, and anhidrosis. [Johann Friedrich Horner, Swiss ophthalmologist. 1831-1886.]

Horton's syndrome: Severe headache due to the release of histamine in the body. To be differentiated from migraine. [Bayard Taylor Horton, American physician. 1895-   .]

hospital: An institution that is devoted to the prevention, diagnosis, treatment, or rehabilitation of persons who are physically or mentally ill or injured. DAY H., one which patients attend daily and return to their homes at night. Recreational and occupational therapy are often provided. Used mostly for psychiatric and geriatric patients. NIGHT H., one for patients who are able to go to work during the day but who return to the hospital at night because they require treatment or some other service that cannot be obtained elsewhere. Used mostly by psychiatric patients. OPEN H., see **open.**

host: 1. An organism that receives a transplant of tissue from another organism. 2. In biology, the organic structure upon which a parasite lives or grows. INTERMEDIATE or INTERMEDIARY H., one in which a parasite passes its larval or cystic stage.

hot: 1. Having a relatively high temperature. 2. Term is used colloquially to describe something that is charged with electricity or that contains dangerous radioactive material. H. FLASH, a phenomenon, usually associated with the menopause, and due to vasodilation of the vessels of the head and neck particularly, accompanied by a visible flush and sweating and sometimes a feeling of suffocation.

hourglass contraction: A circular constriction in the middle of a hollow organ (usually the stomach or uterus), dividing it into two portions.

housemaid's knee: See **bursitis.**

HPFSH: Human pituitary follicle (*q.v.*) stimulating hormone.

hr: Abbreviation for hour.

h.s.: Abbreviation for *hora somni,* hour of sleep; bedtime.

Hubbard tank: A large tank used in physical therapy, especially for underwater exercises.

humerus (hū'-mer-us): The bone of the upper arm, between the elbow and shoulder joint.—humeral, adj.; humeri, pl.

humidity (hū-mid'-it-i): The amount of moisture in the atmosphere as measured by a hygrometer. POSITIVE H., the actual amount of vapor present in the air; expressed in grains per cubic foot. RELATIVE H., the ratio of the amount of moisture present in the air to the amount which would saturate it (at the same temperature).

humor, humour (hū'-mor): Any normal fluid or semi-fluid of the body. AQUEOUS H., the fluid filling the anterior and posterior chambers in front of the optical lens. VITREOUS H., the gelatinous mass filling the interior of the eyeball from the lens to the retina.

humoralism (hū'-mor-al-ism): An ancient doctrine, now obsolete, that the human body is made up of four humors, and that health and temperament are determined by changes in these humors; they were blood, phlegm, choler (yellow bile) and melancholy (black bile).

humpback, hunchback: Kyphosis (*q.v.*).

hunger (hun'-ger): A longing, desire, or urgent need, especially for food. AIR H., see **air.** H. PAIN, epigastric pain which is relieved by taking food; associated with duodenal ulcer.

Hunter-Hurler syndrome: Gargoylism (*q.v.*).

hunterian chancre: The hard sore of primary syphilis. [John Hunter, Scottish surgeon. 1728-1793.]

Huntington's chorea: Hereditary chorea (*q.v.*) which develops in middle age, or later, and is characterized by progressive dementia and random jerking movements of the entire body. [George Huntington, American physician. 1851-1916.]

Hutchinson's teeth: Defect of the upper central incisors which is regarded as part of the facies of the congenital syphilitic person. The central incisors (second dentition)

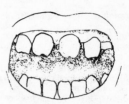

Hutchinson's teeth

are broader at the gum than at the cutting edge and each shows an elliptical notch in the lower edge; the lateral incisors are 'pegged.' [Jonathan Hutchinson, English surgeon. 1828-1913.]

HVP-77: An attenuated vaccine based on a rubella virus strain called HVP-77 (high virus passage of the 77th level); first developed in 1965 and licensed for production in the U.S. in 1969; used to produce active immunity against rubella (German measles).

hyaline (hī'-a-lin): Like glass; transparent. H. MEMBRANE DISEASE, see **respiratory distress syndrome.**

hyalitis (hī-al-ī'-tis): Inflammation of the optical vitreous humor or its enclosing membrane.

hyaloid (hī'-a-loid): Resembling hyaline; glassy. H. MEMBRANE, the transparent capsule enclosing the optical vitreous humor.

hyaluronic acid (hī-al-ūr-on'-ik): A polysaccharide that occurs as a gelatinous substance in the intercellular spaces, especially in the skin; it holds the cells together.

hyaluronidase (hī-al-ū-ron'-i-dās): An enzyme found in some pathogenic bacteria, sperm and some venoms; it breaks down hyaluronic acid (*q.v.*) and thus increases the permeability of tissues. When injected subcutaneously, it promotes the absorption of fluid; given with or immediately before a subcutaneous infusion.

hydatid (hī'-dat-id): 1. Any cyst-like structure. 2. The cyst formed by a tapeworm and found in various parts of the body, especially the liver. It may rupture and give rise to 'daughter' cysts. See **Echinococcus.**

hydatidiform (hī-da-tid'-i-form): Pertaining to or resembling a hydatid. H. MOLE, see **mole.**

hydr-, hydro-: Denotes: (1) water; (2) water-loving organism; (3) hydrogen.

hydragogue (hī'-dra-gog): 1. A purgative which produces a watery evacuation of the bowel. 2. Producing a watery discharge, particularly from the intestines.

hydramnios (hī-dram'-ni-os): An excess of amniotic fluid.

hydrargyrum (hīd-rar'-ji-rum): Mercury or quicksilver.

hydrarthrosis (hī-drar-thrō'-sis): A collection of watery fluid in a joint cavity. INTERMITTENT H., synovitis appears periodically, develops spontaneously, lasts a few days, and disappears as mysteriously. Joint may be normal between attacks. Affects young women mostly; may be due to an allergy.

hydrate (hī'-drāt): 1. A compound made up of water in chemical union with another substance. 2. To combine with or take up water.—hydration, n.

hydration (hī-drā'-shun): The union or combining of water with another substance.

hydremia (hī-drē'-mi-a): A relative excess of plasma volume compared with cell volume of the blood; it is normally present in late pregnancy.—hydremic, adj.

hydroa (hī-drō'-a): A skin condition marked by the eruption of vesicles or bullae; dermatitis herpetiformis (*q.v.*). H. AESTIVALE, a vesicular or bullous skin disease of children; the vesicles appear upon reddened patches of the skin. It may recur every summer; affects exposed parts and probably results from photosensitivity; often associated with porphyrinuria (*q.v.*). H. VACCINIFORME is a more severe form of this in which scarring ensues. Also hydroaestivale.

hydrocarbon (hī-drō-car'-bon): Any compound that contains only hydrogen and carbon.

hydrocele (hī'-drō-sēl): A swelling due to accumulation of serous fluid, especially in the tunica vaginalis of the testis, or along the spermatic cord.

hydrocephalus (hī-drō-sef'-a-lus): 'Water on the brain.' An excess of cerebrospinal fluid inside the skull; usually a congenital condition; results in enlargement of the head, atrophy of the brain and mental weakness. EXTERNAL H., the excess of fluid is mainly in the subarachnoid space. INTERNAL H., the fluid excess is mainly in the ventricles of the brain.—hydrocephalic, adj.

hydrochloric acid (hī-drō-klō'-rik): A colorless compound of hydrogen and chlorine; it is caustic and has an escharotic effect when undiluted. Also secreted by the stomach lining and normally present in gastric juice in a 0.2 percent solution.

hydrocyanic acid (hī-drō-sī-an'-ik): An extremely dangerous acid, obtained from the stones of peaches and other fruits, used as an exterminant for rodents and other insects. Inhalation of very small amounts will cause death. Also called prussic acid.

hydrogen (hī'-drō-jen): A colorless, odorless, combustible gas; found in all organic compounds and water. The lightest element known. H. ION CONCENTRATION, a measure of the acidity or alkalinity of a solution, expressed as pH and ranging from pH 1 to 14, 7 being approximately neutral; the lower numbers denote acidity, the higher ones alkalinity. H. PEROXIDE (H_2O_2), an oxidizing agent used for cleansing wounds.

hydrolabyrinth (hī-drō-lab'-i-rinth): An excess of fluid (endolymph) in the inner ear.

hydrolysis (hī-drol'-is-is): The splitting into more simple substances by the addition of water.—hydrolytic, adj.; hydrolyze, v.

hydrometer (hī-drom'-et-er): An instrument for determining the specific gravity of fluids.—hydrometry, n.

hydrometra (hī-drō-mē'-tra): A collection of watery fluid within the uterus.

hydronephrosis (hī-drō-nē-frō'-sis): Distension of the kidney pelvis with urine, from obstructed outflow. If unrelieved, pressure eventually causes atrophy of kidney tissue.—hydronephrotic, adj.

hydropericarditis (hī-drō-pe-ri-kar-dī'-tis): Pericarditis with effusion.

hydropericardium (hī-drō-pe-ri-kar'-di-um): Fluid in the pericardial sac in the absence of inflammation. Can occur in heart and kidney failure.

hydroperitoneum (hī-drō-pe-ri-tō-nē'-um): Ascites (*q.v.*).

hydrophilia (hī-drō-fil'-i-a): The property of readily absorbing water.—hydrophilic, adj.

hydrophobia (hī-drō-fō'-bi-a): Rabies in man. A once fatal disease caused by a neurotropic virus. Spasm of throat occurs when patient attempts to eat or drink—hence 'hydrophobia.'

hydropneumothorax (hī-drō-nū-mō-thō'-raks): Pneumothorax further complicated by effusion of fluid in the pleural cavity. Often tubercular.

hydrops (hī'-drops): Dropsy; an abnormal accumulation of serous fluid in the body tissues or in a body cavity.—hydropic, adj. H. FETALIS, severe form of erythroblastosis fetalis (*q.v.*).

hydrorrhea (hī-drō-rē'-a): Copious watery discharge from any organ or part.

hydrosalpinx (hī-drō-sal'-pinks): Distension of the fallopian tube with watery fluid.

hydrosis (hī-drō'-sis): Hidrosis (*q.v.*).

hydrotherapist (hī-drō-ther′-a-pist): One trained in the use of hydrotherapy (*q.v.*).

hydrotherapy (hī-drō-ther′-a-pi): Treatment of disease by the scientific application of water, hot or cold, externally or internally.

hydrothorax (hī-drō-thō′-raks); The presence of serous fluid in the pleural cavity.

hydroureter (hī-drō-ū-rē′-ter): Abnormal distension of a ureter with urine; may be caused by stricture, the presence of a stone, or a new growth.

hydrouria (hī-drō-ūr′-i-a); An increase in the water content of urine while the amount of solids remains normal or is reduced.

hydrous (hī′-drus): Describes a substance containing chemically-bound water.

hydroxyl (hī-drok′-sil): The univalent group OH, consisting of a hydrogen atom linked with an oxygen atom; when combined with certain other radicals hydroxides are formed.

hydruria (hī-drū′-ri-a): Polyuria (*q.v.*). See **diabetes insipidus**.

hygiene (hī′-jēn): The science dealing with health and its maintenance. COMMUNITY or PUBLIC H., embraces all measures taken to supply the community with pure food and water, good sanitation, housing, etc. INDUSTRIAL H. (occupational H.), includes all measures taken to preserve the individual's health while he is at work. MENTAL H., deals with the establishment of healthy mental attitudes and emotional reactions. ORAL H., deals with the proper care of the mouth and teeth for the maintenance of health. PERSONAL H., deals with those measures taken by the individual to preserve his own health. SOCIAL H., deals with sex education, marriage, family relations and the promotion of sexual health. —hygienic, adj.

hygienist (hī′-ji-en-ist): One who specializes in the science of health. DENTAL H., one trained to give dental prophylactic treatment.

hygr-, hygro-: Denotes moisture, humidity.

hygroma (hī-grō′-ma): A cyst, bursa or sac filled with watery fluid. CYSTIC H., a cystic swelling containing watery fluid, usually situated in the neck, and present at birth. —hygromata, pl.; hygromatous, adj.

hygrometer (hī-grom′-et-er): An instrument for measuring the amount of moisture in the air. See **humidity**.

hygroscopic (hī-grō-skop′-ik): Readily absorbing water, *e.g.,* glycerin.

hymen (hī′-men): A membranous perforated structure stretching across the vaginal entrance. IMPERFORATE H., a congenital condition leading to hematocolpos. See **cryptomenorrhea**.

hymenectomy (hī men-ek′-to-mi): Surgical excision of the hymen.

hymenotomy (hī-men-ot′-o-mi): Surgical incision of the hymen.

hyoid (hī′-oid): A U-shaped bone at the root of the tongue.

hypacusis (hī-pa-kū′-sis): Slightly impaired hearing. Also hypacusia.

hypalgesia (hī-pal-jē′-zi-a): Decreased sensitiveness to pain. Also hypalgia.

hyper-: Denotes: (1) excessive, above normal; (2) located above.

hyperacidaminuria (hī′-per-as-id-am-i-nū′-ri-a): An excess of amino acids in the urine.

hyperacidity (hī-per-as-id′-it-i): Excessive acidity. See **hyperchlorhydria**.

hyperactivity (hī-per-ak-ti′-vi-ti): Excessive activity.

hyperacusis (hī-per-a-kū′-sis): 1. Abnormal acuteness of hearing. 2. Painful sensitivity to sounds. Also hyperacusia.

hyperadiposis (hī-per-ad-i-pō′-sis): Excessive fatness.

hyperalbuminemia (hī-per-al-bū-mi-nē′-mi-a): Abnormally high percentage of albumin in the blood.

hyperalgesia (hī-per-al-jē′-zi-a): Excessive sensitivity to pain. Also hyperalgia.— hyperalgesic, adj.

hyperalimentation (hī-per-al-i-men-tā′-shun): Administration or ingestion of more than the optimal amount of food. May be given intravenously through an indwelling subclavian catheter into the superior vena cava; the solution given contains the substances necessary for complete nutrition when the patient cannot take these via the usual route; has been used for patients with such conditions as esophageal obstruction, ulcerous conditions, cancer of different parts of the digestive tract and accessory organs, enteritis, ulcerative colitis, burns.

hyperammonuria (hī-per-am-mō-nū′-ri-a): Increased excretion of ammonia in the urine.

hyperaphia (hī-per-ā′-fi-a): Abnormal acuteness of the sense of touch.

hyperasthenia (hī-per-as-thē′-ni-a): Extreme weakness.—hyperasthenic, adj.

hyperbaric (hī-per-bar′-ik): At greater pressure, specific gravity or weight than normal. H. OXYGEN CHAMBER, sealed cylinder containing oxygen under pressure. Accommodates patient, attendant and equipment. In some units surgery can be performed. Anaerobic organisms and their ability to produce toxins are adversely affected by oxygen. O₂ saturated tissues respond better to radiotherapy.

normal sensitiveness to cold. Also hypercryesthesia.

hypercythemia (hī-per-sī-thē′-mi-a): An abnormal number of red blood cells in the circulating blood.

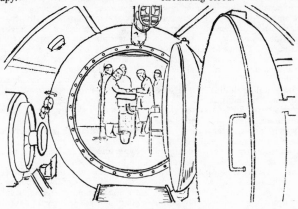

Hyperbaric oxygen chamber

hyperbilirubinemia (hī-per-bi-li-roo-bi-nē′-mi-a): Excessive bilirubin in the blood, resulting in jaundice.—hyperbilirubinemic, adj.

hyperbulia (hī-per-boo′-li-a): Excessive willfulness.

hypercalcemia (hī-per-kal-sē′-mi-a): Excessive calcium in the blood.—hypercalcemic, adj.

hypercalciuria (hī-per-kal-si-ū-ri-a): Greatly increased calcium excretion in urine, as seen in hyperparathyroidism. Of importance in pathogenesis of nephrolithiasis. IDIOPATHIC H., H. for which there is no known metabolic cause.

hypercapnia (hī-per-kap′-ni-a): Excessive CO₂ in the blood.—hypercapnic, adj.

hyperchloremia (hī-per-klō-rē′-mi-a): Excessive amount of chloride in the circulating blood.—hyperchloremic, adj.

hyperchlorhydria (hī-per-klor-hī′-dri-a): Excessive hydrochloric acid in the gastric juice.—hyperchlorhydric, adj.

hypercholesterolemia (hī-per-kol-es-te-rol-ē′-mi-a): Excessive cholesterol in the blood. Predisposes to atheroma and gallstones. Also found in myxedema.—hypercholesterolemic, adj.

hyperchylia (hī-per-kī′-li-a): Excessive secretion of gastric juice.

hypercryalgesia (hī-per-krī-al-jē′-zi-a): Ab-

hypercytosis (hī-per-sī-tō′-sis): An abnormal increase in the number of cells in the circulating blood; term is sometimes used synonymously with leukocytosis (q.v.).

hyperdactylia (hī-per-dak-til′-i-a): The presence of more than the usual number of fingers or toes.

hyperdipsia (hī-per-dip′-si-a): Intense, relatively temporary thirst.

hyperelectrolytemia (hī-per-ē-lek-tro-līt-ē′-mi-a): Dehydration (not manifested clinically) associated with high serum sodium and chloride levels.

hyperemesis (hī-per-em′-e-sis): Excessive vomiting. H. GRAVIDARUM, the pernicious vomiting of pregnancy.

hyperemia (hī-per-ē′-mi-a): Excess of blood in an area. ACTIVE H., caused by an increased flow of blood to a part. PASSIVE H. occurs when there is restricted flow of blood from a part.—hyperemic, adj.

hyperesthesia (hī-per-es-thē′-zi-a): Excessive sensitiveness of the skin or another special sense organ.—hyperesthetic, adj. Cf. **anesthesia**.

hyperextension (hī-per-eks-ten′-shun): Over-extension of a limb or part.

hyperflexion (hī-per-flek′-shun): Excessive flexion of a limb or part.

hypergalactia (hī-per-ga-lak′-shi-a): Excessive secretion of milk.

hypergeusia (hī-per-gū′-zi-a): Abnormal acuteness of the sense of taste.

hyperglycemia (hī-per-glī-sē′-mi-a): An excessive amount of sugar in the blood. —hyperglycemic, adj.

hyperglycinemia (hī-per-glī-sin-ē′-mi-a): Excessive amount of glycine in the serum. Can cause acidosis and mental retardation. —hyperglycinemic, adj.

hyperglycosuria (hī-per-glī-cō-sū′-ri-a): The excretion of glucose in the urine in much greater amounts than is usually observed in glycosuria.

hyperhidrosis (hī-per-hī-drō′-sis): Excessive sweating.—hyperhidrotic, adj.

hyperinsulinism (hī-per-in′-sū-lin-izm): A condition caused by excessive secretion of insulin, which causes an abnormally low blood sugar concentration; may be due to pathology of the pancreas or overdosage of insulin. Characterized by intermittent or continuous loss of consciousness, with or without convulsions. Sometimes called 'insulin shock.'

hyperinvolution (hī-per-in-vo-loo′-shun): Reduction to below normal size, as of the uterus after parturition.

hyperkalemia (hī-per-kal-ē′-mi-a): Excessive potassium in the blood.—hyperkalemic, adj.

hyperkeratosis (hī-per-ker-a-tō′-sis): Hypertrophy of the cornea or of the horny layer of the skin.—hyperkeratotic, adj.

hyperketonuria (hī-per-kē-tō-nū′-ri-a): Excessive secretion of ketone bodies in the urine.

hyperkinesia (hī-per-kī-nē′-si-a): Excessive movement; abnormal restlessness.—hyperkinetic, adj.

hyperleukocytosis (hī-per-lū-kō-sī-tō′-sis): An increase in the number of leukocytes in the blood greater than that usually seen in leukocytosis.

hyperlipemia (hī-per-lī-pē′-mi-a): Excessive fat in the blood.—hyperlipemic, adj.

hypermastia (hī-per-mas′-ti-a): 1. Abnormal increase in the size of the mammary gland. 2. The presence of supernumerary mammary glands.

hypermetabolism (hī-per-me-tab′-ol-izm): An abnormal increase in the utilization of food materials by the body, resulting in the production of excessive heat. Characteristic of thyrotoxicosis.—hypermetabolic, adj.

hypermetropia (hī-per-mē-trō′-pi-a): Hyperopia (*q.v.*).—hypermetropic, adj.

hypermnesia (hī-perm-nē′-zi-a): Unusual power of memory.

hypermobility (hī-per-mō-bil′-i-ti): Excessive mobility.

hypermotility (hī-per-mō-til′-i-ti): Increased movement, as peristalsis.

hypermyotonia (hī-per-mī-ō-tōn′-i-a): Excessive muscle tonus.

hypermyotrophy (hī-per-mī-ot′-rō-fi): Unusual wasting of muscle tissue.

hypernatremia (hī-per-na-trē′-mi-a): An unusually high amount of sodium in the plasma of the blood.—hypernatremic, adj.

hypernephroma (hī-per-ne-frō′-ma): Grawitz tumor. A malignant neoplasm of the kidney.—hypernephromata, pl.; hypernephromatous, adj.

hypernoia (hī-per-noy′-a): Excessive mental activity.

hypernutrition (hī-per-nū-tri′-shun): Overfeeding.

hyperonychia (hī-per-ō-nik′-i-a): Excessive growth of the nails.

hyperopia (hī-per-ō′-pi-a): A condition in which the rays of light entering the eye are focused behind the retina; usually due to a flattening of the eyeball from front to back. Farsightedness.—hyperopic, adj.   Syn., hypermetropia.

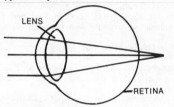

Hyperopia

hyperorexia (hī-per-ō-rek′-si-a): Excessive appetite. Bulimia.

hyperosmia (hī-per-oz′-mi-a): An abnormally high sensitiveness to odors. —hyperosmic, adj.

hyperostosis (hī-per-os-tō′-sis): Thickening or overgrowth of bone. Exostosis.

hyperoxaluria (hī-per-ok-sa-lū′-ri-a): Excessive oxaluria (*q.v.*).—hyperoxaluric, adj.

hyperoxemia (hī-per-ok-sē′-mi-a): A condition in which the blood is excessively acid.

hyperoxia (hī-per-ok′-si-a): An excess of oxygen in the tissues or the system. —hyperoxic, adj.

hyperparathyroidism (hī-per-pa-ra-thī′-roid-izm): A condition due to overaction of the parathyroid glands resulting in loss of calcium from the bones and an increase in serum calcium levels; may result in osteitis fibrosa cystica with decalcification and spontaneous fracture of bones.

hyperperistalsis (hī-per-pe-ri-stal'-sis): Excessive peristalsis.—hyperperistaltic, adj.

hyperphagia (hī-per-fā'-ji-a): Overeating.

hyperphasia (hī-per-fā'-zi-a): Excessive talkativeness.

hyperphosphatemia (hī-per-fos-fa-tē'-mi-a): Excess of phosphates in the blood.

hyperphosphaturia (hī-per-fos-fa-tū'-ri-a): An increased amount of phosphates in the urine.

hyperphrenia (hī-per-frē'-ni-a): 1. Excessive mental activity. 2. An unusually high intellect.

hyperpiesis (hī-per-pī-ē'-sis): High blood pressure of unknown origin, especially essential hypertension (*q.v.*).

hyperpigmentation (hī-per-pig-men-tā'-shun): Increased or excessive pigmentation.

hyperpituitarism (hī-per-pit-ū'-it-ar-izm): Overactivity of the anterior lobe of the pituitary producing gigantism or acromegaly (*q.v.*).

hyperplasia (hī-per-plā'-zi-a): Excessive formation of cells resulting in overgrowth of tissue.—hyperplastic, adj.

hyperplastic (hī-per-plas'-tik): 1. Pertaining to hyperplasia. 2. Overgrown.

hyperpnea (hī-perp-nē'-a): Rapid, deep breathing; panting; gasping.—hyperpneic, adj.

hyperpotassemia (hī-per-pot-a-sē'-mi-a): Increased potassium in the blood, theoretically can cause heart block, cardiac arrest and muscle paralysis.—hyperpotassemic, adj.

hyperpsychosis (hī-per-sī-kō'-sis): Excessive mental activity.

hyperpyrexia (hī-per-pī-rek'-si-a): Extremely high fever.—hyperpyretic, hyperpyrexial, adj.

hyperreflexia (hī-per-rē-flek'-si-a): Exaggeration of the deep tendon reflexes.

hypersecretion (hī-per-se-krē'-shun): Excessive secretion.

hypersensitivity (hī-per-sen-si-tiv'-i-ti): A state of being unduly sensitive to a stimulus or an allergen (*q.v.*).—hypersensitive, adj.

hypersomnia (hī-per-som'-ni-a): A condition in which one sleeps for long periods of time but is normal in the intervals between sleeping.

hypersplenism (hī-per-splen'-izm): A condition in which there is increased hemolytic activity of an enlarged spleen; there may be refractory anemia, leukopenia, or thrombocytopenia, in spite of active bone marrow.

hypersteatosis (hī-per-stē-a-tō'-sis): Excessive secretion by sebaceous glands.

hypersthenia (hī-pers-thē'-ni-a): Excessive or abnormal strength or tonicity of muscles.

hypertelorism (hī-per-tel'-or-izm): 1. Greater than normal width between two paired parts or organs. 2. Genetically determined cranial anomaly (low forehead and pronounced vertex) associated with mental subnormality. OCULAR H., greater than normal space between the eyes.

hypertension (hī-per-ten'-shun): Abnormally high tension, by custom alluding to blood pressure and involving systolic and/or diastolic levels. Hyperpiesis. ESSENTIAL H., that which occurs without preexisting disease or demonstrable change in kidneys, heart, or blood vessels; also sometimes called primary H. or benign H. MALIGNANT H., usually develops at a comparatively early age, runs a rapid course, and has a poor prognosis. PORTAL H., abnormally high blood pressure in the portal venous system; often seen in cirrhosis of the liver. RENAL H., that due to damaged or defective kidney function.—hypertensive, adj.

hyperthelia (hī-per-thē'-li-a): The presence of one or more supernumerary nipples.

hyperthermalgesia (hī-per-ther-mal-jē'-si-a): Abnormal sensitiveness to heat.

hyperthermia (hī-per-ther'-mi-a): 1. Extremely high temperature; hyperpyrexia. 2. A method of treating disease by raising the temperature of the body, either by external applications, the introduction of disease organisms into the body, or the injection of foreign proteins.

hyperthyroidism (hī-per-thī'-roid-izm): Thyrotoxicosis (*q.v.*).

hypertonia (hī-per-tō'-ni-a): Abnormally increased tone in a muscular structure.—hypertonic, adj.; hypertonicity, n.

hypertonic (hī-per-ton'-ik): 1. Having hypertonia (*q.v.*). 2. Having an osmotic pressure greater than a solution used for comparison, *e.g.*, normal saline has a greater osmotic pressure than normal physiological (body) fluids.

hypertoxic (hī-per-tok'-sik): Very poisonous.

hypertrichiasis (hī-per-trik-ī'-a-sis): Excessive hairiness. Also hypertrichosis.

hypertrophy (hī-per'-tro-fi): Increase in the bulk of a tissue or structure, not due to tumor formation; usually the result of functional activity, *e.g.,* the H. of a muscle. May be congenital, compensatory, complementary, or functional.

hyperuresis (hī-per-ū-rē′-sis): Polyuria (*q.v.*).

hyperuricemia (hī-per-ū-ris-ē′-mi-a): Excessive uric acid in the blood. Characteristic of gout.—hyperuricemic, adj.

hyperuricuria (hī-per-ū-rik-ū′-ri-a): Excess of uric acid in the urine.

hyperventilation (hī-per-ven-ti-lā′-shun): Over-breathing. A state in which there is a decrease of carbon dioxide in the blood as a result of rapid and deep breathing; symptoms may include dizziness, confusion and muscle cramps.—Syn., hyperpnea.

hypervitaminosis (hī-per-vī-ta-min-ō′-sis): Any condition arising from an excess of vitamins; large overdoses of vitamins A and D may cause pathological conditions. Water-soluble vitamins apparently do not accumulate in the body in sufficient quantities to cause pathological conditions.

hypervolemia (hī-per-vō-lē′-mi-a): An abnormal increase in the volume of plasma circulating in the body. Plethora (*q.v.*).—hypervolemic, adj.

hypesthesia (hip-es-thē′-zi-a): Hypoesthesia (*q.v.*).

hypha (hī′-fa): One of the filaments that compose a fungus.

hyphema (hī-fē′-ma): Hemorrhage into the anterior chamber of the eye.

hyphidrosis (hip-hid-rō′-sis): Too little perspiration.

hypn-, hypno-: Denotes: (1) sleep; (2) hypnotism.

hypnagogue (hip′-na-gog): An agent that induces sleep. A hypnotic.

hypnoanalysis (hip-nō-an-al′-i-sis): Psychoanalysis with the patient under hypnosis (*q.v.*).

hypnolepsy (hip′-nō-lep-si): Uncontrollable, abnormal drowsiness.

hypnosis (hip-nō′-sis): A state resembling sleep, brought about by the hypnotist utilizing the mental mechanism of suggestion. H. can be used to produce painless labor, dental extractions, and is occasionally utilized in minor surgery and in psychiatric practice.—hypnotic, adj.; hypnotize, v.t.

hypnotherapy (hip-nō-ther′-a-pi): Treatment by prolonged sleep or hypnosis.

hypnotic (hip-not′-ik): 1. Pertaining to hypnotism. 2. A drug which produces a sleep resembling natural sleep.

hypo-: Denotes: (1) deficient, less than normal; (2) located beneath or below.

hypoacidity (hī-pō-as-id′-i-ti): Less than normal acidity; term usually used in reference to acidity of the gastric juice.

hypoactivity (hī-pō-ak-tiv′-i-ti): Abnormally diminished activity; said of glands, nerves, muscles, or of the entire organism.

hypoacusis (hī-pō-a-kū′-sis): Hearing impairment.

hypobaropothy (hī-pō-bar-op′-a-thi): A condition caused by diminished air pressure or decrease in oxygen in the air. Examples are altitude sickness, mountain sickness, aviator's sickness, caisson disease (*q.v.*).

hypobulia (hī-pō-bū′-li-a): Abnormal weakness of the will.

hypocalcemia (hī-pō-kal-sē′-mi-a): Decreased calcium in the blood. See **tetany.** —hypocalcemic, adj.

hypocapnia (hī-pō-kap′-ni-a): Less than the normal amount of carbon dioxide in the circulating blood.

hypochloremia (hī-pō-klō-rē′-mi-a): Less than the normal amount of chlorides in the circulating blood. A form of alkalosis. —hypochloremic, adj.

hypochlorhydria (hī-pō-klor-hī′-dri-a): Decreased hydrochloric acid in the gastric juice.—hypochlorhydric, adj.

hypochlorite (hī-pō-klō′-rīt): Any salt of hypochlorous acid. They are easily decomposed to yield active chlorine, and have been widely used on that account in treating wounds, *e.g.,* Dakin's solution.

hypochloruria (hī-pō-klor-ū′-ri-a): The excretion of abnormally small amounts of chlorides in the urine.

hypocholesteremia (hī-pō-kol-es-ter-ē′-mi-a): Less than the normal amount of cholesterol in the blood.

hypochondria (hī-pō-kon′-dri-a): A fixed mental attitude involving the erroneous conviction that the body or an organ is diseased. Excessive anxiety about one's health; common in depressive and anxiety states.—hypochondriac, adj.; hypochondriasis, n.

hypochondriac (hī-pō-kon′-dri-ak): 1. One suffering from hypochondria (*q.v.*). 2. Pertaining to the hypochondrium (*q.v.*).

hypochondrium (hī-pō-kon′-dri-um): The upper lateral region (left and right) of the abdomen, just below the lower ribs.—hypochondriac, adj.

hypochromia (hī-pō-krō′-mi-a): 1. Deficiency in coloring or pigmentation. 2. Less than the normal percentage of hemoglobin in the red blood cells.

hypochylia (hī-pō-kī′-li-a): Deficiency in the amount of gastric juice secreted.

hypodactyly (hī-pō-dak′-til-i): Less than the normal number of fingers or toes.

hypodermic (hī-pō-der′-mik): 1. Below the skin; subcutaneous. 2. An injection into or under the skin. 3. A small syringe with a hollow needle used for injecting drugs or other agents into or under the skin. —hypodermically, adv.

hypodermis (hī-pō-der′-mis): The layer of tissue lying immediately beneath the corium of the skin (*q.v.*).

hypodermoclysis (hī-pō-der-mok′-li-sis): The injection of a large amount of fluid, usually saline solution, into the subcutaneous tissues.

hypodipsia (hī-pō-dip′-si-a): Abnormally diminished sensation of thirst.

hypoesthesia (hī-pō-es-thē′-zi-a): Abnormally diminished sensitiveness of a part.

hypofibrinogenemia (hī-pō-fī-brin-ō-jen-ē′-mi-a): See **afibrinogenemia.**—hypofibrinogenemic, adj.

hypofunction (hī-pō-fungk′-shun): Diminished performance.

hypogalactia (hī-pō-gal-ak′-shi-a): Deficient secretion of milk.

hypogammaglobulinemia (hī-pō-gam-ma-glob-ū-lin-ē′-mi-a): Decreased gamma globulin in the blood. Lessens resistance to infection.—hypogammaglobulinemic, adj.

hypogastrium (hī-pō-gas′-tri-um): That area of the anterior abdomen which lies immediately below the umbilical region. It is flanked on either side by the iliac fossae.—hypogastric, adj.

hypogeusia (hī-pō-gū′-zi-a): Abnormally diminished sense of taste. Also hypogeusesthesia.

hypoglossal (hī-pō-glos′-al): Under the tongue. H. NERVE, one of the twelfth pair of cranial nerves.

hypoglycemia (hī-pō-glī-sē′-mi-a): Decreased blood sugar, attended by anxiety, excitement, perspiration, delirium or coma (insulin). H. can be produced intentionally (insulin treatment) in schizophrenia. —hypoglycemic, adj.

hypohidrosis (hī-pō-hī-drō′-sis): Abnormally decreased secretion of sweat.

hypoinsulinism (hī-pō-in′-sū-lin-izm): Deficient secretion of insulin by the pancreas; results in hyperglycemia.

hypokalemia (hī-pō-kal-ē′-mi-a): Abnormally low potassium level of the blood. See **potassium deficiency.**—hypokalemic, adj.

hypokinesia (hī-pō-kī-nē′-si-a): Abnormally decreased motor activity or function; paresis (*q.v.*).

hypoleukocytosis (hī-pō-lū-kō-sī-tō′-sis): Less than the normal number of leukocytes in the circulating blood.

hypomagnesemia (hī-pō-mag-nēs-ē′-mi-a): Decreased magnesium in the blood. —hypomagnesemic, adj.

hypomania (hī-pō-mā′-ni-a): A moderate form of mania (*q.v.*), in which the patient is easily distracted.—hypomanic, adj.

hypomastia (hī-pō-mas′-ti-a): Abnormal smallness of the breasts.

hypomenorrhea (hī-pō-men-ō-rē′-a): Less than the normal amount of uterine bleeding at regular intervals; the period of flow may be the same or less than normal time.

hypometabolism (hī-pō-me-tab′-ol-ism): An abnormal decrease in the body's utilization of food materials with resulting diminution in the production of heat; low metabolic rate. Characteristic of myxedema.

hypomnesis (hī-pom-nē′-sis): Defective memory.

hypomotility (hī-po-mō-ti′-li-ti): Decreased movement of any part, *e.g.,* the stomach or intestines.

hypomyotonia (hī-pō-mī-ō-tōn′-i-a): Abnormally decreased muscular tonicity.

hyponatremia (hī-pō-na-trē′-mi-a): Abnormally low concentration of sodium in the blood.—hyponatremic, adj.

hyponatruria (hī-pō-nat-rū′-ri-a): Abnormally low level of sodium in the urine.

hyponychial (hī-pō-nik′-i-al): Beneath a nail.

hypo-osmolarity (hī-pō-oz-mō-lar′-i-ti): Syn., hypotonicity. A solution exerting a lower osmotic pressure than another is said to have hypo-osmolarity with reference to it. In medicine the comparison is usually made with normal plasma.

hypoparathyroidism (hī-pō-pa-ra-thī′-roid-izm): The condition produced by undersecretion or removal of the parathyroid glands; the serum calcium level is decreased, resulting in tetany (*q.v.*).

hypopepsia (hī-pō-pep′-si-a): Impaired digestion, particularly when it is due to deficient secretion of pepsin.

hypopharynx (hī-pō-far′-ingks): That portion of the pharynx lying below and behind the larynx, correctly called the laryngopharynx.

hypophoria (hī-pō-fō′-ri-a): A state in which the visual axis of one eye is lower than that of the other.

hypophosphatemia (hī-pō-fos-fa-tē′-mi-a): Decreased phosphates in the blood.—hypophosphatemic, adj.

hypophosphaturia (hī-pō-fos-fa-tū′-ri-a): Reduced excretion of phosphates in the urine.

hypophrenia (hī-pō-frē′-ni-a): Feeblemindedness.—hypophrenic, adj.

hypophyseal (hī-pō-fiz′-ē-al): Pertaining to a hypophysis, particularly the pituitary gland.

hypophysectomy (hī-pō-fi-sek′-to-mi): Surgical removal of the pituitary gland.

hypophysis (hī-pof′-i-sis): Any outgrowth or process. H. CEREBRI, the small oval-shaped gland lying in the pituitary fossa of the sphenoid bone and connected to the under surface of the brain by a stalk; the pituitary gland.—hypophyseal, adj.

hypopiesis (hī-pō-pī-ē′-sis): Abnormally low pressure. Low blood pressure.

hypopigmentation (hī-pō-pig-men-tā′-shun): Decreased or poor pigmentation.

hypopituitarism (hī-pō-pit-ū′-it-ar-izm): Pituitary gland insufficiency, especially of the anterior lobe. Absence of gonadotrophins leads to failure of ovulation, uterine atrophy, amenorrhea. Loss of trophic hormones to other endocrines produces mental inertia, laziness, weakness, lack of sweating, sensitivity to cold, oliguria, loss of pubic and axillary hair, hypoglycemia, pale skin, depigmentation of mammary areolae and perineum. Can result from postpartum infarction of the pituitary gland.

hypoplasia (hī-pō-plā′-zi-a): Defective or incomplete development of any tissue.—hypoplastic, adj.

hypopnea (hī-pop-nē′-a): Abnormal decrease in the rate and depth of respirations. Opp. to hyperpnea.

hypopotassemia (hī-pō-pot-a-sē′-mi-a): See hypokalemia.

hypoproteinemia (hī-pō-prō-tē-in-ēm′-i-a): A deficiency of protein in the blood plasma, from dietary deficiency or excessive excretion (albuminuria).—hypoproteinemic, adj.

hypoprothrombinemia (hī-pō-prō-throm-bin-ē′-mi-a): Deficiency of prothrombin in the blood which retards its clotting ability. See **vitamin K** and **jaundice**.—hypoprothrombinemic, adj.

hypoptyalism (hī-pō-tī′-al-izm): Deficient secretion of saliva. Also hyposalivation.

hypopyon (hī-pō′-pi-on): A collection of pus in the anterior chamber of the eye.

hyporeactive (hī-pō-rē-ak′-tiv): Having less than normal response to stimuli.

hyporeflexia (hī-pō-rē-flek′-si-a): A condition of weakened reflexes.

hyposecretion (hī-pō-sē-krē′-shun): Deficient rate or amount of secretion.

hyposensitive (hī-pō-sen′-si-tiv): Having a deficient response to stimuli.

hyposensitization (hī-pō-sen-si-tī-zā′-shun): Reduction of the sensitiveness of an individual, especially to allergens.

hyposmia (hī-poz′-mi-a): Abnormally decreased sensitiveness to odors.

hyposomnia (hī-pō-som′-ni-a): Insomnia (q.v.).

hypospadias (hī-pō-spā′-di-as): A congenital malformation in which the male urethra opens on the under surface of the penis; that of the female opens into the vagina instead of externally from the bladder. Also hypospadia.—hypospadiac, adj.

hypostasis (hī-pos′-ta-sis): 1. A sediment. 2. Congestion of blood in a part due to impaired circulation.—hypostatic, adj.

hypostatic (hī-pō-stat′-ik): 1. Caused by or pertinent to hypostasis (q.v.). 2. Abnormally static; said of certain inherited characteristics that are hidden or suppressed by other characteristics. H. CONGESTION, see **congestion**. H. PNEUMONIA, see **pneumonia**.

hyposthenia (hī-pos-thē′-ni-a): Bodily weakness.—hyposthenic, adj.

hyposthenuria (hī-pos-the-nūr′-i-a): The secretion of urine that is of lower than normal specific gravity; often associated with chronic nephritis.

hypostosis (hip-os-tō′-sis): Deficient development of bone.

hypotension (hī-pō-ten′-shun): Lowered tension; lowered blood pressure. May be primary or secondary. A person is considered hypotensive when the systolic pressure is below 110 mm mercury and the diastolic below 70 mm. ESSENTIAL H., may exist without apparent pathologic cause; occurs most frequently in women and the undernourished. ORTHOSTATIC H., low blood pressure which occurs when a person stands up after being in a supine position; also called postural hypotension.

hypotensive (hī-pō-ten′-siv): 1. A drug or agent that lowers blood pressure. 2. A person suffering from hypotension. 3. Characterized by low blood pressure.

hypothalamus (hī-pos-thal′-a-mus): Below the thalamus. The part of the midbrain nearest to the pituitary gland; important because the nuclei of this region control the body temperature, visceral activities, sleep, water balance, and the metabolism of fats and carbohydrates; also important in emotional and motivational behavior.

hypothenar eminence (hī-poth′-e-nar): The eminence on the ulnar side of the palm below the little finger.

hypothermia (hī-pō-therm′-i-a): 1. Below normal body temperature (below 98.6° F, or 37° C). 2. Artificially induced H. (86° F or 30° C) can be used in the treatment of head injuries and in cardiac surgery. It reduces the oxygen consumption of the tissues and thereby allows greater and more prolonged interference of normal blood circulation. H. OF THE NEWBORN, failure of the newborn child to adjust to external cold; may be associated with infection.

hypothesis (hī-poth′-e-sis): A theory or an assumption made for the sake of argument, or as a basis for action to be taken.

hypothrepsia (hī-pō-threp′-si-a): Malnutrition. See **athrepsia.**

hypothrombinemia (hī-pō-throm-bin-ē′-mi-a): A deficiency of thrombin in the blood; results in a tendency toward bleeding.

hypothyroidism (hī-pō-thī′-roid-izm): A group of symptoms caused by deficiency of thyroid secretion. See **cretinism** and **myxedema.**

hypotonic (hī-pō-tōn′-ik): 1. Having a low osmotic pressure; less than isotonic. 2. Lacking in tone, tension, strength.—hypotonia, hypotonicity, n.

hypotrichosis (hī-pō-tri-kō′-sis): Presence of less than the usual amount of hair.

hypotrophy (hī-pot′-ro-fi): Progressive degeneration of cells and tissues with loss of function.

hypouresis (hī-pō-ū-rē′-sis): Reduced output of urine.

hypouricuria (hī-pō-ū-rik-ū′-ri-a): Less than the normal amount of uric acid in the urine.

hypoventilation (hī-pō-ven-ti-lā′-shun): 1. Diminished breathing or underventilation. 2. Less than the normal amount of air entering the lungs; results in elevation of the carbon dioxide content of the blood.

hypovitaminosis (hī-pō-vī-ta-min-ō′-sis): A deficiency of one or more of the essential vitamins. Less severe than avitaminosis (q.v.).

hypovolemia (hī-pō-vō-lē′-mi-a): An abnormal decrease in the amount of blood circulating in the body. Opp. to hypervolemia.—hypovolemic, adj.

hypoxemia (hī-pok-sē′-mi-a): Less than the

normal amount of oxygen in the arterial blood.—hypoxemic, adj.

hypoxia (hī-pok′-si-a): Diminished amount of oxygen in the tissues.—hypoxic, adj.

hypsarrhythmia (hip-sa-rith′-mi-a): Term applied to a condition in infants that is characterized by a distinct abnormality in the electrocardiogram and which is usually associated with mental retardation; often accompanied with spasms or quivering.

hyster-, hystero-: Denotes: (1) the uterus; (2) hysteria.

hysterectomy (his-ter-ek′-to-mi): Surgical removal of the uterus. ABDOMINAL H., effected via a lower abdominal incision. SUBTOTAL H., removal of the uterine body, leaving the cervix in the vaginal vault. TOTAL H., complete removal of the uterine body and the cervix. VAGINAL H., effected through the vagina. WERTHEIM'S H., total removal of the uterus, the adjacent lymphatic vessels and glands, and a cuff of the vagina.

hysteria (his-ter′-i-a): A psychoneurosis or neurosis characterized by a physical disorder such as blindness or paralysis, brought on by psychological rather than organic disorder. Marked by conversion of anxiety into such symptoms as nervousness, uncontrollable laughing, crying, convulsions, intense muscular activity, psychic disorders.—hysterical, hysteric, adj.

hysterical (his-ter′-i-kal): Related to or affected with hysteria (q.v.). H. NEUROSIS, see **hysteria.**

hysterics (his-ter′-iks): An uncontrollable fit of laughing or crying, or both. See **hysteria.**

hysterography (his-ter-og′-ra-fi): 1. X-ray examination of the uterus. 2. The procedure of making a graphic record that shows the strength of uterine contractions during labor.—hysterograph, hysterogram, n.; hysterographical, adj.; hysterographically, adv.

hysteromyoma (his-ter-ō-mī-ō′-ma): A myoma (q.v.) of the uterus.

hysteropexy (his′-ter-ō-pek-si): Fixation of a displaced or abnormally placed uterus; may be fastened to the vaginal or abdominal wall.

hysteroptosis (his-ter-op-tō′-sis): Prolapse of the uterus.

hysterorrhaphy (his-ter-or′-ra-fi): Surgical repair of a lacerated uterus.

hysterosalpingectomy (his-ter-ō-sal-pin-jek′-to-mi): Excision of the uterus and usually both uterine tubes (oviducts).

hysterosalpingography (his-ter-ō-sal-ping-og′-ra-fi): X-ray examination of the uterus and tubes after injection of a contrast medium.

hysterosalpingo-oophorectomy (his-ter-ō-sal-pin-gō-ō-of-o-rek′-to-mi): Removal of the uterus, fallopian tubes and ovaries.

hysterosalpingostomy (his-te-rō-sal-ping-os′-to mi): Anastomosis between an oviduct and the uterus.

hysterotomy (his-ter-ot′-o-mi): Incision into the uterus.

hysterotrachelorrhaphy (his-ter-ō-trā-kel-or′-a-fi): Repair of lacerated cervix uteri.

I

I^{131}, I^{132}: Radioactive isotopes of iodine.

-ia: Word termination often used in naming diseases or pathological conditions, *e.g.,* neuralgia.

-iasis (pl., iases): Denotes: (1) morbid condition, disease; (2) disease having characteristics of a specific thing, *e.g.,* elephantiasis.

-iatric, -iatrics: Denotes medical treatment or healing.

-iatrist: Denotes physician, medicine, healing.

iatro-: Denotes medicine; healing.

iatrogenic (ī-at-rō-jen′-ik): A secondary condition arising from treatment of a primary condition.

-iatry: Denotes medical treatment; healing.

ichor (ī′-kor): A thin, watery discharge, as from a raw wound or ulcer.—ichorous, adj.

ichthyosis (ik-thi-ō′-sis): A congenital chronic condition of the skin which becomes rough, dry and scaly over the entire body; the hair is lusterless. Cold weather causes intense itching. Fish skin. Xeroderma. I. HYSTRIX, a form of congenital nevi with patches of warty excrescences.

ichthyotoxin (ik-thi-ō-tok′-sin): A poisonous substance found in the blood serum of the eel. The term is often applied to any toxic substance derived from fish.

ICN: Abbreviation for International Council of Nurses.

ictal (ik′-tal): Pertaining to a stroke or seizure, *e.g.,* an acute epileptical seizure.

icteric (ik-ter′-ik): Pertaining to or affected with jaundice.

icterus (ik′-ter-us): Jaundice. I. GRAVIS, acute yellow atrophy (see **acute**). I. GRAVIS NEONATORUM, one of the clinical forms of hemolytic disease of the newborn (erythroblastosis fetalis, *q.v.*). I. NEONATORUM is the normal, or physiological jaundice occurring in the first week of life as a result of destruction of hemoglobin in excess of the infant's needs. I. INDEX, an index (expressed in units) representing the bilirubin concentration in the blood plasma; used in diagnosis of jaundice. The normal range is 4-6 units.

ictus (ik′-tus): A stroke or blow; a sudden attack or fit.

ICU: Abbreviation for intensive care unit (*q.v.*).

id: That part of the unconscious mind which consists of a system of primitive urges (instincts) and according to Freud (*q.v.*) persists unrecognized into adult life.

idea: The memory of past perceptions. A mental perception, image, or concept. An I. depends upon an image in the same way that a perception (*q.v.*) depends on a sensation.

ideation (ī-dē-ā′-shun): The process concerned with the highest function of awareness, the formation of ideas. It includes thought, intellect and memory.

idée fixe (ē-dā fēks′): A fixed idea; an obsession.

identical twins: Two offspring developed from a single fertilized egg. They are always of the same sex and commonly much alike in appearance. See **binovular, uniovular.**

identification (ī-den-ti-fi-kā′-shun): Recognition. In psychology, the way in which we form our personality by modeling it on a chosen person, *e.g.,* I. with the parent of same sex—helping to form one's sex role; I. with a person of one's own sex in the hero-worship of adolescence.

Identoband (ī-den′-tō-band): A band placed around the wrist or ankle of a patient for identification purposes; has the patient's name on it and sometimes other information about him.

ideology (id-ē-ol′-o-jē): 1. The science dealing with the development of ideas. 2. The ideas or manner of thinking that characterizes a group or an individual.

ideomotor (ī-dē-o-mō′-tor): Descriptive of automative muscular activity that is aroused by thoughts or ideas. Agitated movements of parts of the body resulting from mental agitation.

idio-: Denotes: (1) self-produced, self-producing, arising within the self; (2) separate, distinct, peculiar.

idiocy (id′-i-ō-si): Extreme mental deficiency, usually congenital but may follow disease or injury during childhood; due to incomplete or abnormal development of the brain. See **amaurotic familial idiocy.**

idiopathic (id-i-ō-path′-ik): Self-originated; of unknown cause. Relating to a peculiar individual characteristic.

idiopathy (id-i-op′-a-thi): A pathologic state of unknown or spontaneous origin.—idiopathic, adj.

idiosyncrasy (id-i-ō-sin′-kra-si): A peculiar variation of constitution or temperament. Unusual individual response to certain drugs, proteins, etc., whether by injection, ingestion, inhalation or contact.

idiot: A person affected with idiocy (*q.v.*); he ranks lowest in the grades of mental deficiency, has an IQ of below 25, is unable to use language meaningfully, protect himself from ordinary dangers, or be a productive member of society. MONGOLIAN I., one who exhibits mongolism (*q.v.*).

idioventricular (id-i-ō-ven-trik′-ū-lar): Pertaining to the cardiac ventricles and not affecting the atria.

IH: Abbreviation for infectious hepatitis (*q.v.*).

il-: See **in-**.

ileectomy (il-ē-ek′-to-mi): Surgical excision of the ileum.

ileitis (il-ē-ī′-tis): Inflammation of the ileum. REGIONAL I. (Crohn's disease), a chronic, stenosing inflammation of the ileum which may give rise to intestinal obstruction.

ileo-: Denotes the ileum.

ileocecal (il-ē-ō-sē′-kal): Pertaining to the ileum and the cecum. I. VALVE, the sphincter muscle that guards the opening between the ileum and the large intestine, allowing material to pass from small to large intestine, but not in the reverse direction.

ileocecostomy (il-ē-ō-sē-kos′-to-mi): The surgical creation of an artifical opening between the ileum and the cecum.

ileocolic (il-ē-ō-kol′-ik): Pertaining to the ileum and the colon.

ileocolitis (il-ē-ō-kō-lī′tis): Inflammation of the ileum and the colon.

ileocolostomy (il-ē-ō-kō-los′-to-mi): A surgically made fistula between the ileum and the colon, usually the transverse colon. Most often used to bypass an obstruction or inflammation in the cecum or ascending colon.

ileocystoplasty (il-ē-ō-sis′-tō-plas-ti): Operation to increase the capacity of the urinary bladder. See **colocystoplasty.**—ileocystoplastic, adj.

ileoproctostomy (il-ē-ō-prok-tos′-to-mi): An anastomosis between the ileum and the rectum; used when disease extends to the sigmoid colon.

ileorectal (il-ē-ō-rek′-tal): Pertaining to the ileum and the rectum.

ileosigmoidostomy (il-ē-ō-sig-moid-os′-to-mi): An anastomosis between the ileum and sigmoid colon; used when most of the colon has to be removed.

ileostomy (il-ē-os′-to-mi): A surgically made fistula between the ileum and the anterior abdominal wall; usually a permanent form of artificial anus when the whole of the large bowel has to be removed, *e.g.,* in severe ulcerative colitis. I. BAGS, rubber or plastic bags used to collect the liquid discharge from an ileostomy.

ileoureterostomy (il-ē-o-ū-rēt-er-os′-to-mi): Transplantation of the lower ends of the ureters from the bladder to an isolated loop of small bowel which, in turn, is made to open on the abdominal wall. See **bladder.**

ileum (il′-ē-um): The lower three-fifths of the small intestine, lying between the jejunum and the cecum; about 12 feet long. —ileal, adj.

ileus (il′-ē-us): Intestinal obstruction. Usually restricted to paralytic as opposed to mechanical obstruction and characterized by abdominal distension, vomiting and the absence of pain.

ili-, ilio-: Denotes the ilium.

iliopectineal (il-i-ō-pek-tin′-ē-al): Pertaining to the ilium and the pubis.

iliosciatic (il-i-ō-sī-at′-ik): Pertaining to the ilium and the ischium.

iliotrochanteric (il-i-ō-trō-kan-ter′-ik): Pertaining to the ilium and a trochanter.

ilium (il′-i-um): The large, flaring, lateral and uppermost of the three bones that compose the innominate (hip) bone; it is a separate bone in fetal life. The flank.—iliac, adj.

illusion (i-lū′-zhun): 1. A misidentification of a sensation, *e.g.,* of sight, a white sheet being mistaken for a ghost; an apparition. 2. The state or fact of being deceived. 3. A false impression or misconception. 4. A perception that does not give the true character of an object; may be normal as in certain optical illusions, or abnormal as occurs in insanity.

IM, im: Abbreviations for intramuscular or intramuscularly.

im-: See **in-**.

image (im′-ij): 1. A reasonably accurate representation or imitation of a person or thing, *e.g.,* a statue. 2. An optical picture transferred to the brain by the optic nerve. 3. A mental representation of a thing not actually present but that is recalled by memory or created by imagination. 4. A revived experience of a percept recalled from memory (smell or taste). See **afterimage.**

imagery (im′-ij-ri): Imagination. The recall of mental images of various types depending upon the special sense organs involved when the images were formed, *e.g.,* auditory I., motor I., visual I. (sight), tactile I. (touch), olfactory I.

imbalance (im-bal'-ans): Want of balance. Lack of equality of power between opposing forces, especially between muscles and particularly the ocular muscles. Term is also used in reference to lack of balance between the endocrine secretions, as well as to describe the condition of an upset of the acid-base relationship and the electrolytes in the body fluids.

imbecile (im'-be-sil): One affected with deficiency of intermediate grade, *i.e.,* between the grades of idiot and moron; the IQ is between 25-50, and the mental age between 3 and 7. Such an individual is weak-minded, yet capable of some education and training.

imbibition (im-bi-bish'-un): The absorption of a liquid by a solid without causing any chemical change.

immersion (i-mer'-shun): The plunging of a limb or part into a fluid.

immiscible (i-mis'-i-b'l): Not capable of being mixed with something else.

immobilization (im-mō-bil-ī-zā'-shun): The act of making immovable. In medicine or surgery, the act of making a normally movable limb or part immovable by splints, bandages, surgical procedures, etc.—immobilize, v.t.

immune (i-mūn'): Not susceptible to a particular infection. I. BODY, antibody (*q.v.*). I. REACTION, that which causes a body to reject a transplanted organ. I. SERUM, a serum containing I. bodies.

immunity (i-mūn'-i-ti): A state of relative resistance to a disease. Immunity can be NATURAL (acquired from inherited qualities) or it can be ACQUIRED, actively or passively, naturally or artificially. ACTIVE IMMUNITY is acquired naturally during a disease (infectious), or artificially by vaccination with dead or living organisms of the disease. Such immunity is long lasting. PASSIVE I. is acquired naturally when maternal antibodies pass to the child via the placenta or the milk, or artificially by administering immune sera containing antibodies obtained from animals or human beings. ARTIFICIAL PASSIVE I. is more temporary than active I. A simple classification, based on the way immunity is produced, lists four types; (1) ARTIFICIAL ACTIVE, produced by the introduction into the body of *antigens;* (2) ARTIFICIAL PASSIVE, produced by the introduction into the body of

antibodies; (3) NATURAL ACTIVE, produced by having the disease; (4) NATURAL PASSIVE, acquired through heredity.

immunization (im-ū-nī-zā'-shun): The process of making an individual immune, or of becoming immune.—immunize, v.t.

immunogenesis (im-ū-nō-jen'-e-sis): The process of production of immunity.—immunogenetic, adj.

immunogenicity (im-ū-nō-jen-is'-i-ti): The ability to produce immunity.

immunoglobulins (im-ū-nō-glob'-ū-lins): Syn., gamma globulins (*q.v.*).

immunology (im-ū-nol'-oj-i): The special study of immunity.—immunological, adj.; immunologically, adv.

immunopathology (im-ū-nō-path-ol'-oj-i): Abnormal immune reaction, as when a person becomes sensitized.

immunosensitivity (im-ū-nō-sen-si-tiv-i-ti): The state produced by immunopathology (*q.v.*).

immunosuppressive (im-ū-nō-sup-res'-iv): That which prevents the occurrence of an immune reaction (*q.v.*).

immunotherapy (im-ū-nō-ther'-a-pi): Any treatment used to produce immunity.

immunotransfusion (im-ū-nō-trans-fū'-zhun): Transfusion of blood from a donor previously rendered immune by repeated inoculations with a given agent from the recipient.

impacted (im-pak'-ted): Firmly wedged or pressed together so as to be immovable; said of a fracture when the jagged ends of bone are wedged together, of feces in the rectum, of a fetus in the uterus, of a tooth in its socket, or of a calculus in a duct.—impaction, n.

impalpable (im-pal'-pa-b'l): Not palpable. Incapable of being felt by touch (palpation).

impatent (im-pā'-tent): Closed or obstructed; not patent.

imperforate (im-per'-for-āt): Lacking a normal opening. I. ANUS, absence of an opening into the rectum. I. HYMEN, a fold of mucous membrane at the vaginal entrance which has no natural outlet for the menstrual fluid.

impermeable (im-per'-mē-a-b'l): Impenetrable; not permitting passage, as of a fluid through a membrane.

impetigo (im-pe-tī'-gō): A common, acute, inflammatory, pustular skin disease. I. CONTAGIOSA, a highly contagious form of I., commonest on the face and scalp; starts with a small red spot, quickly develops into superficial vesicles that rupture; the escaped serum dries into honey-colored gummy crusts; lesions spread rapidly. See **ecthyma**. —impetiginous, adj.

implantation (im-plan-tā′-shun): 1. The insertion of living cells or solid materials into the tissues, *e.g.*, accidental implantation of tumor cells in a wound; implantation of radium or solid drugs. 2. The attachment of the fertilized ovum to the epithelial lining of the uterus.

implants (im′-plantz): Tissues or drugs inserted surgically into the human body, *e.g.*, implantation of pellets of testosterone under the skin in treatment of carcinoma of the breast; implantation of deoxycortone acetate (DOCA) in Addison's disease.

impotence (im′-pō-tens): Lack of sexual power, by custom referring to the male; may be due to a physiological or psychological condition.

impotent (im′-pō-tent): 1. Barren or sterile. 2. Unable to copulate.—impotence, n.

impregnate (im-preg′-nāt): Fill. Saturate. Render pregnant.

impulse (im′-puls): 1. A sudden uncontrollable urge to act without deliberation. 2. A sudden push or communicated force.

in-: Denotes: (1) in, into, within, inside; (2) a sense of negation, *e.g.*, not, non-, -un. Appears as il- before l; im- before b, m, p; ir- before r.

inaccessibility (in-ak-ses-i-bil′-i-ti): In psychiatry, denotes absence of patient response.

inactivate (in-ak′-ti-vāt): To destroy the active principle or the activity of an agent or a substance.—inactivation, n.

inanimate (in-an′-i-mat): 1. Not alive. 2. Bereft of life or consciousness. 3. Dull, inert, stolid.

inanition (in-a-nish′-un): Exhaustion and wasting from lack of food or from lack of proper assimilation of food. I. FEVER, occurs during the first few days of life; high fever with rapid weight loss and restlessness; also called dehydration fever.

inarticulate (in-ar-tik′-ū-lat): 1. Not jointed. 2. Said of speech that is not intelligible. 3. Not able to speak distinctly or clearly.

inassimilable (in-a-sim′-il-a-b'l): Not capable of absorption and appropriation by the body for nourishment.

inborn (in′-born): Descriptive of physical and mental characteristics that are present at birth and that have developed or been implanted while the fetus was in utero, but which are not inherited. Innate.

incarcerated (in-kar′-ser-ā-ted): In medicine, the abnormal imprisonment of a part, as in a hernia which is irreducible, or a pregnant uterus held beneath the sacral promontory.

incendiarism (in-sen′-di-ar-izm): An obsession for setting fires.

incest (in′-sest): Sexual intercourse between near kindred, whose marriage is prohibited by law.

incidence (in′-si-dens): The rate of occurrence of an event or of a condition, *e.g.*, the number of cases of a specific disease occurring in a specified time.

incipient (in-sip′-i-ent): Initial, beginning, in early stages.

incise (in-sīz′): To cut or cut into.

incision (in-sizh′-un): A cut or wound produced by cutting into body tissue, using a sharp instrument.—incise, v.t.; incisional, adj.

incisors (in-sī′-zers): The eight front cutting teeth, four in each jaw.

inclusion bodies: Minute particles found in the cells of tissues that are affected by a virus, *e.g.*, the virus of smallpox or measles. They are stainable and vary in size, appearance and quantity) with different diseases.

incoherent (in-kō-hēr′-ent): The state or fact of being confused, disjointed, inconsistent, rambling, incongruous, or without proper sequence.—incoherence, n.

incompatibility (in-kom-pat-ib-il′-i-ti): In medicine and pharmacology, a situation in which two substances cannot be used together without producing undesirable reaction. Usually refers to the bloods of donor and recipient in transfusion, when antigenic differences in the red cells result in reactions such as hemolysis and agglutination. See **blood groups.**

incompetence (in-kom′-pe-tens): Inadequacy to perform a natural or required function; often said of cardiac valves.—incompetent, adj.

incontinence (in-kon′-tin-ens): Inability to control the evacuation of any excretion, particularly the urine and feces. OVERFLOW I., dribbling from an over-full bladder. STRESS I., occurs when the intra-abdominal pressure is raised as in coughing or sneezing; due to relaxation or incompetence of sphincter muscle of the urethra or injury of the pelvic floor.

incontinent (in-kon′-tin-ent): Unable to resist yielding to normal impulses such as the sexual impulse, or normal urges such as the urge to defecate or urinate.

189   **infection**

incoordination (in-kō-or-din-ā′-shun): Inability to produce smooth, harmonious muscular movements.

incubate (in′-ku-bāt): To promote the growth of microorganisms by placing them in an incubator (q.v.).

incubation (in-ku-bā′-shun): In medicine, the maintenance of organisms in conditions that are optimal for their growth and reproduction. I. PERIOD, the time that elapses between entry of infection and the appearance of the first symptom of disease.

incubator (in′-ku-bā-ter): A temperature-regulated apparatus in which: (1) premature or delicate babies may be placed; (2) microorganisms can be cultivated.

incus (ing′-kus): The central one of the chain of three small bones of the middle ear, taking its name from its shape, i.e., it resembles an anvil.

index: 1. The second finger; the pointer. 2. The ratio of measurement (size, capacity, or function) of one substance, thing, or part of a thing compared with a standard that is fixed after a series of observations and usually represented as 1 or 100.

Indian hemp: Cannabis indica (q.v.). Hashish.

indican (in′-di-kan): A potassium salt formed from the decomposition of tryptophan in the intestinal tract and found in the urine.

indicanuria (in-di-kan-ū′-ri-a): The presence of more than the normal amount of indican in the urine. See indole.

indicator (in′-di-kā-ter): In chemistry, a substance used to make visible the completion of a chemical reaction.

indigenous (in-dij′-e-nus): Native to a certain locality or country.

indigestion (in-di-jes′-chun): Dyspepsia. Lack or failure of digestion (q.v.).

indirect contact: Refers to the transfer of infection by such conveyers as milk, water, air, contaminated hands and inanimate objects.

indisposition (in-dis-pō-zi′-shun): In medicine, a slight or temporary illness; malaise.

indole (in′-dōl): A product of intestinal putrefaction: it is oxidized to indoxyl in the liver and excreted in urine as indican. See indicanuria.

indolent (in′-dō-lent): Lazy, sluggish, inert. In medicine, a sluggish ulcer which is generally painless and slow to heal.

induction (in-duk′-shun): The act of bringing on or causing to occur, as applied to anesthesia and labor.

indurated (in′-dū-rāt-ed): Hardened.

induration (in-dū-rā′-shun): The hardening of tissue as in hyperemia, infiltration by neoplasm, etc.—indurated, adj.

industrial disease: Occupational disease (q.v.).

indwelling (in′-dwel-ling): Pertaining to a drainage or feeding tube, or a catheter, that is fastened in a position and allowed to remain fixed for a period of time. See Foley catheter.

inebriation (in-ē-brē-ā′-shun): Drunkenness.

inert (in-ert′): 1. Slow, sluggish, inactive; having no physical or mental activity. 2. Term used to denote drugs that have no pharmaceutical or therapeutic action.

inertia (in-er′-shi-a): Lack of activity or force, physical or mental. UTERINE I., lack of contraction of parturient uterus. May be primary due to constitutional weakness; secondary due to exhaustion from frequent and forcible contractions.

in extremis (in eks-trē′-mis): At the point of death.

infant (in′-fant): A child less than two years of age; in law, a person under the age of 21. PREMATURE I., one born before term but capable of life; one who weighs less than 5.5 pounds at birth and is born 29-36 weeks after conception.

infanticide (in-fan′-ti-sīd): The killing of an infant.

infantile (in′-fan-tīl): Pertaining to an infant. Childish. I. UTERUS, term used to describe a uterus that is undeveloped or underdeveloped.

infantile paralysis: See poliomyelitis.

infantilism (in-fant′-il-izm): General retardation of physical, intellectual and emotional development with persistence of childish characteristics into adolescence and adult life.

infarct (in′-farkt): Area of tissue affected when end artery supplying it is occluded, e.g., in kidney or heart. Common complication of subacute endocarditis.

infarction (in-fark′-shun): 1. Formation of an infarct. 2. Death of a section of tissue because the blood supply has been shut off.

infect (in-fekt′): To cause infection; to contaminate with disease-producing organisms.

infection (in-fek′-shun): 1. The successful invasion, establishment, and growth of microorganisms in a degree sufficient to cause symptoms of disease in the host. 2. The condition produced by the introduction and growth of microorganisms in the tissues of the body. AIR-BORNE I., one transmitted by the air, *e.g.,* organisms may be transmitted from the respiratory tract of one person to another by droplets discharged in coughing or sneezing. CONTACT I., one caused by direct transmission from one person to another, *e.g.,* by kissing. MASS I., one caused by invasion of large numbers of a disease-producing organism. SECONDARY I., one imposed on another infection. SUBCLINICAL I., one not severe enough to cause clinical symptoms. See **cross infection, droplet, indirect contact.**

infectious (in-fek′-shus): 1. Communicable; capable of being transmitted by direct or indirect contact. 2. Denoting a disease caused by a specific, pathogenic organism and capable of being transmitted to another individual. I. HEPATITIS, an endemic type of hepatitis caused by a virus. I. MONONUCLEOSIS, an infectious fever, of unknown origin, characterized by glandular enlargement, skin eruptions and increased mononuclear leukocytes in the blood.

inferior (in-fēr′-i-or): In anatomy, lower or beneath. I. VENA CAVA, the main vein returning blood to the heart from the trunk and lower extremities.

inferiority complex: See under **complex.**

infertility (in-fer-til′-i-ti): Lack of ability to reproduce.

infestation (in-fes-tā′-shun): The presence of such animal parasites as insects, ticks, fleas, mites, lice, or worms in or on the body.—infest, v.t.

infiltration (in-fil-trā′-shun): Penetration of the surrounding tissues by a fluid or foreign substance; the leaking or oozing of a fluid into the tissues. I. ANESTHESIA, analgesia produced by infiltrating the tissues with a local anesthetic.

infirm in-firm′): Weak or feeble, either physically or mentally, because of old age or illness.

infirmary (in-firm′-ary): A hospital, usually small, especially in a school or other institution.

infirmity (in-firm′-i-ti): An unhealthy or debilitated condition of body or mind.

inflamed (in-flāmd′): Hot and swollen; affected with inflammation (*q.v.*).

inflammation (in-fla-mā′-shun): The protective, characteristic chemical or physical reaction of living tissues to injury, infection or irritation; characterized by pain, swelling, redness and heat.—inflammatory, adj.

inflation (in-flā′-shun): In medicine, the distention of a part with liquid or gas.

influenza (in-floo-en′-za): An acute, highly contagious infection, marked by inflammation of the nasopharynx and respiratory tract, fever, prostration, muscular and neurologic pains, gastrointestinal disturbances, headache, and depression; primarily caused by a filterable virus and occurring in epidemic and pandemic form. Syn., la grippe, the grip, 'flu.'—influenzal, adj.

infra-: Denotes a position or status under or below.

infraclavicular (in-fra-kla-vik′-ū-lar): Below the clavicle.

infraorbital (in-fra-or′-bit-al): Below or on the floor of the orbital cavity.

infrared rays: Long, invisible rays beyond the red end of the visible spectrum. Used therapeutically for the production of heat in the tissues.

infraspinous (in-fra-spī′-nus): Below a spine, *e.g.,* of the scapula.

infriction (in-frik′-shun): The application of a medicated substance to the skin using friction.

infundibulum (in-fun-dib′-ū-lum): Any funnel-shaped passage or structure.—infundibular, adj.; infundibula, pl.

infusion (in-fū′-zhun): 1. An aqueous solution containing the active principle of a drug, made by pouring water on the crude drug. 2. Fluid other than blood flowing by gravity into the body. See **amniotic fluid infusion.**

ingestant (in-jes′-tant): A substance that is taken into the body through the mouth or digestive system.

ingestion (in-jest′-chun): 1. The act of taking food, fluid or medicine into the stomach. 2. The process by which cells take in foreign substances.

ingrowing toenail: A nail whose edges have grown into the tissue on either side of it, causing inflammation and pain.

inguinal (ing′-gwi-nal): Pertaining to the groin. I. CANAL, a tubular opening through the lower part of the anterior abdominal wall, parallel to and a little above the I. (Poupart's) ligament. It measures 1.5 in. In the male it contains the spermatic cord; in the female, the uterine round ligaments. I. HERNIA, one occurring through the internal abdominal ring of the I. canal.

inhalant (in-hā′-lant): A substance that may be taken into the body by inhalation into the lungs.

inhalation (in-ha-lā′-shun): 1. The breathing in of air, or other vapor, etc. 2. A medicinal substance which is inhaled.

inhaler (in-hā′-ler): 1. An apparatus that provides for the breathing in of medicinal substances. 2. An apparatus that can be worn to prevent breathing in dust, smoke, dirt, etc.

inherent (in-hir′-rent): Innate; inborn.

inheritance (in-her′-i-tans): The process of acquiring characters or qualities by transmission from parent to offspring, or the characters and qualities so acquired.

inherited (in-her′-i-ted): Descriptive of mental and physical characteristics that one has received from one's ancestors.

inhibition (in-hi-bish′-un): Loss or partial loss of function or activity. In psychiatry, the restraint of a function or activity as a result of mental (psychic) influences.

inhibitor (in-hib′-i-tor): A substance or agent that interferes with a physiological function or a chemical reaction.

inject (in-jekt′): To force in. In medicine, to force fluid, gas, air, or other substance into tissue, a cavity, or an organ of the body.

injected (in-jek′-ted): 1. Congested; with full vessels. 2. Thrown in by injection (*q.v.*).

injection (in-jek′-shun): 1. The act of introducing a fluid (under pressure) into the tissues, a vessel, cavity or hollow organ. (Air can be injected into a cavity. See **pneumothorax.**) 2. The substance injected. See **hypodermic, intra-arterial, intracutaneous, intradermal, intramuscular, intrathecal, intravascular, intravenous, subcutaneous.**

injury (in′-jer-i): A wound or damage to a person or thing, specifically any disruption to the continuity of body tissue which may or may not involve the skin. BIRTH I., the impairment of a body function as a result of some damage to the child during the birth process.

inkblot test: See **Rorschach test.**

innate (in-āt′): Inborn, dependent on genetic constitution.

inner ear: See **ear.**

innervation (in-er-vā′-shun): The nerve supply to or in a part.

innocent (in′-ō-sent): Benign; not malignant.

innocuous (in-ok′-ū-us): Harmless.

innominate (in-nom′-in-at): 1. Unnamed. I. ARTERY, the largest branch of the aortic arch; it divides into the right common carotid and the right subclavian arteries. I. BONE, one of the bones forming the pelvis;

it is composed of the ilium, ischium and pubis; the os innominatum. I. VEINS, formed by the union of the subclavian and internal jugular veins on either side.

inoculate (in-ok′-ū-lāt): To introduce a disease-producing agent or an antigenic material into the body for the purpose of creating immunity, treating a disease, or making a diagnosis.

inoculation (in-ok-ū-lā′-shun): 1. Introduction of material (usually vaccine) into the tissues, often done to create immunity by giving the person a mild form of the disease. 2. Introduction of microorganisms into culture medium for propagation.

inoperable (in-op′-er-a-b'l): Describes a condition that under other circumstances could be relieved or cured by surgery, but because of the location or advanced stage of the pathology surgery would be either ineffective or unsafe.

inorganic (in-or-gan′-ik): Neither animal nor vegetable in origin. In chemistry, the term refers to compounds that do not contain carbon.

inositol (in-ō′-si-tol): A member of the vitamin B_2 complex.

inquest (in′-qwest): A legal inquiry, held by a coroner, into the cause of sudden or unexpected death.

insane (in-sān′): Of unsound or deranged mind. Usually implies inability to manage one's own affairs or conduct oneself in a socially acceptable manner.

insanity (in-san′-i-ti): The condition of being insane (*q.v.*).

insecticide (in-sek′-ti-sīd): An agent which kills insects.—insecticidal, adj.

insemination (in-sem-in-ā′-shun): Introduction of semen into the vagina, normally by sexual intercourse. ARTIFICIAL I., instrumental injection of semen into the female genital tract.

insensible (in-sen′-si-b'l): Without sensation or consciousness. Too small or gradual to be perceived, as I. perspiration (*q.v.*).

insertion (in-ser′-shun): 1. The act of setting or placing in. 2. The attachment of a muscle to the bone it moves.

insidious (in-sid′-i-us): Having an imperceptible commencement, as of a disease with a late manifestation of definite symptoms.

insight (in′-sīt): Ability to accept one's limitations but at the same time to develop one's potentialities; clear and immediate understanding; keen discernment. In psychiatry, means: (1) knowing that one is ill; (2) a developing knowledge of one's present attitudes and past experiences and the connection between them.

in situ (in sī'-tū): In the normal or natural place; in the correct position; undisturbed by neighboring tissues.

insolation (in-sō-lā'-shun): 1. Sunstroke. 2. Treatment of disease by exposure to the sun's rays.

insoluble (in-sol'-ū-b'l): Incapable of being dissolved.

insomnia (in-som'-ni-a): Sleeplessness, especially when chronic.

inspection (in-spek'-shun): Examination of persons or things by the eye.

inspersion (in-sper'-shun): The act of sprinkling, as with a powder or a fluid.

inspiration (in-spi-rā'-shun): The drawing of air into the lungs; inhalation.—inspire, v.t.; inspiratory, adj.

inspissated (in-spis'-āt-ed): Thickened by evaporation, absorption, or dehydration.

instep (in'-step): The arch of the foot on the dorsal surface.

instillation (in-sti-lā'-shun): Insertion of fluid into a cavity, drop by drop, *e.g.,* conjunctival sac, external auditory meatus.

instinct (in'-stingt): An inborn tendency to act in a certain way that is usually helpful and beneficial, *e.g.,* PATERNAL I., to protect children. HERD I., the urge to copy the standards of thinking and behavior of a group.—instinctive, adj.; instinctively, adv.

insufficiency (in-su-fish'-en-sē): The condition of being unable to perform an allotted duty or function. Term is used to describe failure to function properly of such organs and parts as the heart, cardiac valves, liver, stomach, kidney, adrenal or thyroid glands, muscles.

insufflation (in-su-flā'-shun): The blowing of air along a tube (eustachian, fallopian) to establish patency. The blowing of powder, gas or vapor into a body cavity.

insula (in'-sū-la): An island, particularly the islands of Langerhans in the pancreas or the island of Reil, a triangular area of the cerebral cortex. See **island.**

insulation (in-sū-lā'-shun): The surrounding of a body or a space with non-conducting material to prevent the escape or entrance of radiant energy, electricity, sound or heat; also, the material so used.

insulin (in'-sū-lin): A pancreatic hormone made in the islet cells of Langerhans, secreted into the blood, and having a profound effect on carbohydrate metabolism. The hormone is prepared commercially in various forms and strengths which vary in their speed, length and potency of action, and which are used in the treatment of diabetes mellitus (*q.v.*). I. SHOCK, treatment used in some mental diseases whereby insulin is injected to produce convulsions; followed by psychotherapy.

insulinoma (in-sū-lin-ō'-ma): Adenoma of the islets of Langerhans in the pancreas. Also insuloma.

insult (in'-sult): An injury or trauma. To injure or traumatize.

insusceptibility (in-su-sep-ti-bil'-i-ti): Immunity. The incapability of becoming infected with a specific pathogenic agent.

intake (in'-tāk): In medicine, usually refers to substances taken into the body, by mouth or otherwise, and expressed in amounts such as cc's of fluid intake, or caloric content of food intake.

integument (in-teg'-ū-ment): A covering, especially the skin.—integumentary, adj.

intellect (in'-te-lekt): The power or faculty of reasoning, thinking and understanding.

intelligence (in-tel'-i-jens): The ability to comprehend or understand relationships, to think, to solve problems, and to adjust to new situations. Inborn mental ability. I. TESTS, designed to determine the level of intelligence or mental age. I. QUOTIENT, or IQ, the ratio of mental age to chronological age; mental age is divided by chronological age and the result is multiplied by 100.

intensive care unit: A specially equipped and staffed area in a hospital that provides concentrated, intensive and specialized nursing care to critically ill patients who need close observation and frequent ministrations.

intention: A natural process of healing involving union of the edges of a wound. FIRST I., healing of a wound by immediate union and without granulation or suppuration. SECOND I., healing of a wound, after suppuration, by union of the two granulated surfaces. THIRD I., healing of a wound by extensive granulation followed by scar formation. I. TREMOR, see **tremor.**

inter-: Denotes among, between, together, within, in the midst.

interarticular (in-ter-ar-tik'-ū-lar): Between two articulating surfaces.

interatrial (in-ter-ā'-tri-al): Between the two atria of the heart. Previously interauricular.

interauricular (in-ter-aw-rik'-ū-lar): See **interatrial.**

intercellular (in-ter-sel'-ū-lar): Between the cells of a structure.

interclavicular (in-ter-kla-vik'-ū-lar): Between the clavicles.

intercondylar (in-ter-kon'-di-lar): Between condyles, *e.g.,* the intercondylar notch at the lower posterior end of the femur.

intercostal (in-ter-kos'-tal): Between the ribs.

intercourse (in'-ter-kōrs): Communication; interchange or exchange. SEXUAL I., coitus.

intercurrent (in-ter-kur'-ent): Intervening, interrupting or occurring in the midst of a process. Said of a second disease arising in a person already suffering from one disease.

interdisciplinary (in-ter-dis'-i-plin-ar-i): Denoting an overlapping of interests or responsibilities among two or more representatives of different fields of medicine or medical science.

interferon (in-ter-fēr'-on): An antiviral agent, the cell's response to virus invasion. I. protects the cell against further attack.

interictal (in-ter-ik'-tal): Between attacks or paroxysms, *e.g.,* epileptic seizures.

interlobar (in-ter-lō'-bar): Between the lobes of an organ, *e.g.,* interlobar pleurisy.

interlobular (in-ter-lob'-ū-lar): Located or occurring between lobules of an organ.

intermenstrual (in-ter-men'-stroo-al): Between the menstrual periods.

intermittent (in-ter-mit'-ent): Occurring at intervals; characterized by periods of complete cessation of activity. I. CLAUDICATION, see **claudication.** I. FEVER, one in which the symptoms of the disease disappear between attacks of fever, *e.g.,* malaria, undulant fever. I. POSITIVE PRESSURE BREATHING, breathing with the help of an apparatus that can supply gas under positive pressure during inhalation, or exhalation, or both; it may supply negative pressure at the termination of an exhalation; assists in ventilation and may be used to apply aerosol. I. PULSE, one in which there is an absence of beat at intervals.

intern (in'-tern): A recently graduated medical student who lives within the hospital and assists in the care of medical and surgical patients preliminary to becoming licensed to practice. Cf. **extern.**

internal (in-ter'-nal): Inside. I. EAR, that part of the ear which comprises the vestibule, semicircular canals and the cochlea. I. HEMORRHAGE, bleeding into a cavity or organ of the body. I. SECRETIONS, those produced by the ductless or endocrine glands and passed directly into the blood stream; hormones.

International Council of Nurses: Founded in London, 1900. 63 nations of the world are now members. Meets every four years. Purpose is to assist in attaining the highest level of health possible for all peoples of the world.

International Nursing Index: A quarterly index of nursing literature that lists publications from the entire world; published by the American Journal of Nursing Company in cooperation with the National Library of Medicine.

International Red Cross: A worldwide humanitarian organization founded in Switzerland in 1864. Its original purpose was to aid the wounded and other victims of war but its activities now include disaster relief and the sponsorship of many health-related and social programs. The national Red Cross societies, and the Turkish Red Crescent, make up the International Red Cross. The American Red Cross was founded in 1882, largely through the efforts of Clara Barton, and it was officially recognized by Congress in 1905. See **Red Cross.**

internist (in-tern'-ist): A physician who is a specialist in internal medicine, as differentiated from surgery, obstetrics, etc.

internuncial (in-ter-nun'-shi-al): Acting as a connecting medium. I. NEURON, one located between two other neurons in a neural pathway and which transmits impressions from one to the other.

interoceptor (in-ter-ō-sep'-tor): A sensory nerve terminal or end organ situated in the walls of organs or in viscera and which responds to stimuli that arise within the body.

interosseous (in-ter-os'-ē-us): Lying between bones, as some muscles and ligaments.

interphalangeal (in-ter-fa-lan'-jē-al): Between two phalanges.

interrupted: Lacking continuity; broken at intervals. I. STERILIZATION, that which is done at intervals in order to allow any spores to develop in the periods between applications of the procedure. I. SUTURES, a technique of closing a wound with stitches that are each made with a separate piece of suture material.

interseptum (in-ter-sep'-tum): The diaphragm.

intersexuality (in-ter-seks-ū-al'-i-ti): The possession of both male and female characteristics. See **Turner's** and **Klinefelter's syndrome.**

interspinous (in-ter-spī'-nus): Between spinous processes, especially those of the vertebrae.

interstices (in-ter′-sti-sez): Small spaces or gaps in tissues or structures.

interstitial (in-ter-stish′-al): Relating to or situated in the interstices of a tissue or part; distributed through the connective tissue.

intertrigo (in-ter-trī′-gō): A superficial, irritating inflammation occurring on the skin where the folds of moist skin overlap and resulting from chafing and lack of evaporation of sweat.

intertrochanteric (in-ter-trō-kan-ter′-ik): Between trochanters, particularly the greater and lesser trochanters of the femur.

interval (in′-ter-val): The space between two objects or the time between two occurrences.

interventricular (in-ter-ven-trik′-ū-lar): Between ventricles, as those of the brain or heart.

intervertebral (in-ter-ver′-te-bral): Between two adjacent vertebrae, as disks and foramina. I. DISK, a flattened cartilaginous disk lying between vertebrae and that prevents friction and absorbs shock; it is spoken of as 'ruptured' when accident or strain causes the soft central part of the disk to protrude through the surrounding ligament. See **nucleus, prolapse.**

intestine (in-tes′-tin): The bowel; that part of the alimentary canal that extends from the pyloric end of the stomach to the anus. The SMALL I. is separated from the stomach by the pyloric valve, is about 20 ft. in length, and consists of the duodenum, jejunum, and ileum, in that order. Between the small I. and the large I. is the ileocecal valve. LARGE I., about 6 ft. in length, is composed of the cecum, colon (ascending, transverse, and descending), and rectum, in that order. The function of the intestine is to complete digestion of foods and to eliminate waste products.—intestinal, adj.

intima (in′-tim-a): The internal coat of a blood vessel.—intimal, adj.

intolerance (in-tol′-er-ans): 1. Inability to bear pain or discomfort. 2. Idiosyncrasy (*q.v.*) to certain drugs, etc.

intoxication(in-tok-si-kā′-shun): 1. Poisoning. 2. Acute alcoholism; drunkenness.

intra-: Denotes within, on the inside, internal, between the layers of.

intra-abdominal (in-tra-ab-dom′-in-al): Inside the abdomen.

intra-amniotic (in-tra-am-ni-ot′-ik): Within, or into the amniotic fluid or the amnion.

intra-arterial (in-tra-ar-tēr′-i-al): Within an artery.—intra-arterially, adv.

intra-articular (in-tra-ar-tik′-ū-lar): Within a joint.

intrabronchial (in-tra-brong′-ki-al): Within a bronchus.

intracanalicular (in-tra-kan-a-lik′-ū-lar): Within a canaliculus.

intracapsular (in-tra-kap′-sū-lar): Within a capsule, *e.g.,* that of the lens or a joint. Opp. to extracapsular.

intracardiac (in-tra-kar′-di-ak): Within the heart.

intracellular (in-tra-sel′-ū-lar): Within a cell. Opp. to extracellular.

intracerebral (in-tra-ser′-i-bral): Within the cerebrum.

intracorpuscular (in-tra-kor-pus′-kū-lar): Within a corpuscle.

intracranial (in-tra-krā′-ni-al): Within the skull.

intractable (in-trak′-ta-b′l): Obstinate; refractory. Resistant to treatment; not easily cured.

intracutaneous (in-tra-kū-tā′-nē-us): Within the skin tissues.—intracutaneously, adv.

intradermal (in-tra-der′-mal): Within the skin.—intradermally, adv.

intradural (in-tra-dū′-ral): Within the dura mater, *e.g.,* hemorrhage.

intragastric (in-tra-gas′-trik): Within the stomach.

intrahepatic (in-tra-he-pat′-ik): Within the liver.

intralobular (in-tra-lob′-ū-lar): Within a lobule, as the vein draining a hepatic lobule.

intraluminal (in-tra-lū′-min-al): Within the hollow of a tubelike structure.—intraluminally, adv.

intramedullary (in-tra-med′-ū-lar-i): 1. Within the medulla oblongata or the spinal cord. 2. Within the marrow cavity of a bone or the bone marrow.

intramembranous (in-tra-mem′-bran-ous): Within a membrane or between membranes. Descriptive of a type of bone formation that differs from endochondral bone formation.

intramural (in-tra-mūr′-al): Within the layers of the wall of a hollow tube or organ. —intramurally, adv.

intramuscular (in-tra-mus′-kū-lar): Within or into the substance of a muscle, as an intramuscular injection.—intramuscularly, adj.

intranasal (in-tra-nā′-zal): Within the nasal cavity.—intranasally, adv.

intranatal (in-tra-nā′-tal): At the time of birth. Syn., intrapartum (*q.v.*). —intranatally, adv.

intraocular (in-tra-ok′-ū-lar): Within the globe of the eye. I. PRESSURE, the pressure of the fluid within the eye; is measured by a tonometer.

intraoral (in-tra-ō′-ral): Within the mouth, as an I. appliance.—intraorally, adv.

intraorbital (in-tra-or′-bi-tal): Within the orbit.

intraosseous (in-tra-os′-ē-us): Within or into the substance of a bone.

intrapartum (in-tra-par′-tum): During labor or delivery, as asphyxia, hemorrhage, or infection.

intraperitoneal (in-tra-per-i-tō-nē′-al): Within, or going into, the peritoneal cavity. —intraperitoneally, adv.

intrapleural (in-tra-ploo′-ral): Within, or going into, the pleural cavity.—intrapleurally, adv.

intrapsychic (in-tra-sī′-kik): Refers to that which takes place within the psyche or mind of the individual.

intrapulmonary (in-tra-pul′-mo-nar-i): Within the lungs, as I. pressure.

intraretinal (in-tra-ret′-i-nal): Within the retina.

intraspinal (in-tra-spī′-nal): Within, or going into, the spinal canal, as I. anesthesia.—intraspinally, adv.

intrasplenic (in-tra-splen′-ik): Within the spleen.

intrastitial (in-tra-stish′-al): Within the cells of a tissue.

intrasynovial (in-tra-si-nō′-vi-al): Within a synovial membrane or cavity.

intrathecal (in-tra-thē′-kal): Within a sheath. Within, or going under or between the meninges of the brain or spinal cord, as an injection.—intrathecally, adv.

intrathoracic (in-tra-thō-ras′-ik): Within, or occurring within, the cavity of the thorax.

intratracheal (in-tra-trāk′-ē-al): Within, or going into or through the trachea. I. ANESTHESIA, the administration of an anesthetic through a special tube passed through the nose or mouth into and down the trachea.—intratracheally, adv.

intrauterine (in-tra-ū′-ter-in): Being or occurring within the uterus. I. CONTRACEPTIVE DEVICE, a device, usually a metal coil, placed within the uterus to prevent conception. Abbreviated IUCD or IUD.

intravaginal (in-tra-vaj′-i-nal): Within the vagina.—intravaginally, adv.

intravasation (in-trav-a-zā′-shun): The entrance of foreign or abnormal matter into a blood vessel.

intravascular (in-tra-vas′-kū-lar): Within a vessel, especially a blood vessel or lymphatic.

intravenous (in-tra-vē′-nus): Within, or going into a vein or veins.—intravenously, adv.

intraventricular (in-tra-ven-trik′-ū-lar): Within, or going into, a ventricle of the brain or heart.

intra vitam (vī′-tam): During life.

intrinsic (in-trin′-sik): Inherent or inside; from within; real; innate; natural. Often used in reference to certain muscles, *e.g.*, certain eye muscles. I. FACTOR, a substance that is present in the wall of the normal stomach, and which is essential for the satisfactory absorption of the extrinsic factor (*q.v.*).

intro-: Denotes in, into, within, inward, inwardly, to or on the inside.

introitus (in-trō′-it-us): Any opening in the body; an entrance to a cavity, particularly the vagina.

introjection (in-trō-jek′-shun): A mental process whereby a person identifies himself with another person or object; usually someone or something that is greatly loved or admired.

intromission (in-trō-mish′-un): The insertion of a thing or part into another thing or part, as the insertion of a catheter into the bladder or of the penis into the vagina during sexual intercourse.

introspection (in-trō-spek′-shun): Self-examination. The study by a person of his own thoughts and feelings.—introspective, adj.

introversion (in-trō-ver′-zhun): 1. The direction of thoughts and interests inward to the world of ideas, instead of outward to the external world. 2. The turning outside in of a part, more or less completely; invagination (*q.v.*).—introvert, n.; introverted, adj.

introvert (in′-trō-vert): 1. To turn one's thoughts inward toward one's own mental processes. 2. A person who is self-centered and introspective, and who tends to be thoughtful, self-sufficient, and interested more in his own thoughts and feelings than in those of others. Tends to withdraw in social situations and to be a poor mixer. Opp. to extrovert (*q.v.*).

intubation (in-tū-bā′-shun): The insertion of a tube, usually through the nose or mouth, into a part of the body, especially a canal and particularly the trachea or intestine.

DUODENAL I., a procedure for instilling barium into the duodenum prior to fluoroscopy. ENDOTRACHEAL I., done to maintain an airway by keeping the trachea open or to restore patency in cases of obstruction. —intubate, v.t. See **intratracheal anesthesia.**

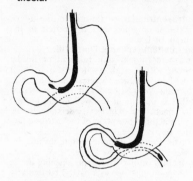

Duodenal Intubation

intumescence (in-tū-mes′-ens): 1. A swelling or prominence on the body. 2. The enlarging or swelling of a part, particularly as a reaction to heat.—intumesce, v.i.; intumescent, adj.

intussusception (in-tus-sus-sep′-shun): A condition in which one part of the bowel slips or telescopes into the part immediately adjacent (invaginates). It occurs most commonly in infants and most frequently at the junction of the ileum and the cecum; causes obstruction. Usual therapy is surgery.

intussusceptum (in-tus-sus-sep′-tum): The invaginated portion of an intussusception.

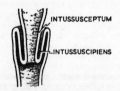

INTUSSUSCEPTUM

INTUSSUSCIPIENS

intussuscipiens (in-tus-sus-sip′-i-ens): The receiving portion of an intussusception.

inulin (in′-ū-lin): A tasteless vegetable starch that occurs in some plants; yields levulose on hydrolysis; is used as a diagnostic agent in some kidney function tests.

inunction (in-ungk′-shun): Annointing. The act of rubbing an oily or fatty substance that contains a drug into the skin for therapeutic purposes, or a substance so used.—inunct, v.t.

in utero: Within the uterus; unborn.

invagination (in-vaj-i-nā′-shun): The act or conditon of being ensheathed; a pushing inward; telescoping; forming a pouch.—invaginate, v.t.

invalid (in′-va-lid): Weak, sickly. A person who is chronically disabled by some infirmity but not completely incapacitated.

invasion (in-vā′-zhun): 1. The entry of bacteria into the body. 2. The beginning or onset of a disease.

inversion (in-ver′-zhun): 1. A turning inside out, upside down, outside in, or in any direction that is the reverse of normal, as I. of the uterus. See **procidentia.** 2. Homosexuality.

invertase (in-ver′-tās): A sugar-splitting enzyme in intestinal juice. Also called sucrase.

invertebrate (in-ver′-te-brāt): An animal without a backbone.

invertin (in-ver′-tin): Invertase (q.v.).

invest (in-vest′): To surround or enclose in a membrane or sheath.

inveterate (in-vet′-er-at): Chronic, recurring; obstinate or resistant to therapy.

in vitro (vī′-trō): In glass, as in a test tube. Outside of the living body.

in vivo (vī′-vō): In living tissue or in a living body.

involucrum (in-vo-lū′-krum): 1. An enveloping membrane or sheath. 2. A sheath of new bone, which forms around necrosed bone, in such conditions as osteomyelitis.

involuntary (in-vol′-un-ta-ri): Independent of the will, as muscle of the chest and abdominal organs. Not volitional.

involution (in-vō-lū′-shun): 1. The normal shrinkage of an organ after fulfilling its functional purpose, e.g., the uterus after labor. 2. The period of progressive alteration in the body after middle age when glandular activity lessens and degenerative changes set in.—involutional, adj.

I & O: Abbreviation for intake and output.

iodide (ī′-ō-dīd): A compound of iodine with another element or radical, e.g., potassium iodide.

iodine (ī′-ō-dēn): A non-metallic element, obtained mostly from seaweed, with several medicinal and industrial uses. TINCTURE OF I., a 2-7% solution of iodine in alcohol, used as an antiseptic and disinfectant for skin and small wounds. LUGOL'S SOLU-

TION, a 5% aqueous solution of iodine given orally in thyrotoxicosis for preoperative stabilization. PROTEIN-BOUND I., (PBI) estimated in thyroid investigations. RADIOACTIVE I., (I^{131}) is used in investigation and treatment of thyrotoxicosis. I. TEST, a test for starch. When iodine is added to a compound containing starch a deep blue color is produced; the color disappears when the substance is heated and reappears when it is cooled.

iodism (ī'-ō-dizm): Poisoning by prolonged or excessive use of iodine or iodides; symptoms are those of a common cold, excessive secretion of saliva, sore gums, rash. Treated by withdrawing the medication.

iodized (ī'-ō-dīzd): 1. Treated with iodine or an iodide. 2. Impregnated with iodine, as table salt.

iodoform (ī-ō'-dō-form): A lemon-yellow, volatile, crystalline, chemically produced substance containing iodine; used as a topical antiseptic for skin and mucous membrane, usually in the form of impregnated gauze.

iodopsin (ī-ō-dop'-sin): A protein substance which, with vitamin A, is a constituent of visual purple present in the retinal cones and important in daylight vision.

ion (ī'-on): An atom, or group of atoms, that has either a positive or negative charge of electricity and which, in electrolysis, passes to one pole or the other.

ionization (ī-on-ī-zā'-shun): 1. The breaking up of a substance into its component ions when in solution. 2. Treatment whereby ions of various substances, *e.g.,* zinc, chlorine, iodine, histamine, are introduced into the skin by means of a constant electrical current.

iontophoresis (ī-on-tō-fō-rē'-sis): The introduction, through the skin, of ions of various salts for therapeutic purposes; accomplished by electrical means.

IPPB: Abbreviation for intermittent positive pressure breathing (*q.v.*).

ipsilateral (ip-si-lat'-er-al): Situated or appearing on the same side, or affecting the same side.—ipsilaterally, adv.

IQ: Intelligence (*q.v.*) quotient.

ir-: See **in-**.

irid-, irido-: Denotes the iris of the eye.

iridectomy (ir-i-dek'-to-mi): Excision of part of the iris, thus enlarging the pupil or creating an artificial one.

iridencleisis (ir-i-den-klī'-sis): An operation for decreasing the intraocular pressure in glaucoma.

iridocele (i-rid'-ō-sēl): Protrusion of part of the iris through a corneal wound.

iridocyclitis (ir-i-dō-sī-klī'-tis): Inflammation of the iris and ciliary body.

iridodialysis (ir-i-dō-dī-al'-i-sis): A separation of the iris from its ciliary attachment, often a result of trauma.

iridokinesis (ir-i-dō-kī-nē'-sis): Contraction and expansion of the iris of the eye.

iridoplegia (ir-i-dō-plē'-ji-a): Paralysis of the sphincter of the iris, with resulting inability of the pupil to contract or dilate.

iridoptosis (ir-i-dop-tō'-sis): Prolapse of the iris.

iridotomy (ir-i-dot'-om-i): An incision into the iris, as in the operation to create an artificial pupil.

iris (ī'-ris): The colored circular membrane forming the anterior one-sixth of the middle coat of the eyeball. It consists of two layers of muscle and is perforated in the center by an opening called the pupil. Contraction of its muscle fibers regulates the amount of light entering the eye. I. BOMBE, bulging forward of the iris due to pressure of aqueous behind, when posterior adhesions are present.—irides, pl.; iridal, iridian, iridic, adj.

iritis (ī-rī'-tis): Inflammation of the iris.

iron: A common metallic element found in some soils and waters and in certain minerals. Present in the body in small amounts, most of it in the red blood cells; important in the physiological process of transporting oxygen to the tissues. Some of it is stored in liver, spleen, bone marrow, but since a certain amount is excreted in feces, it must be supplied daily in the diet. Some of its salts are used in treating various forms of anemia. I. LUNG, a device used to force air in and out of the lungs when the nerves controlling chest muscles fail to act, as occurs in poliomyelitis. See **respirator**.

irradiation (ir-rā-dē-ā'-shun): 1. Subjection of a patient to the action of such rays as those of heat, light, radium, etc., for diagnostic or therapeutic purposes. 2. Subjection of a substance, especially a food, to certain rays, *e.g.,* ultraviolet, to increase its vitamin potency. 3. A spreading out, as of nerve impulses.—irradiate, v.t.

irrational (ir-rash'-un-al): Term applied to one who lacks his usual clarity of thought and speech, and control of his actions.

irreducible (ir-rē-dūs'-i-b'l): 1. Cannot be brought to desired condition. I. HERNIA, when the contents of the sac cannot be returned to the appropriate cavity, without surgical intervention. 2. Incapable of being made smaller or less in amount. 3. In chemistry, incapable of being made simpler or reduced.

irrigation (ir-i-gā′-shun): In medicine, the washing out of a body cavity or part with a continuous stream of water, or other fluid, for therapeutic purposes.—irrigate, v.t.

irritable (ir′-i-ta-b′l): In medicine, capable of responding to stimuli; responding easily to stimuli.—irritability, n.

irritant (ir′-i-tant): Any agent that causes irritation (q.v.).—irritative, adj.

irritation (ir-i-tā′-shun): 1. The normal response of a muscle or nerve to a stimulus. 2. An exaggerated response of a nerve or tissue to stimulus. 3. Greater than normal response of tissues to injury or trauma; may be evidence of the beginning of inflammation.

ischemia (is-kē′-mi-a): Local temporary anemia of an area due to obstruction in the blood vessels supplying the area. MYOCARDIAL I., see **angina.** See also **Volkmann.** —ischemic, adj.

ischi-, ischio-: Denotes the ischium.

ischiorectal (is-ki-ō-rek′-tal): Pertaining to the ischium and the rectum, as an I. abscess which occurs between these two structures.

ischium (is′-ki-um): The lower heavy, posterior part of the innominate bone of the pelvis; the bone on which the body rests when sitting.—ischia, pl.; ischial, adj.

ischo-: Denotes suppression or deficiency.

ischocholia (is-kō-kō′-li-a): Suppression of bile formation or failure of the bile to reach the intestine. Also ischolia.

ischuria (is-kū′-ri-a): Retention or suppression of urine.

island: In anatomy, a group of cells or a mass of tissue, separated in some way or marked off from surrounding tissue. I.'S OF LANGERHANS, clusters of special cells scattered throughout the pancreas; they secrete insulin (q.v.) which pours directly into the bloodstream. I. OF REIL, see insula.

islet (ī′-let): Island (q.v.).

iso-, is-: Denotes equal, like, uniform, homogeneous.

isochronous (ī-sok′-ron-us): Occurring during the same period of time or passing through the same phases at the same time.

isocoria (ī-sō-kō′-ri-a): Equality in the size of the two pupils.

isodactylism (ī-sō-dak′-til-izm): A condition in which all of the fingers are of approximately the same length.

isograft (ī′-sō-graft): A graft of tissue that has been obtained from another individual of the same species. Also called isotransplant.

isoimmunization (ī-sō-im-ū-nī-zā′-shun): The development in an individual of antibodies in response to antigens from another individual of the same species, e.g., the development of anti Rh agglutinins in the blood of an Rh negative person who has been given an Rh positive transfusion, or who is carrying an Rh positive fetus.

isolate (ī′-sō-lāt): To set apart by oneself, separate, or place alone.—isolation, n.

isolation (ī-sō-lā′-shun): The act of setting a person with an infectious disease apart from those who do not have the disease. I. TECHNIQUE, measures and precautions taken to prevent the spread of infection from a patient in isolation to others.

isolette (ī-sō-let′): An incubator for premature babies; provides for accurate control of humidity, temperature, and oxygen supply and is made so that the infant can be cared for without taking him out of it.

isometric (ī-sō-met′-rik): Of equal dimensions. In physiology, a muscle contraction that occurs without shortening of the muscle as it is fixed at both ends, but with increase in tone of the muscle fibers.

isometropia (ī-sō-met-rō′-pi-a): The condition of having equal and like refraction in both eyes.

isomorphous (ī-sō-mor′-fus): Having the same form or shape.

isotherapy (ī-sō-ther′-a-pi): Treatment of a disease by administering its active causal agent, as is done in the treatment for prevention of rabies. Term also used to describe treatment of a diseased organ with that organ or extract of it, e.g., liver disease treated with liver extract. Called also isopathy.

isotonic (ī-sō-ton′-ik): 1. Having equal tension; applied to any solution that has the same osmotic pressure as blood. I. SALINE, (syn., normal saline), 0.9 percent solution of salt in water. 2. Descriptive of muscular contraction that takes place without significant increase in tone but with shortening of the fibers. Opp. to isometric.

isotope (ī′-sō-tōp): One of two or more forms of the same element that have identical chemical properties but differing physical properties. Isotopes with radioactive properties are used in medicine for research, diagnosis, and treatment of disease.

isthmus (is′-mus): In anatomy, a connecting part between two parts, usually a contracted part between two larger parts.

itch: A name given to a wide variety of skin conditions that arouse a sensation of prickling or stinging and an intense desire to scratch or rub the affected part. May be caused by the itch mite, by exposure to irritating plant oils or substances handled in certain occupations; allergic or neurogenic reactions are among many other causes. —itch, v.t., v.i.; itchiness, n.; itchy, itching, adj. See **scabies.**

-ite: Denotes: (1) 'of the nature of'; (2) a salt or an ester of an acid with name ending in -ous.

-itis: Denotes disease, usually inflammatory. —itises, itides, pl.

IU: Abbreviation for International Unit.

IUCD, IUD: Abbreviation for intrauterine contraceptive device.

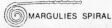

Intrauterine contraceptive devices

IV: Abbreviation for intravenous or intravenously.

ivy poisoning: Dermatitis caused by exposure to a toxic oil contained in the 'poison ivy' plant. Also often used to describe dermatitis caused by exposure to such plant oils as those of of 'poison' oak and sumac.

J

jacket: In medicine, a fixed bandage or covering for a part of the body, especially the thorax or trunk; sometimes made of plaster of paris. STRAIT J., a shirt-like garment with long sleeves used to restrain an irrational or violently disturbed person.

jacksonian epilepsy: See **epilepsy.** [John Hughlings Jackson, English neurologist. 1835-1911.]

Jacquemier's sign (zhak′-mē-ās): Blueness of the vaginal muscosa seen in early pregnancy. [Jean Marie Jacquemier, French obstetrician. 1806-1879.]

jactitation (jak-ti-tā′-shun): Excessive restlessness; constant turning or tossing about as seen in patients with high fever or serious illness.

jargon (jar′-gon): 1. Unintelligible or confused speech. 2. The technical terms used by specialists working in a particular field of knowledge.

jaundice (jawn′-dis): Syn., icterus. A condition characterized by a raised bilirubin level in the blood (hyperbilirubinemia). Minor degrees are detectable only chemically and are most often referred to as LATENT J. Major degrees are recognized by yellow skin, sclera, and muscosae and are referred to as OVERT or CLINICAL J. J. may may be due to (1) obstruction anywhere in the bilary tract (obstructive J.); (2) excessive hemolysis of red blood cells (hemolytic J.); (3) toxic or infective damage of liver cells (hepatocellular J.). ACHOLURIC J., J. without bile in the urine; usually reserved for congenital hemolytic anemia, a familial disease characterized by abnormally fragile, small, spheroidal red cells that hemolyze readily. Congenital spherocytosis. INFECTIOUS or INFECTIVE J., most commonly due to a virus; infectious or infective hepatitis (*q.v.*). MALIGNANT J., acute yellow atrophy of the liver. See **acute.** J. OF THE NEWBORN, icterus neonatorum (*q.v.*).

jawbone: Either the maxilla (upper jaw) or mandible (lower jaw).

jejunectomy (jē-joo-nek′-to-mi): Surgical excision of the jejunum, or part of it.

jejunitis (jē-joo-nī′-tis): Inflammation of the jejunum.

jejuno-ileostomy (jē-joo-nō-il-ē-os′-to-mi): The surgical creation of a passage between the jejunum and a noncontinuous part of the ileum.

jejunostomy (jē-joo-nos′-to-mi): A surgically made fistula between the jejunum and the anterior abdominal wall; used temporarily for feeding in cases where passage of food through the stomach is impossible or undesirable.

jejunum (jē-joo′-num): That part of the small intestine between the duodenum and the ileum. It is about 8 ft. in length.—jejunal, adj.

jelly: A semi-solid gelatinous substance. K. Y. JELLY, trade name for a lubricating jelly. WHARTON'S J., the gelatinous substance that makes up the basic substance of the umbilical cord.

jerk: A sudden involuntary muscular movement; a reflex. Describes certain reflex actions that follow tapping or striking a muscle or tendon, *e.g.*, knee jerk.

jigger (jig′-ger): (*Tunga penetrans*) A flea, prevalent in the tropics. It burrows under the skin to lay its eggs, causing intense irritation. Secondary infection is usual.

joint: The articulation of two or more bones (arthrosis). There are three main classes, designated according to the amount of movement they permit: (1) fibrous (synarthrosis), *e.g.*, the sutures of the skull; (2) cartilaginous (synchondrosis), *e.g.*, between the manubrium and the body of the sternum; (3) synovial, *e.g.*, elbow or hip. CHARCOT'S J., syphilitic degeneration of joint surfaces and surrounding structures. See **Charcot.** J. MOUSE, a loose, small, usually calcified body within a joint.

jugular (jug′-ū-lar): Pertaining to the throat. J. VEINS, two veins passing down either side of the neck.

Jukes: A fictitious name given to a family that was the subject of a sociological study covering five generations that produced a total of over 500 social misfits.

junket (jun′-ket): Milk predigested by the addition of rennet. Curds and whey.

juxtaposition (juks′-ta-pō-zish′-un): Side by side; adjacent; apposition; close at hand.

K

K: Chemical symbol for potassium.
Kahn test: A serological test for the diagnosis of syphilis. [Reuben Leon Kahn, American bacteriologist. 1887-   .]
kala-azar (ka-la az′-ar): An often fatal generalized form of leishmaniasis occurring in the tropics. There is anemia, fever, splenomegaly and wasting. It is caused by the parasite *Leishmania donovani* and is spread by the sand fly.
kalemia (ka-lē′-mi-a): The presence of potassium in the blood.
Kallikak: Fictitious name for a family whose two lines of descendants were subjects of sociological analysis in a study of the influence of hereditary factors on human nature. The female antecedent in one line was feebleminded and that of the other line normal or superior.
kary-, karyo-: Denotes the nucleus of a cell.
karyokinesis (kar-i-ō-kī-nē′-sis): The breaking or division of the nucleus of a cell during the process of mitosis.
karyon (kar′-i-on): Nucleus of a cell.
katabolism (ka-tab′-ō-lizm): Catabolism (*q.v.*).
katatonia (kat-a-tōn′-i-a): Catatonia (*q.v.*).
Keeley cure: A method of treatment for the alcohol or opium habit. [Leslie E. Keeley, American physician. 1834-1900.]
Kelly pad: A special pad of fabric and rubber which is placed under a patient to protect a chair, bed or operating table.
keloid (kē′-loid): An overgrowth of scar tissue, which may produce a contraction deformity; most common in Negroes.
Kenny method, treatment: A method of treating patients with anterior poliomyelitis to prevent paralysis; involves the use of hot wet packs, positioning, and muscle reeducation. [Sister Elizabeth Kenny, Australian nurse. 1886-1952.]
kerat-, kerato-: Denotes: (1) the cornea; (2) horny tissue.
keratectasia (ker-a-tek-tā′-zi-a): Protrusion of the cornea.
keratectomy (ker-a-tek′-to-mi): Removal of a portion of the cornea.
keratin (ker′-a-tin): A relatively insoluble protein found in all horny tissue. In pharmacology, used to coat pills given for their intestinal effect, since K. can withstand gastric juice.

keratinization (ker-a-tin-ī-zā′-shun): Conversion into horny tissue. Occurs as a pathological process in vitamin A deficiency.
keratitis (ker-a-tī′-tis): Inflammation of the cornea.
keratoconjunctivitis (ker-a-tō-kon-jungktiv-ī′-tis): Inflammation of the cornea and the conjunctiva. EPIDEMIC K., due to an adenovirus (*q.v.*). Presents as an acute follicular conjunctivitis with preauricular and submaxillary adenitis. K. SICCA, a form of K. that is associated with lacrimal deficiency. See **Sjögren's syndrome.**
keratoconus (ker-a-tō-kō′-nus): A conical protrusion of the cornea.
keratoderma (ker-a-tō-der′-ma): A condition in which an excess of keratin (*q.v.*) exists in the superficial layers of the skin causing it to become horny.
kerato-iritis (ker-a-tō-ī-rī′-tis): Inflammation of the cornea and iris.
keratolysis (ker-a-tol′-i-sis): Shedding of the epidermis.—keratolytic, adj.
keratoma (ker-a-tō′-ma): An overgrowth of horny tissue. Callosity.—keratomata, pl.
keratomalacia (ker-a-tō-ma-lā′-shi-a): Softening of the cornea; ulceration may occur; frequently caused by lack of vitamin A.
keratopathy (ker-a-top′-a-thi): Any disease of the cornea.—keratopathic, adj.
keratoplasty (ker′-a-tō-plas-ti): Corneal grafting. Replacing of unhealthy corneal tissue with healthy tissue obtained from a donor.—keratoplastic, adj.
keratosis (ker-a-tō′-sis): Thickening of the horny layer of the skin. Also referred to as 'hyperkeratosis.' Has appearance of callus or warty excrescences. K. FOLLICULARIS, a rare congenital condition characterized by areas of crusting papular growths and appearing symmetrically on the trunk, axillae, neck, face, scalp. K. PALMARIS ET PLANTARIS (tylosis), a congenital thickening of the horny layer of the palms and soles. K. SENILIS, dry, harsh condition of the skin seen in the aged; also descriptive of the pigmented, elevated papules seen in the skin of persons who have been long exposed to the sunlight, as well as in the aged. SPLAR K. (peasant's neck) is a form of chronic dermatitis on the exposed areas and is a reaction to excessive sunlight.

kerion (kē′-ri-on): A boggy suppurative mass of the scalp associated with ringworm of the scalp.

kernicterus (ker-nik′-ter-us): A serious form of icterus neonatorum characterized by bile staining and widespread destructive lesions in various parts of the brain. See **icterus.**

Kernig's sign (ker′-nigs): Inability to straighten the leg at the knee joint when the thigh is flexed at right angles to the trunk. Occurs in meningitis. [Vladimir Kernig, Russian physician. 1840-1917.]

ketogenic diet (kē-tō-jen′-ik): A high fat diet that produces ketosis (acidosis).

ketone (kē′-tōn): Any organic compound that contains the carbonyl group CO. The product of incomplete oxidation of fat in the body; when present in the bloodstream K.'s upset the acid-base balance of the body and produce ketosis. See **acetone bodies.**

ketonemia (kē-tō-nē′-mi-a): Ketone bodies in the blood.—ketonemic, adj.

ketonuria (kē-tō-nū′-ri-a): Ketone bodies in the urine.—ketonuric, adj.

ketosis (kē-tō′-sis): A clinical picture that arises when incomplete oxidation of fatty acids results in an accumulation of ketone bodies in the blood. Syndrome includes drowsiness, headache, and deep respirations.—ketotic, adj.

ketosteroids (kē-tō-stē′-roidz): Steroid hormones which contain a keto group, formed by the addition of an oxygen molecule to the basic ring structure. The 17-K. (which have this oxygen at carbon 17) are excreted in normal urine, and are present in excess in overactivity of the adrenal glands and the gonads.

kg: Abbreviation for kilogram.

kidney (kid′-ni): One of two bean-shaped organs, situated on the posterior abdominal wall, behind the peritoneum, in the lumbar region, one on either side of the vertebral column. Function is to secrete urine. ARTIFICIAL K., a popular name for an apparatus that is used for removing from the blood, while it is circulating outside of the body, the same elements normally removed by the kidneys. FLOATING K., one that is misplaced and more or less freely movable. K. STONE, a calculus (*q.v.*) that forms usually in the pelvis of the kidney, composed mostly of calcium oxalate. When small, they may pass down the ureters and through the bladder and urethra causing agonizing colicky pain.

kidney function tests: Various tests are

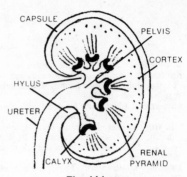

The kidney

available for measuring renal function. All require careful collection of urine specimens. Some of those in common use are: paraaminohippuric acid clearance test for measuring renal blood flow; creatinine clearance test for measuring glomerular filtration rate; ammonium chloride test for measuring tubular ability to excrete hydrogen ions; urinary concentration and dilution tests for measuring tubular function.

kilo-: Denotes one thousand; used chiefly in names of units in the metric system.

kilocalorie (kil′-ō-kal-o-ri): A large calorie. See **calorie.**

kilogram (kil′-ō-gram): One thousand grams; equivalent to 2.2 pounds avoirdupois. Abbreviation, kg.

kin-, kine-, kinesi-, kinesio-, kino-: Denotes motion, action.

kinanesthesia (kin-an-es-thē′-zi-a): Loss of the sense of movement.

kinase (kī′-nās): An enzyme activator. Syn., coenzyme. See **enterokinase, thrombokinase.**

kinematics (kin-e-mat′-iks): The science of motion.

kineplastic surgery (kin′-e-plas-tik sur′-jer-i): Operative measures, whereby certain muscle groups are isolated, and utilized to work certain modified prostheses.

kinesia (kī-nē′-si-a): Motion sickness.

kinesiology (kī-nē-si-ol′-o-ji): The science or study of human motion.

kinesthesia (kin-es-thē′-zi-a): Muscle sense; perception of movement, weight, and position.—kinesthetic, adj. Also kinesthesis.

kinetic (kin′-et-ik): Pertaining to, or producing motion.

Kirschner wire (kirsch′-ner): A wire drilled

into a bone to apply skeletal traction. [Martin Kirschner, German surgeon. 1879-1942.]

kiss of life: A method of artificial respiration in which the exhaled breath of the operator inflates the patient's lungs. Mouth-to-mouth; mouth-to-nose; mouth to nose and mouth are the methods used. Also called mouth-to-mouth resuscitation.

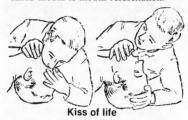

Kiss of life

Klebsiella pneumoniae: See Friedländer's bacillus.

Klebs-Loeffler bacillus: (*Corynebacterium diphtheriae*) A clinicolaboratory term for the diphtheria bacillus named after the discoverers of the organism. [Edwin Klebs, German bacteriologist. 1834-1913. Friederich A. J. Loeffler, German bacteriologist. 1852-1915.]

kleptomania (klep-tō-mā'-ni-a): Compulsive stealing due to mental disturbance, usually of the obsessional neurosis type.

Klinefelter's syndrome: A condition associated with abnormality of the sex chromosomes. The individual appears to be male but has large breasts, small genitalia, atrophied testes, and is sterile. Genetic female, pragmatic male. Commonly recognized in adult life in sterility clinics. [Harry F. Klinefelter, American physician. 1912- .]

Klumpke's paralysis: Paralysis and atrophy of muscles of forearm and hand with sensory and pupillary disturbances due to injury to cervical sympathetic nerves. Clawhand results. [Madame Klumpke, French neurologist. 1859-1927.]

kneading (nēd'-ing): A movement used in massage.

knee: The hinge joint formed by the lower end of the femur and the head of the tibia. K. JERK, a reflex contraction of the relaxed quadriceps muscle elicited by a tap on the patellar tendon; usually performed with the lower femur supported behind, the knee bent and the leg limp. Persistent variation from normal usually signifies organic nerv-

ous disorder. HOUSEMAID'S K., inflammation of the prepatellar bursa. KNOCK-K., abnormal closeness of the knees while the ankles are abnormally far apart; genu valgum. See **valgus.**

kneecap: The patella (*q.v.*).

knee-chest position: The patient rests on the chest and the knees with the face turned to one side. He supports himself on his elbows. Genupectoral position.

knife: In surgery, any cutting instrument.

knit (nit): Term used to describe the growing together of the ends of bones after a fracture.

knock-knee: A condition in which the legs curve inward at the knees; often the result of rickets in childhood. See **genu valgum.**

knuckle (nuk'-l): The dorsal aspect of any of the joints between the phalanges and the metacarpal bones, or between the phalanges.

Koch's bacillus: (*Mycobacterium tuberculosis*) A term used for the tubercle bacillus in clinicolaboratory parlance and named after Koch, who first described the bacillus.

Koch's postulates: A list of requirements that a microorganism must meet before it can be considered the cause of a disease.

Koch-Weeks bacillus: A small, gram-negative rod; the cause of infective conjunctivitis (pinkeye). [Robert Koch, German bacteriologist. 1843-1910. John E. Weeks, American ophthalmologist. 1853-1949.]

Köhler's disease: Osteochondritis of the navicular bone. Confined to children of 3 to 5 years. [Alban Köhler, German physician. 1874-1947.]

koilonychia (koi-lō-nik'-i-a): Spoon-shaped nails, characteristic of iron deficiency anemia.

Kolmer's test: 1. A modification of the Wassermann blood test for syphilis. 2. A complement-fixation test for certain bacteria-caused diseases.

kolp-, kolpo-: See **colp-, colpo-.**

kolpitis (kol-pī'-tis): See **colpitis.**

kolpotomy (kol-pot'-o-mi): See **colpotomy.**

koniosis (kō-ni-ō'-sis): See **coniosis.**

Koplik's spots: Small, bluish-white spots, each surrounded by a bright red ring, that appear on the mucous membrane inside the mouth, opposite the juncture of the teeth, during the first few days of measles; they appear before the rash and are diagnostic. [Henry Koplik, American pediatrician. 1858-1927.]

Kopp's asthma (kops az'-ma): Spasm of the

glottis in children under two; thought to be due to enlarged thymus gland.

kopr-, kopra-: See **copr-, copra-.**

Korsakoff's psychosis or syndrome: A condition which follows delirium and toxic states. Often due to alcoholism or dietary deficiencies. The consciousness is clear and alert, but the patient is disorientated for time and place. His memory is grossly impaired, especially for recent events. Often he confabulates to fill the gaps in his memory. Alcoholic dementia. Polyneuritic psychosis. Afflicts more men than women in the 45-55 age group. [Sergei S. Korsakoff, Russian neurologist. 1854-1900.]

kosher (kō′-shur): Literally, according to Jewish law. Term is used to describe food that is prepared for use according to Jewish law.

koumiss (koo′-mis): Fermented milk. Also kumiss, kumyss.

Krabbe's disease: Genetically determined degenerative disease associated with mental subnormality. [Knud H. Krabbe, Danish neurologist. 1885-1961.]

kraurosis vulvae (kraw-rō′-sis vul′-vē): A degenerative condition of the vaginal introitus associated with postmenopausal lack of estrogen.

Kretschmer's personality types: 1. Pyknic—round body and head, small hands and feet, liable to manic-depressive illnesses. 2. Asthenic—tall, thin, long headed, narrow chested, liable to schizophrenia. [Ernst Kretschmer, German psychiatrist. 1888- .]

Krukenberg's tumor (kroo′-ken-berg): A secondary malignant tumor of the ovary. The primary growth is usually in the stomach. [Friedrich Ernst Krukenberg, German pathologist. 1871-1946.]

kry, kryo-: See **cry-, cryo-.**

krymotherapy (krī-mō-ther′-a-pi): See **crymotherapy.**

kuru (koo′-roo): A chronic, progressive degenerative disorder of the central nervous system found among natives of certain areas of New Guinea; most cases occur in women and children; characterized by tremor, ataxia, strabismus and usually death within a year of onset.

Kveim test: An intradermal test for sarcoidosis using tissue prepared from person known to be suffering from the condition. [Morten Ansgar Kveim, Norwegian physician. 1892- .]

kwashiorkor (kwash-ē-or′-kor): A nutritional disorder of infants and young children when the diet is persistently deficient in essential protein; commonest in primitive tropical races where maize is the staple diet. Characteristic features are anemia, wasting, dependent edema and a fatty liver. Untreated, it progresses to death.

K.Y. jelly: A sterile, lubricating jelly.

kyllosis (kil-lō′-sis): Clubfoot or other foot deformity.

kymograph (kī′-mō-graf): An apparatus for recording movements, *e.g.,* of muscles, columns of blood. Used in physiological experiments.—kymographic, adj.; kymographically, adv.

kyphoscoliosis (kī-fō-skōl-i-ō′-sis): Coexistence of kyphosis and scoliosis (*q.v.*); backward and lateral curvature of the spine.

kyphosis (kī-fō′-sis): An excessive backward curvature of the spine, as occurs in Pott's disease. Humpback.

L

L & A: Abbreviation for light and accommodation, referring to reactions of the pupils of the eyes.

la belle indifference: Lack of concern for the implications of one's disability; seen in patients with hysterical neuroses. See **hysteria.**

labia (lā'-bi-a): Lips. L. MAJORA, two large lip-like folds extending from the mons veneris to encircle the vaginal opening. L. MINORA, two smaller folds lying within the L. majora.—labium, sing.; labial, adj.

labile (lā'-bīl): Unstable; readily changed, as many drugs when in solution. In psychiatry, emotionally unstable.

lability (la-bil'-i-ti): Instability. EMOTIONAL LABILITY, rapid change in mood. Occurs especially in the mental disorders of old age.

labio-: Relates to a lip.

labioglossolaryngeal (lā-bi-ō-glos-ō-lar-in'-jē-al): Relating to the lips, tongue and larynx. L. PARALYSIS, a nervous disease characterized by progressive paralysis of the lips, tongue and larynx.

labioglossopharyngeal (la-bi-ō-glos-ō-far-in'-jē-al): Relating to the lips, tongue and pharynx.

labiomancy (lā'-bi-ō-man-si): Lip reading.

labium (lā'-bi-um): Lip. In anatomy, a term descriptive of a fleshy structure that forms a border or edge of a part. Sing. of labia (*q.v.*).

labor: The act of giving birth to a child; parturition. The first stage lasts from onset until there is full dilatation of the cervical os; the second stage until the baby is delivered; the third stage until the placenta is expelled. COMPLICATED L., in which convulsions, hemorrhage or some other untoward event occurs. DRY L., that which occurs after most of the amniotic fluid has been expelled. INDUCED L., that which is brought on by mechanical or other extraneous means. FALSE L., uterine contractions that occur before the onset of true L. PREMATURE L., that which occurs after the fetus is viable but before the gestation period is complete, that is, between the 28th and 37th weeks of pregnancy.

labyrinth (lab'-i-rinth): An intricate communicating passageway, particularly the tortuous cavities of the internal ear. BONY L., that part which is directly hollowed out of the temporal bone. MEMBRANOUS L., the membrane which loosely lines the bony labyrinth.—labyrinthine, adj.

labyrinthectomy (lab-i-rin-thek'-to-mi): Surgical removal of part or the whole of the labyrinth of the internal ear.

labyrinthitis (lab-i-rin-thī'-tis): Inflammation of the labyrinth of the ear. Syn., otitis interna (*q.v.*).

lacerated (las'-er-āt-ed): Torn.—lacerate, v.t.

laceration (las-er-ā'-shun): A wound made by tearing, as with a blunt object; the edges are torn and ragged.—lacerate, v.t.

lachrymal (lak'-ri-mal): See **lacrimal.**

lacrimal (lak'-ri-mal): Pertaining to tears. L. APPARATUS consists of the structures that secrete tears and drain them from the surface of the eyeball; lacrimal glands, ducts, sac, and nasolacrimal ducts. L. BONE, a tiny bone at the inner side of the orbital cavity. L. DUCT, connects L. gland to upper conjunctival sac. L. GLAND, situated above the upper outer canthus of the eye; secretes tears. L. SAC, situated in a groove in the L. bone at the upper end of the nasolacrimal duct. NASOLACRIMAL DUCT extends from the L. sac to the inferior meatus of the nose.

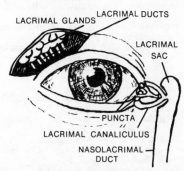

Lacrimal apparatus

lacrimation (lak-ri-mā'-shun): An outflow of tears; weeping.

lacrimonasal (lak-ri-mō-nā'-zal): Pertaining to the lacrimal and nasal bones and ducts.

lact-, lacti-, lacto-: Relates to: (1) milk; (2) lactose.

lactagogue (lak'-ta-gog): Galactagogue (q.v.).

lactalbumin (lakt-al-bū'-min): The more easily digested of the two milk proteins. See caseinogen.

lactase (lak'-tās): A sugar-splitting enzyme of intestinal juice; it splits lactose into glucose (dextrose) and galactose.

lactation (lak-tā'-shun): Secretion of milk. Suckling; the period during which the child is nourished from the breast.

lacteal (lak'-tē-al): 1. Resembling or pertaining to milk. 2. Any one of the beginning lymphatic ducts in the intestinal villi that take up split fats and convey them to the cisterna chyli (q.v.).

lactic (lak'-tik): Pertaining to milk. L. ACID, formed by the action of certain bacteria on lactose and is responsible for the souring of milk. In the body this acid is found in muscles during exercise.

lactiferous (lak-tif'-er-us): Conveying or secreting milk.

lactifuge (lak'-ti-fūj): Any agent that suppresses milk secretion.

Lactobacillus (lak-tō-ba-sil'-us): A genus of bacteria. A large gram-positive rod that is active in fermenting carbohydrates, producing acid. No members are pathogenic. L. ACIDOPHILUS, used in preparing acidophilus milk (q.v.). L. BULGARICUS, ferments milk to produce yoghurt.

lactocele (lak'-tō-sēl): Galactocele (q.v.).

lactoflavin (lak'-tō-flā-vin): Riboflavin (q.v.).

lactogenic (lak-tō-jen'-ik): Stimulating milk production; milk producing.

lactose (lak'-tōs): Milk sugar; a disaccharide that is less soluble and less sweet than ordinary sugar. Used in infant feeding to increase the carbohydrate content of diluted cow's milk.

lactosuria (lak-tō-sū'-ri-a): Lactose in the urine.—lactosuric, adj.

lactotherapy(lak-tō-ther'-a-pi): Treatment by milk diet.

lacuna (la-kū'-na): A small depression or hollow, or a space between cells; sinus. —lacunae, pl.; lacunar, adj.

lag: The time that elapses between the application of a stimulus and the response.

la grippe (la grip): Influenza (q.v.).

laking of blood (lā'-king): Hemolysis (q.v.).

lambdoidal suture (lam-doid'-al): The union between the occipital and parietal bones.

Lamblia intestinalis: Giardia lamblia (q.v.).

lambliasis (lam-blī'-a-sis): Infestation with the parasite Giardia lamblia (q.v.). Can be symptomless, or can produce persistent dysentery and occasionally steatorrhea.

lamella (la-mel'-a): A thin plate-like scale or partition. A gelatin-coated disk containing a drug; it is inserted under the eyelid. —lamellae, pl.; lamellar, adj.

lamina (lam'-in-a): A thin plate or layer, usually of bone.—laminae, pl.

laminectomy (lam-i-nek'-to-mi): Removal of laminae of one or more vertebrae—to expose the spinal cord and meninges. Most often performed in lumbar region, for removal of degenerated intervertebral disk.

lance (lans): 1. A short, two-edged knife; also called lancet. 2. To incise with a knife, as a boil or abscess.

Lancefield's groups: The classification of streptococci into 13 groups according to their pathological actions. The majority of streptococci of epidemiological importance to man belong to Group A. [Rebecca Lancefield, American bacteriologist. 1895- .]

lancinating (lan'-si-nāt-ing): Sharp, cutting, tearing; term used to describe a certain type of pain.

Landsteiner's classification: Classification of blood types as A, O, B, and AB based on the presence or absence of agglutinogens A and B in the red blood cells. See blood groups. [Karl Landsteiner, Austrian biologist in the U.S. 1868-1943.]

Langerhans' islands: See island. [Paul Langerhans, German pathologist. 1847-1888.]

languor (lan'-ger): Listlessness; lack of vigor.

lanolin (lan'-ō-lin): Wool fat containing 30 percent of water. ANHYDROUS L. is the fat obtained from sheep's wool. It is used in ointment bases, as such bases can form water-in-oil emulsions with aqueous constituents, and are readily absorbed by the skin.

lanugo (lan-ū'-gō): The fine down or hair on the fetus from about the fifth month until birth. Also sometimes used to describe fine, downy hair on a child or adult.

laparo-: Relates to: (1) the loin or flank; (2) the abdominal wall, particularly an incision into it.

laparohysterectomy (lap-a-rō-his-ter-ek'-to-mi): Removal of the uterus through an incision in the abdominal wall.

laparoscopy (lap-ar-os'-ko-pi): See peritoneoscopy.—laparoscopic, adj.; laparoscopically, adv.

laparotomy (lap-a-rot'-o-mi): Surgical

opening into the flank; term commonly used to describe any opening into the abdominal wall.

larva (lar'-va): An embryo which is independent before it has assumed the characteristic features of its parents.—larvae, pl.; larval, adj.

larvicide (lar'-vi-sīd): Any agent that destroys larvae.—larvicidal, adj.

laryngeal (lar-in'-jē-al): Pertaining to the larynx.

laryngectomee (lar-in-jek'-to-mē): A person who has had his larynx removed.

laryngectomy (lar-in-jek'-to-mi): Excision of the larynx.

laryngismus stridulus (lar-in-jiz'-mus strid'-ū-lus): Momentary attack of laryngeal spasm; inspiration produces a crowing sound and is followed by a period of apnea caused by the spasmodic closure of the glottis. Associated with low blood calcium in infantile rickets.

laryngitis (lar-in-jī'-tis): Inflammation of the larynx. Usual symptoms are dryness and soreness of the throat, hoarseness of the voice, difficulty in swallowing, sometimes cough.

laryngo-: Denotes the larynx.

laryngofissure (lar-in-gō-fish'-ur): The operation of opening the larynx in midline.

laryngologist (lar-in-gol'-o-jist): A specialist in laryngeal diseases.

laryngology (lar-in-gol'-o-ji): The study of diseases affecting the larynx.

laryngoparalysis (la-rin-gō-par-al'-i-sis): Paralysis of the larynx.

laryngopharyngectomy (lar-in-gō-far-in-jek'-to-mi): Excision of the larynx and lower part of pharynx.

laryngopharynx (la-rin-gō-far'-ingks): The lower portion of the pharynx.—laryngopharyngeal, adj.

laryngoscope (la-rin-gō-skōp): Instrument for exposure and visualization of larynx. —laryngoscophy, n.; laryngoscopic, adj.

laryngospasm (la-rin-gō-spazm): Convulsive involuntary muscular contraction of the larynx, usually accompanied by spasmodic closure of the glottis.

laryngostenosis (lar-in-gō-stē-nō'-sis): Narrowing of the glottic aperture, or of the larynx.

laryngostomy (lar-in-gos'-to-mi): The surgical creation of an artificial opening from the neck into the larynx.

laryngotomy (lar-in-got'-o-mi): The operation of opening the larynx.

laryngotracheal (lar-in-gō-trā'-kē-al): Pertaining to the larynx and trachea.

laryngotracheitis (lar-in-gō-trāk-ē-ī'-tis): Inflammation of the larynx and trachea.

laryngotracheobronchitis (lar-in-gō-trā-kē-ō-brong-kī'-tis): Inflammation of the larynx, trachea and bronchi. Usually refers to an acute respiratory condition in young children; attended by fever, toxemia and laryngeal obstruction. Croup (q.v.).

larynx (lar'-inks): The organ of voice situated below and in front of the pharynx and at the upper end of the trachea. It is composed of muscular and cartilaginous tissue and is lined with mucous membrane. The vocal cords pass from front to back across the lumen of the structure. It also serves as a passageway for air entering the trachea.— laryngeal, adj.

lascivia (las-siv'-i-a): Abnormal degree of sexual desire.

laser (lā'-zer): A device that produces a precisely aimed high intensity beam of light that transmits energy as heat and can coagulate tissue. It has been used in the treatment of detached retina.

Lassa fever: Named for the Nigerian town in which several fatal cases occurred among American missionary nurses in 1969. Caused by an exceptionally virulent virus isolated and identified during that same year. Symptoms vary widely and include very high fever, skin rash with tiny hemorrhages, mouth ulcers, pneumonia, kidney damage, infection of the heart leading to heart failure. Not limited to the tropics or Africa; some cases have occurred in scientists in research laboratories where the virus was being studied.

lassitude (las'-i-tūd): Exhaustion; lack of energy.

latent (lā'-tent): Concealed, hidden, not active.

lateral (lat'-e-ral): At or belonging to the side; away from the median line.—laterally, adv.

laughing gas: Nitrous oxide (q.v.).

lavage (lav-azh'): Irrigation of, or washing out a body cavity.

laxative (laks'-a-tiv): A mild cathartic (q.v.); an aperient.

lb: Abbreviation for pound.

LD: Abbreviation for lethal dose.

LE cells: Characteristic cells found in the bone marrow of patients with lupus erythematosus, together with a special globulin in the plasma.

lead (lēd): One of the records made in electrocardiography; the pattern of the lead varies with the body site to which the electrode is attached.

lead (led): A metal, the salts of which are astringent when applied externally. L. POISONING, acute poisoning is unusual, but chronic poisoning due to absorption of small amounts over a period is fairly common. This can happen to young children who suck articles made of lead alloys or painted with lead paint. Also an industrial hazard. Anemia, loss of appetite, abdominal pains, metallic taste and the formation of a blue line around the gums are characteristic symptoms.

lecithin (les'-i-thin): A nitrogenous, fatty substance in cell protoplasm; widely distributed throughout the body, being found in nerve tissue, semen, bile, and blood. Also found in egg yolk, soy beans, and other seeds.

leech (lēch): *Hirudo medicinalis.* A blood-sucking aquatic worm formerly much used for sucking blood from local areas. Its saliva contains hirudin, an anticoagulant.

leg: The lower leg from the knee to the ankle. BANDY L., bowleg. MILK L., thrombophlebitis of a femoral vein; phlegmasia alba dolens (*q.v.*).

Legg's disease: Quiet hip disease; osteochondritis deformans juvenilis or arthritis of the hip.

Legg-Calvé-Perthes disease: Osteochondritis (*q.v.*) of the head of the femur.

legume (leg'-ūm): A class of plant foods containing the protein legumin, *e.g.,* peas, beans, lentils, peanuts.

legumin (leg'-ū-min): A protein resembling casein, found in plant foods classified as legumes (*q.v.*).

leiomyoma (lī-ō-mī-ō'-ma): A benign tumor originating in smooth muscle tissue.

Leishman-Donovan bodies: The rounded forms of the protozoa Leishmania found in the liver, spleen, and macrophages of patients suffering from the visceral form of leishmaniasis (*q.v.*).

Leishmania (lēsh-mā'-ni-a): Flagellated protozoon which is responsible for leishmaniasis (*q.v.*).

leishmaniasis (lēsh-ma-nī'-a-sis): A communicable protozoan disease, caused by Leishmania (*q.v.*); spread by sand flies. Generalized (or visceral) manifestation is kala-azar (*q.v.*). Cutaneous manifestation is caused by *Leishmania tropica;* also called Aleppo boil, Delhi boil, or oriental sore; characterized by nodules and ulcerating lesions on the skin. The nasopharyngeal manifestation causes ulceration of the nose and throat; espundia. The disease occurs in the Mediterranean and Near East areas, China, and some parts of Africa, and is occasionally brought to the U.S. by persons who have visited in these areas.

lemniscus (lem-nis'-kus): A band of longitudinal fibers, specifically in the central nervous system.

lens (lenz): 1. The small, transparent, biconvex crystalline body which is supported in the suspensory ligament immediately behind the iris of the eye. On account of its elasticity, the lens can alter in shape, enabling light rays to focus exactly on the retina. 2. A piece of transparent material, usually glass, with a regular curvature of one or both surfaces, used for conveying or diffusing light rays, as in a camera, microscope or eyeglasses. CONTACT L., a thin, curved lens that fits over the cornea and is used instead of an eyeglass.

lentectomy (len-tek'-to-mi): Surgical removal of the lens of the eye.

lenticular (len-tik'-ū-lar): Pertaining to or shaped like a lens.

lentigo (len-tī'-gō): A brownish pigmented spot on the skin caused by changes in the skin rather than exposure to sunlight. A freckle.

lentil (len'-til): A widely cultivated European plant whose seeds and stalks furnish a cheap and nutritious legume containing a large amount of protein.

leontiasis (lē-on-tī'-a-sis): Enlargement of face and head giving a lion-like appearance, in such diseases as elephantiasis and leprosy.

leper (lep'-er): A person who has leprosy.

lepromata (lep-rō'-ma-ta): The granulomatous cutaneous nodules of leprosy. —leproma, sing.; lepromatous, adj.

leprosarium (lep-rō-sa'-ri-um): A colony or hospital for persons with leprosy. Also leprosary.

leprosy (lep'-ro-si): A chronic, progressive, communicable disease; endemic in warmer climates; infrequently seen in the U.S. Caused by *Mycobacterium leprae* (Hansen's bacillus) and very resistant to treatment. One of the two types of the disease affects the peripheral nerves, resulting in anesthesia in areas of the skin; the other type affects the skin causing the formation of nodules in skin and mucous membrane that become granulomatous. Transmission of the disease results only from prolonged and intimate contact with an infected person; the incubation period is estimated at two to four years.—leprous, adj.

lept-, lepto-: Denotes small, thin, weak, fine.

leptocytosis (lep-tō-sī-tō'-sis): Thin, flattened red cells circulating in the blood (leptocytes). Characteristic of Cooley's anemia (*q.v.*). Also seen in jaundice, hepatic disease, and sometimes after splenectomy.

leptodermic (lep-tō-der'-mik): Having a thin skin.

leptomeninges (lep-tō-me-nin'-jēz): The pia mater and the arachnoid membranes considered together.

leptomeningitis (lep-tō-men-in-jī'-tis): Inflammation of the two inner covering membranes of the brain or spinal cord. See **leptomeninges.**

Leptospira (lep-tō-spī'-ra): A genus of bacteria. Very thin, coiled spirochetes. Common in water as saprophytes; many pathogenic species may infect both man and animals producing leptospirosis. *L. icterohaemorrhagiae* causes Weil's disease in man. *L. canicola* causes 'yellows' in dogs and pigs; transmissible to man. See **canicola fever.**

leptospirosis (lep-tō-spī-rō'-sis): Spirochetal disease. L. ICTEROHAEMORRHAGICA, Weil's disease (*q.v.*).

lesbian (lez'-bi-an): A female homosexual (*q.v.*).

lesbianism (lez'-bi-an-izm): Homosexuality between women.

lesion (lē'-zhun): Any pathological change in the continuity or structure of a bodily tissue; may be caused by trauma or disease.

lethal (lē'-thal): Deadly, fatal. L. DOSAGE, the amount of a drug or other agent that will cause death.

lethargy (leth'-ar-jē): Abnormal drowsiness; torpor; apathy. Characteristic of certain diseases, *e.g.,* encephalitis.

lethe (lē'-thē): Loss of memory; amnesia.

leuc-, leuco-: See **leuk-, leuko-.**

leucine (lū'-sēn): One of the essential amino acids (*q.v.*).

leucocyte (lū'-kō-sīt): Leukocyte (*q.v.*).

leucotomy (lū-kot'-o-mi): See **leukotomy.**

leuk-, leuko-: Denotes: (1) white; (2) a type of blood cell; (3) white matter of the brain.

leukemia (lū-kē'-mi-a): A fatal disease of the blood-forming organs; of unknown cause. Chief symptom is abnormality in number or type of white blood cells. Other symptoms include poor appetite; lesions in the mouth; enlarged spleen, lymphatics; and bone marrow changes. The disease is classified according to the kind of leukocyte found and whether the condition is acute or chronic. ALEUKEMIC L., refers to a leukemic condition in which the white cell count remains normal or is below normal. —leukemic, adj.

leukocyte (lū'-kō-sīt): A white corpuscle of the blood; a spherical, colorless, nucleated mass that has ameboid movement; chief function is to act as a scavenger in protecting the body from invading organisms. —leukocytic, adj. See **basophil, eosinophil, lymphocyte, mononuclear, polymorphonuclear.**

leukocythemia (lū-kō-sī-thē'-mi-a): An increase in the number of white blood cells; leukemia.

leukocytolysis (lū-kō-sī-tol'-i-sis): Destruction and disintegration of white blood cells. —leukocytolytic, adj.

leukocytometer (lū-kō-sī-tom'-e-ter): An instrument for counting white blood cells.

leukocytosis (lū-kō-sī-tō'-sis): Increased number of leukocytes in the blood. Often a physiological response to infection.—leukocytotic, adj.

leukocyturia (lū-kō-sī-tū'-ri-a): Presence of leukocytes in the urine.

leukoderma (lū-kō-der'-ma): Defective skin pigmentation, especially when it occurs in patches or bands.

leukoma (lū-kō'-ma): White opaque spot on the cornea.—leukomata, pl.; leukomatous, adj.

leukonychia (lū-kō-nik'-i-a): White spots on the nails.

leukopenia (lū-kō-pē'-ni-a): A white blood cell count that is below normal; less than 5000 per cu mm.—leukopenic, adj.

leukoplakia (lū-kō-plā'-ki-a): A disease characterized by the occurrence of white, thickened patches on mucous membrane, usually on the lips and inside of mouth; may also occur on genitalia. Often seen in smokers, but also due to bad fitting dentures, vitamin A deficiency, or uncleanliness. Sometimes becomes malignant.

leukopoiesis (lū-kō-poi-ē'-sis): The formation of white blood cells.—leukopoietic, adj.

leukorrhea (lū-kō-rē'-a): A sticky, whitish vaginal discharge containing mucus and pus cells.—leukorrheal, adj.

leukotomy (lū-kot'-o-mi): PREFRONTAL L., an operation for the treatment of certain forms of chronic insanity by cutting the connection fibers in the white matter of the frontal lobe of the brain. May produce a state of irreversible apathy and inertia; it is usually reserved for chronic schizophrenics and patients in whom there is gross behavior disorder such as prolonged violence, self-mutilation and extreme restlessness.

levator (le-vā'-tor): A muscle which acts by raising a part. An instrument for lifting a depressed part.—levatores, pl.

Levin's tube (le-vēnz'): A tube inserted through the nose into the upper alimentary tract for continuous gastric suction, especially after operations, or for use in making gastric acid tests. [Abraham Louis Levin, American physician. 1880-1940.]

levitation (lev-i-tā'-shun): 1. The sensation of rising or floating in the air. 2. The act of supporting a patient on a cushion of air.

levulose (lev'-ū-lōs): Fructose or fruit sugar. Sweeter and more easily digested than ordinary sugar; useful in diabetes.

lewisite (lū'-i-sīt): A lethal war gas resembling mustard gas. It causes blisters on the skin, tearing, and irritation of the lungs. [W. Lee Lewis, American chemist. 1879-1943.]

-lexis, -lexy: Denotes: (1) speech; (2) a kind of reading.

libido (li-bē'-dō): The vital force or energy that results in purposeful actions. Freud's name for the urge to obtain sensual satisfaction which he believed to be the mainspring of human behavior. Sometimes more loosely associated with the meaning of sexual urge. Freud's meaning was satisfaction through all the senses.—libidinal, adj.

lice: Pl. of louse. See **Pediculus.**

lichen (lī'-ken): In medicine, aggregates of papular skin lesions. L. NITIDUS, characterized by minute, shiny, flat-topped, pink papules of pinhead size. L. PLANUS, aggregates of small, persistent papules, polygonal in shape, flat-topped and of reddish-purple hue. L. SCROFULOSORUM, small, flat-topped papules that occur as an allergic phenomenon in tuberculosis. L. SIMPLEX, a psychosomatic condition which produces areas of irritating, leathery, shiny papules (lichenification). Syn., neurodermatitis. L. SPINULOSUS, a disease of children characterized by very small spines protruding from the follicular openings of the skin and resulting from vitamin A deficiency. L. URTICATUS, papular urticaria (q.v.).—lichenoid, adj.

lichenification (lī-ken-i-fik-ā'-shun): Thickening of the skin, usually secondary to scratching. Striae become more prominent, forming a criss-cross pattern so that the area affected appears to be composed of a great many small, shiny rhomboids.

Lieberkühn's crypts, glands or follicles

(lē'-ber-kēnz): Simple tubular glands in the mucous membrane of the small intestine. [Johann Nathaniel Lieberkühn, German physician and anatomist. 1711-1756.]

lie detector: An apparatus that records changes in breathing rate, pulse rate, blood pressure and sweating of the hands—symptoms thought to be indicative of emotional reactions to certain words or questions when one is not telling the truth.

lien (lī'-en): The spleen.—lienal, adj.

lien-, lieno-: Denotes the spleen. See also splen-, spleno-.

lienculus (lī-en'-kū-lus): A small accessory spleen.

lienitis (lī-en-ī'-tis): Inflammation of the spleen.

lienorenal (lī-en-ō-rē'-nal): Pertaining to the spleen and kidney.

ligament (lig'-a-ment): A strong band of fibrous tissue serving to bind bones or other parts together, or to support a structure or an organ.—ligamentous, adj.

ligate (lī'-gāt): To apply a ligature (q.v.). To tie off blood vessels, etc., with a ligature during an operation.

ligation (lī-gā'-shun): The application of a ligature (q.v.).

ligature (lig'-a-tūr): The material used for tying vessels or sewing the tissues. Silk, horsehair, catgut, kangaroo tendon, silver wire, nylon, linen, and fascia can be used. See **suture.**

lightening: Term used to denote the relief of pressure on the diaphragm by the abdominal viscera when the presenting part of the fetus descends into the pelvis in the last two to three weeks of pregnancy.

lightning (līt'-ning): Descriptive of paroxysmal, stabbing pains, as those that occur in the lower limbs in tabes dorsalis.

limbus (lim'-bus): A border. In anatomy, a border or edge of certain organs, e.g., the edge where the cornea joins the sclera.

lime water: Solution of calcium hydroxide (about 0.15 percent). It is used in a number of skin lotions, and with an equal volume of linseed or olive oil it forms a soothing application. It is also used in infant feeding as it hinders the formation of large curds.

liminal (lim'-i-nal): The lowest intensity of a stimulus which can be perceived by the human sense. See **subliminal.**

linctus (lingk'-tus): A sweet, syrupy liquid; it should be slowly sipped.

linea (lin'-ē-a): A line.—Lineae, pl. L. ALBA, the white line visible after removal of skin from the center of the abdumen, stretching from the ensiform cartilage to the pubis, its position being indicated by a slight depression on the surface. The transversalis and parts of the oblique muscles are inserted into it. L. ALBICANTES, white lines that appear on the abdomen after reduction of tension caused by stretching such as occurs in tumors, pregnancy, edema, etc. L. ASPERA, roughened line on posterior aspect of the femur. L. NIGRA, a pigmented line from umbilicus to pubis that appears in pregnancy.

lingua (ling′-gwa): The tongue.—lingual, adj.

liniment (lin′-i-ment): An oily liquid to be applied to the skin by friction.

linin (lĭn′-in): The substance that makes up the thread-like network in a cell and on which the granules of chromatin are situated.

linked (linkt): In genetics, descriptive of characters that are so united to each other that they are always inherited together.

linoleic acid (lin-ō-lē′-ik): An unsaturated, essential fatty acid. Found in vegetable fats.

lint: A soft, absorbent material used for surgical dressings. It is fluffy on one side and smooth on the other.

lip: labium (*q.v.*).

lip-, lipo-: Denotes: (1) fat; (2) fatty tissue.

lipase (lī′-pās): Any fat-splitting enzyme. PANCREATIC L., steapsin (*q.v.*).

lipemia (lip-ē′-mi-a): Increased lipids (especially cholesterol) in the circulating blood.—lipemic, adj.

lipid (lip′-id): Any one of a group of compound substances that are insoluble, or only slightly so, in water but are soluble in alcohol, ether, chloroform or other such substances, and that can be metabolized in the body. Along with carbohydrates and proteins, lipids are the chief constituents of living cells.

lipiduria (lip-i-dū′-ri-a): The presence of lipids in the urine.

lipocardiac (lip-ō-kar′-di-ak): Pertaining to fatty degeneration of the heart muscle, or to a person affected with this condition.

lipochondrodystrophy (lip-ō-kon-drō-dis′-tro-fi): A congenital abnormality of fat metabolism involving the bones, skin, cartilage, brain and other organs; characterized by short stature, kyphosis, and possibly mental deficiency.

lipogenous (lip-oj′-e-nus): Producing fat or fatness.

lipoid (lip′-oid): 1. Resembling fat. 2. A lipid.

lipoidosis (lip-oi-dō′-sis): Disease that is due to disorder of fat metabolism.

lipolysis (li-pol′-i-sis): The chemical breaking down of fat.

lipoma (lip-ō′-ma): A benign tumor containing fatty tissue.—lipomata, pl.; lipomatous, adj.

lipomatosis (lip-ō-ma-tō′-sis): A condition marked by an abnormal accumulation of fat in a localized area.

lipoprotein (lip-ō-prō′-tē-in): A conjugated protein formed by the combination of a lipid and a simple protein.

lipuria (lip-ū′-ri-a): Fat in the urine. Adiposuria.—lipuric, adj.

Liq: Abbreviation for liquor.

liquefaction (lik-we-fak′-shun): The conversion of a solid or gas into a liquid.

liquid (lik′-wid): A substance that flows freely, is neither a solid nor a gas, has no definite shape but takes the shape of its container.

liquor (lik′-er): A solution. In anatomy, refers to certain body fluids; in pharmacology, refers to an aqueous solution. L. AMNII, the fluid surrounding the fetus. L. FOLLICULI, the fluid surrounding a developing ovum in a graafian follicle. L. SANGUINIS, the fluid part of the blood (plasma).

lisp: To pronounce the letters s and z with the sound of th.

liter (lē′-ter): A unit of liquid measurement in the metric system, being 1000 cc or 1000 ml. Equivalent to 1.0567 quarts U.S. liquid measure. Also litre.

lith-, litho-, -lith: Denotes calculi (stones).

lithagogue (lith′-a-gog): An agent that promotes the expulsion of calculi, especially urinary calculi.

lithiasis (lith-ī′-a-sis): Formation of calculi.

lithicosis (lith-i-kō′-sis): Pneumoconiosis (*q.v.*).

litholapaxy (lith-ol′-a-pak-si): Crushing a stone within the urinary bladder and removing the fragments by irrigation.

litholysis (lith-ol′-i-sis): The dissolving of calculi, especially urinary calculi in the bladder.

lithonephrotomy (lith-ō-ne-frot′-ō-mi): Surgical incision of the kidney for the removal of a calculus.

lithopedion (lith-ō-pē′-di-on): A dead fetus that has been retained in the uterus and has become calcified.

lithotomy (lith-ot′-o-mi): An operation on a duct or organ for the removal of a calculus, especially from the urinary bladder. L. PO-

SITION, that in which the patient lies on his back with the thighs raised and the knees supported and widely separated.

lithotripsy (lith'-ō-trip-si): An operation for crushing calculi in the bladder or urethra.

lithotrite (lith'-ō-trīt): An instrument for crushing a stone in the urinary bladder, or in the urethra.

lithous (lith'-us): Pertaining to or resembling a calculus.

lithuresis (lith-ū-rē'-sis): Voiding of gravel in the urine.

litmus (lit'-mus): A vegetable pigment, obtained from lichen, used as an indicator of acidity or alkalinity. Blue L. paper turns red when in contact with an acid. Red L. paper turns blue when in contact with an alkali.

litter: A portable stretcher or couch used for transporting the sick or wounded.

Little's disease: Diplegia of spastic type causing 'scissor leg' deformity. Congenital disease in which there is cerebral atrophy or agenesis. [William John Little, English surgeon. 1810-1894.]

liver: The largest gland in the body, lobular in structure, weighing from 3 to 4 pounds in the adult male, less in women. It is dark red in color and is situated in the upper right section of the abdomen; dome-shaped from fitting closely under the diaphragm. It produces bile, converts most sugars into glycogen which it also stores, and is essential to life. The liver of some animals is used as a food and as the source of pharmaceutical preparations used in treatment of certain anemias. L. SPOTS, yellowish-brown patches or spots on the skin. See **cirrhosis, hobnail.**

livid (liv'-id): Ashen, cyanotic. Blue discoloration due to bruising, congestion of blood, or insufficient oxygenation; black and blue.

lobar pneumonia: See **pneumonia.**

lobate (lō'-bāt): Divided into or made up of lobes.

lobe (lōb): 1. The lower part of the external ear. 2. A more or less well-defined section of an organ, separated from neighboring sections by a fissure, sulcus, or connective tissue.—lobar, adj.

lobectomy (lō-bek'-to-mi): Excision of a lobe, as of the lung.

lobotomy (lō-bot'-o-mi): Incision into a lobe. FRONTAL or PREFRONTAL L., cutting through the nerve fibers that pass from the frontal lobe of the cerebrum to the thalamus; done to relieve certain mental states or intractable pain.

lobule (lob'-ūl): A small lobe or a subdivision of a lobe.—lobular, lobulated, adj.

local: Not general; restricted to one part or area of the body. L. ANESTHETIC, see **anesthetic.** L. INFECTION, one restricted to a relatively small area, *e.g.,* a boil.

localize (lō'-kal-īz): 1. To limit the spread. 2. To determine the site of a lesion.—localization, n.

localized: Restricted to one area or spot; not spread throughout the body. Opp. to systemic.

lochia (lō'-ki-a): The vaginal discharge of blood and tissue debris which occurs during the puerperium. At first pure blood, it later becomes paler, diminishes in quantity and finally ceases.—lochial, adj.

lockjaw: Tonic muscle spasm making it impossible to open the jaws. See **tetanus.**

locomotor (lō-kō-mō'-tor): Can be applied to any tissue or system used in human movement. Most usually refers to nerves and muscles. Sometimes includes the bones and joints. L. ATAXIA, the disordered gait and loss of sense of position in the lower limbs which occurs in tabes dorsalis (*q.v.*). Tabes dorsalis is sometimes referred to, still, as 'locomotor ataxia.'

loculated (lok'-ū-lā-ted): Divided into numerous cavities.

loculus (lok'-ū-lus): A small depression, cavity or space.—loculi, pl.; locular, adj.

locus (lō'-kus): Place.—loci, pl

log-, logo-, -log, -logue: Denotes: (1) speech; (2) discourse.

logopathy (log-op'-ath-i): Any speech disorder of central nervous system origin.

logopedics (log-ō-pē'-diks): The study and treatment of speech defects.

logorrhea (log-ō-rē'-a): Excessive talkativeness.

-logy: Denotes the science, theory, or doctrine of the subject named in the stem.

loin: The lower part of the back, between the lower ribs and the iliac crest; the area immediately above the buttocks.

longevity (lon-jev'-i-ti): 1. Length of life. 2. A long individual life.

longsightedness: Hyperopia (*q.v.*).

loop: 1. A curve or bend. HENLE'S L., a loop in the uriniferous tubule of the kidney. 2. A heat-resisting wire set into a handle and used in the laboratory for transferring bacteriological material. 3. Lay term for a commonly used intrauterine contraceptive device; may be of metal or plastic.

lordosis (lor-dō'-sis): An exaggerated forward, convex curve of the lumbar spine.

lotion (lō′-shun): A liquid preparation, usually medicated, used externally on the skin.

loupe (loop): A magnifying lens used in ophthalmology.

louse (lows): A small parasitic insect; there are three varieties affecting man.—lice, pl. See **Pediculus.**

lozenge (loz′-enj): A medicated, sweetened tablet that is held in the mouth until it is dissolved; a troche.

L.P.N.: Abbreviation for licensed practical nurse.

LSD: Lysergic acid diethylamide. Derivative of an alkaloid found in ergot. Has potent hallucinogenic action. Sometimes used to produce abreaction (*q.v.*).

lubb-dupp (lubb-dupp′): The sounds heard through the stethoscope when listening to the normal heartbeat. *Lubb* is heard when the atrioventricular valves close and *dupp* when the semilunar valves close. The first sound is longer and of lower pitch than the second. Also called lupp-dupp.

lucid (loo′-sid): Clear, particularly in reference to the mind.—lucidity, n; lucidly, adv.

Ludwig's angina: See **angina.**

Luer syringe: A glass syringe for injecting substances hypodermically or intravenously.

lues (lū′-ēz): Syphilis.—luetic, adj.

lumb-, lumbo-: Refers to: (1) the loin; (2) the lumbar area.

lumbago (lum-bā′-gō): Incapacitating low back pain, usually of muscular origin.

lumbar: Pertaining to the loins. L. PUNCTURE, puncture into the subarachnoid space of the spinal cord, usually between the fourth and fifth lumbar vertebrae, to remove an excess of fluid, to obtain fluid for examination, or to inject a medicament. L. SYMPATHECTOMY, surgical removal of the sympathetic chain in the lumbar region; used to improve the blood supply to the lower limbs by allowing the blood vessels to dilate.

lumbocostal (lum-bō-kos′-tal): Pertaining to the loins and ribs.

lumbosacral (lum-bō-sā′-kral): Pertaining to the loin or lumbar vertebrae and the sacrum.

lumen (loo′-men): The channel of a tubular structure.—lumina, pl.; luminal, adj.

lunacy (lū′-na-si): Insanity; so called because in olden times it was thought to be due to the moon's influence.

lunatic (lū′-na-tik): A term formerly much used to describe an insane person.

lung: One of the two main organs of respiration which occupy the greater part of the thoracic cavity. They are made up of an arrangement of air tubes terminating in air vesicles; connect with the outside by the bronchi and the trachea; are divided into lobes, the right lung being composed of the superior, middle, and inferior lobes and the left lung of the superior and inferior lobes. The lungs are separated from each other by the heart and other organs in the mediastinum. Together they weigh about 42 oz., and they are concerned with the oxygenation of the blood.

lungmotor: A respiratory apparatus similar to a pulmotor (*q.v.*), used to force air into the lungs in cases of asphyxia.

lunula (lū′-nū-la): A small semicircular area, especially the semilunar pale area seen at the root of the nail.

lupus (loo′-pus): A destructive, chronic, nodular skin condition with many manifestations. L. ERYTHEMATOSUS; see **collagen, LE cells.** The discoid variety is characterized by a superficial inflammation of the skin with disk-like patches that have reddish edges and depressed centers; commonest on the nose where the eruption appears in a butterfly pattern extending over the adjoining cheeks. The disseminated type is characterized by large areas of erythema on the skin, pyrexia, toxemia, enlargement of lymph nodes, involvement of serous membranes (pleurisy, pericarditis), and renal damage; may be an auto-immune process. L. PERNIO, a form of sarcoidosis (*q.v.*); lesions on the hands and ears resemble those of frostbite. L. VULGARIS, the commonest form of skin tuberculosis; ulceration occurs over cartilage (nose or ear) with necrosis and facial disfigurement. —lupiform, lupous, adj.

lutein (loo′-tē-in): Yellow pigment in the corpus luteum (*q.v.*); also in egg yolk and fat cells.

luteotrophin (loo-tē-ō-trō′-fin): Hormone secreted by the anterior pituitary gland; it assists the formation of the corpus luteum in the ovary. Stimulates milk production after parturition. Previously called lactogenic hormone, prolactin. Also luteotropin.

luteum (loo′-tē-um): Yellow. CORPUS L., see **corpus.**

luxation (luks-ā′-shun): Dislocation.

L.V.N.: Abbreviation for licensed vocational nurse.

lying-in: L. PERIOD, the puerperium (*q.v.*). The term postnatal is now preferred. L. HOSPITAL, a maternity hospital.

lymph (limf): The pale, colorless or slightly yellow fluid that exudes from the blood through the capillaries, bathes the cells, and passes into lymphatic ducts which return the fluid to the bloodstream. Its function is to serve as the medium of exchange of nutrients and wastes between the blood and the cells. It resembles plasma, but contains only one type of blood cell, the lymphocyte.—lymphous, adj.

lymph-, lympho-: Denotes: (1) lymph; (2) lymphatic tissue; (3) lymphocytes.

lymphadenectasis (lim-fad-e-nek′-ta-sis): Enlargement of one or more lymph nodes.

lymphadenectomy (lim-fad-e-nek′-to-mi): Excision of one or more lymph nodes.

lymphadenitis (lim-fad-e-nī′-tis): Inflammation of one or more lymph nodes; usually produced by bacteria or their products; may be acute or chronic. The gland swells and there may be suppuration; the surrounding area may be red, hot, and tender to the touch.

lymphadenoid (lim-fad′-e-noid): Pertaining to or having the characteristics of a lymph gland.

lymphadenoma (lim-fad-e-nō′-ma): 1. An enlarged lymph node. MULTIPLE L., Hodgkin's disease.

lymphadenopathy (lim-fad-e-nop′-a-thi): Any disease of the lymph glands.—lymphadenopathic, adj.

lymphangiectasis (lim-fan-ji-ek′-ta-sis): Dilation of the lymph vessels; results from some obstruction in the flow of lymph. May cause formation of lymphangioma.—lymphangiectatic, adj.

lymphangiectomy (lim-fan-ji-ek′-to-mi): The surgical removal of a lymph vessel.

lymphangiogram (lim-fan′-ji-ō-gram): Radiograph demonstrating the lymphatic system after injection of an opaque medium.—lymphangiography, n.; lymphangiographical, adj.; lymphangiographically, adv.

lymphangioma (lim-fan-ji-ō′-ma): A fairly well circumscribed swelling or simple tumor consisting of lymph vessels; frequently associated with similar formation of blood vessels. May be present at birth or soon afterwards; occurs most commonly on the head, neck, axilla.—lymphangiomata, pl.; lymphangiomatous, adj.

lymphangioplasty (lim-fan′-ji-ō-plas-ti): Replacement of lymphatics by artificial channels (buried silk or nylon threads) to drain the tissues. Relieves the 'brawny arm' after radical mastectomy.—lymphangioplastic, adj.

lymphangitis (lim-fan-ji′-tis): Inflammation of lymph vessel or vessels. May be due to infection through the skin, usually by streptococci; in fingertip infections a red line may be seen running up the arm. The condition usually terminates at the lymph node into which the vessel empties, but may result in septicemia. Symptoms include headache, chills, fever, malaise, increased white blood cell count.

lymphatic (lim-fat′-ik): 1. Pertaining to, or conveying or containing lymph. 2. A vessel that conveys lymph. L. SYSTEM, the vessels and glands (nodes) through which the lymph passes as it returns to the blood stream.

lymphedema (lim-fe-dē′-ma): Swelling of the subcutaneous tissues with excess lymph fluid due to faulty lymph drainage. May be congenital or hereditary, or may result from trauma or excision of lymph nodes. L. PRAECOX, gradual enlargement of the lower extremities of girls, starting in the feet; begins between the age of 10 and 25. See **elephantiasis.**

lymphoblast (lim′-fō-blast): An immature lymphocyte (*q.v.*).

lymphoblastoma (lim-fō-blas-tō′-ma): Any one of several types of malignant lymphoma in which single or multiple tumors arise from lymphoblasts in lymph nodes. Sometimes associated with acute lymphatic leukemia. Term is sometimes used synonymously with lymphosarcoma (*q.v.*). L. MALIGNUM, Hodgkin's disease (*q.v.*).

lymphocyte (lim′-fō-sīt): A variety of white blood cell formed in the lymphoid tissues of the body; round, colorless, somewhat motile, have a single nucleus and no cytoplasmic granules. Classified as large and small. They make up 20 to 30 percent of the total white blood cells.

lymphocythemia (lim-fō-sī-thē′-mi-a): Excess of lymphocytes in the blood. Seen in such infectious diseases as infectious mononucleosis, undulant fever, measles, mumps, whooping cough.

lymphocytopenia (lim-fō-sī-tō-pē′-ni-a): A reduction in the normal number of lymphocytes in the blood.

lymphocytopoiesis (lim-fō-sī-tō-poi-ē′-sis): The formation of lymphocytes.

lymphocytosis (lim-fō-sī-tō′-sis): Lymphocythemia (*q.v.*).

lymphoepithelioma (lim-fō-ep-i-thēl-i-ō'-ma): A rapidly growing malignant tumor arising in the modified epithelial tissue in the area of the tonsil and nasopharynx. Often has metastases in cervical lymph nodes.—lymphoepitheliomata, pl.

lymphogranuloma (lim-fō-gran-ū-lō'-ma): Term descriptive of several diseases in which the chief pathological change is the development of lesions resembling granulomas (*q.v.*). L. VENEREUM, an important contagious venereal disease, caused by a virus, transmitted by sexual contact; primary lesion on genitalia may go unnoticed; later regional lymph nodes enlarge and typical buboes form followed by formation of draining sinuses that leave thick scars when they heal. General symptoms are fever, malaise, joint pains. May cause elephantiasis of genitalia, ischiorectal abscesses and rectal stricture, the latter particularly in women. Also called lymphogranuloma inguinale.

lymphography (lim-fog'-ra-fi): X-ray examination of the lymphatic system after it has been rendered radiopaque.—lymphographical, adj.; lymphographically, adv.

lymphoid (lim-foid'): Pertaining to or resembling lymph.

lymphoma (lim-fō'-ma): Term includes several tumors of lymphatic tissue. Of unknown cause, tumor starts as enlargement of lymph nodes, usually cervical or inguinal; later extends to adjacent chains and liver and spleen. May be transformed into one of the malignant types, including Hodgkin's disease. The benign form remains localized and does not recur after surgical removal.

lymphopenia (lim-fō-pē'-ni-a): A reduction in the proportion of lymphocytes in the circulating blood.

lymphorrhagia (lim-fō-rā'-ji-a): An outpouring of lymph from a severed lymphatic vessel.

lymphosarcoma (lim-fō-sar-kō'-ma): A malignant tumor of unknown cause, arising in the lymphatic tissue and tending to metastasize freely.—lymphosarcomata, pl.; lymphosarcomatous, adj.

lymph-vascular (limf-vas'-kū-lar): Relating to lymphatic vessels.

lys-, lysi-, lyso-, -lysis: Denotes: (1) disintegration, decomposition, dissolution; (2) loosening.

lysergic acid: See **LSD.**

lyse, lyze: To produce, cause, or undergo lysis (*q.v.*).

lysin (lī'-sin): A cell dissolving substance in blood. See **bacteriolysin, hemolysin.**

lysine (lī'-sēn): An essential amino acid necessary for growth in infants and to maintain nitrogen balance in adults. Deficiency may cause nausea, dizziness and anemia. It is destroyed by dry heating, *e.g.*, toasted bread and cereals such as puffed wheat.

lysis (lī'-sis): 1. A gradual return to normal, used especially in relation to pyrexia. Opp., crisis. 2. Dissolution and disintegration of bacteria and cells by the action of a lysin. 3. Loosening of an organ from adhesions. —lytic, adj.

Lysol: Well-known disinfectant containing 50 percent creosol in soap solution. It has a wide range of activity, but the preparation is caustic and this limits its use.

lysozyme (lī'-sō-zīm): A bacteriolytic enzyme present in tears, saliva, nasal mucus, and many animal fluids; also found in egg white.

M

M: Abbreviation for thousand, mixture, meter, and molar (solution).

m: Abbreviation for minim (min is preferred); and for meter (M is preferred).

μ: Symbol used for micron; the Greek letter mu.

MA: Abbreviation for mental age.

Macaca mulatta: A genus of monkey, much used in physiologic experimentation.

maceration (mas-e-rā′-shun): The softening of a solid by moisture, *e.g.*, the softening of the horny layer of the skin by moisture around the toes in tinea pedis (*q.v.*). In obstetrics, term is applied to the changes in the tissues of a fetus that is retained in the uterus after it has died.

macr-, macro-: Denotes: (1) large size (opp. to micro-); (2) abnormally large, *e.g.*, macrocolon; (3) visible to the naked eye.

macrocephalous (mak-rō-sef′-a-lus): Having an excessively large or long head.—macrocephalic, adj.

macrocheilia (mak-rō-kī′-li-a): Excessive development of the lips.

macrocnemia (mak-rok-nē′-mi-a): Excessive development of the legs below the knees.

macrocyte (mak′-rō-sīt): A large red blood cell, found in the blood in some forms of anemia, especially pernicious anemia.—macrocytic, adj.

macrocytosis (mak-rō-sī-tō′-sis): The presence in the circulating blood of abnormally large red blood cells.

macrodactyly (mak-rō-dak′-ti-li): Excessive development of the fingers or toes.

macroesthesia (mak-rō-es-thē′-zi-a): A sensation that things seen or felt are larger than they really are.

macrogenesy (mak-rō-jen′-e-si): Gigantism.

macrogenitosomia (mak-rō-jen-i-tō-sō′-mi-a): Excessive development of the body in general, and especially of the sex organs. When this occurs at an early age it is called M. PRAECOX.

macroglossia (mak-rō-glos′-i-a): Abnormally large tongue.

macrognathia (mak-rō-nā′-thi-a): Abnormally large jaw.

macromastia (mak-rō-mas′-ti-a): Abnormally large breasts.

macrophage (mak′-rō-fāj): A 'wandering' phagocytic cell; plays an important part in organization and repair of tissue.

macroplasia (mak-rō-plā′-zi-a): Overgrowth of a tissue or part. Gigantism.

macropodia (mak-rō-pōd′-i-a): Abnormally large feet.

macropsia (mak-rop′-si-a): A disorder of vision in which things appear larger than they really are.

macroscopic (mak-rō-skop′-ik): Visible to the naked eye; gross. Opp. to microscopic.

macrosomia (mak-rō-sō′-mi-a): Abnormally large body size. Also megasomia.

macula (mak′-ū-la): A spot or stain on a body tissue, not elevated but differentiated from the surrounding area.—maculae, pl.; macular, adj.; maculation, n. M. LUTEA, the yellow spot on the retina, the area of clearest vision. M. SOLARIS, a sunspot; a freckle.

macule (mak′-ūl): A discolored spot, not raised above the skin's surface.—macular, adj.

maculopapular (mak′-ū-lō-pap′-ū-lar): The presence of macules and raised palpable spots (papules) on the skin.

Madura foot: A fungus disease of the foot found in India and the tropics. Characterized by swelling and the development of nodules and sinuses from which there is a characteristic exudate containing granules that may be white, yellow, red, brown, orchid or black. See **mycetoma.**

maduromycosis (ma-dū-rō-mī-kō′-sis): Madura foot (*q.v.*).

magma: 1. A substance made up of finely divided particles suspended in a small amount of fluid. 2. A paste-like substance or salve.

magnesium (mag-nē′-zi-um): A silvery metallic substance found in bone, muscle, and blood; considered essential to nutrition and growth. Present in many animal and vegetable foods; deficiency in the diet causes disturbance in bone development and irritability of the nervous system that may result in convulsions and tetany. Chemical symbol is Mg.

magnum (mag′-num): Large or great, as foramen M. in the occipital bone.

maidenhead: The hymen.

maim (mām): To disable or wound by violence.

main (mān): Hand.

mainlining: Slang term used to describe the injection of a drug directly into a vein.

mal: Disease or disorder. M. DE MER, seasickness. GRAND M., major epilepsy. PETIT M., minor epilepsy.

mal-: Denotes: (1) ill, bad, badly, poor, poorly, inadequate; (2) abnormal, irregular.

mala (mā'-la): The cheek or cheek bone.—malar, adj.

malabsorption (mal-ab-sorp'-shun): Poor or disordered absorption.

malac-, malaco-: Denotes a condition of abnormal softness.

malacia (ma-lā'-shi-a): 1. Abnormal softening of a part. See **keratomalacia, osteomalacia.** 2. Abnormal craving for certain foods, especially spicy foods.

maladjustment (mal-ad-just'-ment): Bad or poor adjustment to environment socially, mentally, emotionally, or physically; often results in conflict-producing behavior.

malady (mal'-a-di): A disease, disorder or indisposition.

malaise (mal-āz'): A feeling of illness and discomfort.

malalignment (mal-a-līn'-ment): Faulty alignment, as of the teeth, or a fracture.

malar (māl'-ar): Relating to the cheek. M. or ZYGOMATIC BONE forms the prominence of the cheek.

malaria (ma-lā'-ri-a): An infectious, febrile, tropical disease caused by one of the genus *Plasmodium,* and carried by mosquitoes of the genus *Anopheles.* Characterized by anemia, toxemia, and splenomegaly, and intermittent paroxysms of fever, chills, and sweating that occur at intervals corresponding to the time it takes for a new generation of the parasites to develop in the blood. If the paroxysms occur every 24 hrs. the malaria is known as 'quotidian'; if every 48 hrs., 'tertian'; if every 72 hrs., 'quartan.'—malarial, adj.

malariotherapy (ma-lā-ri-ō-ther'-a-pi): The introduction of hyperpyrexia by inoculation with a benign form of malaria. Used in treatment of neurosyphilis and certain other affections. Pyretotherapy.

malassimilation (mal-a-sim-il-ā'-shun): Poor or disordered assimilation.

malformation (mal-for-mā'-shun): Abnormal shape or structure; deformity.

malignant (ma-lig'-nant): Virulent and dangerous; that which is likely to become progressively worse and to have a fatal termination. M. GROWTH or TUMOR, cancer or sarcoma. M. PUSTULE, anthrax.—malignancy, n.

malinger (ma-ling'-er): To feign, induce, or deliberately prolong an illness or incapacitation to avoid work or a duty or to excite sympathy.—malingerer, n.; malingering, v.i.

malleolus (mal-lē'-o-lus): A part or process of a bone shaped like a hammer. EXTERNAL M., at the lower end of the fibula. INTERNAL M., situated at the lower end of the tibia.—malleoli, pl.; malleolar, adj.

malleus (mal'-ē-us): The hammer-shaped lateral bone of the middle ear.

malnutrition (mal-nū-trish'-un): The state of being poorly nourished. May be caused by inadequate intake of food, or of one or more of the essential nutrients, or by malassimilation.

malocclusion (mal-o-kloo'-zhun): Failure of the upper and lower teeth to meet properly when the jaws are closed.

malodorous (mal-ō'-dor-us): Having an offensive or unpleasant odor.

malpighian (mal-pig'-i-an): 1. M. CORPUSCLES or CAPSULES, the renal glomeruli with Bowman's capsule enclosing them (see **glomerulus**). 2. Name given to certain small lymphoid bodies or patches distributed throughout the spleen. [Marcello Malpighi, Italian anatomist, founder of microscopic anatomy. 1628-1694.]

malposition (mal-pō-zish'-un): Any abnormal position of a part.

malpractice (mal-prak'-tis): Unethical, improper or injurious treatment by a physician or surgeon. Also now used to describe such treatment by a professional nurse.

malpresentation (mal-prē-zen-tā'-shun): Any unusual presentation of the fetus in the pelvis.

Malta fever: See **Brucella, brucellosis.**

maltase (mawl'-tās): A sugar-splitting (saccharolytic) enzyme found in the body, especially in intestinal juice.

maltose (mawl'-tōs): Malt sugar, a disaccharide; produced by the hydrolysis of starch during digestion.

malunion (mal-ūn'-yon): Union of a fracture in faulty position.

mamma (ma'-ma): The breast; milk-secreting gland.—mammae, pl.; mammary, adj.

mammal (mam'-al): An individual belonging to the highest class of vertebrates; a warm-blooded animal that suckles its young and whose body is covered with skin that is more or less hairy.

mammectomy (mam-ek'-to-mi): Surgical

removal of one or both breasts; mastectomy.

mammilla (ma-mil′-a): 1. The nipple. 2. A small papilla or nipple-like structure.—mammillae, pl.; mammillated, mammillary, adj.

mammitis (mam-ī′-tis): Mastitis (*q. v.*).

mammography (mam-og′-ra-fi): X-ray examination of the breast after injection of an opaque agent. Syn., mastography.—mammographic, adj.; mammographically, adv.

mammoplasty (mam′-ō-plas-ti): Any plastic operation on the breast.—mammoplastic, adj.

mammose (mam-mōs′): Having large breasts.

mammotrophic (mam-o-trō′-fik): Having an effect upon the breast.

mandible (man′-dib′l): The lower jawbone.—mandibular, adj.

mania (mā′-ni-a): 1. One phase of manic-depressive psychoses in which the prevailing mood is one of undue elation, pronounced psychomotor overactivity, and often pathological excitement. 2. Excessive or obsessive enthusiasm for a thing or an activity; in this sense often used as a combining form, *e.g.,* erotomania.—manic, adj.

-mania: Formerly denoted any kind of madness. Currently used to denote a morbid preoccupation with some idea or activity, or a compulsive need to carry out a certain kind of behavior.

maniac (mā′-ni-ak): A person affected with mania (*q. v.*). A person who is insane or violently disturbed.—maniacal, adj.

manic (man′-ik): Pertaining to or affected with mania (*q. v.*).

manic depressive psychosis (man′-ik dē-pres′-iv sī-kō′-sis): A type of mental disorder characterized by mood swings from the normal in the direction of either excitement and elation, or depression, despondency, fatigue. Not all patients exhibit both moods, and often there are periods of complete normality between the two phases.

manikin (man′-i-kin): A model of the human body, used in teaching anatomy and also for demonstrating and teaching nursing procedures.

manipulation (ma-nip-ū-lā′-shun): Using the hands skillfully as in reducing a fracture or hernia, or changing the fetal position. In physical therapy, the movement of a joint beyond the limit to which the individual can move it voluntarily.

mannerism (man′-er-izm): A way of speaking, acting, or behaving that is unusual or peculiar, and characterizes a particular person.

manometer (man-om′-et-er): An instrument for measuring the pressure exerted by liquids or gases. See **sphygmomanometer; tonometer.**

Mantoux test (man-too′): A test for tuberculosis; a minute amount of diluted tuberculin (PPD) (*q. v.*) is injected intradermally. If the person has, or has had tuberculosis, hyperemia and a wheal will develop at the site of the injection.

manubrium (man-ū′-bri-um): A handle-shaped structure; the upper part of the breast bone or sternum.

manus (mā′-nus): The hand, including the fingers.

maple syrup urine disease: A familial metabolic disorder, of unknown origin, with urine smelling of maple syrup, and affliction of the central nervous system sometimes resulting in mental subnormality. Usually fatal within the first few months of life.

marasmus (mar-az′-mus): Wasting away of the body, especially that of a baby, without apparent cause.—marasmic, adj.

Marfan's syndrome: Hereditary congenital disorder of unknown cause. There is dislocation of the lens, congenital heart disease and arachnodactyly with hypotonic musculature and lax ligaments, occasionally excessive height and abnormalities of the iris. [B. J. A. Marfan, French physician. 1858-1942.]

margin: An edge or border, as of an organ or structure.—marginal, adj.

marihuana, marijuana (mar-i-wah′-na): Cannabis (*q. v.*).

marrow: The highly vascular soft pulpy tissue that fills the cavities of most bones. YELLOW M., found in cavities of long bones; contains fat cells. RED M., found at the ends of long bones and throughout the cancellous parts of flat and irregular bones such as vertebrae, ribs, sternum; principal function is manufacture of red blood cells.

masculinize (mas′-kū-lin-īz): To confer or produce male characteristics in a female.—masculinization, n.

mask: 1. A covering for the face, used to protect either the wearer or a patient; also used to apply medications, especially those in gas form to be inhaled. 2. An expression characteristic of a certain disorder or condition. M. OF PREGNANCY, a brownish, patchy discoloration on the face and neck; occurs during pregnancy and disappears after delivery. PARKINSON'S M., a fixed expression with staring and infrequent winking, characteristic of patients with Parkinson's disease.

masochism (mas'-ō-kizm): A form of sexual perversion in which one has a pathological desire to inflict pain upon himself or to suffer pain, abuse, or humiliation at the hands of another. Opp. to sadism. [Leopold von Sacher-Masoch, Austrian historian. 1836-1895.]

masochist (mas'-ō-kist): One who practices masochism (*q.v.*).

mass: 1. A lump. 2. A mixture so prepared that it can be made up into pills.

massage (ma-sahzh'): Physical therapy that consists of manipulating the tissues of the body by the use of friction, stroking, kneading, etc.

masseter (mas-ē'-ter): The chief muscle of mastication; situated at the side of the face. It raises the lower jaw.

masseur (ma-ser'): A man who gives massage.

masseuse (ma-sūz'): A woman who gives massage.

mast-, masto-: Denotes: (1) breast; (2) mastoid.

mastadenoma (mast-ad-e-nō'-ma): A benign tumor of the breast.

mastalgia (mas-tal'-ji-a): Pain in the breast.

mastatrophia (mas-ta-trō'-fi-a): Atrophy or shrinking of the breasts.

mast cell: A large, round or ovoid, plump, granulated cell found normally in connective tissues; specific functions unknown.

mastectomy (mas-tek'-to-mi): Surgical removal of the breast. SIMPLE M., removal of the breast with the overlying skin. RADICAL M., removal of the breast with the skin and underlying pectoral muscle together with all the lymphatic tissue of the axilla. Combined with radiotherapy this operation is the usual treatment for carcinoma of the breast.

mastication (mas-ti-kā'-shun): The act of chewing.

mastitis (mas-tī'-tis): Inflammation of the mammary gland. CHRONIC CYSTIC M., the name formerly applied to nodular changes in the breast, now usually called fibrocystic disease.

mastocarcinoma (mas-tō-kar-si-nō'-ma): Carcinoma of the breast.

mastography (mas-tog'-ra-fi): See **mammography.**—mastographic, adj.;

mastoid (mas'-toid): Nipple-shaped. M. AIR CELLS extend in a backward and downward direction from the antrum. M. ANTRUM, the air space within the mastoid process, lined by mucous membrane continuous with that of the tympanum and mastoid cells. M. PROCESS, the rounded prominence on the mastoid portion of the temporal bone just behind the ear.

mastoidectomy (mas-toid-ek'-to-mi): Drainage of the mastoid air cells and excision of diseased tissue.

mastoiditis (mas-toid-ī'-tis): Inflammation of any part of the mastoid process; usually the result of an extension of a middle ear infection.

mastoidotomy (mas-toid-ot'-o-mi): Incision into the mastoid process of the temporal bone.

mastoptosis (mas-to-tō'-sis): Sagging or pendulous breasts.

masturbation (mas-tur-bā'-shun): Self-stimulation of the genital organs, manually or by other body contact, but not sexual intercourse, usually resulting in orgasm.

match test: A rough test of respiratory function. If a person is unable to blow out a lighted match held four inches from a fully open mouth there is significant reduction of respiratory function.

mater (mā'-ter): The Latin word for mother. DURA M., the fibrous outer covering of the brain and spinal cord. PIA M., the vascular, delicate membrane that immediately invests the brain and spinal cord. Between it and the dura M. lies the arachnoid (*q.v.*).

materia medica (mat-ē'-ri-a med'-i-ka): The science dealing with the origin, preparation, action and dosage of drugs.

maternal (ma-ter'-nal): Pertaining to the female parent.

maternity (ma-ter'-ni-ti): Motherhood.

matrix (mā'-triks): The foundation substance in which the tissue cells are embedded. The basic material from which a thing develops.

matter: 1. Any substance that occupies space. 2. Pus. GRAY M., composed mainly of nerve cells, found in the brain cortex. WHITE M., composed mainly of medullated nerve fibers.

maturation (mat-ū-rā'-shun): The process of attaining full development.—maturate, v.i.

mature (ma-tūr'): To be fully developed, or to reach full development; to ripen.

maxilla (mak-sil'-a): The jawbone; in particular the upper jaw.—maxillary, adj.; maxillae, pl.

maxillofacial (mak-sil-ō-fā'-shal): Pertaining to the maxilla and the face. A subdivision in plastic surgery.

maximum (mak′-si-mum): The largest; utmost; the greatest possible size, quantity, value or degree.—maximal, adj.

maze: A labyrinth consisting of blind alleys and one correct path, used in the study of animal and human learning processes.

μ**c:** Abbreviation for microcurie (*q.v.*).

McBurney's point: A point about one-third of the way between the anterior superior iliac spine and the umbilicus, the site of maximum tenderness in cases of acute appendicitis. [Charles McBurney, American surgeon. 1845-1913.]

McDowell's operation: The operation for removal of an ovarian cyst through an abdominal incision. Named for the surgeon who first performed it in 1809. [Ephraim McDowell, American surgeon. 1771-1830.]

mcg: Abbreviation for microgram (*q.v.*).

M.D.: Abbreviation for Doctor of Medicine.

measles (mē′-zelz): Rubeola. Morbilli. An acute infectious disease caused by a virus and spread by droplets; characterized by fever, a blotchy rash, and catarrhal inflammation of the mucous membranes. Endemic and worldwide in distribution. See **Koplik's spots, German measles (rubella).**

meatus (mē-ā′-tus): An opening or channel, usually referring to the opening into a passageway into the body. AUDITORY M., the external opening into the auditory canal. URINARY M., the opening from the exterior into the urethra.

mechanoreceptors (mek-an-ō-rē-sep′-tors): Receptors that are sensitive to differences in pressure, such as those experienced through the sense of touch or hearing.

mechanotherapy (mek-an-ō-ther′-a-pi): The treatment of disease by the use of various kinds of mechanical apparatus, especially as in physiotherapeutics.

Meckel's diverticulum (mek′-els dī-vertik′-ū-lum): A blind, pouch-like sac sometimes arising from the free border of the ileum. It may be 2 to 3 in. in length and is a remnant of the duct which, in the embryo, connects the yolk sac with the primitive alimentary canal. [Johann Friedrich Meckel, German anatomist and gynecologist. [1781-1833.]

meconium (mē-kō′-ni-um): The discharge from the bowel of a newly born baby. It is greenish-black, viscid, and contains epithelial cells, mucus and bile. M. ILEUS, impaction of M. in the bowel. Associated with smelly, fatty stools and chest infection. Earliest sign of mucoviscidosis (*q.v.*).

media (mē′-di-a): In anatomy, the middle coat of an artery. Pl. of medium (*q.v.*).

mediad (mē′-di-ad): Toward the middle; toward a median line or plane of the body.

medial (mē′-di-al): Pertaining to or near the middle.—medially, adv.

median (mē′-di-an): The middle. M. LINE, an imaginary line passing through the center of the body from a point between the eyes to between the closed feet. In statistics, the value midway in a distribution of frequencies, that is, half of the observations fall above and half below the median value.

mediastinum (mē-di-as-tī′-num): The space between the lungs; bounded by the lungs on either side, the sternum in front, the vertebrae in back, and the diaphragm at the bottom; contains all the organs of the chest except the lungs.—mediastinal, adj.

medical (med′-i-kal): Pertinent to medicine or the treatment of disease. M. JURISPRUDENCE, the application of medical science and facts to legal problems. Forensic medicine.

medicament (med-ik′-a-ment): A remedy or medicine.

medicate (med′-i-kāt): 1. To impregnate with a drug or medicine. 2. To treat disease by administering a drug or drugs. —medicated, adj.

medication (med-i-kā′-shun): Administration of a medicine.

medicinal (med-is′-in-al): 1. Pertaining to a medicine. 2. Having healing or curing effects or properties.

medicine (med′-i-sin): 1. The science or art of treating or preventing disease. 2. That branch of the healing art that deals with the treatment of disease by the administration of internal remedies as distinguished from such specialties as surgery. 3. A drug. 4. A therapeutic agent.

Mediterranean fever: See **Brucella, brucellosis.**

medium (mē′-di-um): A substance used in bacteriology for the growth of organisms. —media, pl.

medulla (me-dul′-a): 1. The marrow in the center of a long bone. 2. The soft internal portion of glands, as distinguished from the outer part, *e.g.,* kidneys, adrenals, lymph nodes, etc.—medullary, adj. M. OBLONGATA, the upper part of the spinal cord between the foramen magnum of the occipital bone and the pons varolii.

medullated (med′-ū-lā′-ted): Containing or surrounded by a covering or sheath, particularly referring to nerve fibers.

medulloblastoma (med-ū-lō-blas-tō′-ma):

Malignant, rapidly growing tumor, seen mostly in children; appears in the midline of the cerebellum.

meg-, mega-, megal-, megalo-: Denotes: (1) great size, powerful, enlarged; (2) mega denotes one million units (metric system).

megacephalic (meg-a-se-fal′-ik): Large-headed. Syn., macrocephalic, megalocephalic.

megacolon (meg-a-kō′-lon): Condition of dilated and elongated colon. In an adult the cause is unknown. In a child the parasympathetic ganglion cells are absent in the distal part of the colon; Hirschsprung's disease (*q.v.*).

megacurie (meg′-a-kū-ri): A unit of radioactivity; 1,000,000 curies (*q.v.*).

megakaryocyte (meg-a-kar′-i-ō-sīt): Large, multinucleated cells of the marrow that are generally thought to produce blood platelets.

megaloblast (meg′-a-lō-blast): A large, nucleated, primitive red blood cell.

megalocardia (meg-a-lō-kar′-di-a): Cardiomegaly (*q.v.*).

megalocephalic (meg-al-ō-se-fal′-ik): See **megacephalic.**

megalokaryocyte (meg-al-ō-ka′-ri-ō-sīt): Syn., megakaryocyte (*q.v.*).

megalomania (meg-a-lō-mā′-ni-a): Delusions of grandeur or self-importance, characteristic of general paralysis of the insane. See **general.**

megalopsia (meg-a-lop′-si-a): Macropsia (*q.v.*).

megaphonia (meg-a-fōn′-i-a): Abnormal loudness of voice.

meibomian (mī-bō′-mi-an): M. GLANDS, sebaceous glands lying in grooves on the inner surface of the eyelids, their ducts opening on the free margins of the lids. M. CYST, chalazion (*q.v.*). [Heinrich Meibom, German anatomist. 1638-1700.]

Meigs's syndrome (meg′-zes): Benign, solid ovarian tumor associated with hydroperitoneum and hydrothorax. [Joe V. Meigs, American anatomist. 1892- .]

Meissner's corpuscles: Important receptors for the sense of touch; consist of elongated bodies enclosing the terminal ends of several afferent nerve fibers; lie just beneath the epidermis. Most numerous on the finger tips, palms of the hands and soles of the feet, tip of the tongue, and in the skin around the mouth and nipples. Sensitive to light touch and pressure.

melan-, melano-: Denotes: (1) melanin; (2) black, dark.

melancholia (mel-an-kō′-li-a): Extremely unhappy state, usually accompanied by inhibition of mental and physical activity. In psychiatry the term is reserved to mean severe forms of depression.—melancholic, adj. INVOLUTIONAL M., a major affective disorder, chiefly of the middle-aged and elderly; marked by anxiety, agitation, insomnia, feelings of guilt and hypochondria.

melanin (mel′-a-nin): A dark brown or black pigment found normally in hair, skin, choroid and retina of the eye, pia mater, cardiac muscle, and in some tumors. Accounts for racial differences in skin color.

melanism (mel′-a-nizm): Excessive deposit of pigment in tissues or the skin.

melanocarcinoma (mel′-a-nō-kar-si-nō′-ma): A malignant tumor believed to be of epithelial origin. A malignant melanoma (*q.v.*).

melanoderma (mel-a-nō-der′-ma): An abnormal amount of melanin in the skin as evidenced by the formation of pigmented spots.

melanoglossia (mel-a-nō-glos′-i-a): Black tongue.

melanosarcoma (mel-an-ō-sar-kō′-ma): One form of malignant melanoma. —melanosarcomata, pl.; melanosarcomatous, adj.

melanosis (mel-a-nō′-sis): A condition characterized by the appearance of dark brown or brownish-black pigmentation in tissues of the body, as in the skin in sunburn or Addison's disease, or around the nipples and elsewhere during pregnancy.—melanotic, adj.

melanous (mel′-a-nus): Dark-complexioned.

melanuria (mel-a-nū′-ri-a): The presence of melanin in the urine. The voiding of dark-colored urine or urine that turns dark upon standing.—melanuric, adj.

melasma (me-laz′-ma): Any dark discoloration of the skin, as in Addison's disease.

melena (mel′-e-na): 1. Black vomit. 2. Dark, tarry stools resulting from the action of intestinal juices on free blood. M. NEONATORUM, melena of the newborn, resulting from the extravasation of blood into the alimentary canal during the first few hours after birth.

melenemesis (mel-e-nem′-e-sis): The vomiting of dark material that has been colored as a result of the action of gastric juices on blood.

meli-: Denotes: (1) sweetness; (2) honey.

-melia: Denotes a condition of the limbs.

melioidosis (me-li-oi-dō′-sis): A disease

melitensis

with symptoms resembling those of glanders (*q.v.*); affects rats and transmissible to man by the rat flea; occurs in certain parts of Asia and the Far East.

melitensis (mel-i-ten′-sis): Brucellosis (*q.v.*).

melitis (me-lī′-tis): Inflammation of the cheek.

melituria (mel-i-tū′-ri-a): The presence of sugar in the urine; diabetes mellitus.

melodiotherapy (mel-ō-di-ō-ther′-a-pi): Treatment by music. Syn., musicotherapy.

melomania (mel-ō-mā′-ni-a): Excessive fondness for music.

meloplasty (mel′-ō-plas-ti): 1. Plastic surgery of the cheek. 2. Plastic surgery of an extremity.

member: An organ or a part of the body, particularly a limb.

membrane (mem′-brān): A thin, soft, pliable sheet of tissue that lines a tube or cavity, covers an organ or structure, or divides a space or organ. There are four major types in the body: cutaneous, mucous, serous, synovial. All are protective in function and secrete a fluid.—membranous, adj. BASEMENT M., a thin layer beneath the epithelium of mucous surfaces. CROUPOUS M., a yellow-white M. that forms on the tracheal surfaces in laryngotracheobronchitis. CUTANEOUS M., the skin. DIPHTHERITIC M., a thick, tough fibrinous M. that forms on mucous surfaces, characteristic of diphtheria. HYALINE M., a thin sheet of material lining the alveoli, alveolar ducts and bronchioles, sometimes found in postmortem examination of infants whose death was due to idiopathic respiratory distress. HYALOID M., that surrounding the vitreous humor of the eye. MUCOUS M., contains glands that secrete mucus. Lines cavities and passages that communicate with the exterior of the body. SEMIPERMEABLE M., one that allows the passage through it of a solvent such as water, but not any of the substances held in solution. SEROUS M., a lubricating M., lining closed cavities, and reflected over their enclosed organs. SYNOVIAL M., that lining the intra-articular parts of bones and ligaments; secretes synovial fluid for lubrication. TYMPANIC M., that which separates the middle ear from the external auditory canal; the ear drum.

membranous croup: A lay term for diphtheria (*q.v.*).

memory (mem′-o-ri): The mental faculty of being able to retain and consciously or unconsciously recall or relive that which has been learned or experienced in the past.

men-, meno-: Denotes menstruation; the menses.

menacme (me-nak′-mi): The period of a woman's life during which menstruation persists.

menarche (me-nar′-kē): When the menstrual periods commence and other bodily changes occur.

Mendel's law: A theory of heredity, evolved by an Austrian monk, which deals with the interaction of dominant and recessive characters in crossbreeding. Foundation of the present theory of heredity. [Gregor Johann Mendel. 1822-1884.]

mendelian (men-dēl′-i-an): Pertaining to Mendel's theory. See **Mendel's law.**

Ménière's disease, syndrome (mān-yers′): A disorder of the membranous labyrinth of the inner ear; occurs in adult life. May accompany such disorders as drug poisoning, blood dyscrasias, circulatory disorders, neuritis or tumor, although the exact cause of the symptoms may be unknown. The most characteristic and disturbing symptom is dizziness; tinnitus, nausea, vomiting, and progressive deafness may also occur. [Prosper Ménière, French otologist. 1799-1862.]

mening-, meningi-, meningo-: Denotes a membrane, particularly one of the membranes (meninges) that cover the brain and spinal cord.

meninges (men-in′-jēs): Membranes, specifically the three protective and nutritive membranes surrounding the brain and spinal cord: the dura mater (outer); the arachnoid (middle); the pia mater (inner).—meninx, sing.; meningeal, adj.

meningioma (men-in-ji-ō′-ma): A slowly growing fibrous tumor arising from the meninges, usually occurring in adults over 30 years of age; may cause damage by pressing on the brain or adjacent parts.

meningism, meningismus (men′-in-jism, men-in-jis′-mus): Condition presenting with signs and symptoms of meningitis (*e.g.*, neck stiffness); meningitis does not develop. It may be hysterical in origin; may also result from irritation of the meninges at the onset of acute febrile diseases, particularly in children.

meningitis (men-in-jī′-tis): Inflammation of the meninges. Inflammation of the dura mater is called **pachymeningitis.** The arachnoid and pia mater are most commonly affected and the condition is known as **leptomeningitis.** May be caused by any one of several microorganisms, the most common being meningococcus, pneumococcus, streptococcus, and the tubercle bacillus. Presence of the organism in the spinal fluid is diagnostic. Fever, malaise, stiff neck, vomiting, severe headache, stupor, confusion, delirium, convulsions, and unconsciousness are among the symptoms. Sometimes only the cerebral meninges are involved, sometimes only those of the spinal cord, and sometimes both. See **leptomeningitis, pachymeningitis.** An epidemic form of M. is known as 'cerebrospinal fever'; the infecting organism is *Neisseria meningitidis* (meningococcus).—meningitides, pl.; meningitic, adj.

meningocele (men-ing′-gō-sēl): Protrusion of the meninges through a bony defect in the skull or spinal column. It forms a cyst filled with cerebrospinal fluid. See **spina bifida.**

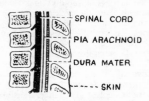

SPINAL CORD

PIA ARACHNOID

DURA MATER

SKIN

Meningocele   Meningomyelocele

meningococcus (men-ing-gō-kok′-us): Syn., *Neisseria meningitidis.*—meningococcal, adj.

meningoencephalitis (men-ing′-gō-en-sef-al-ī′-tis): Inflammation of the brain and the meninges. May follow such infections as measles, mumps, tularemia, influenza, and some types of pneumonia.—meningoencephalitic, adj.

meningomyelocele (men-ing′-gō-mī′-el-ō-sēl): Protrusion of a portion of the spinal cord and its enclosing membranes through a bony defect in the vertebral column. Syn., myelomeningocele.

meninx (mē′-ninks): Singular of meninges (*q.v.*).

meniscectomy (men-i-sek′-to-mi): The removal of a semilunar cartilage, especially from the knee joint, following injury and displacement. The medial cartilage is damaged most commonly.

meniscus (men-is′-kus): 1. A semilunar cartilage, particularly in the knee joint. 2. The curved upper surface of a column of liquid; may be concave or convex. —menisci, pl.

menopause (men′-ō-pawz): The permanent cessation of menstruation; occurring normally between the ages of 45 and 50. The change of life. Climacteric. ARTIFICAL M., an earlier menopause induced by radiotherapy or surgery for some pathological condition.—menopausal, adj.

menorrhagia (men-ō-rā′-ji-a): An excessive regular menstrual flow.

menses (men′-sēz): The sanguineous fluid discharged from the uterus during menstruation; menstrual flow.

menstrual (men′-stroo-al): Relating to the menses. M. CYCLE, the cyclical chain of uterine and ovarian changes that result from hormonal influence and that occur in women in the time from the beginning of one menstrual period to that of the next.

menstruation (men-stroo-ā′-shun): The periodic physiologic discharge of blood, secretions, and tissue debris from the nonpregnant uterus at approximately 4-week intervals; lasts 4-5 days; commences at about age 13 and ceases at about age 45.—menstruate, v.i.; menstrual, menstruous, adj.

mental: 1. Pertaining to the chin. 2. Pertaining to the mind or intellect. M. AGE, see under **age.** M. DEFICIENCY, feeblemindedness; failure of or incomplete mental development, usually considered to be of nervous system origin and not curable; classified according to degree of intellectual capacity. M. DISEASE, one that affects the mind or intellect; insanity. M. HYGIENE, the science of maintaining mental health and preventing development of mental disorders such as neuroses and psychoses. M. INCOMPETENCE, inability to manage one's own life, affairs or property. M. RETARDATION, subnormal intellectual functioning; may be evident at birth; varies in degree from mild to severe, with IQ's from as low as 20 to as high as 68; may be accompanied by emotional disturbances and there is usually social and maturational impairment. M. TELEPATHY, ESP; mind reading. M. TEST, one given to determine one's mental capacity.

mentality (men-tal'-i-ti): Mental power or learning ability.

mentoplasty (men'-tō-plas-ti): Plastic surgery on the chin.

mer-, mero-: Denotes: (1) the thigh; (2) part, partial, or division into segments.

mercurialism (mer-kū'-ri-al-izm): Chronic poisoning from misuse of mercury as a drug or from industrial exposure to the metal or its fumes. Symptoms include stomatitis with ulceration and sloughing of the mucous membrane of the mouth, salivation, loosening of the teeth, gastroenteritis with griping and diarrhea, sometimes bloody stools, skin eruptions. In severe cases prognosis is grave.

Mercurochrome (mer-kū'-ro-krōm): A red dye containing about 25 percent of mercury in combination; formerly much used for its local antiseptic properties.

mercury (mer'-kū-ri): Quicksilver. A heavy metallic element, liquid at ordinary temperatures. M. and its salts formerly much used as purgatives, antisyphilitics, intestinal antiseptics and astringents. An important medical use is in the manufacture of various types of manometers and thermometers. Symbol is Hg.

mercy death: Euthanasia (q.v.).

mes-, meso-: Denotes: (1) in or toward the middle; (2) an intermediate connecting part: (3) the mesentery or a membrane that supports a specific part.

mesarteritis (mes-ar-ter-ī'-tis): Inflammation of the middle coat of an artery.

mescaline (mes'-ka-lēn): A hallucinogenic agent derived from small tubercles on the mescal cactus, native to Mexico and southwestern U.S. Peyote. Produces hallucinations; useful in experimental psychiatry.

mesencephalon (mes-en-sef'-a-lon): The midbrain (q.v.).

mesenteritis (mes-en-te-rī'-tis); Inflammation of the mesentery (q.v.).

mesentery (mes'-en-ter-i): A large fold of peritoneum that invests the intestines and attaches them to the posterior abdominal wall; it holds the organs in place and carries blood vessels, nerves and lymphatics to them. Usually refers specifically to the fan-shaped fold of peritoneum that encircles the small intestine (particularly the jejunum and the ileum) and attaches it to the posterior abdominal wall.

mesial (mē'-zi-al): Situated at the middle. Toward the midline of the body.

mesmerism (mes'-mer-izm): 1. The induction of hypnosis by the method practiced by Mesmer and believed to involve animal magnetism; broadly, hypnotism. 2. Intense fascination.—mesmerize, v.t. [Franz A. Mesmer, Austrian physician. 1733-1815.]

mesocolon (mes-ō-kō'-lon): The fold of peritoneum that attaches the colon to the posterior abdominal wall.

mesoderm (mes'-ō-derm): The middle one of the three primary germ layers of the embryo; from it are developed all connective tissues, bone, muscle, cartilage, circulatory and lymphatic tissues, the lining of serous cavities and of the organs of the genitourinary tract. It lies between the ectoderm and the entoderm (q.v.).—mesodermal, adj.

mesothelioma (mes-ō-thē-li-ō'-ma): A tumor originating in the mesothelium (q.v.). One type is a rapidly fatal tumor that spreads over the pleural covering of the lung; of current interest because of its association with the asbestos industry.

mesothelium (mes-ō-thē'-li-um): Tissue that develops from the mesoderm (q.v.) of the embryo and forms the epithelial layer covering of all serous membranes, e.g., peritoneum. See **epithelium.**

meta-: Denotes: (1) change, transformation in: (2) between, among, after, over, along with.

metabolic (met-a-bol'-ik); Pertaining to metabolism. BASAL M. RATE (BMR), the figure that expresses the amount of energy (heat) released in the body, based on the amount of oxygen utilized and carbon dioxide produced in a given period of time when the body is at complete rest in a warm atmosphere at least 12 hours after the ingestion of food.—metabolically, adv. See **metabolism.**

metabolism (me-tab'-ō-lizm): The series of physical and chemical changes in the body by which nutrition is effected, energy is provided for life processes, and life is maintained. The tissues are broken down by wear and tear (catabolism) and rebuilt (anabolism) continuously.—metabolic, adj. BASAL M., the energy used by a body at complete rest, being the minimum necessary to maintain life.

metabolite (me-tab'-ō-līt): Any product of metabolism. ESSENTIAL M., a substance necessary for proper metabolism, e.g., vitamins.

metacarpal (met-a-kar'-pal): 1. Pertaining to that part of the hand called the metacarpus (*q. v.*). 2. Any one of the five bones of the metacarpus.

metacarpophalangeal (met-a-kar-pō-fal-an′-jē-al): Pertaining to the metacarpus and the phalanges.

metacarpus (met-a-kar′-pus): The five bones which form that part of the hand between the wrist and fingers.—metacarpal, adj.

metamorphopsia (met-a-mor-fop′-si-a): A disturbance of vision in which the shapes of objects seen are distorted.

metamorphosis (met-a-mor′-fo-sis): 1. A change in the shape, size, function or structure of a substance. 2. A transition from one stage of development to another.

metaphase (met′-a-fāz): The middle stage in mitotic cell division; it is the stage at which the chromosomes separate in a particular manner. See **mitosis.**

metaphysis (me-taf′-i-sis): That part of a long bone that lies between the shaft (diaphysis) and the extremity (epiphysis). During the growth period it consists of spongy bone; after growth is completed, it is continuous with the epiphysis.—metaphyses, pl.; metaphyseal, adj.

metaplasia (met-a-plā′-zi-a): Conversion of one type of tissue into another, *e.g.,* cartilage into bone.—metaplastic, adj.

metastasis (me-tas′-ta-sis): 1. The transference of disease from the original site to another part of the body, usually by blood or lymph, and resulting in development of a similar lesion at the new site. 2. A secondary growth that results from the transference of disease to a site distant from the original lesion. Term is used particularly with reference to malignant growths.—metastases, pl.; metastatic, adj.; metastasize, v.

metatarsal (met-a-tar′-sal): 1. Pertaining to that part of the foot called the metatarsus (*q. v.*). 2. Any one of the five bones of the metatarsus.

metatarsalgia (met-a-tar-sal′-ji-a): Pain under the heads of the metatarsal bones where they articulate with the phalanges.

metatarsophalangeal (met-a-tar-sō-fal-an′-jē-al): Pertaining to the metatarsus and the phalanges.

metatarsus (met-a-tar′-sus): The five bones that form the skeleton of that part of the foot between the ankle and toes.—metatarsal, adj.

Metchnikoff's theory: The theory that invading bacteria or other disease-producing agents are attacked and destroyed by the phagocytes (*q. v.*) and that this activity produces inflammation. [Elie Metchnikoff, Russian zoologist in Paris. 1845-1916.]

meteorism (mē′-tē-or-izm): Excessive accumulation of gas in the intestines. Tympanites.

meter, metre (mē′-ter): 1. Basic unit of length in the metric system; equivalent to approximately 39.37 inches. 2. An apparatus for measuring the quantity of anything passing through it.

-meter: Refers to: (1) a measurement; (2) an instrument used in making a measurement.

methadone treatment: The treatment of a person addicted to a drug, usually heroin, with methadone, a narcotic which is also addicting but less socially disabling than heroin.

methane (meth′-ān): Marsh gas; the colorless, odorless, flammable gas that is given off by decomposing organic matter.

methemoglobin (met-hē-mō-glō′-bin): A form of hemoglobin consisting of a combination of globin with an oxidized heme, containing ferric iron. This pigment is unable to transport oxygen. M. may be formed following the administration of a wide variety of drugs, including the sulfonamides. M. may be present in blood as a result of a congenital abnormality.

methemoglobinemia (met-hē-mō-glō-bin-ē′-mi-a): Methemoglobin in the blood. If large quantities are present, individuals may show cyanosis, but otherwise no abnormality except, in severe cases, breathlessness on exertion, because the methemoglobin cannot transport oxygen.—methemoglobinemic, adj.

methemoglobinuria (met-hē-mō-glō-bin-ūr′-i-a): Methemoglobin in the urine.—methemoglobinuric, adj.

methionine (me-thī′-o-nēn): One of the sulphur-containing amino acids; essential for growth in infants and for maintenance of nitrogen equilibrium in adults. Occasionally used therapeutically in hepatitis and other conditions associated with liver damage.

methyl alcohol: Wood alcohol. See **alcohol.**

metr-, metro-: Denotes the uterus.

metra: The uterus.

metratonia (mē-tra-tō′-ni-a): Atony of the uterus.

metratrophia (mē-tra-trō′-fi-a): Atrophy of the uterus.

metric system: A system of weights and measures, invented and first used in France in the late 18th century. Now used in most countries except English-speaking ones but even in these it is now used for scientific purposes. Employs a decimal scale. The unit of weight is the gram, of length is the meter, and of capacity is the liter.

metritis (mē-trī′-tis): Inflammation of the uterus.

metrocele (mē′-trō-sēl): Hernia of the uterus.

metrocolpocele (mē-trō-kol′-pō-sēl): A hernia of the uterus into the vagina; prolapse of the uterus.

metrodynia (mē-trō-din′-i-a): Pain in the uterus.

metrofibroma (mē-trō-fī-brō′-ma): A fibroma of the uterus.

metropathia hemorrhagica (mē-trō-path′-i-a hem-or-aj′-ik-a): Irregular episodes of uterine bleeding due to excessive and unopposed estrin in the bloodstream. Usually associated with a follicular cyst in the ovary.

metroptosis (mē-trop-tō′-sis): Prolapse (falling) of the uterus.

metrorrhagia (mē-trō-rā′-ji-a): Uterine bleeding between the menstrual periods.

metrorrhexis (mē-tro-rek′-is): Rupture of the uterus.

mg: Abbreviation for milligram (*q.v.*).

mi-, mio-: Denotes less, fewer, slightly.

Michel's clips (mi′-shels): Small metal clips used instead of sutures for the closure of a wound.

micr-, micro-: Denotes: (1) small or minute size or amount (opp. to macro-); (2) abnormal smallness, *e.g.*, microcephalia; (3) instruments or objects used in dealing with minute objects, *e.g.*, microscope, microtome; (4) one one-millionth part (metric system).

micrencephaly (mī-kren-sef′-a-li): Abnormal smallness of the brain.—micrencephalic, adj. Also micrencephalia, microencephaly.

microanatomy (mī-krō-a-nat′-o-mi): Histology (*q.v.*).

microangiopathy (mī-krō-an-ji-op′-a-thi): Disease of the small blood vessels.

microbe (mī′-krōb): A microscopic organism, especially one capable of causing disease. Syn., microorganism.—microbial, microbic, adj.

microbiology (mī-krō-bī-ol′-o-ji): The science of microorganisms.

microbrachia (mī-krō-brā′-ki-a): Abnormal smallness of the arms.

microcephalic (mī-krō-sef-al′-ik): 1. Pertaining to an abnormally small head. 2. An individual with an unusually small head.

microcephaly (mī-krō-sef′-a-li): Abnormal smallness of the head.—microcephalic, adj.

Micrococcus (mī-krō-kok′-us): A genus of bacteria. Gram-positive spherical bacteria occurring in irregular masses. They comprise saprophytes, parasites and pathogens.

microcurie (mī-krō-kū′-rē): A unit of radioactivity; one one-millionth of a curie.

microcyte (mī′-krō-sīt): An undersized red blood cell found in anemic blood.—microcytic, adj.

microcytosis (mī-krō-sī-tō′-sis): An abnormal number of microcytes in the circulating blood.

microdissection (mī-krō-di-sek′-shun): Dissection of cells or tissues under the microscope.

Microfilaria: The embryos of **Filaria** (*q.v.*). Cause filariasis (*q.v.*).

micrognathia (mī-krō-nā′-thi-a): Small jaw, especially the lower one.

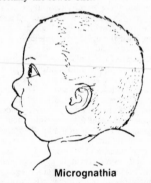

Micrognathia

microgram (mī′-krō-gram): One one-thousandth of a milligram; one one-millionth of a gram. Represented by the symbol μg. Abbreviated mcg.

micron (mī′-kron): A unit of length in the metric system; used for measuring blood cell diameters and bacteria, one one-thousandth of a millimeter or one one-millionth of a meter. Approximately 1/25,000 of an inch. Represented by the Greek letter μ.

microorganism (mī-krō-or′-gan-izm): A microscopic cell. (Often synonymous with bacterium but includes virus, protozoon, rickettsia, fungus, alga, and lichen.)

microphage (mī′-krō-fāj): A very small phagocyte (*q.v.*).

microphotograph (mī-krō-fō′-tō-graf): A small photograph of a microscopic object;

it is usually magnified for viewing and interpreting. See **photomicrograph.**

microphysics (mī-krō-fiz′-iks): That branch of physics that deals with molecules, atoms, and elementary particles of matter.

microplasia (mī-krō-plā′-zi-a): Dwarfism.

micropodia (mī-krō-pō′-di-a): Abnormal smallness of the feet.

micropsia (mī-krop′-si-a): A pathological condition in which objects appear to be smaller than they actually are. Micropia.—microptic, adj.

microscope (mī′-krō-skōp): An instrument consisting of a lens or an arrangement of lenses for making enlarged images of minute cells or objects. BINOCULAR M., one that has two eyepieces. COMPOUND M., one that has two lens systems. ELECTRON M., one in which an electric beam causes an image to be projected on a fluorescent screen where it may be viewed or photographed. SIMPLE M., one that has only one lens; a magnifying glass.

microscopic (mī-krō-skop′-ik): Extremely small; visible only with the aid of a microscope.

Microsporum (mī-krō-spō′-rum): A genus of fungi which causes various superficial cutaneous infections. Parasitic, living in keratin-containing tissues of man and animals. Cause of ringworm. *M. audouini* is the commonest cause of scalp ringworm.

microsurgery (mī-krō-ser′-jer-i): Dissection or the performance of surgery under a microscope or magnifying lens. Micromanipulation.

microtome (mī′-krō-tōm): An instrument for making thin sections of tissue for microscopic study.

microwave (mī′-krō-wāv): An electromagnetic wave of very short length and high frequency.

micturiton (mik-tū-rish′-un): The act of passing urine.—micturate, v.

midbrain: The mesencephalon; that short portion of the brain stem that lies just above the pons and just below the cerebrum; it connects the cerebrum with the pons and the cerebellum.

midget (mij′-et): An individual who is smaller than normal, but whose organs and parts are perfectly formed.

midriff (mid′-rif): 1. The diaphragm (*q.v.*). 2. The middle region of the human torso, particularly the front external aspect.

midwife (mid′-wīf): A woman who attends women in childbirth. Accoucheuse (*q.v.*).

midwifery (mid′-wīf-ri): The practice of delivering babies or of assisting women in childbirth, by women who are not physicians but who are trained in obstetrical procedures.

migraine (mī′-grān): Hemicrania. A syndrome characterized by recurring throbbing headache, usually unilateral initially; of unknown cause. Symptoms include photophobia, nausea, vomiting. More common in women than men; often there is a family history of M.; may result from unconscious emotional conflicts; when severe may result in incapacitation.

migration (mī-grā′-shun): In physiology, the passage of leukocytes through the walls of vessels into tissue spaces in order to combat organisms that have invaded tissues.

Mikulicz's disease: Chronic hypertrophic enlargement of the lacrimal and salivary glands. Of unknown etiology, but now thought to be an auto-immune process. [Johannes von Mikulicz-Radecki, Rumanian surgeon. 1850-1905.]

miliaria (mil-i-ā′-ri-a): An inflammatory skin condition characterized by vesicular and erythematous eruption caused by blocking of sweat ducts, and their subsequent rupture, or their infection by bacteria or fungi. Often accompanied by burning, itching, prickling sensation. Common in the tropics. Prickly heat.

miliary (mil′-i-a-ri): Resembling a millet seed. M. TUBERCULOSIS, a form in which minute tuberculous nodules are widely disseminated throughout the organs and tissues of the body.

milieu (mē-lyuh′): Environment; surroundings. M. THERAPY, treatment, usually psychiatric, in a carefully structured environment in which all elements such as furnishings, equipment, staff, etc. enhance the medical therapy and help the patient toward rehabilitation.

milium (mil′-i-um): A condition in which small, pearly nodules or papules form in the skin, especially of the face and particularly about the eyelids; due to retention of secretion from a sebaceous gland.— milia, pl.

milk leg: Phlegmasia alba dolens (*q.v.*).

milk sugar: Lactose.

Miller-Abbott tube: A double-lumen rubber tube with an inflatable balloon at the distal end; used in diagnosis and treatment of obstructive lesions of the small intestine. [Thomas Grier Miller, American physician. 1886- . William Osler Abbott, American physician. 1902-1943.]

milli-: Denotes one one-thousandth part (metric system).

millicurie (mil-li-kū′-rē): A unit of radioactivity; one one-thousandth of a curie. Abbreviated mc.

milligram (mil′-li-gram): One one-thousandth of a gram. Approximately 0.015 grains. Abbreviated mg.

milliliter (mil′-li-lē-ter): One one-thousandth of a liter or 1 cc. Approximately 16 minims. Abbreviated ml.

millimeter (mil′-li-mē-ter): One one-thousandth of a meter. Approximately 1/25 of an inch. Abbreviated mm.

millimicron (mil-li-mī′-kron): One one-thousandth of a micron (q.v.). Abbreviated mμ.

mineralocorticoid (min-er-al-ō-kor′-ti-koid): A secretion of the adrenal cortex that affects the fluid and electrolyte balance of the body chiefly through its influence on sodium retention and potassium loss from the body. See **aldosterone.**

miner's anemia: Ancylostomiasis (q.v.).

miner's elbow: Inflammation of the bursa over the point of the elbow. Syn., student's elbow.

min: Abbreviation for minim. Also m. (Should be written out because min may be confused with minute and m with meter.)

minim (min′-im); A unit of capacity in the apothecaries' system, being one-sixtieth of a fluid dram. Abbreviated min. or m., but often written out to avoid confusion.

minimum lethal dose: The smallest dose that will cause death. Abbreviated MLD.

minor: In surgery, an operation in which the risk of death and the death rate are negligible.

miosis (mī-ō′-sis); Contraction of the pupil of the eye.

miotic (mī-ot′-ik): Pertaining to or producing miosis.

miscarriage (mis-kar′-ij): Expulsion of the fetus before it is viable, i.e., before the 28th week.

miscegenation (mis-e-je-nā′-shun): Intermarriage or cohabitation between persons of different races.

mistura (mis-tū′-ra): A mixture.

mit-, mito-: Denotes: (1) thread or thread-like: (2) mitosis.

mite (mīt): Minute animal that is parasitic on man and that produces various skin irritations.

mitochondria (mī-tō-kon′-dri-a): Filament-like structures and granules in the cytoplasm of the cell, disclosed by differential staining.

mitosis (mī-tō′-sis): A complicated method of indirect cell division occurring in specialized cells.—mitotic, adj.

mitral (mī′-tral): 1. Mitre-shaped. 2. Pertaining to the bicuspid valve between the left atrium and the left ventricle of the heart. M. INCOMPETENCE, a defect in the closure of the mitral valve whereby blood tends to flow backward into the left atrium when the valve is closed. M. STENOSIS, narrowing of the mitral orifice, usually due to the formation of fibrous tissue as a result of rheumatic fever. M. VALVULOTOMY (VALVOTOMY), an operation for splitting the cusps of a stenosed mitral valve.

mixture (miks′-tūr): A combination of two or more substances, usually in liquid form, with each substance retaining its particular physical characteristics.

ml: Abbreviation for milliliter (q.v.).

MLD: Minimum lethal dose (q.v.).

mm: Abbreviation for millimeter (q.v.).

MMPI: Abbreviation for Minnesota Multiphasic Personality Inventory. A device for self-rating. It measures various aspects of personality. Used often to test patients over 16 years of age who have various kinds of psychological disorders.

mnemonics (nē-mon′-iks): The science of improving the memory, or the techniques used for this purpose. M. DEVICE, a scheme for aiding the memory by establishing an artificial relationship between two things that are normally not related.

mobilization (mō-bi-li-zā′-shun): The process by which a fixed part is made movable, or motion is restored to an ankylosed joint. STAPES M., surgery to correct immobility of the stapes; used in treating certain types of deafness.

modiolus (mō-dī′-ō-lus): The central, bony pillar of the cochlea, around which the spiral canal winds.

modus (mō′-dus): Manner. M. OPERANDI, a way of performing an operation or of working.

molar teeth (mō′-lar): The double teeth or grinders, three on either side of each jaw.

mold (mōld): Multicellular fungus. Often used synonymously with fungus. Member of the plant kingdom with no differentiation into root, stem or leaf, and without chlorophyll. Structurally consists of filaments or hyphae, which aggregate into a mass of cobwebby filaments called mycelium. Propagation is by means of spores. Occurs in infinite variety, as common saprophytes contaminating foodstuffs, and more rarely as pathogens.

mole (mōl): Lay term for a nevus; a circumscribed, pigmented, elevated area on the skin. CARNEOUS M., the dead and organized remains of a fetus that has died in utero. HYDATIDIFORM M., a condition in which the chorionic villi of the placenta undergo cystic degeneration and the fetus is absorbed; may be a harmless condition safely corrected, but a proportion of these moles are active and if remnants are left in the uterus after abortion of the mole, malignant changes may ensue, giving rise to a chorionepithelioma (q.v.).

molecule (mol′-e-kūl): The smallest particle into which matter can be divided and still retain its identity.—molecular, adj.

mollities (mol-ish′-i-ēz): Softness. M. OSSIUM, osteomalacia (q.v.).

molluscum (mol-us′-kum): A soft tumor. M. CONTAGIOSUM, a mildly contagious type of wart that appears especially on the face, buttocks, and perineum as a waxy papule, often umbilicated; spread is by autoinoculation. M. FIBROSUM, the superficial tumors of Recklinghausen's disease (q.v.).

mon-, mono-: Denotes: (1) involving, affecting, or having a single element or part; (2) restricted to one.

monarticular (mon-ar-tik′-ū-lar): Relating to or affecting only one joint.

monaural (mon-aw′-al): 1. Pertaining to one ear. 2. One ear functioning alone. 3. Hearing with one ear.

Mönckeberg's sclerosis: Senile degenerative change resulting in calcification of the medial coat in arteries, especially of the limbs; leads to intermittent claudication or gangrene. [Johann Georg Mönckeberg, German pathologist. 1877-1925.]

mongol (mong′-gol): A person affected with mongolism (q.v.).—mongoloid, adj.

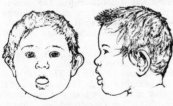

Mongolism

mongolism (mong′-gol-izm): Down's syndrome. Refers to a type of congenital mentally subnormal child, with facial characteristics resembling the Mongolian races. Stigmata include oval tilted eyes, short,

flat-bridged nose, flattened occiput, broad hands and feet with widened space between first and second digits, stubby fingers, and generally retarded growth. Results from abnormality of chromosome 21. Two types: (1) Failure of division of chromosome 21 results in an extra chromosome instead of the normal pair. The infant has 47 chromosomes. Usually born of elderly mothers. (2) Abnormality of chromosome 21, total number of 46 being normal. Usually born of young mothers. High risk of recurrence in subsequent pregnancies.

Monilia (mo-nil′-i-a): The generic name for a large group of fungi or molds; those that are pathogenic are now more commonly called Candida (q.v.).

moniliasis (mon-il-ī′-a-sis): Disease caused by infection with species of Monilia (Candida). Candidiasis (q.v.).

moniliform (mo-nil′-i-form): Like a string of beads; beaded. Used to describe the arrangement of microorganisms, or clinical features such as a skin rash.

monitor (mon′-i-tor): 1. To constantly watch, observe or check on a state or condition. 2. An electronic apparatus that is attached to the patient and automatically records such physical signs as respiration, pulse and blood pressure; may be employed in caring for an anesthetized person who is undergoing or recuperating from surgery or some other procedure.

monoblepsia (mon-ō-blep′-si-a): A condition of vision in which one is able to see better with only one eye than with two. The term is also applied to color blindness in which all colors appear to be the same.

monochromatic (mon-ō-krō-mat′-ik): 1. Existing in one color only. 2. Staining with only one dye at a time. 3. A person who exhibits monochromatism (q.v.).

monochromatism (mon-ō-krō′-ma-tizm): Complete color blindness; all colors appear as shades of gray. A rare disorder.

monococcus (mon-ō-kok′-us): A coccus that occurs singly, not in pairs, chains, or groups.

monocular (mon-ok′-ū-lar): Pertaining to or affecting one eye only. See **microscope.**

monocyte (mon′-ō-sīt): A large mononuclear leukocyte.—monocytic, adj.

monocytopenia (mon-ō-sī-tō-pē′-ni-a): Less than the normal number of monocytes in the circulating blood.

monocytosis (mon-ō-sī-tō′-sis): An abnormal increase in the proportion of leukocytes in the circulating blood. The normal value is 3-8% of the total leukocyte count.

monogenesis (mon-ō-jen′-e-sis): Nonsexual reproduction.

monomania (mon-ō-mā′-ni-a): Obsessed with a single idea or group of ideas.

mononuclear (mon-ō-nū′-klē-ar): With a single nucleus. Usually refers to a type of blood cell (monocyte), the largest of the cells in the normal blood with a round, oval or indented nucleus.

mononucleosis (mon-ō-nū-klē-ō′-sis): An increase in the number of circulating monocytes (mononuclear cells) in the blood. IN-FECTIOUS M. is an acute infectious type of M., probably caused by a virus; characterized by sudden onset, fever, malaise, sore throat, enlargement of lymph nodes and spleen. Occurs most frequently between the ages of 20 and 30 and is usually self-limited and benign.

monophasia (mon-ō-fā′-zi-a): Aphasia in which the individual is able to utter only one word or phrase and repeats it constantly.

monoplegia (mon-ō-plē′-ji-a): Paralysis of only one limb, or of one muscle or group of muscles.—monoplegic, adj.

monorchidism (mon-or′-ki-dizm): Having only one testis, or the condition of only one testis having descended into the scrotum. Monorchism.

monosaccharide (mon-ō-sak′-a-rīd): A simple sugar ($C_6H_{12}O_6$). Examples are glucose, fructose and galactose.

monosexual (mon-ō-seks′-ū-al): Having the characteristics of only one sex.

monovular (mon-ov′-ū-lar): Pertaining to a single ovum; or derived from a single ovum, as identical twins.

monoxide (mon-ok′-sīd): An oxide in which the molecules have only one atom of oxygen. Commonly used by the laity instead of 'carbon monoxide.'

monster (mon′-ster): Term formerly much used to describe an infant grossly malformed at birth as a result of faulty development. Many are born dead or die soon after birth; in a few cases surgery can be performed to correct the anomaly.

mons veneris (mons ven′-er-is): The eminence formed by the pad of fat which lies over the pubic bone in the female.

mood: A prevailing attitude or state of mind. In psychiatry, a sustained emotional state such as melancholia or mania.

morbid (mor′-bid): Diseased. Pertaining to, affected by, or productive of disease. Grisly or gruesome. M. ANATOMY, that branch of anatomy that is concerned with the study of diseased tissues and organs.

morbidity (mor-bid′-i-ti): 1. The state of being sick or diseased. 2. The sick rate; the ratio of sick persons or of cases of disease to the number of well persons in a specified community.

morbific (mor-bif′-ik): Causing disease; pathogenic.

morbilli (mor-bil′-lī): Measles (q.v.).

morbilliform (mor-bil′-i-form): Describes a rash resembling that of measles.

morbus (mor′-bus): Disease.

mores (mō′-rēz): The fixed customs of a particular group. Habits; manners; moral code.

morgue (morg): A place where dead bodies are placed temporarily until they are identified or claimed for burial.

moribund (mor′-i-bund): In a dying state.

morning sickness: Nausea and vomiting when arising in the morning, especially that which occurs during the first 4 to 16 weeks of pregnancy.

moron (mō′-ron): A feebleminded person with a potential mental age of 8 to 12 years and an IQ of 50 to 70, thus ranking him below normal and highest in the group of mental defectives (the other two grades are imbecile and idiot).

morph-, morpho-: Denotes form, shape, type, structure.

-morph, -morphous: Denotes shape or form.

morphea (mor′-fē-a): Localized scleroderma (q.v.).

morphine (mor′-fēn): The active principle of opium and a valuable narcotic, hypnotic, and analgesic. Habit-forming, thus its sale and distribution are controlled by federal law.

morphinism (mor′-fin-izm): Addiction to morphine.

morphology (mor-fol′-o-ji): The science that deals with the form and structure of living things, apart from their functions.—morphological, adj.; morphologically, adv.

mortal: 1. Fatal; causing or resulting in death. 2. Human.

mortality (mor-tal′-i-ti): 1. The quality of being mortal (q.v.). 2. The death rate; the number of deaths in a unit of population occurring within a prescribed time. Mortality rates for deaths from all causes are usually expressed as number of deaths per 1000 population.

mortician (mor-tish′-an): A funeral director. An undertaker; one who is trained to care for the dead.

mortification (mor-ti-fi-kā′-shun): Local death of tissue. See **gangrene.**

mother complex: Oedipus complex (*q.v.*).

motile (mō′-til): Capable of spontaneous movement.—motility, n.

motion sickness: Nausea and usually vomiting due to stimulation of the semicircular canals caused by the irregular or rhythmic motion of an airplane, car or boat, or by swinging.

motivation (mō-ti-vā′-shun): Drive; incentive.

motor: Pertaining to action or motion. See **neuron.**

mottling (mot′-ling): Discoloration of the skin with patches of varying size, shape and color.

mould (mōld): Mold (*q.v.*).

moulding (mōld′-ing): The shaping of the fetal head in adjustment to the shape and size of the birth canal during the passage of the fetus through the canal in labor.

mountain sickness: Symptoms of sickness, tachycardia and dyspnea, due to low oxygen content of rarefied air at a high altitude.

mouth: An aperture or opening into a cavity; specifically the opening through which food passes into the body.

mouth-to-mouth resuscitation: See **resuscitation.**

movement: 1. Motion; the act of moving. 2. The act of emptying the colon; defecation. 3. The material evacuated from the rectum during one bowel movement; the stool.

mucin (mū′-sin): A mixture of glycoproteins found in or secreted by many cells and glands. The chief constituent of mucus.—mucinous, adj.

mucinolysis (mū-sin-ol′-i-sis): Dissolution of mucin.—mucinolytic, adj.

mucocele (mū′-kō-sēl): 1. Distension of a cavity with mucus. 2. A cyst or cyst-like structure that contains mucus.

mucocutaneous (mū-kō-kū-tā′-nē-us): Pertaining to mucous membrane and skin.

mucoid (mū′-koid): Resembling mucus.

mucolysis (mū-kol′-i-sis): Dissolution of mucus.—mucolytic, adj.

mucoprotein (mū-kō-prō′-tē-in): One of a group of complex protein compounds that occur in body tissues and fluids; has chemical characteristics of a protein but does not coagulate when heated.

mucopurulent (mū-kō-pū′-rū-lent): Containing mucus and pus.

mucopus (mū′-kō-pus): Mucus containing pus.

mucor (mū′-kor): A general name for a variety of molds that are frequently found on dead or decaying vegetable matter; some of them are pathogenic to man.

mucosa (mū-kō′-sa): A mucous membrane (*q.v.*).—mucosal, adj.; mucosae, pl.

mucosanguineous (mū-kō-sang-gwin′-ē-us): Composed of both mucus and blood.

mucous (mū′-kus): Pertaining to, secreting or containing mucus. See **membrane.** M. COLITIS, mucomembranous colitis; possibly a functional disorder, manifested by passage of mucus in the stool, obstinate constipation and occasional colic. M. POLYPUS, condition in which the mucous membrane becomes pedunculated and projects from the surface in polypoid masses.

mucoviscidosis (mū-kō-vis-id-ō′-sis): A congenital hereditary disease with failure of development of normal mucus-secreting glands, sweat glands and pancreas. May be present in a baby as meconium ileus; in infancy with septic bronchitis and steatorrhea. Stools contain excess fat; trypsin is absent from stool and duodenal juice. See **cystic, fibrosis.**

mucus (mū′-kus): The viscid fluid secreted by the mucous glands. Contains mucin and such other substances as inorganic salts, epithelial cells, leukocytes, and water.

multi-: Denotes: (1) multiple, many, much; (2) affecting many parts.

multiarticular (mul-ti-ar-tik′-ū-lar): Pertaining to or affecting several joints.

multicellular (mul-ti-sel′-ū-lar): Constructed of many cells.

multiglandular (mul-ti-gland′-ū-lar): Pertaining to or affecting several glands.

multigravida (mul-ti-grav′-id-a): A woman who has been pregnant more than once.—multigravidae, pl.

multilobar (mul-ti-lō′-bar): Possessing several lobes.

multilobular (mul-ti-lob′-ū-lar): Possessing many lobules.

multilocular (mul-ti-lok′-ū-lar): Possessing many small cysts, loculi or pockets.

multinuclear (mul-ti-nūk′-lē-ar): Possessing many nuclei.—multinucleate, adj.

multipara (mul-tip′-a-ra): A woman who has had two or more pregnancies resulting in viable children. Written Para II, III, etc.—multiparae, pl.; multiparous, adj.

multiple sclerosis: See **sclerosis.**

multivalent (mul-ti-vā′-lent): 1. In chemistry, having the power of combining with three or more univalent atoms. 2. Pertaining to an agent that is effective against sev-

mumps

eral varieties or strains of a certain microorganism.

mumps: An acute, infectious disease, characterized by inflammation of one or both parotid (*q.v.*) glands; caused by a filterable virus. The chief symptom is a sensitive swelling below and in front of the ear and edema of the surrounding tissues, distorting the features. The most common complication in the adult male is orchitis, in the female, ovaritis and mastitis. Syn., epidemic parotitis.

mummification (mum-i-fi-kā′-shun): 1. Dry gangrene. 2. The drying up of a dead fetus in the uterus. 3. Restraining a patient by wrapping in a sheet; used to keep mental patients from injuring themselves and others and to restrain a restive child during an operation or other procedure.

mummy restraint: A type of physical restraint in which the entire body is wrapped in a sheet or blanket and only the head is exposed.

mural (mū′-ral): Pertaining to or occurring in the wall of a cavity, organ or vessel.

muriatic acid (mū-ri-at′-ik as′-id): Hydrochloric acid (*q.v.*).

murmur: An abnormal, usually soft, blowing sound, not necessarily significant, sometimes heard on auscultation of the heart and great vessels, in addition to the normal heart sounds. May be heard during systole or diastole, or both, and may be functional or organic. PRESYSTOLIC M., occurs just before the systole and is usually due to stenosis of one of the atrioventricular orifices. SYSTOLIC M., abnormal quality of the first heart sound usually related to the area of one of the heart valves, *e.g.*, systolic mitral murmur.

Murphy drip: The continual slow drip of a fluid into the body, usually into the rectum, or the apparatus used for administering fluid in this way.

Musca domestica (mus′-ka dom-es′-ti-ka): The common house fly, capable of transmitting many organisms pathogenic to man.

muscae volitantes (mus′-kē vol-i-tan′-tēz): The sensation of moving spots before the eyes. Caused by the presence of cells or cell fragments in the vitreous humor.

muscle (mus′l): Strong, contractile tissue that produces movement in or of the body. Classified according to structure, muscle tissue is striated (striped), nonstriated (smooth), and indistinctly striated. Also classified according to whether it is voluntary (under conscious control) or involuntary (under control of the autonomic nervous system). Characteristics of muscle tissue are contractility, excitability, extensibility and elasticity. CARDIAC M. forms the walls of the heart, is indistinctly striated and involuntary. SKELETAL M. surrounds the skeleton, is striated and voluntary. VISCERAL M. (internal) is nonstriated (except for the heart) and involuntary.—muscular, adj.

muscle-bound: Having some of one's muscles enlarged, tense, and lacking in elasticity; usually due to overexercise.

muscul-, musculo-: Denotes muscle, muscular.

muscular (mus′-kū-lar): 1. Pertaining to a muscle or muscles. 2. Descriptive of an individual with well-developed muscles.

muscular dystrophy (mus-kū-lar dis′-trō-fē): A hereditary disease characterized by progressive atrophy and wasting away of muscles. Affects primarily children or young adults. Of unknown cause; several types are identified. **Pseudohypertrophic** or **Duchenne** type is the most severe; onset usually before five years of age; runs a malignant course; characterized by such symptoms as pseudohypertrophy of muscles followed by atrophy, skeletal deformities, lordosis, protruding abdomen, congestive heart failure; respiratory infections are a common complication.

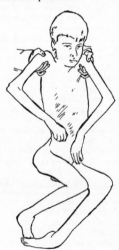

Muscular dystrophy

musculature (mus'-kū-la-tūr): The muscular system or any part of it.

musculocutaneous (mus'-kū-lō-kū-tā'-nē-us): Pertaining to both muscle and skin.

musculomembranous (mus-kū-lō-mem'-bran-us): Pertaining to both muscle and membrane. Descriptive of such muscles as the occipitofrontalis which is largely membranous.

musculoskeletal (mus-kū-lō-skel'-e-tal): Pertaining to the muscular and skeletal systems.

musculotendinous (mus-kū-lō-ten'-din-us): Pertaining to or composed of muscle and tendon.

musicomania (mū-zi-kō-mā'-ni-a): An insane love of music.

musicotherapy (mū-zi-kō-ther'-a-pi): The use of music in the treatment of disease; most frequently used for patients with nervous or mental disorders.

mussitation (mus-i-tā'-shun): Movement of the lips without producing sound; sometimes seen in delirious patients.

mutant (mū'-tant): A cell which is the result of a genetic change. It has characteristics that are different from those of its parents and that can be passed on to its offspring. A sport.

mutation (mū-tā'-shun): 1. A transformation or change in form, quality, or some other characteristic. 2. A genetic change in the germ plasm of a cell which results in a change of the characters of the cell. This change is heritable, remaining until further mutation occurs. INDUCED M., a gene mutation produced by a known agent outside the cell, *e.g.,* ultraviolet radiation. NATURAL M., a gene mutation taking place without apparent influence from outside the cell.

mute (mūt): 1. Unable to speak. 2. A person who is unable to speak. DEAF-M., a person who is unable to speak or to hear.

mutilate (mū'-ti-lāt): To maim or disfigure the body by removing, destroying or deforming some essential and conspicuous part.—mutilation, n.

mutism (mū'-tizm): In psychiatry, refusal to speak; may be conscious or unconscious; often seen in psychotic patients.

my-, myo-: Denotes muscle.

myalgia (mī-al'-ji-a): Pain in the muscles.—myalgic, adj.

myasthenia (mī-as-thē'-ni-a): Muscular weakness. M. GRAVIS, a progressive disorder, seen mostly in adults 20 to 50 years of age; characterized by marked fatigability of voluntary muscles, especially those of the face, lip, tongue, throat and neck, and eye. The patient has a characteristic sleepy expression due to ptosis of the eyelids and weakness of the facial muscles.

myatonia (mī-a-tō'-ni-a): Absence of tone in muscle. M. CONGENITA, a form of congenital muscular dystrophy in infancy. Child is unable to bear the weight of the head on the shoulders.—myatonic, adj.

myatrophy (mī-at'-rō-fi): Atrophy of muscle.

myc-, myceto-, myco-: Denotes fungus.

mycelium (mī-sē'-li-um): The tangled mass of branching filaments (hyphae) that represents the body of a mold or fungus.—mycelial, mycelian, mycelioid, adj.

mycetoma (mī-sē-tō'-ma): A fungus infection, usually of the feet, occurring in tropical and subtropical regions. Similar to actinomycosis and aspergillosis (*q.v.*). Syn., Madura foot, maduromycosis.

Mycobacterium (mī-kō-bak-tē'-ri-um): Small slender rod bacteria, gram-positive and acid-fast, both to a varying degree. Saprophytic, commensal and pathogenic species. *M. tuberculosis* causes tuberculosis; *M. leprae,* leprosy.

mycology (mī-kol'-o-ji): The study of fungi.—mycologist, n.; mycological, adj.; mycologically, adv.

Mycoplasma (mī-kō-plaz'-ma): A genus of microorganisms intermediate in size between viruses and bacteria; includes the pleuropneumonia-like organisms (PPLO); important in respiratory diseases. One type is associated with acute leukemia.

mycoprotein (mī-kō-prō'-te-in): The protein in fungi or bacteria.

mycosis (mī-kō'-sis): Any disease caused by a fungus. May be superficial affecting only the skin and its appendages, or systemic.—mycotic, adj. M. FUNGOIDES is a chronic and usually fatal disease; not fungal in origin. It is manifested by general pruritus, followed by skin eruptions of diverse character which become infiltrated and finally develop into granulomatous ulcerating tumors. A form of reticulo-endothelial disease.

mydriasis (mid-rī'-a-sis): Abnormal dilatation of the pupil of the eye.

mydriatics (mid-ri-at'-iks): Drugs which cause mydriasis (*q.v.*).

myectomy (mī-ek'-to-mi): Surgical removal of part of a muscle.

myel-, myelo-: Denotes: (1) bone marrow; (2) spinal cord.

myelencephalitis (mī-el-en-sef′-a-lī-tis): In-flammation of the brain and spinal cord.

myelic (mī-el′-ik): Pertaining or refer-ring to (1) bone marrow; (2) the spinal cord.

myelin (mī′-e-lin): The white, fatty sub-stance constituting the medullary sheath of certain nerve fibers.

myelitis (mī-e-lī′-tis): Inflammation of (1) the spinal cord; (2) bone marrow.

myeloblast (mī′-el-ō-blast): An immature cell in the bone marrow; it develops into a granular leukocyte.

myeloblastoma (mī-el-ō-blas-tō′-ma): A fairly well circumscribed malignant tumor consisting of a mass of myeloblasts (q.v.).

myeloblastosis (mī-e-lō-blast-tō-sis): Ab-normally large number of myeloblasts in the blood or in the tissues, sometimes seen in acute leukemia.

myelocele (mī′-el-ō-sēl): A form of spina bifida (q.v.); the development of the spinal cord itself has been arrested, and the central canal of the cord opens on the skin surface discharging cerebrospinal fluid. Incompati-ble with life.

myelocytes (mī′-el-ō-sīts): Bone marrow cells from which leucocytes develop. Pres-ent in the blood in some pathological condi-tions, e.g., leukemia.—myelocytic, adj.

myeloencephalitis (mī-el-ō-en-sef-a-lī′-tis): Acute inflammation of the brain and spinal cord. EPIDEMIC M., acute anterior poli-omyelitis (q.v.).

myelogenous (mī-el-oj′-en-us): Produced in or by the bone marrow.

myelography (mī-el-og′-ra-fi): Visualization of the spinal cord after the injection of a contrast medium into the subarachnoid space.—myelographic, adj.; myelograph-ically, adv.

myeloid (mī′-el-oid): 1. Pertaining to or derived from bone marrow. 2. Pertaining to the spinal cord.

myeloma (mī-el-ō′-ma): 1. A tumor of the medullary canal. 2. A tumor containing cells of the type normally found in bone marrow.—myelomata, pl.; myelomatous, adj. MULTIPLE M., a primary malignant tu-mor of bone marrow; associated with hyperplasia of the bone marrow, Bence Jones protein in the urine, neuralgic pain, sometimes spontaneous fractures.

myelomalacia (mī-el-ō-mal-ā′-shi-a): Soft-ening of the spinal cord.

myelomatosis (mī-el-ō-ma-tō′-sis): Multi-ple myeloma (q.v.). See **Bence Jones protein.**

myelomeningocele (mī-el-ō-men-ing′-gō-sēl): Meningomyelocele (q.v.).

myelopathy (mī-el-op′-ath-i): Any disease of the spinal cord.—myelopathic, adj.

myocardia (mī-ō-kar′-di-a): A noninflam-matory disease of the myocardium; term is often used to describe heart failure when the cause is unknown.

myocardial (mī-ō-kar′-di-al): Pertaining to the myocardium. M. INFARCTION, the for-mation of an infarct (q.v.) in the myocar-dium.

myocarditis (mī-ō-kar-dī′-tis): Inflamma-tion of the myocardium.

myocardium (mī-ō-kar′-di-um): The middle and thickest of the layers of the heart wall; composed of indistinctly striated, involun-tary muscle tissue.—myocardial, adj.

myocele (mī′-ō-sēl): Protrusion of a muscle through its ruptured sheath.

myoclonus (mī-ok′-lō-nus): Clonic contrac-tions of individual or groups of muscles. Twitching.—myoclonic, adj.

myodegeneration (mī-ō-dē-jen-er-ā′-shun): Degeneration of muscle.

myodynia (mī-ō-din′-i-a): Pain in a muscle; myalgia.

myoelectric (mī-ō-ē-lek′-trik): Pertaining to the electrical properties of muscle.

myoendocarditis (mī-ō-en-dō-kar-dī′-tis): Inflammation of the heart muscle and the endocardium.

myofibrosis (mī-ō-fi-brō′-sis): Excessive connective tissue in muscle. Leads to inade-quate functioning of part.—myofibroses, pl.

myogenic (mī-ō-jen′-ik): Originating in, starting from, muscle.

myoglobin (mī-ō-glō′-bin): Oxygen-trans-porting muscle protein. Syn., myohemo-globin.

myoglobinuria (mī-ō-glō-bin-ū′-ri-a): Ex-cretion of myoglobin in the urine as in crush syndrome. Syn., myohemoglobinuria.

myohemoglobin (mī-ō-hēm-ō-glōb′-in): A hemoglobin present in muscle; of much lower molecular weight than blood hemo-globin. It is liberated from muscle and ap-pears in the urine in the 'crush syndrome.'

myohemoglobinuria (mī-ō-hēm-ō-glōb-in-ūr′-i-a): Myohemoglobin in the urine.

myoma (mī-ō′-ma): A tumor of muscle tis-sue.—myomata, pl.; myomatous, adj.

myomalacia (mī-ō-mal-ā′-shi-a): Softening of muscle, as occurs in the myocardium af-ter coronary occlusion.

myomectomy (mī-ō-mek′-to-mi): Surgical removal of a myoma, specifically a uterine myoma.

myometritis (mī-ō-mē-trī′-tis): Inflammation of the muscular wall of the uterus.

myometrium (mī-ō-mē′-tri-um): The thick muscular wall of the uterus.

myoneural (mī-ō-nūr′-al): Pertaining to muscle and nerve. M. JUNCTION, the place where a nerve ending terminates in muscle tissue.

myopalmus (mī-ō-pal′-mus): Muscle twitching.

myopathy (mī-op′-a-thi): Any disease or abnormal condition of muscle tissue.

myope (mī′-ōp): A nearsighted person.—myopic, adj.

myopia (mī-ō′-pi-a): Nearsightedness. The light rays come to a focus in front, instead of on, the retina.—myopic, adj.

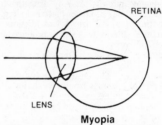

RETINA

LENS

Myopia

myoplasty (mī′-ō-plas-ti): Plastic surgery of muscles, or the use of muscle tissue in plastic surgery.—myoplastic, adj.

myorrhaphy (mī-or′-a-fi): Suturing of a wound in muscle, or of a divided muscle.

myorrhexis (mī-ō-rek′-sis): Rupture of a muscle.

myosarcoma (mī-ō-sar-kō′-ma): A malignant tumor derived from muscle.—myosarcomata, pl.; myosarcomatous, adj.

myosin (mī′-ō-sin): The main protein of muscle. Thought to be important in the contraction and relaxation of muscle.

myosis (mī-ō′-sis): Excessive contraction of the pupil of the eye. Miosis.—myotic, adj.

myositis (mī-ō-sī′-tis): Inflammation of a voluntary muscle. M. OSSIFICANS, deposition of active bone cells in muscle, resulting in hard swellings.

myospasm (mī′-ō-spazm): Spasmodic contraction of a muscle.

myotics (mī-ot′-iks): Drugs that cause myosis (q.v.).

myotomy (mī-ot′-om-i): Cutting or dissection of muscle tissue.

myotonia (mī-ō-tō′-ni-a): A disorder characterized by increased muscular contractions and decreased relaxation; tonic muscle spasm.

myringa (mi-ring′-ga): The eardrum or tympanic membrane.

myringitis (mir-in-jī′-tis): Inflammation of the eardrum (tympanic membrane).

myringoplasty (mir-ing′-ō-plas-ti): Any plastic operation on the eardrum (tympanic membrane).—myringoplastic, adj.

myringotome (mir-ing′-ō-tōm): A delicate instrument for incising the eardrum (tympanic membrane).

myringotomy (mir-ing-ot′-o-mi): Incision of the eardrum (tympanic membrane).

mysophobia (mī-sō-fō′-bi-a): A morbid fear of dirt or germs, or of touching familiar objects, e.g., doorknobs.

myxadenitis (miks-ad-en-ī′-tis): Inflammation of a mucous gland or glands.

myxadenoma (miks-ad-en-ō′-ma): A benign tumor with the structure of a mucous gland, or one that contains mucous elements.

myxedema (mik-sē-dē′-ma): Clinical syndrome of hypothyroidism. Patient becomes slow in movement and dull mentally; there is bradycardia, low temperature, dry skin and swelling of limbs and face. The BMR (q.v.) is low, and the blood cholesterol is raised. No enlargement of gland as in Hashimoto's disease. CONGENITAL M., cretinism (q.v.).

myxoma (mik-sō′-ma): A connective tissue tumor composed largely of mucoid material.—myxomata, pl.; myxomatous, adj.

myxosarcoma (mik-sō-sar-kō′-ma): A malignant tumor of connective tissue with a soft, mucoid consistency.—myxosarcomata, pl.; myxosarcomatous, adj.

myxovirus (mik-sō-vī′-rus): Name proposed by the International Congress of Microbiology, 1953, for the influenza group of viruses. They infect mucus-secreting tissue and include the parainfluenza viruses, measles virus, respiratory syncytial virus.

N

Na: Chemical symbol for sodium (natrium).

nabothian follicles: Tiny cysts that form in the cervical glands of the uterus when these become inflamed and their secretions are retained because of obstruction in the ducts. [Martin Naboth, German anatomist. 1675-1721.]

NaCl: Chemical abbreviation for sodium chloride.

nacreous (nāk′-rē-us): Having a lustrous, mother-of-pearl appearance; said of bacterial colonies.

nail: 1. A piece of material (usually bone or metal) used to hold pieces of a fractured bone together. 2. The horny, cutaneous plate that covers the dorsal surface of the distal ends of fingers and toes. The root is that part that is imbedded in a deep fold of skin at the base. The bed, or matrix, is that part of the corium of the skin on which the nail lies and from which the new substance develops.

nailing: The operation of fastening the ends of a fractured bone together with a nail.

nape: The back of the neck; the nucha.

narc-, narco-: Denotes: (1) stupor, deep sleep; (2) numbness.

narcissism (nar-sis′-izm): Self-love; absorption with one's own perfections. In psychiatry, the narcissistic personality is one in which the sexual love-object is the self; named for a character in Greek mythology who fell in love with his own image reflected in a fountain.

narcoanalysis (nar-kō-a-nal′-i-sis): Psychoanalysis with the patient under sedation; the purpose is to recover repressed memories along with the emotion that accompanied the experience, with the idea of integrating the experience into the patient's personality.

narcohypnosis (nar-kō-hip-nō′-sis): A hypnotic state produced by some drugs and used sometimes in psychotherapy.

narcolepsy (nar′-kō-lep-si): An irresistible tendency to attacks of deep sleep, occurring in the daytime; seen in diverse clinical conditions.—narcoleptic, adj.

narcomania (nar-kō-mā′-ni-a): 1. Insane craving for narcotics. 2. Insanity resulting from alcoholism or from a narcotic drug habit.

narcose (nar′-kōs): Stuporous.

narcosis (nar-kō′-sis): Unconsciousness, stupor, or insensibility produced by a drug and from which recovery is possible. BASAL N., a state of unconsciousness produced by drugs prior to giving an anesthetic.

narcosynthesis (nar-kō-sin′-the-sis): The building up of a clearer mental picture of an incident involving the patient by reviving memories of it under semi-narcosis, so that both he and the therapist can examine the incident in clearer perspective.

narcotic (nar-kot′-ik): 1. Pertinent to or producing narcosis. 2. Any drug that in moderate doses produces profound sleep.

narcotism (nar′-kō-tizm): 1. Addiction to narcotics. 2. A state of stupor produced by a narcotic drug.

narcotize (nar′-kō-tīz): To put a person under the influence of a narcotic drug.

nares (nār-ēz): The nostrils. ANTERIOR N., the pair of openings from the exterior into the nasal cavities. POSTERIOR N., the pair of openings from the nasal cavities into the nasopharynx. Syn., choanae.—naris, sing.

nas-, nasi-, naso-: Denotes the nose; nasal.

nasal (nā′-zal): Pertaining to the nose.

nasogastric (nā-zō-gas′-trik): Pertaining to the nose and stomach, as passing a tube via this route.

nasolacrimal (nā-zō-lak′-ri-mal): Pertaining to the nose and lacrimal apparatus.

nasopharyngitis (nā-zō-far-in-jī′-tis): Inflammation of the nasopharynx.

nasopharyngoscope (nā-zō-far-in′-gō-skōp): An endoscope for viewing the nasal passages and postnasal space.—nasopharyngoscopic, adj.

nasopharynx (nā-zō-far′-inks): The portion of the pharynx above the soft palate.—nasopharyngeal, adj.

nasosinusitis (nā-zō-sī-nū-sī′-tis): Inflammation of the nasal cavities and adjacent sinuses.

natal (nā′-tal): Pertaining to: (1) birth; (2) the buttocks.

nates (nā′-tēz): The buttocks.

National Formulary: A drug compendium published by the American Pharmaceutical Association. Contains drugs not included in the U.S. Pharmacopoeia and, with it, recognized by the courts as an official reference book. Abbreviated NF. It is revised every five years.

National Institutes of Health: The principal research division of the United States Public Health Service. Sponsors, conducts, and supports research and scientific investigation in medicine and related sciences.

National League for Nursing: A national organization formed in 1952 by the fusion of seven groups: The National League for Nursing Education; The National Organization for Public Health Nursing; The Association of Collegiate Schools of Nursing; The Joint Committee on Careers in Nursing; The National Committee for Improvement of Nursing Services; The National Accrediting Service; and The Joint Committee on Practical Nurses and Auxiliary Workers in Nursing Services. Its objectives are the improvement of nursing services and nursing education and it works to improve the standards of educational programs for both professional and practical nurses. There are Leagues in almost all states and in many local communities.

natrium (nā′-tri-um): Sodium.

natriuresis (nā-tri-ū-rē′-sis): A condition in which there is an unusually large amount of sodium in the urine; occurs in some kidney disorders.

natural (nat′-ū-ral): 1. Neither artificial nor pathological. 2. Being born with. 3. Normal. N. CHILDBIRTH, a system of management for normal childbirth in which anesthesia, sedation, and surgical intervention are replaced by prenatal reeducation and psychological preparation for delivery.

naturopathy (nā-tūr-op′-a-thi): A system of treatment that makes use of such physical forces as light, heat, water, and massage; surgical procedures are not used and only such medications as those derived from herbs, vitamins, etc. are used.

nausea (naw′-sē-a): 1. A sensation of discomfort or sickness in the area of the stomach; usually precedes vomiting but not always. 2. Extreme disgust; loathing.— nauseating, adj.; nauseate, v.t.; v.i.

nauseant (naw′-sē-ent): A drug that produces nausea.

nauseous (naw′-sē-us): Producing nausea, disgust, or loathing.

navel (nā′-vel): The umbilicus. The depression in the center of the abdomen marking the place where the umbilical cord is attached to the fetus.

navicular (nav-ik′-ū-lar): 1. Shaped like a boat or canoe. 2. Pertaining to a bone in the wrist and one in the ankle.

ne-, neo-: Denotes new, recent, different.

nearsightedness: Lay term for myopia (q.v.).

nebula (neb′-ū-la): 1. A greyish, corneal opacity. 2. An oily mixture for use in a nebulizer (q.v.).

nebulizer (neb-ū-līz-er): An apparatus for converting a liquid into a fine spray. Syn., atomizer.

neck: 1. The part between the head and the shoulders. 2. The constricted portion of a bone or an organ, e.g., the neck of the femur, the neck of the uterus.

necr-, necro-: Denotes: (1) death; (2) a dead body.

necrectomy (nek-rek′-to-mi): Surgical removal of necrosed tissue.

necrobiosis (nek-rō-bī-ō′-sis): The degeneration or death of cells followed by replacement; may be normal as in red blood cells and epithelial cells, or abnormal as in a pathological progress.

necromania (nek-rō-mā′-ni-a): 1. Morbid interest in death or in corpses. 2. A form of insanity in which one wishes to die.

necropsy (nek′-rop-si): The examination of a dead body.

necrose (nek′-rōs): 1. To become necrotic. 2. To be necrotic.

necrosis (ne-krō′-sis): Localized death of tissue.—necrotic, adj.

needling (nēd′-ling): Puncturing with a needle as in discission of the lens capsule in surgical treatment of cataract. Discission.

negative: Indicates that a substance or microorganism tested for is not present in the material examined.

negativism (neg′-a-tiv-izm): 1. Habitual skepticism. 2. Tendency to do the opposite of what one is asked or expected to do. Occurs commonly in children at the age of two, but not usual in adults. Often associated with schizophrenia.

Negri bodies: Microscopic bodies found in the cytoplasm of certain nerve cells of animals or persons with rabies. Of diagnostic importance.

Neisseria (nīs-ēr′-i-a): A genus of coccus microorganisms; gram-negative, nonmotile, usually found in pairs with their adjacent sides slightly flattened. N. catarrhalis, found in sputum normally and also in the respiratory tract during infections. N. gonorrhoeae, the causative agent of gonorrhea and ophthalmia neonatorum. N. meningitidis, also called N. intracellularis, the causative agent of meningitis.

Nemathelminthes (nem-a-thel-min′-thēz): The roundworms.

Nematoda (nem-a-tō-da): A class of Nemathelminthes (*q.v.*) that includes the true roundworms; many are parasitic in man.—nematode, sing.

neoarthrosis (nē-ō-ar-thrō′-sis): Abnormal articulation; a false joint as at the site of a fracture.

neocyte (nē′-ō-sīt): An immature leukocyte.

neologism (nē-ol′-ō-jizm): A specially coined word, often nonsensical; may express a thought disorder.

neonatal (nē-ō-nā′-tal): Pertaining to the period immediately following birth and continuing through the first month of life. N. MORTALITY, the death rate of babies in the first month of life.

neonate (nē′-ō-nāt): A newborn baby up to one month old.

neonatologist (nē-ō-nā-tol′-o-jist): A physician who specializes in the care and treatment of the newborn.

neonatology (nē-ō-nā-tol′-o-ji): That branch of medicine that is concerned with the care and treatment of the newborn.

neonatorum (nē-ō-nat-or′-um): Pertaining to the newborn.

neoplasia (nē-ō-plā′-zi-a): Literally the formation of new tissue. By custom refers to the pathological process in tumor formation.—neoplastic, adj.

neoplasm (nē′-ō-plazm): Any abnormal new growth of cells or tissues that serves no useful purpose; a tumor. May be benign, malignant, or potentially malignant.—neoplastic, adj.

nephr-, nephro-: Denotes the kidney.

nephralgia (nef-ral′-ji-a): Pain in the kidney.

nephrectasia (nef-rek-tā′-zi-a): Distention of the pelvis of the kidney.

nephrectomy (nef-rek′-to-mi): Removal of a kidney.

nephredema (nef-re-dē′-ma): Edema caused by disease of the kidney. Rarely, edema of the kidney.

nephric (nef′-rik): Pertaining to the kidney.

nephritic (nef-rit′-ik): 1. Pertaining to: (1) nephritis; (2) the kidney. 2. A person affected with nephritis.

nephritis (nef-rī′-tis): A term embracing a group of conditions in which there is either an inflammatory or an inflammatory-like condition, focal or diffuse, in the kidneys. ACUTE N., Bright's disease. A diffuse inflammatory reaction of both kidneys, usually following a streptococcal infection, and classically manifest by puffiness of the face and scanty blood-stained urine. Other symptoms are fever, pain in the lumbar region, frequent painful urination. CHRONIC N., a chronic condition in which there is widespread fibrous replacement of functioning kidney tissue, resulting in progressive renal failure and an arterial hypertension and terminating ultimately in death. NEPHROTIC N., a chronic condition of unknown cause characterized by massive edema and heavy proteinuria.

nephroblastoma (nef′-rō-blas-tō′-ma): A malignant tumor of the kidney; occurs almost exclusively in children. Thought to develop from embryonic structures. Also called embryoma and Wilms' tumor.

nephrocalcinosis (nef-rō-kal-sin-ō′-sis): A condition characterized by development of multiple areas of calcification in the kidney tubules, resulting in renal insufficiency.

nephrocapsectomy (nef-rō-kap-sek′-to-mi): Surgical removal of the kidney capsule. Usually done for chronic nephritis. Also nephrocapsulectomy.

nephrocystitis (nef-rō-sis-tī′-tis): Inflammation of the kidney and the urinary bladder.

nephrogenic (nef-rō-jen′-ik): Arising in or produced by the kidney.

nephrogram (nef′-rō-gram): X-ray of renal shadow following injection of opaque medium.—nephrography, n.; nephrographical, adj.; nephrographically, adv.

nephrohydrosis (nef-rō-hī-drō′-sis): Hydronephrosis (*q.v.*).

nephrohypertrophy (nef-rō-hī-per′-tro-fi): Hypertrophy of the kidney.

nephrolith (nef′-rō-lith): A kidney stone.

nephrolithiasis (nef-rō-lith-ī′-a-sis): The presence of stones in the kidney.

nephrolithotomy (nef-rō-lith-ot′-o-mi): Removal of a stone from the kidney by an incision through the kidney substance.

nephrology (nef-rol′-o-ji): Scientific study of the kidneys and the diseases that affect them.

nephromegaly (nef-rō-meg′-a-li): Enlargement of one or both kidneys.

nephron (nef′-ron): The basic functional unit of the kidney, comprising a glomerulus, Bowman's capsule, proximal and distal convoluted tubules, with loop of Henle connecting them; a straight collecting tubule follows via which urine is conveyed to the renal pelvis.

nephropathy (nef-rop′-a-thi): Kidney disease.—nephropathic, adj.

nephropexy (nef′-rō-pek-si): Surgical fixation of a floating kidney.

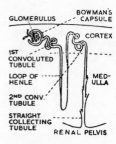

Diagram of nephron

nephrophthisis (nef-rof′-ti-sis): Tuberculosis of the kidney.

nephroptosis (nef-rop-tō′-sis): Downward displacement of the kidney.

nephropyelitis (nef-rō-pī-e-lī′-tis): Inflammation of the pelvis of the kidney.

nephropyosis (nef-rō-pī′-ō-sis): Pus formation in the kidney.

nephrorrhaphy (nef-ror′-a-fi): Suturing a kidney or fixing a kidney in place by suturing. Nephropexy.

nephrosclerosis (nef-rō-skler-ō′-sis): Hardening or sclerosis of the kidney. Seen in cardiovascular-renal disease. May be benign or malignant. ARTERIOLAR N., caused by sclerosis of the small arteries of the kidney.—nephrosclerotic, adj.

nephrosis (nef-rō′-sis): Any degenerative, noninflammatory change in the kidney.—nephrotic, adj.

nephrostomy (nef-ros′-to-mi): A surgically established fistula from the pelvis of the kidney to the body surface.

nephrotic (nef-rot′-ik): Resembling, pertaining to, or caused by nephrosis.

nephrotomy (nef-rot′-o-mi): An incision into the kidney substance.

nephroureterectomy (nef-rō-ū-rē′-ter-ek′-to-mi): Removal of the kidney along with a part or the whole of the ureter.

nerve: An elongated bundle of fibers that serves for the transmission of impulses between various parts of the body and the nerve centers. AFFERENT N., one conveying impulses from the tissues to a nerve center; also known as 'receptor' and 'sensory N.' EFFERENT N., one that conveys impulses outward from the nerve centers; also known as 'effector,' 'motor,' 'secretory,' 'trophic,' 'vasoconstrictor,' 'vasodilator,' etc., according to function and location. See **ganglion, neuron, plexus.**

nervous (ner′-vus): 1. Relating to nerves or N. tissue. 2. Referring to a state of restlessness or timidity. 3. Easily excited or agitated. N. SYSTEM, the structures controlling the actions and functions of the body; it comprises the brain and spinal cord and their nerves, and the ganglia and fibers forming the autonomic system.

nervous breakdown: A common nonmedical term for an emotional illness or psychosis.

nettle rash (net′-t'l): Popular term to describe urticaria; wheals of the skin.

neur-, neuro-: Denotes: (1) nerve; (2) neural tissue; (3) nervous system.

neural (nū′-ral): Pertaining to a nerve or nerves.

neuralgia (nū-ral′-ji-a): Severe, paroxysmal pain occurring along the course of one or more nerves. Many varieties are distinguished and named according to the part affected or the nerve that supplies the part affected.—neuralgic, adj.

neurapraxia (nū-ra-praks′-i-a): Temporary loss of function in peripheral nerve fibers. Most commonly due to crushing or prolonged pressure.

neurasthenia (nū-ras-thē′-ni-a): A frequently misused term, the precise meaning of which is an uncommon nervous condition consisting of lassitude, inertia, fatigue and loss of initiative. Restless fidgeting, oversensitivity, undue irritability and often an asthenic physique are also present. Nervous exhaustion.—neurasthenic, adj.

neurasthenic (nū-ras-then′-ik): 1. One suffering from neurasthenia (q.v.). 2. Pertaining to neurasthenia.

neuraxis (nū-rak′-sis): An axon. Also neuraxon.

neurectomy (nū-rek′-to-mi): Excision of part of a nerve.

neurilemma (nū-ri-lem′-a): Neurolemma (q.v.).

neuritis (nū-rī′-tis): Inflammation of a nerve.—neuritic, adj.

neuroanastomosis (nū-rō-an-as′-to-mō-sis): The operation of joining or making a junction between nerves.

neuroanatomy (nū-rō-a-nat′-o-mi): The anatomy of the nervous system.

neuroblast (nū′-rō-blast): A primitive nerve cell.

neuroblastoma (nū-rō-blas-tō′-ma): A malignant tumor composed chiefly of cells resembling neuroblasts; occurs most often in the adrenal medulla.—neuroblastomata, pl.; neuroblastomatous, adj.

neurodendrite (nū-rō-den-drīt): A dendrite.

neurodermatitis (nū-rō-der-ma-tī'-tis): Lichen simplex (*q.v.*). Leathery, thickened patches of skin secondary to pruritus and scratching. As the skin thickens, irritation increases, scratching causes further thickening and so a vicious circle is set up. The appearance of the patch develops characteristically as a thickened sheet dissected into small, shiny, flat-topped papules.

neuroepithelium (nū-rō-ep-i-thē'-li-um): Simple columnar epithelium made up of cells that act as receptors for external stimuli, as in the nose, tongue, and cochlea.

neurofibril (nū-rō-fī'-bril): One of the many fine fibrils that run through the cytoplasm and the axons and dendrites of a nerve cell. It is thought that they form the conducting element of the neuron.

neurofibroma (nū-rō-fī-brō'-ma): A tumor arising from the connective tissue of nerves. See **Recklinghausen's disease.**

neurofibromatosis (nū-rō-fī-brō-ma-tō'-sis): A condition characterized by the formation of multiple fibromata. Recklinghausen's disease (*q.v.*).

neurogenic (nū-rō-jen'-ik): 1. Originating within or forming nervous tissue. 2. Stimulating nervous energy. N. BLADDER, any defect in the functioning of the urinary bladder that is the result of damage to the nerve supply to that organ.

neuroglia (nū-rog'-li-a): The supporting tissue of the brain and cord.—neuroglial, adj.

neurogram (nū'-rō-gram): The imprint that a mental experience makes on the brain; important in the development of memory and of personality.

neurohormone (nū'-rō-hor-mōn): A hormone that stimulates neuronal activity, *e.g.,* adrenaline.

neurohumor (nū-rō-hū'-mor): A chemical substance that is formed in the neuron and liberated at the nerve endings; participates in the transmission of nerve impulses.

neurolemma (nū-rō-lem'-a): The thin membranous outer covering of a myelinated nerve or of the axon of a nonmyelinated nerve. Neurilemma.

neuroleptics (nū-rō-lep'-tiks): Drugs acting on the nervous system. Includes the tranquilizers and antidepressants.

neurologic (nū-rō-log'-ik): Pertaining to neurology or to the nervous system.

neurologist (nū-rol'-o-jist): A specialist in neurology.

neurology (nū-rol'-o-ji): The science and study of nerves—their structure, function and pathology; the branch of medicine dealing with diseases of the nervous system.—neurological, adj.

neurolymph (nū'-rō-limf): Cerebrospinal fluid.

neurolysis (nū-rol'-i-sis): 1. The breaking down of nerve substance. 2. The operation of freeing a nerve from adhesions. 3. Exhaustion of a nerve from overstimulation.

neuroma (nū-rō'-ma): A tumor made up of nerve cells and nerve tissue. An old general term for many neoplasms of the nervous system.

neuromuscular (nū-rō-mus'-kū-lar): Pertaining to nerves and muscles.

neuromyositis (nū-rō-mī-ō-sī'-tis): Inflammation of both the nerves and muscles of a part.

neuron (nū'-ron): The structural unit of the nervous system comprising fibers (dendrites) that convey impulses to the nerve cell; the nerve cell itself; and the fibers (axons) that convey impulses from the cell. LOWER MOTOR N., the cell is in the spinal cord and the axon passes to skeletal muscle. UPPER MOTOR N., the cell is in the cerebral cortex and the axon passes down the spinal cord to arborize with a lower motor N.—neuronal, neural, adj.

neuroparalysis (nū-rō-pa-ral'-i-sis): Paralysis caused by disease of the nerve(s) supplying the affected part.

neuropathic (nū-rō-path'-ik): 1. Relating to disease of the nervous system. 2. Having a nervous disease.

neuropathology (nū-rō-path-ol'-oj-i): A branch of medicine dealing with diseases of the nervous system.

neuropharmacology (nū-rō-far-ma-kol'-o-ji): The branch of pharmacology dealing with the drugs that affect the nervous system.

neuroplasm (nū'-rō-plazm): The cytoplasm of a nerve cell.

neuroplasty (nū'-rō-plas-ti): Surgical repair of nerves.—neuroplastic, adj.

neuropsychiatry (nū-rō-sī-kī'-a-tri): The combination of neurology and psychiatry. Specialty dealing with organic and functional disease.—neuropsychiatric, adj.

neuropsychosis (nū-rō-sī-kō'-sis): Psychosis of neurologic origin.

neurorrhaphy (nū-ror'-a-fi): Suturing the ends of a divided nerve.

neurosis (nū-rō'-sis): A functional (*i.e.,* psychogenic) disorder consisting of a symptom or symptoms caused, though usually unknown to the patient, by mental disorder. The four commonest are anxiety state, reactive depression, hysteria and obsessional N. (*q.v.*). Distinguished from a psychosis (*q.v.*) by the fact that a neurosis arises as a result of stresses and anxieties in the patient's environment. INSTITUTIONAL N., apathy, withdrawal, and non-participation occurring in long-term patients as a result of environment; may be distinguished from the signs and symptoms for which the patient was admitted to the institution. —neuroses, pl.; neurotic, adj.

neurospasm (nū'-rō-spazm): Twitching of a muscle due to a disorder of the nerve supplying the muscle.

neurosurgery (nū-rō-sur'-jer-i): Surgery of the nervous system.—neurosurgical, adj.

neurosyphilis (nū-rō-sif'-i-lis): Infection of brain or spinal cord, or both, by *Treponema pallidum*. The variety of clinical pictures produced is large, but the two common syndromes encountered are tabes dorsalis and general paralysis of the insane (GPI). The basic pathology is disease of the blood vessels, with later development of pathological changes in the meninges and the underlying nervous tissue. Very often symptoms of the disease do not arise until 20 years or more after the date of primary infection. See **Argyll Robertson pupil**.—neurosyphilitic, adj.

neurothlipsis (nū-rō-thlip'-sis): Irritation or pressure on one or more nerves.

neurotic (nū-rot'-ik): 1. Pertaining to neurosis. 2. Nervous. 3. A person suffering from a neurosis or from instability of the nervous system.

neurotomy (nū-rot'-o-mi): Surgical cutting of a nerve.

neurotoxin (nū-rō-toks'-in): Any substance that is poisonous or destructive to nervous tissue.—neurotoxic, adj.

neurotripsy (nū-rō-trip'-si): The surgical crushing of a nerve.

neurotropic (nū-rō-trō'-pik): With predilection for the nervous system, used especially of *Treponema pallidum*, some forms of which seem always to produce neurosyphilitic complications. N. viruses (rabies, poliomyelitis, etc.) make their major attack on the cells of the nervous system.

neutral (nū'-tral): Having no positive properties or characteristics. In chemistry, neither acid nor basic in reaction.

neutralization (nū-tral-ī-zā'-shun): 1. The conversion of an acid or basic substance into a neutral one. 2. The process of render-

ing any action or process ineffective.—neutralize, v.t.

neutrocyte (nū-trō-sīt): A neutrophil (*q.v.*).

neutron (nū'-tron): One of the basic particles of the nucleus of the atom; it breaks down into a proton and an electron. N. CAPTURE THEORY, a new concept of treatment for carcinoma.

neutropenia (nū-trō-pē'-ni-a): Shortage of neutrophils, not sufficient to warrant the term 'agranulocytosis.'—neutropenic, adj.

neutrophil (nū'-trō-fil): One form of polymorphonuclear leucocyte (*q.v.*).

neutrophilia (nū-trō-fil'-i-a): An increase in the number of neutrophils in the blood.

nevus (nē'-vus): A general term used to describe any congenital circumscribed pigmented lesion on the skin; may be of epidermal or connective tissue origin or of vascular origin. A mole; a birthmark.—nevi, pl.; nevoid, adj.

New and Nonofficial Drugs: Annual publication of the American Medical Association; lists drugs that have been accepted by the Association's Council on Drugs. Abbreviated NND.

NF: Abbreviation for National Formulary (*q.v.*).

niacin (nī-a'-sin): One of the essential food factors of the vitamin B complex. Found in high protein diets, vegetables, enriched or whole grain flour and cereals, milk. Deficiency may result in rough skin, loss of strength, general weakness, mental depression.

nicotinic acid: Niacin (*q.v.*).

nictitation (nik-ti-tā'-shun): Rapid and involuntary blinking of the eyelids.

nidation (nī-dā'-shun): Implantation of the early embryo in the uterine mucosa.

nidus (nī'-dus): 1. The focus of an infection. Septic focus. 2. A group of cells within the central nervous system.

Niemann-Pick disease: A lipoid metabolic disturbance, chiefly in female Jewish infants. There is enlargement of the liver, spleen and lymph nodes with mental subnormality. [Albert Niemann, German pediatrician. 1880-1921. Ludwig Pick, German pediatrician. 1868-1935.]

night blindness: Nyctalopia. Sometimes occurs in vitamin A deficiency and is a maladaptation of vision to darkness.

night cry: A shrill noise, uttered during sleep. May be of significance in hip disease, when pain occurs in the relaxed joint.

nightmare: A terrifying dream in which the person is unable to help himself or get out of a frightening situation; usually accompanied by a feeling of suffocation.

night sweat: Profuse sweating, usually during sleep; typical of tuberculosis.

nightwalking: Walking during sleep. Somnambulism.

NIH: National Institues of Health (*q.v.*).

nihilism (nī′-hil-izm): In medicine, a form of delusion in which the patient denies the reality of everything; the denial of existence. THERAPEUTIC N., a disbelief in the therapeutic value of drugs.

Nikolsky's sign: A condition in which the external layer of skin 'slips' or rubs off with slight friction or injury; seen in pemphigus vulgaris (*q.v.*). [Pyotr V. Nikolsky, Russian dermatologist. 1885- .]

niphablepsia (nif-a-blep′-si-a): Snow blindness. Also niphotyphlosis.

nipple (nip′-l): 1. The conical eminence in the center of each breast, containing the outlets of the milk ducts; a teat. 2. An artificial substitute for the human nipple used on an infant's nursing bottle.

Nissl('s) bodies: Granular stainable protein bodies within the cytoplasm of nerve cells.

nit: The egg of a louse. The nit of the head louse is found firmly attached to the shaft of a hair.

nitric acid (nī′-trik as′-id): A colorless, corrosive inorganic acid that gives off choking fumes. It is exceedingly caustic; sometimes used for removing warts. Also used in certain tests for albumin in the urine.

nitrogen (nī′-trō-jen): A colorless, tasteless, odorless gaseous element; chief constituent of air; essential constituent of protein food. N. is excreted mainly as urea in the urine; ammonia, creatine and uric acid account for a further small amount; less than 10% total N. is excreted in feces.—nitrogenous, adj. N. BALANCE, the difference between the intake and output of N. by the body; a person is in positive N. balance when the intake exceeds the output, in negative balance when the intake of N. is less than the output. N. EQUILIBRIUM, the condition that exists when the amount of N. excreted equals the amount taken into the body in foods. NONPROTEIN N. (NPN), nitrogenous constituents of the blood that are not protein, *i.e.*, urea, uric acid, creatine, creatinine, amino acids, ammonia.

nitrogenous (nī-troj′-en-us): Relating to or containing nitrogen.

nitrous oxide (nī′-trus ok′-sīd): A colorless sweet-tasting gas with a not unpleasant odor; widely used in obstetrics, dental surgery and for induction anesthesia. Laughing gas.

NLN: Abbreviation for The National League for Nursing (*q.v.*).

NND: New and Nonofficial Drugs (*q.v.*).

Noct: Abbreviation for *nocte,* meaning night.

noct-, nocti-, nocto-: Denotes night or during the night.

nocturia (nok-tū′-ri-a): Excessive urination during the night.

nocturnal (nok-tur′-nal): Nightly; during the night. N. ENURESIS, bed-wetting during sleep.

node (nōd): A protuberance, knob, swelling. A constriction.—nodal, nodular, adj. ATRIOVENTRICULAR N., the commencement of the bundle of His (*q.v.*) in the right atrium of the heart. LYMPH N., a mass of lymphoid tissue resembling a gland, found along the course of lymph vessels. N. OF RANVIER, a constriction in the neurilemma of a nerve fiber. [Louis Antoine Ranvier, French pathologist. 1835-1922.] SINOATRIAL N., situated at the opening of the superior vena cava into the right atrium; the wave of contraction begins here, then spreads over the heart; called the pacemaker of the heart.

nodose (nō′-dōs): Characterized by the presence of nodes.

nodule (nod′-ūl): A small node or tubercle.—nodular, adj.

noma (nō′-ma): Gangrenous stomatitis, usually observed in malnourished children or debilitated adults. See **cancrum oris.**

nomenclature (nō′-men-klā-tūr): A system of words and terms used in a particular science or discipline.

non-: Denotes not, without, absence of.

non compos mentis (non kom′-pos men′-tis): Of unsound mind.

nonconductor (non-kon-duk′-tor): A substance that does not readily conduct heat, light, sound or electricity.

nonpathogenic (non-path-ō-jen′-ik): Not productive of or causing disease.

non repetat.: Do not repeat. Term used in ordering medications.

nonunion (non-ūn′-yun): Failure of the ends of a fractured bone to unite or knit together.

nonviable (non-vī′-a-b'l): Not capable of life, or of living independently. Often said of a fetus that is born before it is capable of living outside the uterus.

NOPHN: Abbreviation for The National Organization for Public Health Nursing.

norepinephrine (nor-ep-i-nef′-rin): A hormone secreted by the adrenal medulla. Noradrenalin.

norm: A fixed standard or model.

norm-, normo-: Denotes normal.

normal: Natural; average; regular; healthy. N. SALINE or SALT SOLUTION, solution of distilled water with sodium chloride dissolved in it in the same concentration as occurs in the blood.

normoblast (nor′-mō-blast): A normal sized nucleated red blood cell, the precursor of the erythrocyte. Normally present in the bone marrow, but appears in the blood in certain types of anemia.

normocyte (nor′-mō-sīt): A nucleated red blood cell of normal size and hemoglobin content.—normocytic, adj.

normoglycemia (nor-mō-glī-sē′-mi-a): The condition of having the normal amount of glucose in the blood.

normotension (nor-mō-ten′-shun): Normal tension, by current custom alluding to blood pressure.—normotensive, adj.

normothermia (nor-mō-ther′-mi-a): Normal body temperature, as opposed to hyperthermia and hypothermia.—normothermic, adj.

normotonic (nor-mō-ton′-ik): Normal strength, tension, tone, by current custom referring to muscle tissue.—normotonicity, n.

normovolemia (nor-mō-vō-lē′-mi-a): Having the normal volume of blood.

nos-, noso-: Denotes disease, pathology.

nose: The prominent structure in the middle of the face; the organ of smell and the beginning of the respiratory tract; it warms and filters the inspired air.

nosebleed: Hemorrhage from the nose. Syn., epistaxis.

nosology (nō-sol′-o-je): The science of the systematic classification of diseases.

nosomania (nos-ō-mā′-ni-a): The unfounded and insane belief that one is afflicted with a particular disease.

nostalgia (nos-tal′-ji-a): Homesickness. —nostalgic, adj.

nostrils (nos′-trils): The anterior openings in the nose; the anterior nares.

nostrum (nos′-trum): A quack or patent remedy; or secret remedy that is recommended by its maker.

notch: A rather deep impression or indentation; usually refers to such an indentation on the surface of a bone or organ.

notochord (nō′-tō-kord): The long rod of cells that forms the longitudinal supportive structure in an embryo. Traces of it remain in the adult in the central portion of the intervertebral disks.

noxious (nok′-shus): Harmful; not wholesome.

NREM: Abbreviation for no rapid eye movements. NREM sleep is that which begins as the person passes from wakefulness to deep sleep and no rapid eye movements occur. NREM sleep is interrupted by periods of REM sleep (q.v.), and represents about three-fourths to four-fifths of one's total sleeping time.

nucha (nū′-ka): The nape of the neck.—nuchal, adj.

nucleated (nū′-klē-āt-ed): Possessing one or more nuclei.

nucleolus (nū-klē′-ō-lus): A rounded body within the cell nucleus.

nucleoplasm (nū′-klē-ō-plazm): The protoplasm that makes up the nucleus of the cell.

nucleoproteins (nū-klē-ō-prō′-tē-inz): Proteins found especially in the nuclei of plant and animal cells. They consist of a protein conjugated with nucleic acid and are broken down during digestion. Among the products are the purine and pyrimidine bases. An end product of nucleoprotein metabolism is uric acid which is excreted in the urine.

nucleotoxin (nū-klē-ō-tok′-sin): Any agent that is toxic to cell nuclei including drugs, toxins and viruses.—nucleotoxic, adj.

nucleus (nū′-klē-us): 1. The inner essential part of a living cell, being necessary for the growth, nourishment and reproduction of the cell, and for the transmission of hereditary characteristics. 2. A circumscribed accumulation of nerve cells with a particular function. 3. The central core of an atom.—nuclei, pl.; nuclear, adj. N. PULPOSIS, the soft core of an intervertebral disk which can prolapse (q.v.) into the spinal cord and/or nerve roots. Most common in the lumbar region where it causes low back pain and/or sciatica.

nullipara (nul-lip′-a-ra): A woman who has not borne a child.—nulliparous, adj.; nulliparity, n.

nummular (num′-ū-lar): Coin shaped; resembling rolls of coins, as the sputum in phthisis.

nurse: 1. One who cares for the sick, wounded or helpless, under the direction of a physician; usually implies one specially trained to give such care. 2. To care for the sick, wounded or helpless. 3. To feed an infant at the breast. GRADUATE N., one who has graduated from a professional school of nursing. PRACTICAL N., one who cares for the sick, under the direction of a graduate N., but is not a graduate of a professional school of nursing. REGISTERED N., a graduate N. who has been registered and licensed to practice nursing by a Board of Examiners for the state in which she lives or works. OCCUPATIONAL HEALTH N., one who works in a factory, mill, department store, office, hotel, or other place of employment; her function is to give immediate and expert care to injuries received by employees or others in these places, to follow up on sick and injured employees, and to help develop accident prevention programs. PRIVATE DUTY N., one who cares for a single patient in his home or the hospital. PUBLIC HEALTH N., one who performs her services for patients in their homes, schools or outpatient clinics; works for an agency and is not self-employed; works with other health workers on community health programs; is concerned with keeping the people of the country physically and mentally healthy. Also called community nurse. Visiting nurses function in public health capacities. SCHOOL N., one employed by the school to participate in health programs for school children. STAFF N., one who gives bedside care to patients in a hospital.

nurses' aide: A person who assists nurses to care for the sick, wounded or helpless; may be a paid employee or a volunteer; may have a brief period of instruction before starting work or may be given on-the-job instruction in tasks that are less technical than those performed by nurses.

nursing: Strictly, the activities that are involved in giving physical and emotional care to the sick, wounded, and helpless. Broadly, all activities performed by nurses and that are concerned with restoration or maintenance of community health as well as personal physical and mental health.

nursing audit: A systematic, formal, written appraisal, by nurses, of the quality of nursing care given to patients (as shown by the nursing records and by observation) as compared with the standards of care that have been set up as acceptable to the individual institution.

nursing diagnosis: A critical determination of the patient's nursing needs either for the purpose of reporting to the physician or planning for the patient's nursing care. Also sometimes defined as a scientific approach to solving the problems associated with the patient's nursing needs.

Nursing Outlook: The official publication of the National League for Nursing. Published monthly.

nutation (nū-tā'-shun): Nodding; applied to uncontrollable head shaking.

nutrient (nū'-tri-ent): 1. Food that supplies the elements necessary to nourish the body. 2. Nourishing. 3. Serving as or providing nourishment. N. ARTERY, one that enters a long bone. N. FORAMEN, hole in a long bone that admits the N. artery.

nutriment (nū'-tri-ment): Nourishment.

nutrition (nū-tri'-shun): 1. The sum total of the processes by which the living organism receives and utilizes the materials necessary for survival, growth and repair of worn-out tissues. 2. The science that deals with the food requirements of the body.

nutritious (nū-trish'-us): Containing elements needed for growth, development and health. Syn., nutritive.

nutritive (nū'-tri-tiv): Pertaining to or supplying nutrition to the body.

nyct-, nycti-, nycto-: Denotes: (1) night; (2) darkness.

nyctalgia (nik-tal'-ji-a): Pain that occurs only during sleep.

nyctalopia (nik-tal-ō'-pi-a): Night blindness.

nyctophobia (nik-tō-fō'-bi-a): Abnormal fear of the night and darkness.

nycturia (nik-tū'-ri-a): Nocturia (*q.v.*).

nymphae (nim'-fē): The labia minora.

nymphomania (nim-fō-mā'-ni-a): Excessive sexual desire in a female.—nymphomaniac, adj., n.

nystagmus (nis-tag'-mus): Involuntary and jerky repetitive movement of the eyeballs.

O

O: In chemistry, the symbol for oxygen. In optics, the abbreviation for *oculus,* meaning eye; *e.g.,* oculus sinister (OS), left eye.

o-, oo-: Denotes ovum.

oat cell sarcoma: A sarcoma (*q.v.*) in which the cells have long, oval nuclei and the cells themselves are elongated and blunted at the ends.

OB, Obs: Abbreviations for obstetric, obstetrical.

ob-: Denotes: (1) toward, against, over; (2) inward; (3) completely; (4) in reverse order; (5) in the way of (something).

obese (ō-bēs'): Excessively fat. A person whose weight is more than 20% above the average for his body build is considered obese. Syn., fat, corpulent.

obesity (ō-bēs'-it-i): The condition of excessive accumulation and storage of fat in the body. Syn., corpulence.

obfuscate (ob'-fus-kāt): To becloud, dim, confuse; to make obscure or unnecessarily complicated.—obfuscated, adj.; obfuscation, n.

obfuscation (ob-fus-kā'-shun): 1. Clouding, as of the cornea. 2. Mental confusion.

obicularis (ō-bik-ū-lar'-is): Descriptive of a muscle that encircles an opening of the body. O. OCULI, surrounds the eye. O. ORIS, surrounds the mouth.

objective (ob-jek'-tiv): 1. An aim or purpose. 2. A lens or series of lenses in a microscope. 3. Pertaining to things external to one's self. Opp. subjective (*q.v.*). O. SIGNS, those which the observer notes, as distinct from the symptoms of which the patient complains.

obligate (ob'-li-gāt): No alternative. Used to describe functions of cells which are essential, *e.g.,* O. parasite, cannot exist other than as a parasite.

obliteration (ob-lit-er-ā'-shun): Complete removal of a part, whether by surgery, disease, or degeneration.—obliterative, adj.

obsession (ob-sesh'-un): A persistent, pathological concern with an idea or set of ideas that dominate the mind, often suggesting irrational actions. A symptom of mental illness, especially paranoia.—obsessional, adj.

obsessional neurosis (ob-sesh'-un-al nū-rō'-sis): Two types. 1. Obsessive compulsive thoughts: constant preoccupation with a constantly recurring morbid thought which cannot be kept out of the mind, and enters against the wishes of the patient who tries to eliminate it. The thought is almost always painful and out of keeping with the person's normal personality. 2. Obsessive compulsive action: consists of a feeling of compulsion to perform repeatedly a simple act, *e.g.,* hand-washing, touching door knobs, etc. Ideas of guilt frequently form the basis of an obsessional state.

obsessive compulsive: Name given to a type of neurosis in which there is constant recurrence of thoughts, ideas, or actions that the individual does not want or initiate, but which he is unable to prevent.

obstetrician (ob-ste-trish'-un): A qualified doctor who practices the science and art of obstetrics.

obstetrics (ob-stet'-riks): The science dealing with the care of the pregnant woman during the antenatal, parturient and puerperal stages; midwifery.—obstetric, obstetrical, adj.

obstipation (ob-sti-pā'-shun): Obstinate constipation.

obstruction (ob-struk'-shun): 1. Blocking, clogging or closing of a passageway. 2. An obstacle that blocks a passageway. 3. The condition of being blocked or clogged.

obtund (ob-tund'): To blunt or to dull, said especially of pain or of sensation.—obtundent, adj.; n.

obturation (ob-tū-rā'-shun): Closure; occlusion. Usually said of an opening or a passageway.—obturate, v.t.

obturator (ob'-tū-rāt-or): That which closes an aperture. O. FORAMEN, the opening in the innominate bone which is largely closed by muscles and fascia.

obtuse (ob-tūs'): Dense, stupid, dull, blunted; lacking awareness of perception or sensation.—obtuseness, adj.; obtusely, adv.

obtusion (ob-tū'-zhun): A blunting or the condition of being blunted.

occipital (ok-sip'-it-al): Pertaining to the back part of the head. O. BONE, the bone at the back of the head, characterized by the large hole (foramen magnum) through which the cranial cavity communicates with the spinal canal. O. LOBE, the portion of the cerebral hemisphere that lies behind the parietal and temporal lobes.

occipitoanterior (ok-sip-it-ō-an-tē′-ri-or): Denoting the position of the fetus when the occiput lies in the anterior half of the maternal pelvis.

occipitofrontal (ok-sip-i-tō-fron′-tal): Pertaining to the occiput and forehead.

occipitoposterior (ok-sip-it-ō-pos-tē′-ri-or): Denoting the position of the fetus when the occiput is in the posterior half of the maternal pelvis.

occiput (ok′-si-put): The posterior region of the skull.

occlude (o-klood′): 1. To shut, close, or stop up so as to prevent the normal passage of something. 2. To bring together, as the upper and lower teeth.

occlusion (o-kloo′-zhun): The closure of an opening, especially of ducts or blood vessels. In dentistry, the fit of the teeth as the two jaws meet.

occult (o-kult′): 1. Hidden, concealed, obscure. 2. In medicine, not detectable except by microscopic or chemical means; used especially to describe conditions such as blood in the urine or feces, but also to describe certain infections, lesions or neoplasms. O. BLOOD, see **blood.**

occupational: O. DELIRIUM, psychiatric term for a condition occurring in dementia and consisting of purposeless over-activity relating to a patient's occupation. O. DERMATITIS, see **dermatitis.** O. DISEASE, one contracted by reason of occupational exposure to an agent known to be hazardous to health, *e.g.,* dust, fumes, chemicals, radiation, etc. Also called industrial disease. O. HEALTH NURSE, see **nurse.** O. NEUROSIS, a functional disorder of a part of the body caused by occupational activity, *e.g.,* writer's cramp. O. THERAPY, see **therapy.**

ocul-, oculo-: Denotes: (1) the eye; (2) ocular.

ocular (ok′-ū-lar): 1. Pertaining to the eye, or the sense of sight. 2. The eyepiece of a microscope.

oculist (ok′-ū-list): Older term for ophthalmologist (*q.v.*).

oculogyric (ok-ū-lō-jī′-rik): Referring to rotary movements of the eyeball. O. CRISIS, a spasm of eye muscles that occurs in some neurological disorders; the eyeballs become fixed in one position, usually upwards; seen in parkinsonism.

oculomotor (ok-ū-lō-mō′-tor): Pertaining to or causing movements of the eyeball. O. NERVE, the third cranial nerve which moves the eye and supplies the upper eyelid.

oculus (ok′-ū-lus): The organ of vision; the eye.—oculi, pl.; ocular, adj.

OD: Abbreviation for *oculus dexter,* meaning right eye.

o.d.: Abbreviation for *omni die,* meaning every day.

odditis (ō′-dī′-tis): Inflammation of the sphincter of Oddi at the junction of the duodenum and the common bile duct.

odont-, odonto-: Denotes a tooth or teeth.

odontalgia (ō-don-tal′-ji-a): Toothache.

odontectomy (ō-don-tek′-to-mi): Surgical removal of a tooth or teeth.

odonterism (ō-don′-ter-izm): Chattering of the teeth.

odontitis (ō-don-tī′-tis): Inflammation of a tooth or of the teeth.

odontoid (ō-don′-toid): Resembling a tooth. O. PEG OR PROCESS, the toothlike projection from the upper surface of the body of the second cervical vertebra or axis.

odontolith (ō-don′-to-lith): Tartar; the concretions which are deposited around teeth.

odontology (ō-don-tol′-o-ji): Dentistry.

odontoma (ō-don-tō′-ma): A tumor developing from or containing tooth structures. —odontomata, pl.; odontomatous, adj.

odontoprisis (ō-don-tō-prī′-sis): Grinding of the teeth. Bruxism (*q.v.*).

odontotherapy (ō-don-tō-ther′-a-pi): The treatment given for diseases of the teeth.

-odynia: Denotes pain.

oedipism (ed′-i-pizm): 1. Infliction of injury to one's own eyes. 2. Manifestation of the Oedipus complex (*q.v.*).

Oedipus complex (ed′-i-pus kom′-pleks): [Oedipus, King of Thebes, unwittingly killed his father and married his own mother. When he discovered the true relationship he tore out his own eyes.] An unconscious attachment of a child for the opposite parent resulting in a feeling of jealousy towards the other parent and then guilt, producing emotional conflict; usually said of male offspring. This process was described by Freud as part of his theory of infantile sexuality and considered to be normal in male infants.

oes-: For words beginning thus and not found here, see words beginning with es-.

OH: The symbol that represents the hydroxyl ion in solution. When one or more OH groups unite with a metallic element, a base is formed.

o.h.: Abbreviation for *omni hora,* meaning every hour.

-oid: Denotes having the quality, form, or appearance of; resembling.

Oidium (ō-id′-i-um): A genus of fungi widely distributed in nature, now usually called *Candida* (*q. v.*).

ointment (oynt′-ment): A semisolid fatty mixture that is applied externally as a protective covering or as a vehicle for a medicinal substance that is to be absorbed.

old tuberculin: See **tuberculin.**

ole-, olei-, oleo-: Denotes oil.

oleaginous (ō-lē-aj′-i-nus): Greasy; oily.

olecranon (ō-lek′-ra-non): The large process at the upper end of the ulna; it forms the tip of the elbow when the arm is flexed.

oleum (ōl′-ē-um): Oil. O. RICINI, castor oil, a purgative.

olfactory (ol-fak′-to-ri): Pertaining to the sense of smell. O. NERVE, nerve of the sense of smell, terminating in the nasal mucosa; it is the first cranial nerve. O. ORGAN, the nose.—olfaction, n.

olig-, oligo-: Denotes: (1) deficiency, insufficiency; (2) little, few.

oligemia (ol-i-gē′-mi-a): Diminished total quantity of blood in the body.—oligemic, adj.

olighydria (ol-ig-hid′-ri-a): Scanty perspiration. Also oligidria.

oligoamnios (ol-i-gō-am′-ni-os): Oligohydramnios (*q.v.*).

oligocythemia (ol-i-gō-sī-thē′-mi-a): Deficiency in the cellular elements in the blood.

oligodactylia (ol-i-gō-dak-til′-i-a): Fewer than the normal number of fingers or toes.

oligoerythrocythemia (ol-i-gō-e-rith-rō-sī-thē′-mi-a): A deficiency of red blood cells or of coloring matter in these cells.

oligohemia (ol-i-gō-hē′-mi-a): Oligemia (*q.v.*).

oligohydramnios (ol-i-gō-hī-dram′-ni-os): Deficient amount of amniotic fluid.

oligohydruria (ol-i-gō-hī-drū′-ri-a): Excretion of small amount of highly concentrated urine.

oligohypermenorrhea (ol-i-gō-hī-per-men-ō-rē′-a): Infrequent menstruation but with excessive flow.

oligohypomenorrhea (ol-i-gō-hī-pō-men-ō-rē′-a): Infrequent menstruation with less than normal flow.

oligoleukocythemia (ol-i-gō-lū-kō-sī-thē′-mi-a): Leukopenia (*q.v.*).

oligomenorrhea (ol-i-gō-men-ō-rē′-a): Infrequent menstruation; normal cycle is prolonged beyond 35 days.

oligophrenia (ol-i-gō-frē′-ni-a): Mental deficiency due to faulty development. PHENYLPYRUVIC O., O. characterized by excretion of phenylpyruvic acid in the urine; see **phenylketonuria.**

oligospermia (ol-i-gō-sper′-mi-a): Deficiency in the number of spermatozoa in the semen.

oliguria (ol-i-gū′-ri-a): Deficient urine secretion in relation to amount of fluid intake.—oliguric, adj.

olive oil: The oil of the olive; used externally as an emollient and lubricant, internally as a lubricant, and as a food.

o.m.: Abbreviation for *omni mane,* meaning every morning.

om-, omo-: Denotes shoulder.

-oma: Denotes tumor or neoplasm of the part named in the stem.

omentum (ō-men′-tum): A single or double fold of peritoneum that passes from the stomach to another abdominal organ. The functions of the O. are protection, repair and fat storage. GREATER O., the fold which hangs from the lower border of the stomach and covers the front of the intestines. LESSER O., a smaller fold, passing between the transverse fissure of the liver and the lesser curvature of the stomach. —omental, adj.

omodynia (ō-mō-din′-i-a): Pain in the shoulder.

omphal-, omphalo-: Denotes the umbilicus.

omphalitis (om-fa-lī′-tis): Inflammation of the umbilicus.

omphalocele (om′-fal-ō-sēl): Congenital umbilical hernia.

omphaloncus (om-fa-long′-kus): A swelling or tumor of the umbilicus.

omphalus (om′-fa-lus): The umbilicus.

o.n.: Abbreviation for *omni nocte,* meaning every night.

onanism (ō′-nan-izm): Incomplete sexual intercourse with withdrawal before the emission of semen.

onc-, onco-: Denotes: (1) tumor, swelling, mass; (2) barb or hook.

Onchocerca (on-kō-ser′-ka): Filarial worm.

onchocerciasis (on-kō-ser-kī′-a-sis): Infestation of man with Onchocerca. Adult worms encapsulated in subcutaneous connective tissue. Can cause cataract.

oncogenic (on-kō-jen′-ik): 1. Capable of tumor production. 2. Pertaining to the origin and growth of a neoplasm: often used to describe the carcinogenic viruses.

oncology (on-kol′-o-ji): The scientific study of tumors.—oncological, adj.; oncologically, adv.

oncolysis (on-kol′-i-sis): Destruction of a neoplasm. Sometimes used to describe reduction in size of a tumor.—oncolytic, adj.

onych-, onycho-: Denotes the nails.

onychectomy (on-i-kek'-to-mi): Surgical removal of a nail.

onychia (ō-nik'-i-a): Acute inflammation of the nail matrix; suppuration may spread beneath the nail, causing it to become detached and fall off.

onychocryptosis (on-ik-ō-krip-tō'-sis): Ingrowing of the nail.

onychogryposis (on-ik-ō-gri-pō'-sis): A deformity of the nails in which they become ridged, thickened, sometimes with an inward curvature.

onycholysis (on-i-kol'-i-sis): Loosening of toe- or fingernail.—onycholytic, adj.

onychomycosis (on-ik-ō-mī-kō'-sis): A fungal infection of the nails. Called also ringworm of the nails.

onychophagy (on-i-kof'-a-ji): Nailbiting.

onyx (on'-iks): A finger- or toenail.

onyxis (ō-nik'-sis): Ingrowing of a nail or nails.

oocyte (ō'-ō-sīt): An immature ovum.

oogenesis (ō-ō-jen'-e-sis): The production and formation of ova in the ovary.—oogenetic, adj.

oophor-, oophoro-: Denotes: (1) ovary; (2) ovarian.

oophoralgia (ō-of-or-al'-ji-a): Pain in an ovary.

oophorectomy (ō-of-ō-rek'-to-mi): Excision of an ovary.—oophorectomize, n.

oophoritis (ō-of-or-ī'-tis): Inflammation of an ovary.

oophorocystectomy (ō-of-or-ō-sis-tek'-to-mi): Removal of an ovarian cyst.

oophoron (ō-of'-or-on): The ovary.

oophorosalpingectomy (ō-of-or-ō-sal-pin-jek'-to-mi): Excision of an ovary and its associated fallopian tube.

oosperm (ō'-ō-sperm): A fertilized ovum.

opacity (ō-pas'-i-ti): Non-transparency; cloudiness; an opaque spot, as on the cornea or lens.

opaque (ō-pāk'): Not transparent.

OPD: Abbreviation for outpatient department.

open: 1. Exposed to the air. 2. Not covered by skin. O. FRACTURE, one in which an external wound leads to the fractured bone. O. HOSPITAL, a mental hospital with unbarred windows and unlocked doors. O. REDUCTION, reduction of a fracture after incision into the site of the fracture. O. WOUND, one that opens to the surface of the body.

operable (op'-er-a-b'l): Descriptive of a condition that it is thought can be cured or improved by surgery which will not endanger the patient's life or general health.

operation (op-er-ā'-shun): A procedure in which a surgeon uses his hands or instruments for correcting or altering a pathological condition or state, or for removing a tumor, limb, etc. ELECTIVE O., one for which haste is not required; can be performed at the patient's and surgeon's convenience. EMERGENCY O., one that must be done immediately in order to save the patient's life. EXPLORATORY O., one done for diagnostic purposes. MAJOR O., one involving risk to the patient's life. MINOR O., a relatively simple one that usually does not involve risk to the patient's life. RADICAL O., one done to effect a complete cure. SUBTOTAL O., one in which not all of the involved organ is removed.

ophthalm-, ophthalmo-: Denotes: (1) the eye; (2) the eyeball.

ophthalmalgia (of-thal-mal'-ji-a): Pain in the eye.

ophthalmectomy (of-thal-mek'-to-mi): Surgical removal of the eyeball by enucleation.

ophthalmia (of-thal'-mi-a): Inflammation of the eye involving especially the conjunctiva. O. NEONATORUM, purulent infection of the eyes of an infant at birth as it passes through the genital tract; may be caused by the gonococcus. SYMPATHETIC O., iridocyclitis of one eye secondary to injury or disease of the other.

ophthalmic (of-thal'-mik): Pertaining to the eye.

ophthalmitis (of-thal-mī'-tis): Syn., ophthalmia (q.v.).

ophthalmologist (of-thal-mol'-o-jist): A physician who specializes in the diseases and refractive errors of the eye.

ophthalmology (of-thal-mol'-o-ji): The science that deals with the structure, function and diseases of the eye.—ophthalmological, adj.; ophthalmologically, adv.

ophthalmoplegia (of-thal-mō-plē'-ji-a): Paralysis of either the extrinsic or intrinsic muscles of the eye.—ophthalmoplegic, adj.

ophthalmoptosis (of-thal-mop-tō'-sis): Protrusion of the eyeball; exophthalmos (q.v.).

ophthalmoscope (of-thal'-mō-skōp): An instrument fitted with a lens and illumination for examining the interior of the eye.—ophthalmoscopic, adj.

ophthalmotomy (of-thal-mot'-o-mi): Incision into the eyeball.

ophthalmotonometer (of-thal-mō-tō-nom'-

et-er): Instrument for determining the intraocular tension.

-opia: Refers to sightedness, *e.g.,* myopia.

opiate (ō'-pi-āt): 1. Any drug derived from opium. 2. In a broad sense sometimes used to describe any drug that produces sleep.

opisthotonos (op-is-thot'-on-os): Extreme extension of the body occurring in tetanic spasm. Patient may be supported on his head and heels alone. Symptom may be present in meningitis and strychnine poisoning as well as in tetanus.—opisthotonic, adj.

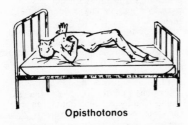

Opisthotonos

opium (ō'-pi-um): Dried juice of O. poppy capsules; long used as a narcotic and analgesic; habit-forming. Contains valuable alkaloids such as morphine, codeine, papaverine.

opiumism (ō'-pi-um-izm): The habit of using opium or the physiological condition resulting from the habitual use of opium.

opodidymus (ō-pō-did'-i-mus): A fetus with a single body but two heads that are partly fused.

opotherapy (ō-pō-ther'-a-pi): The use of animals' organs in the treatment of disease.

oppilation (op-i-lā'-shun): Constipation.—oppilative, adj.

opponens (ō-pō'-nenz): 1. Opposing. 2. The name given to several small muscles of the hand or foot which act to draw the lateral digits across the palm or sole.

opportunistic infection: A serious infection with a microorganism that normally has little or no pathogenic activity but which has been activated by a serious disease or a modern method of treatment.

opsoclonia (op-sō-klō'-ni-a): A condition characterized by irregular, jerking horizontal and vertical movements of the eyeball. Opsoclonus.

opsonic index (op-son'-ik in'-deks): A figure obtained by experiment which indicates the ability of phagocytes to ingest foreign bodies such as bacteria.

opsonin (op'-son-in): An antibody which unites with antigen, usually part of intact cells, and renders the cells more susceptible to phagocytosis. See **antibodies.**—opsonic, opsoniferous, adj.; opsonification, n.

-opsy: Denotes examination of.

optic (op'-tik): Pertaining to sight or to the eye. O. CHIASM, CHIASMA, the X-shaped crossing on the ventral surface of the brain where some of the fibers of the two optic nerves cross to the opposite sides and continue in the optic tracts of those sides. O. DISK, the point at the back of the retina where the O. nerve enters the eyeball. O. NERVES, the second pair of cranial nerves; conduct visual stimuli from the retina to the brain.

optical (op'-ti-kal): Related to vision or the science of optics.

optician (op-tish'-an): One who makes and dispenses lenses to correct refractive errors in vision.

optics (op'-tiks): That branch of physics that deals with light, its sources, transmission, refraction, absorption, etc., particularly as these phenomena relate to vision.

optimum (op'-ti-mum): The quality of being the best or most favorable; conducive to the most favorable activity or result. In bacteriology, the temperature at which bacteria grow best. O. POSITION, that which will be the least awkward and most useful should a limb remain permanently paralyzed.

opto-: Denotes: (1) vision; (2) the eye; (3) optic.

optokinetic (op-tō-kī-net'-ik): Pertaining to or involving movements of the eyeball.

optometer (op-tom'-et-er): An instrument used for measuring the power and range of vision.

optometrist (op-tom'-e-trist): One who practices optometry (*q.v.*).

optometry (op-tom'-e-tri): 1. Measurement of visual acuity with an optometer. 2. An occupation consisting of examining the eye for refractive errors and prescribing lenses or any other means except drugs, for the correction of these errors; non-medical visual care.

OPV: Abbreviation for oral poliovaccine (Sabin's vaccine, *q.v.*).

OR: Abbreviation for operating room.

orad (ō'-rad): Toward the mouth.

oral: Pertaining to the mouth.—orally, adj. O. PHASE, the earliest phase of psychosexual development (*q.v.*) in which the child derives pleasure from sucking or biting; persists into adult life in sublimated form.

orb: A sphere. In medicine, the eyeball.

orbicular (or-bik′-ū-lar): Resembling a globe; spherical or circular.

orbit (or′-bit): In anatomy, the bony socket that encloses and protects the eyeball and its appendages.—orbital, adj. Also eye socket.

orchi-, orchid-, orchio-: Denotes the testes.

orchialgia (or-ki-al′-ji-a): Pain in a testis. Also orchidalgia.

orchidectomy (or-ki-dek′-to-mi): Excision of one or both testes; castration. Also orchectomy, orchiectomy.

orchidopexy (or-ki-dō-pek′-si): The operation of bringing an undescended testis into the scrotum, and fixing it in this position. Also orchiopexy, orchiorrhaphy.

orchidotherapy (or-ki-dō-ther′-a-pi): Treatment of disease with testicular extract. Orchiotherapy.

orchiepididymitis (or-ki-ep-i-did-i-mī′-tis): Inflammation of a testis and an epididymis.

orchioncus (or-ki-ong′-kus): Tumor of the testis.

orchis (or′-kis): The testis.—orchitic, adj.

orchitis (or-kī′-tis): Inflammation of a testis.

orderly: A male attendant in a hospital or other institution.

ordure (or′-dūr): Excrement.

orf: A disease of sheep, transmissible to man; caused by a filterable virus; characterized by dark red papules that become indurated, fever, rheumatic pains.

organ: A differentiated part of the body that may or may not be grouped with other parts to perform a specific function. O. OF CORTI, see **Corti.**

organic: 1. Pertaining to an organ. 2. Associated with life. O. CHEMISTRY, the study of substances that contain carbon. O. DISEASE, one in which there is structural change. O. PSYCHOSIS, a psychosis, usually severe, that results from disturbance of brain function due to some physical disorder such as tumor, injury, or infection.

organism (or′-gan-izm): A living cell or group of cells differentiated into functionally distinct parts which are interdependent. Any living individual, either plant or animal.

organization (or-gan-ī-zā′-shun): 1. The process of providing or assuming a structure. 2. The change in the structure of a blood clot in a vein whereby it becomes fibrous.

organopathy (or-ga-nop′-a-thi): Organic disease. See **organ.**

organotherapy (or-ga-nō-ther′-a-pi): Treatment of disease by administration of animal organs or the extracts of these organs.

organ transplant: The replacement of a diseased or malfunctioning organ or part with one from another individual, either living or recently deceased. Organs that have been transplanted include kidney, heart, liver, lung, pancreas, spleen, and recently, an entire human eye. The principal problem in transplants is the rejection of the organ by the immunological defenses of the donee which treat the transplanted organ as foreign and try to destroy it. Corneal transplants are frequently successful.

orgasm (or′-gazm): The crisis of sexual excitement.

oriental sore (o-ri-en′-tal sōr′): Delhi boil. A form of cutaneous leishmaniasis producing papular, crusted, granulomatous eruptions of the skin. A disease of the tropics and sub-tropics.

orientation (or-i-en-tā′-shun): Clear awareness of one's position relative to the environment. In mental conditions o. 'in space and time' means that the patient knows where he is and recognizes the passage of time, i.e., can give the correct date. Disorientation means the reverse.

orifice (or′-i-fis): A mouth or opening.

origin (or′-i-jin): The commencement or source of anything. O. OF A MUSCLE, the end that remains relatively fixed during contraction of the muscle.

ornithine (or′-ni-thēn): An amino acid, obtained from arginine by splitting off urea.

Ornithodoros (or-ni-thod′-o-rōs): A genus of ticks which are the vectors of the organisms causing such diseases as spotted fever, Q fever, tick fever, tularemia, relapsing fever, and certain types of encephalitis.

ornithosis (or-ni-thō′-sis): A contagious virus disease of wild birds and some domestic fowl, sometimes transmitted to man. Disease closely resembles psittacosis but is usually less severe.

oropharynx (or-ō-far′-inks): 1. That portion of the pharynx that is below the level of the hyoid bone. 2. Pertaining to the mouth and pharynx.—oropharyngeal, adj.

orrhorrhea (or-ro-rē′-a): A copious serous or waterly discharge.

orth-, ortho-: Denotes: (1) straight, normal, in proper order; (2) correct, corrective.

orthodontics (or-thō-don′-tiks): A branch of dentistry dealing with prevention and correction of irregularities and malocclusion of the teeth.

orthodontist (or-thō-don′-tist): A dentist who specializes in orthodontics (q.v.).

orthopedics (or-thō-pē'-diks): A branch of surgery dealing with deformities and diseases of the skeleton and its associated structures and their correction, whether by apparatus, manipulation, or surgery.

orthopedist (or-tho-pē'-dist): A physician who specializes in orthopedics (*q.v.*).

orthopnea (or-thop-nē'-a): Inability to breathe except in an upright, sitting position.—orthopneic, adj.

orthopsychiatry (or-thō-sī-kī'-a-tri): That branch of psychiatry that deals with the amelioration of disorders of personality and behavior in normal or near-normal persons, particularly in children and young adults.

orthoptic (or-thop'-tik): Relating to orthoptics (*q.v.*). O. EXERCISES, a system of eye exercises designed to strengthen the eye muscles and prescribed to help correct such conditions as strabismus (*q.v.*) or squint.

orthoptics (or-thop'-tiks): Study and treatment of muscle imbalances of the eye, or of faulty visual habits, *e.g.,* squint.

orthostatic (or-thō-stat'-ik): Caused by or related to the upright stance. O. ALBUMINURIA, occurs in some healthy subjects only when they take the upright position. When lying in bed the urine is normal.

orthotist (or'-thō-tist): One who makes and fits orthopedic appliances.

OS: Abbreviation for *oculus sinister,* meaning left eye.

os: A mouth. EXTERNAL O., the opening of the cervix into the vagina. INTERNAL O., the opening of the cervix into the uterine cavity.—ora, pl.

os: A bone.—ossa, pl. O. CALCIS, the heel bone; the calcaneus. O. COXAE, the hip bone. O. INNOMINATUM, os coxae.

osche-, oscheo-: Denotes the scrotum.

oscheitis (os-kē-ī'-tis): Inflammation of the scrotum.

oscheocele (os'-kē-ō-sēl): Swelling, tumor, or hernia of the scrotum.

oscheoncus (os-kē-ong'-kus): Tumor of the scrotum.

oscillating bed (os'-il-āt-ing): A mechanical bed so designed that it may be tilted at regular intervals thus changing the patient's posture and allowing for the alternate filling and draining of the blood vessels of the lower extremities.

oscillation (os-il-ā'-shun): A swinging or moving to and fro; a vibration.

oscillometry (os-il-om'-et-ri): Measurement of vibration, using a special apparatus (oscillometer, oscilloscope). Measures the

magnitude of the pulse wave more precisely than palpation.

-ose: Denotes: (1) full of, having the qualities of; (2) a carbohydrate substance.

-osis (pl., oses): Denotes: (1) action, process, condition; (2) increase, formation; (3) disease caused by a specific fungus.

Osler's nodes: Small painful areas (due to emboli) in pulp of fingers or toes, or palms and soles, occurring in subacute bacterial endocarditis. [William Osler, English physician (Canadian birth). 1849-1919.]

osmesis (oz-mē'-sis): The sense of smell; the act of smelling.

osmidrosis (oz-mi-drō'-sis): Bromhidrosis (*q.v.*).

osmolarity (os-mō-lar'-i-ti): The osmotic pressure exerted by a substance in aqueous solution, defined in terms of the number of active particles per unit volume.

osmoreceptor (oz-mō-re-sep'-tor): 1. A sensory nerve ending that is responsive to stimulation by odors. 2. A sensory nerve ending that is responsive to changes in the osmotic pressure of the surrounding medium.

osmosis (os-mō'-sis): The passage of fluid across a membrane under the influence of osmotic pressure (*q.v.*).

osmotic pressure (os-mot'-ik): The force with which the fluid part of a solution is drawn across a semipermeable membrane that separates two solutions of different concentrations and that permits passage of the fluid but not of the solutes, the direction of flow being from the solution of lesser to the solution of greater concentration.

osseous (os'-ē-us): Pertaining to, composed of, or resembling bone.

ossi-: Denotes bone.

ossicle (os'-ik'l): A small bone, particularly one of those contained in the middle ear: the malleus, incus, and stapes.

ossification (os-i-fi-kā'-shun): The formation of bone; the conversion of cartilage, etc., into bone.—ossify, v.t., v.i.

ostalgia (os-tal'-ji-a): Pain in a bone. Ostealgia.

oste-, osteo-: Denotes bone.

ostearthritis (os-tē-ar-thrī'-tis): Osteoarthritis (*q.v.*).

ostectomy (os-tek'-to-mi): Surgical removal of a bone or part of a bone. Osteectomy.

osteitis (os-tē-ī'-tis): Inflammation of bone. O. DEFORMANS, rarefaction occurs, leading to bowing of long bones and deformity of flat bones. Paget's disease. O. FIBROSA, cavities form in the interior of bone. Cysts may be solitary or the disease generalized. This second condition is the result of excessive parathyroid secretion and absorption of calcium from bone.

osteoarthritis (os-tē-ō-ar-thrī'-tis): Degenerative arthritis. A chronic disease of joints occurring mostly in middle or old age, characterized by degenerative changes in the bone and cartilage of one, several, or all of the joints. The articular cartilage becomes worn and osteophytes may form at the periphery of the joint surface and loose bodies result. Apparently no specific cause; may be primary, or follow disease or injury involving the articular surfaces of synovial joints; other factors may be heredity, occupation, overweight, faulty posture.—osteoarthritic, adj.

osteoblast (os'-tē-ō-blast): A bone-forming cell.

osteoblastoma (os-tē-ō-blas-tō'-ma): An uncommon tumor of osteoblasts; occurs chiefly in the spine in young people.

osteochondritis (os-tē-ō-kon-drī'-tis): Inflammation of both bone and cartilage. Term most often applied to non-septic conditions, especially avascular necrosis involving a joint surface. O. DEFORMANS JUVENILIS, a form of O. occurring most often in boys 5-10 years of age; disturbance of growth at the epiphyseal cartilage results in flattening of the head of the femur causing muscle spasm, limitation of movement, limping and sometimes shortening of the leg. Syn., Legg's disease. Legg-Calvé-Perthes disease. O. DISSECANS, a form of O. in which small pieces of an articular joint may separate to form loose bodies in the joint; seen most often in the knee and shoulder. See **Scheuermann's disease.**

osteochondroma (os-tē-ō-kon-drō'-ma): A benign tumor made up of osseous and cartilaginous tissue.

osteochondrosis (os-tē-ō-kon-drō'-sis): A disease of the ossification centers in the bones of children. Usually begins with a degeneration that is followed by regeneration and calcification. May affect the femur, tibia, vertebrae, bones of the wrist or hand.

osteoclasia (os-tē-ō-klā'-zi-a): The destruction and absorption of bony tissue by osteoclasts.

osteoclasis (os-tē-ok'-la-sis): The therapeutic fracture of a bone in a closed operation; performed to correct a deformity or to reset a bone that has healed incorrectly.

osteoclast (os'-tē-ō-klast): A large multinucleated cell that is formed in the bone marrow; its function is to dissolve or remove unwanted or dead bone.

osteoclastoma (os-tē-ō-klas-tō'-ma): A tumor made up of cells resembling osteoclasts. May be benign, recurrent, or frankly malignant. The usual site is near the end of a long bone. See **myeloma.**

osteocystoma (os-tē-ō-sis-tō'-ma): A cystic tumor of bone usually occurring in childhood or early adolescence. Site is most often the shaft of a long bone, particularly the upper part of the humerus.

osteocyte (os'-tē-ō-sīt): A bone cell.

osteodystrophy (os-tē-ō-dis'-tro-fi): Faulty formation or growth of bone. Osteodystrophia.

osteofibroma (os-tē-ō-fi-brō'-ma): A tumor made up mostly of fibrous tissue but which has small foci of bony tissue.

osteogenesis (os-tē-ō-jen'-e-sis): Formation of bone; development of bones.—osteogenic, adj. O. IMPERFECTA, an inherited condition in which the bones are brittle and subject to fracture. Sometimes fractures occur in intrauterine life, and sometimes they do not occur until the child is old enough to walk. Also called brittle bones, fragilitas ossium.

osteogenic (os-tē-ō-jen'-ik): Bone producing. O. SARCOMA, a general term for a malignant tumor arising in cells whose normal function is the production of bone; usually occurring in children and young adults; characterized by pain, swelling, and early metastases especially to the lung.

osteoid (os'-tē-oid): Resembling bone.

osteolysis (os-tē-ol'-i-sis): Softening or dissolution of bone, especially that caused by loss of calcium.

osteolytic (os-tē-ō-lit'-ik): Relating to osteolysis. Destructive of bone.

osteoma (os-tē-ō'-ma): A bony tumor; usually developing on a bone, but may also be on some other organ, e.g., lung or pleura; may be single or multiple.

osteomalacia (os-tē-ō-ma-lā'-shi-a): A condition of adult life in which there is a softening of bone due to deficiency of vitamin D, calcium, and phosphate, or excessive absorption of calcium and phosphorus from the bones. May occur in malnutrition or pregnancy; often referred to as 'adult rickets.'

osteomyelitis (os-tē-ō-mī-e-lī'-tis): Inflammation of bone caused by a pyogenic organism such as staphylococcus, streptococcus, pneumococcus or meningococcus; usually begins in the bone marrow and may remain localized or spread to other parts of the bone; may follow injury to the bone, a skin infection, or an abscess in another part of the body.

osteoncus (os-tē-ong′-kus): A bone tumor. Osteoma.

osteonecrosis (os-tē-ō-nē-krō′-sis): Death (necrosis) of bone when it occurs in areas considered large as compared with such small foci of necrosis as occur in dental caries.

osteopath (os′-tē-ō-path): One who practices osteopathy.

osteopathy (os-tē-op′-a-thi): 1. Any disease of bone. 2. A theory that attributes a wide range of disorders to mechanical derangements of the skeletal system, which it claims can be rectified by suitable manipulations along with adequate nutrition and favorable environment.—osteopathic, adj.

osteoperiostitis (os-tē-ō-per-i-os-tī′-tis): Inflammation of periosteum and the bone under it.

osteopetrosis (os-tē-ō-pē-trō′-sis): A condition in which there is an increase in the density of bones, clubbing of the ends of long bones, retarded growth, anemia, and a strong tendency to spontaneous fractures. Called also 'marble bones' and Albers-Schönberg disease (*q.v.*).

osteophage (os′-tē-ō-fāj): Syn., osteoclast (*q.v.*).

osteophone (os′-tē-ō-fōn): A device for helping the deaf to hear. An audiophone.

osteophony (os-tē-of′-on-i): The conduction of sound waves to the inner ear by bone.

osteophyte (os′-tē-ō-fīt): A bony outgrowth or spur, usually at the margins of joint surfaces, *e.g.,* in osteoarthritis.—osteophytic, adj.

osteoplasty (os′-tē-ō-plas-ti): Any plastic operation on bone.—osteoplastic, adj.

osteopoikilosis (os-tē-ō-poi-ki-lō′-sis): A congenital condition of the bones in which there are multiple areas of sclerosis throughout the bones; usually asymptomatic but the bones are subject to easy fracture.

osteoporosis (os-tē-ō-po-rō′-sis): Loss of density of bone and enlargement of the bone spaces due to disturbance of mineral metabolism and failure of the osteoclasts to lay down sufficient matrix; characterized by abnormal porousness, fragility, and reduction in quantity of bone. Most often seen in women after menopause; may also accompany pathologic conditions, *e.g.,*

parathyroid tumor.—osteoporotic, adj.

osteosarcoma (os-tē-ō-sar-kō′-ma): A malignant tumor originating in bone cells or containing bony tissue.—osteosarcomata, pl.; osteosarcomatous, adj.

osteosclerosis (os-tē-ō-skler-ō′-sis): Abnormal density or hardness of bone.—osteosclerotic, adj.

osteotome (os′-tē-ō-tōm): An instrument for cutting bone; it is similar to a chisel, but it is bevelled on both sides of its cutting edge.

osteotomy (os-tē-ot′-o-mi): The surgical division or cutting of bone.

ostitis (os-tī′-tis): Osteitis (*q.v.*).

ostium (os′-ti-um): The opening or mouth of any tubular passage.—ostial, adj.; ostia, pl.

Ostomies Anonymous: A national organization of persons who have had mutilating or traumatic surgery for treatment of cancer. Its purpose is to assist such persons to express their fears and anxieties and to adjust to their condition.

-ostomy: Denotes the formation of an opening or outlet, usually surgical.

OT: Abbreviation for (1) old tuberculin (*q.v.*); (2) occupational therapy. See **therapy.**

ot-, oto-: Denotes the ear.

otalgia (ō-tal′-ji-a): Earache.

otic (ō′-tik): Pertaining to the ear.

otitis (ō-tī′-tis): Inflammation of the ear. O. EXTERNA, O. of the external auditory canal. O. INTERNA, O. of inner ear, usually caused by extension of inflammation from the middle ear; main symptoms are dizziness, nausea, nystagmus, headache and possibly deafness. O. MEDIA, O. of the middle ear; may be acute or chronic; may follow infectious disease such as measles or scarlet fever; chief symptoms are pain, fever, tinnitis, bulging of the tympanic membrane, possibly deafness.

otoblennorrhea (ō-tō-blen-ō-rē′-a): A mucous discharge from the ear.

otocleisis (ō-tō-klī′-sis): Closure of the eustachian tube or of the external auditory canal; may be caused by a new growth or by collection of cerumen in the external canal.

otodynia (ō-tō-din′-i-a): Earache. Otalgia.

otoencephalitis (ō-tō-en-sef-a-lī′-tis): Inflammation of the brain resulting from an extention of inflammation of the middle ear.

otolaryngology (ō-tō-lar-in-gol′-o-ji): The branch of medical science that deals with the structure, function, and diseases of the ear and the larynx.

otoliths (ō'-tō-līths): Tiny dustlike deposits of calcium carbonate within the membranous labyrinth of the inner ear.

otologist (ō-tol'-ō-jist): One specializing in the functions and diseases of the ear.

otology (ō-tol'-ō-ji): The branch of medical science that deals with the structure, functions, and diseases of the ear.

-otomy: Refers to a surgical incision.

otomycosis (ō-tō-mī-kō'-sis): A fungal (Aspergillus, Candida) infection of the external auditory meatus and canal.—otomycotic, adj.

otoplasty (ō'-tō-plas-ti): Plastic surgery for the correction of deformed, flattened, or protruding ears; done preferably during childhood.

otopyorrhea (ō-tō-pī-o-rē'-a): Flow of purulent discharge from the ear; often results from chronic otitis media with perforation of the ear drum.

otorhinolaryngology (ō-tō-rī-nō-lar-in-gol'-o-ji): The branch of medical science that deals with the structure, function, and diseases of the ear, nose and throat.

otorrhea (ō-tō-rē'-a): A discharge from the external auditory meatus, especially one that is mucopurulent.

otosclerosis (ō-tō-skler-ō'-sis): A condition of progressive deafness marked by new bone formation affecting primarily the labyrinth of the inner ear and causing ankylosis of the stapes to the margin of the round window. Of unknown origin; heredity may be a factor.—otosclerotic, adj.

otoscope (ō'-tō-skōp): An instrument for examining the ear; auriscope (q.v.).—otoscopic, adj.

otosis(ō-tō'-sis): Mishearing spoken words.

OU: Abbreviation for *oculus uterque,* meaning each eye or both eyes.

ounce: A measure of weight. In the avoirdupois system it is 1/16 of a pound, or 437.5 grains. In the apothecaries' system it is 1/12 of a pound, or 480 grains. A fluid ounce is equal to 8 fluidrams in the apothecaries' system, 29.57 ml in the metric system. Abbreviation oz.

outlet: An opening, usually in the nature of a passageway, by means of which something escapes.

outpatient: An ambulatory patient who lives outside the hospital but comes to the hospital clinic or dispensary for treatment.

output: 1. The quantity of waste substance produced by a process such as metabolism and excreted from the body, *e.g.,* the amount of urine voided in a given time. Opp. of intake. 2. The amount of a substance ejected from a given place, *e.g.,* the cardiac output of blood.

ov-, ovi-, ovo-: Denotes ovum.

oval window: Fenestra ovalis (q.v.).

ovar-, ovari-, ovario-: Denotes: (1) ovary; (2) ovarian.

ovarian (ō-var-'i-an): Pertaining to the ovaries. O. CYST, an ovarian tumor containing fluid—may be benign or malignant.

ovariectomy (ō-var-i-ek'-to-mi): Excision of an ovary. Oophorectomy.

ovariocentesis (ō-var-i-ō-sen-tē'-sis): Surgical puncture of an ovary usually for the drainage of an ovarian cyst.

ovarioncus (ō-var-i-ong'-kus): Tumor of the ovary.

ovariotomy (ō-var-i-ot'-om-i): Literally means incision of an ovary, but is the term usually applied to the removal of an ovary. Also oophorectomy.

ovaritis (ō-var-i'-tis): Oophoritis (q.v.).

ovary (ō'-var-i): One of the paired sex glands of the female; an oval, flattened gland, about 1½ inches long, suspended on the posterior surface of the broad ligament, one on either side of the uterus. The substance is vascular and fibrous and contains the egg cells one of which matures and is expelled periodically. Function of the gland is to develop the egg cells and also to produce the female sex hormones. CYSTIC O., retention cysts in the ovarian follicles.

overcompensation (ō-ver-kom-pen-sā'-shun): Name given any type of behavior a person adopts in order to cover up a deficiency in his personality, of which he is aware. Thus a person who is afraid may react by becoming arrogant or boastful or quarrelsome.

overflow: Continuous escape of fluid such as tears or urine.

overhydration (ō-ver-hī-drā'-shun): The presence of excess fluids in the body.

overriding: 1. The slipping of one end of a fractured bone past the other end 2. The molding of the fetus's head during delivery.

overtoe: A condition in which the great toe lies over the adjacent toes. Hallux varus.

oviduct (ō'-vi-dukt): Syn., fallopian tube

(*q.v.*). Also called uterine tube.

ovotherapy (ō-vō-ther′-a-pi): Therapeutic use of ovarian secretion, particularly that from the corpus luteum.

ovulation (ov-ū-lā′-shun): The maturation and rupture of a graafian follicle with the discharge of an ovum.

ovule (ō′-vūl): The ovum before it has been expelled from the ovary.

ovum (ō′-vum): The female reproductive cell; a round cell about 0.1 mm in diameter that develops in the graafian follicle and, when mature, is expelled by the follicle into the abdominal cavity whence it enters the fallopian tube; unless fertilized is cast off; this occurs approximately every 28 days during a female's life from puberty to menopause.—ova, pl.; ovarian, adj.

oxalate(ok′-sa-lāt): Any salt of oxalic acid.

oxalemia (ok-sa-lē′-mi-a): Presence of abnormally large amounts of oxalates in the blood.

oxalic acid (ok-sal′-ik): An organic acid found in many plants that are used as foods.

oxaluria (ok-sa-lū′-ri-a): The excretion of urine containing calcium oxalate crystals; often associated with dyspepsia (*q.v.*).

oxidase (ok′-si-dās): Any enzyme which promotes oxidation.

oxidation (ok-si-dā′-shun): The process of converting a substance into an oxide by the addition of oxygen. The carbon in organic compounds undergoes o. with the formation of carbon dioxide when they are combusted in air, or when they are metabolized in living material in the presence of oxygen. Also used in biochemistry for the process of the removal of hydrogen from a molecule (*e.g.*, in the presence of air, ascorbic acid undergoes o. with the formation of dehydroascorbic acid). The loss of an electron with an increase in valency (*e.g.*, the conversion of ferrous to ferric iron) is also an o. The greater part of the energy present in foods is made available to the body by the process of o. in the tissues.

oxide (ok′-sīd): Any compound of oxygen with another element or radical, usually a metal.

oxidize (ok′-si-dīz): To combine oxygen with an element or a radical, or to cause such combination to take place.

oxidosis (ok-si-dō′-sis): Acidosis (*q.v.*).

oxy-: Denotes: (1) the presence of oxygen in

a substance; (2) pointed; (3) sharp, sour, quick.

oxyblepsia (ok-sē-blep′-si-a): Unusual acuteness of vision.

oxycephaly (ok-sē-sef′-a-li): A congenital deformity in which the head is more pointed than rounded.

oxygen (ok′-si-jen): A colorless, odorless, gaseous element; necessary for life and combustion. The most abundant element on earth; constitutes 20% by weight of air. Used medically as an inhalation; supplied in cylinders in which the gas is at a high pressure. See **hyperbaric.**

oxygenation (ok-si-je-nā′-shun): The saturation of a substance (particularly blood) with oxygen.—oxygenated, adj.

oxygenator (ok-si-je-nā′-tor): A device for oxygenating the blood outside of the body. The 'artificial lung' as used in heart surgery.

oxygeusia (ok-si-gū′-si-a): Abnormally keen sense of taste.

oxyhemoglobin (ok-si-hē-mō-glō′-bin): Oxygenated hemoglobin, an unstable compound.

oxylalia (ok-se-lā′-li-a): Abnormally fast speech.

oxyntic (oks-in′-tik): Producing acid. o. CELLS, the cells in the gastric mucosa which produce hydrochloric acid.

oxyopia (ok-si-ō′-pi-a): Abnormally acute vision.

oxyosmia (ok-si-os′-mi-a): Abnormally acute sense of smell.

oxytocic (ok-si-tō′-sik): Hastening parturition; an agent promoting uterine contractions.

oxyuriasis (ok-si-ūr-ī′-a-sis): Infestation with pinworms or threadworms.

oz: Abbreviation for ounce.

ozena (ō-zē′-na): An atrophic condition of the nasal mucous membrane with associated crusting and an offensive-smelling discharge.

ozone (ō′-zōn): A modified and condensed form of oxygen; a slightly blue irritating gas, generated naturally by the action of ultraviolet light rays on oxygen; also made commercially. Has stronger oxidizing properties than oxygen; is used as an antiseptic and disinfectant, *e.g.*, in the purification of water.

ozostomia (ō-zō-stō′-mi-a): Foul breath; halitosis.

P: Chemical symbol for phosphorus. P³², radioactive phosphorus.

Pablum: Trade name for a precooked cereal food for infants; contains wheat, oat, and corn meals in addition to iron, sodium chloride, wheat embryo, alfalfa leaves.

pabulum (pab′-ū-lum): Food or nourishment.

pacemaker: In anatomy, a body part that establishes and maintains a rhythmic activity, in particular, the sinoatrial node (*q.v.*). ARTIFICIAL P., an emergency electrical device used to reestablish the muscular contractions of an arrested heart or to steady the heart beat; consists of an electrode that is fitted to the epicardium and attached to an electrical source that is either implanted within the body or located externally to the body. It increases the ventricular rate by supplying a current pulse that initiates a rate of contraction of the ventricle resulting in output that is adequate for allowing the patient to participate in his usual life activities.

pachy-: Denotes massive, heavy, thick, dense.

pachyblepharon (pak-i-blef′-a-ron): Thickening of an eyelid, especially near the edge.

pachycephalia (pak-i-sef-ā′-li-a): Abnormal thickness of the skull bones.—pachycephalic, pachycephalous, adj.

pachychilia (pak-i-kī′-li-a): Abnormal thickness of the lips. Also pachycheilia.

pachydactyly (pak-i-dak′-ti-li): Enlargement or thickening of the fingers or toes, especially at their ends.

pachyderma (pak-i-der′-ma): Abnormal thickness of the skin. See **elephantiasis.** Also pachydermia.

pachyglossia (pak-i-glos′-i-a): Abnormal thickness of the tongue.

pachymeningitis (pak-i-men-in-jī′-tis): Inflammation of the dura mater (or pachymeninx).

pachyonychia (pak-i-ō-nik′-i-a): Abnormal thickening of the fingernails or toenails, often congenital.

pachypleuritis (pak-i-plū-rī′-tis): Inflammation of the pleura accompanied by thickening of the membrane. Productive pleurisy.

pachysomia (pak-i-sō′mi-a): Abnormal thickening of parts of the body, especially of the soft parts, as seen in acromegaly.

pacifier (pas′-i-fi-er): 1. A rubber nipple-shaped device for babies to suck or bite upon. 2. A tranquilizer.

Pacini's corpuscles: Oval bodies in the deep parts of the corium of the skin that act as end organs for the sense of pressure; found especially in the skin of the hands and feet, but also in tendon and some internal structures. [Filippo Pacini, Italian anatomist. 1812-1883.]

paed-, paedo-: See **ped-, pedo-.**

Paget's disease: 1. Osteitis deformans. A chronic disease of the bone, seen usually in the elderly; of unknown cause. There is softening and thickening of the bone with consequent distortion, and bowing deformity of the long bones. 2. A progressive, inflammatory, eczematous dermatosis of the nipple and surrounding area, seen most often in older women. There is itching, soreness, ulceration and retraction of the nipple. May be precancerous or associated with cancer of the breast. [Sir James Paget, English surgeon. 1814-1899.]

Paget-Schroeffer syndrome: Axillary or subclavian vein thrombosis, often associated with effort, in fit young persons.

pain: Physical or mental suffering. A state of localized or generalized discomfort that ranges from mild distress to acute agony; usually caused by injury to a part or disturbance of the normal condition or functioning of a part of the body. In the plural usually refers to the pains experienced during childbirth. AFTERPAINS, those due to the contraction of the uterus following the birth of a child. FALSE P'S., occur late in pregnancy and resemble labor pains but do not result in labor. GROWING P'S., those that sometimes occur in muscles and joints of adolescents and children; may be manifestation of rheumatic fever. HUNGER P'S., those that occur in the stomach when it is time for a meal; sometimes a sign of gastric disorder. LABOR P'S., the progressively severe, involuntary, rhythmic pains that occur during childbirth. PHANTOM LIMB P., that which is felt as being in a limb although the limb has been amputated. REFERRED P., that which is felt in a part other than the part where it is produced.

painter's colic: Lead colic (*q.v.*). See **lead poisoning.**

palatable (pal′-a-tab′l): Pleasant or agreeable to the taste; savory.

palate (pal′-at): The roof of the mouth, consisting of the structures that separate the mouth from the nasal cavity. ARTIFICIAL P., prosthesis for use in cleft palate. CLEFT P., a congenital cleft between the palatal bones which leaves a gap in the roof of the mouth, opening directly into the nose. Usually associated with harelip. SOFT P., situated at the posterior end of the palate and consisting of muscle covered with mucous membrane; forms the pillars of the fauces and the uvula.—palatal, palatine, adj.

palatine (pal′-a-tīn): Pertaining to the palate. P. ARCHES, the bilateral double pillars or arch-like folds formed by the descent of the soft palate as it meets the pharynx.

palatoplasty (pal′-a-tō-plas-ti): Plastic surgery of the palate, including operations to correct cleft palate. Uraniscoplasty.

palatoplegia (pal-at-ō-plē′-ji-a): Paralysis of the muscles of the soft palate.—palatoplegic, adj.

palatorrhaphy (pal-a-tor′-a-fi): An operation for the repair of a cleft palate. Syn., staphylorrhaphy, uraniscoplasty.

palikinesia (pal-i-kī-nē′-si-a): Pathological, involuntary repetition of certain movements.

palilalia (pal-i-lā′-li-a): The constant repetition of a word or phrase with increasing rapidity.

palliate (pal′-ē-āt): To reduce the severity of; allay; abate; mitigate; lessen. To ease pain or symptoms without curing the condition.

palliative (pal′-ē-ā-tive): 1. Anything which serves to alleviate but cannot cure a disease. 2. Providing relief but not curing.

pallid (pal′-id): Lacking the normal amount of color; wan.

pallidectomy (pal-i-dek′-to-mi): Destruction of a predetermined section of globus pallidus. See **chemopallidectomy** and **sterotactic surgery**.

pallidotomy (pal-i-dot′-o-mi): Surgical severance of the fibers from the cerebral cortex to the corpus striatum. Done to relieve the tremor in Parkinson's disease.

pallor (pal′-lor): Absence of normal color in the skin, especially of the face; paleness.

palm: The anterior, somewhat concave, flexor surface of the human hand; extends from the wrist to the bases of the fingers. The flat of the hand.

palmar (pal′-mar): Pertaining to the palm of the hand. P. ARCHES, superficial and deep, are formed by the anastomosis of the radial and ulnar arteries.

palpable (pal′-pa-b′l): 1. Evident, plain. 2. Capable of being felt or touched.

palpation (pal-pā′-shun): The act of feeling or touching the external surface of the body in order to determine the condition of a part or organ lying underneath: a procedure used in making physical diagnoses.

palpebra (pal′-pe-bra): The eyelid. INFERIOR P., the lower eyelid. SUPERIOR P., the upper eyelid.—palpebral, adj.; palpebrae, pl.

palpebral (pal′-pe-bral): Pertaining to the eyelids. P. CARTILAGES, the thin, cartilage-like plates of tissue that make up the framework of the eyelids. P. COMMISSURE, the union of the upper and lower eyelid, either medial or lateral. P. FISSURE, the opening between the two eyelids.

palpebration (pal-pe-brā′-shun): 1. Winking. 2. Abnormally frequent winking.

palpitation (pal-pi-tā′-shun): Rapid forceful beating of the heart of which the patient is conscious.

palsy (pawl′-zi): Paralysis, temporary or permanent. Term most often used in combination. BELL'S P., facial hemiparalysis from a lesion of the seventh (facial) nerve, resulting in distortion of the facial features; cause unknown. [Charles Bell, Scottish physician. 1774-1842.] BIRTH P., that due to injury received at birth. CEREBRAL P., non-progressive, persistent disorder of motor power and coordination, due to damage to brain. ERB'S P., also ERB-DUCHENNE PARALYSIS, involves the shoulder and arm muscles; caused by a lesion of the fifth and sixth cervical nerve roots. The arm hangs loosely at the side, with the forearm pronated ('waiter's tip' position). Most commonly a birth injury. SCRIVENER'S P., writer's cramp. SHAKING P., paralysis agitans (q.v.). WASTING P., progressive muscular atrophy.

pan-, pant-, panta-, pano-, panto-: Denotes: (1) all, completely, whole; (2) general.

panacea (pan-a-sē′-a): A universal remedy;

a cure-all. Term derived from Panacea, the daughter of Aesculapius and who, along with her sister Hygiea, assisted in caring for the sacred serpents and in carrying out rites in early Greek temples of healing.

panarteritis (pan-ar-ter-ī′-tis): Periarteritis nodosa (*q.v.*).

panarthritis (pan-arth-rī′-tis): Inflammation of all the structures of a joint, or of all of the joints.

pancarditis (pan-kar-dī′-tis): Inflammation of all the structures of the heart.

pancreas (pan′-krē-as): A long, narrow, tongue-shaped glandular organ lying below and behind the stomach. Its head or right end is encircled by the duodenum and its tail often touches the spleen. It is about 7 in. long and weighs about 3.5 oz. It secretes pancreatic juice which passes into the duodenum via the pancreatic duct which joins the common bile duct, and which acts on all classes of foods. It also secretes, in the Islands of Langerhans (*q.v.*), insulin which is necessary for the regulation of carbohydrate metabolism.—pancreatic, adj.

pancreatalgia (pan-krē-a-tal′-ji-a): Pain in the pancreas.

pancreatectomy (pan-krē′-at-ek′-to-mi): Excision of part or the whole of the pancreas.

pancreatic function test: Levin's tubes are positioned in the stomach and second part of duodenum. The response of the pancreatic gland to various hormonal stimuli can be measured by analysing the duodenal aspirate.

pancreatitis (pan-krē-a-tī′-tis): Inflammation of the pancreas, characterized by pain and tenderness of the abdomen, nausea, vomiting, and tympanites.

pancreatolith (pan-krē-at′-ō-lith): A stone in the pancreas.

pandemic (pan-dem′-ik): 1. An infection spreading over a whole country or the world. 2. Widely epidemic.

pang: A sudden piercing physical pain or feeling of mental anguish.

panhysterectomy (pan-his-ter-ek′-to-mi): Removal of the entire uterus, including the cervix.

panhysterosalpingo-oophorectomy (pan-his-ter-ō-sal-ping′-ō ō-of-o-rek⁴-to-mi): Surgical removal of the uterus, cervix, fallopian tubes and ovaries.

panic (pan′-ik): Sudden overpowering fear, brought on by a trifling cause or a misapprehension of danger, usually accompanied by unreasonable behavior and frantic efforts to escape. In psychiatry, an attack of intense anxiety, often with considerable disintegration of the personality.

panniculitis (pa-nik′-ū-lī-tis): Inflammation of the thin sheet of fatty subcutaneous connective tissue of the abdomen.

panniculus (pan-nik′-ū-lus): A layer or sheet of tissue. P. ADIPOSUS, a sheet of superficial fascia that contains deposits of fat.

pannus (pan′-us): Vascularization of the cornea, usually the upper half, resulting in thickening and opacity and causing dimness of vision; often caused by conjunctival irritation; frequently also a complication of trachoma.

panphobia (pan-fō′-bi-a): Morbid fear of everything.

panophthalmitis (pan-of-thal-mī′-tis): Inflammation of all the tissues of the eyeball.

panoptosis (pan-op-tō′-sis): General prolapse or ptosis of all of the abdominal organs.

panosteitis (pan-os-tē-ī′-tis): Inflammation of all constituents of a bone—medulla, bony tissue and periosteum.

panotitis (pan-ō-tī′-tis): Inflammation of all the parts of the ear.

pant: 1. A short, quick, labored breath. 2. To breathe quickly or with difficulty; to gasp for breath.

panty-girdle syndrome: Occurs in women of sedentary occupation when they wear a panty-girdle type of foundation garment; by the end of the day the ankles have become swollen.

pantothenic acid (pan-tō-then′-ik as′-id): A constituent of the vitamin B complex. Widely distributed in plant and animal tissues; found in yeast, liver, heart, salmon eggs, various grains.

pap: Any soft, pulpy food for infants or invalids; *e.g.,* bread soaked in milk or water.

Papanicolaou (pa-pa-nik′-o-low): P. TEST, a cytological test of secretions from the cervix or vagina for early detection of the presence of cancer cells. [George N. Papanicolaou, Greek physician, anatomist and cytologist in the U.S. 1883-1962.]

papilla (pa-pil′-a): A small, nipple-shaped eminence.—papillae, pl.; papillary, papillate, adj. CIRCUMVALLATE P., the large papillae found at the base of the tongue; arranged in a V shape; contain taste buds. FILIFORM P., fine hairlike papillae at the tip of the tongue. FUNGIFORM P., fungus-shaped papillae found chiefly on the dorso-central area of the tongue. MAMMARY P., the pigmented projection on the anterior aspect of the mammary gland into which the milk ducts open. OPTIC P., the terminus of the optic nerve at the point where it enters the eyeball. RENAL P., the summit of one of the renal pyramids. TACTILE P., one that projects into the true skin and contains an end organ for touch. VALLATE P., a circumvallate P.

papilledema (pap-il-ē-dē′-ma): Edema of the optic disk; indicative of increased intracranial pressure. Choked disk (*q.v.*).

papillitis (pap-i-lī′-tis): Inflammation of a papilla (*q.v.*).

papilloma (pap-i-lō′-ma): A usually benign tumor arising from a nonglandular epithelial surface. Frequently occurs on the skin as a wart, and as a polyp on the mucous membrane of the nose, throat, and bladder. —papillomatous, adj.; papillomata, pl.

Pap test: Papanicolaou (*q.v.*) test.

papule (pap′-ūl): A small, solid, usually round or conical, circumscribed elevation on the skin. A pimple.—papular, adj.

papulopustular (pap-ū-lō-pus′-tū-lar): Pertaining to, or showing both papules and pustules (*q.v.*).

par-, para-: Denotes: (1) beside, alongside, parallel; (2) closely resembling a true form, *e.g.*, paratyphoid; (3) faulty, irregular, abnormal, a perversion.

Para: A word used to designate the number of pregnancies a woman has had that have resulted in viable births. It is combined with the proper numeral, *e.g.*, Para I, II, etc.

para-aminobenzoic acid (par-a-am-i-nō-ben-zō′-ik): A member of the vitamin B complex. Deficiency associated with premature graying of dark colored rats. No value in restoring natural hair color in man.

paracentesis (par-a-sen-tē′-sis): Surgical puncture of the wall of a body cavity (thoracic or abdominal wall, tympanic membrane) with a needle, trocar, or other hollow instrument for the purpose of drawing off fluid. Aspiration. Also called tapping.—paracenteses, pl.

parachromatopsia (par-a-krō-ma-top′-si-a): Color blindness.

paracolpitis (par-a-kōl-pī′-tis): Inflammation of the tissues surrounding the vagina.

paracusia (par-a-kū′-si-a): Impaired or disordered hearing. Paracusis.

paracyesis (par-a-sī-ē′-sis): Extrauterine pregnancy.

paradipsia (par-a-dip′-si-a): A perverted and exaggerated appetite for fluids out of proportion to the needs of the body.

paraganglioma (par-a-gang-li-ō′-ma): A benign neoplasm that occurs in the medullary portion of the adrenal gland.

parageusia (par-a-gū′-si-a): 1. A disorder or perversion of the sense of taste. 2. An unpleasant taste in the mouth.

paralalia (par-a-lā′-li-a): A disorder of speech in which sounds are distorted or one letter is substituted for another.

paralexia (par-a-lek′-si-a): An impairment of reading ability, characterized by the transposition of words and syllables so that the resulting combinations are meaningless.

paralogia (par-a-lō′-ji-a): Inability to reason, marked by illogical speech and self-deception.

paralysis (pa-ral′-i-sis): Complete or incomplete loss of nervous function to a part of the body. This may be sensory or motor or both. P. AGITANS (Parkinson's disease) results from lack of muscular control. There is a mask-like expression, shuffling gait, tremor of the limbs and pill-rolling movements of the fingers. The mind remains clear. See **basal ganglia**. BULBAR P., involves the labioglossopharyngeal region and results from degeneration of motor nuclei in the medulla oblongata. DIVER'S P., see **caisson disease**. INFANTILE P., see **poliomyelitis**. FLACCID P. results mainly from lower motor neuron lesions. There are diminished or absent tendon reflexes. LANDRY'S (ACUTE ASCENDING) P. is accompanied by fever, is rapidly progressive; begins in the feet and ascends slowly. Many terminate in respiratory stasis and death. PSEUDOBULBAR P., affects chiefly the facial muscles; there is gross disturbance in control of the tongue, bilateral hemiplegia and mental changes following a succession of 'strokes'; resembles bulbar P. SPASTIC P., results mainly from upper motor neuron lesions. There are exaggerated tendon reflexes, rigidity of muscles of the extremities with atrophy. See **palsy**.

paralytic (par-a-lit′-ik): 1. A person afflicted with paralysis. 2. Pertaining to paralysis. P. ILEUS, paralysis of the intestinal muscle so that the bowel content cannot pass onward even though there is no mechanical obstruction. See **aperistalsis**.

paralyze (par′-a-līz): To produce a state of paralysis (*q.v.*).

paramedian (par-a-mē′-di-an): Situated near the midline.

paramedical (par-a-med′-i-kal): Having an

parametritis

260

indirect or secondary relationship to the medical profession. P. WORKERS include pharmacists, technicians, physical and speech therapists, social workers.

parametritis (par-a-me-trī/-tis): Inflammation of the parametrium (*q.v.*).

parametrium (par-a-me/-tri-um): The connective tissues immediately surrounding the uterus.—parametrial, adj.

paramnesia (par-am-ne/-zi-a): A disorder of memory in which the person believes that he remembers events that never took place; it is involuntary falsification. Also sometimes denotes a person who remembers words but forgets their meanings so that his use of them results in incomprehensible speech.

paranasal (par-a-nā/-zal): Near the nasal cavities, as the various sinuses.

paranoia (par-a-noi/-a): A chronic, slowly progressvie psychiatric disorder characterized by well organized delusions of grandeur or of persecution, attitudes of suspicion, excessive ambition. Mental powers, including clear, orderly thinking are preserved. True paranoia occurs rarely but many other psychotic conditions resemble it.—paranoid, adj.

paranoiac (par-a-noi/-ak): 1. Resembling, pertaining to, or suffering from paranoia. 2. A person suffering from paranoia. P. BEHAVIOR, characterized by extreme suspicion of others, delusions of persecution, megalomania.

paranoid (par/-a-noid): Resembling paranoia.

paranomia (par-a-nō/-mi-a): A type of aphasia characterized by inability to properly name objects seen or touched.

paraparesis (par-a-par/-e-sis): Partial paralysis affecting particularly the lower extremities.

paraphasia (par-a-fā/-zi-a): A speech disorder characterized by inablty to use the right words, or to arrange words correctly in sentences; the result is unintelligible speech. Jargon.

paraphilia (par-a-fil/-i-a): Preference for sexual practices that are unsual, aberrant, prohibited, or for some other reason unacceptable.

paraphimosis (par-a-fī-mō/-sis): A condition in which the prepuce has been retracted behind the glans penis and cannot be replaced; the tight ring of skin interferes with the flow of blood in the glans.

paraphonia (par-a-fō/-ni-a): Partial loss of the voice or any change in its quality. P. PUBERUM, the harsh, deep, irregular quality that develops in boys' voices at puberty.

paraphrenia (par-a-fre/-ni-a): A paranoid state characterized by delusions of grandeur but in which the person's thinking processes are not disturbed.

paraplegia (par-a-plē/-ji-a): Paralysis of the lower half of the body, including the lower trunk and both legs; usually due to disease or injury of the spinal cord.—paraplegic, paraplectic, adi.

paraplegic (par-a-plē/-jik): Pertaining to paraplegia. Also sometimes used to denote a person suffering from paraplegia.

parapraxia (par-a-prak/-si-a): A term used to describe such minor errors of behavior as forgetfulness, a tendency to misplace things, or slips of the tongue or pen.

pararectal (par-a-rek/-tal): Near the rectum.

parasigmatism (par-a-sig/-ma-tizm): Imperfect pronunication of the letter *s*, resulting in a lisp.

parasite (par/-a-sīt): Any organism that lives in or on another organism and obtains all or part of its nourishment from its host.—parasitic, adj.

parasitemia (par-a-sī-te/-mi-a): A condition in which parasites are present in the blood.—parasitemic, adj.

parasiticide (par-a-sit/-i-sīd): Any agent that destroys parasites.

parasitology (par-a-si-tol/-o-ji): The science that treats of parasites and their effects on other living organisms, especially the human body.

paraspadias (par-a-spād/-i-as): A developmental anomaly in which the urethra opens on one side of the penis.

parasympathetic (par-a-sim-path-et/-ik): Refers to part of the autonomic nervous system; consists of some of the cranial and sacral nerves that are concerned with the innervation of smooth and cardiac muscle and glands.

parasympatholytic (par-a-sim-path-ō-lit/-ik): Opposing or blocking the action of parasympathetic nerve fibers, or an agent that has this physiological effect.

parasympathomimetic (par-a-sim-path-ō-mī-met/-ik): Producing effects similar to those produced by stimulation of parasympathetic nerve fibers, or an agent that has this physiological action.

parathormone (par-a-thor/-mōn): A hormone secreted by the parathyroid glands; controls the metabolism of calcium and phosphorus. Excess hormone causes mobilization of calcium from the bones, which become rarefied.

parathyroid (par-a-thī/-roid): Any one of

several, usually four, small endocrine glands lying close to or embedded in the posterior surface of the thyroid gland. They secrete a hormone, parathormone (*q.v.*).

parathyroidectomy (par-a-thĭ-roid-ek′-to-mi): Excision of one or more parathyroid glands.

paratyphoid fever (par-a-tī′-foid): Descriptive of a variety of enteric fevers that closely resemble typhoid fever but which are less prolonged and severe. Usually contracted by eating food that has become contaminated with bacteria of the genus *Salmonella*. See **TAB.**

paraurethral (par-a-ū-rē′-thral): Near the urethra.

paravaginal (par-a-vaj′-in-al): Near the vagina.

paravertebral (par-a-ver′-te-bral): Alongside or near the vertebral column. P. BLOCK ANESTHESIA is induced by infiltration of local anesthetic around the spinal nerve roots as they emerge from the intervertebral foramina. P. INJECTION of local anesthetic into sympathetic chain can be used as a test in ischemic limbs to see if sympathectomy will be of value.

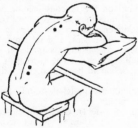

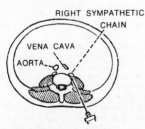

RIGHT SYMPATHETIC CHAIN

VENA CAVA

AORTA

Paravertebral injection

paregoric (par-e-gor′-ik): Camphorated tincture of opium frequently used in cough syrups and mixtures; also used in treatment of diarrhea.

parencephalocele (par-en-sef′-al-ō-sēl): Protrusion of part of the cerebellum through a defect in the structure of the cranium.

parencephalon (par-en-sef′-a-lon): The cerebellum.

parenchyma (par-eng′-ki-ma): The specialized tissue of an organ that, in contradistinction to its interstitial tissue, is concerned with its function.—parenchymal, parenchymatous, adj.

parenteral (par-en′-ter-al): Refers to the administration of a substance by some manner other than via the intestinal tract.

paresis (par′-e-sis), (pa-rē′-sis): 1. Slight or partial paralysis. 2. General paralysis of the insane; the result of syphilitic infection of brain and meninges; onset insidious beginning with headache and fatigability with slowly progressing deterioration, involving personality changes as well as tremor, speech disturbances, Argyll Robertson pupil (*q.v.*), increasing muscular weakness. Dementia paralytica.

paresthesia (par-es-thē′-zi-a): Abnormal tactile sensation such as burning, tingling, pricking, creeping; may be a symptom of psychosis or neurological disease.

paretic (pa-ret′-ik): 1. Pertaining to paresis. 2. A person afflicted with paresis.

paries (pa′-ri-ēz): A wall; by common usage refers to the wall of a hollow organ or cavity.—parietes, pl.; parietal, adj.

parietal (par-ī′-et-al): Pertaining to a wall. P. BONES, the two bones which form the sides and vault of the skull. P. LOBE, one of the five lobes of each hemisphere of the cerebrum; lies over the parietal bone.

parietofrontal (par-ī-et-ō-fron′-tal): Pertaining to the parietal and frontal bones or the part of the cerebral cortex that lies under them.

parietooccipital (par-ī′-et-ō-ok-sip′-it-al): Pertaining to the parietal and occipital bones or region.

parity (par′-i-ti): Condition of a woman with regard to the number of children she has borne.

parkinsonian (par-kin-sōn′-i-an): 1. Of, like, or referring to Parkinson's disease. 2. A person afflicted with Parkinson's disease. P. MASK, a fixed, staring expression with eyebrows raised, infrequent winking and immobility of facial muscles, characteristic feature of Parkinsonism.

parkinsonism: See **paralysis** and **postencephalitic.**

Parkinson's disease: Paralysis agitans (*q.v.*). [James Parkinson, English physician. 1755-1854.]

parodynia (par-ō-din/-i-a): Abnormal or difficult labor.

paronychia (par-ō-nik/-i-a): Suppurative inflammation around a fingernail. A whitlow (*q.v.*).

parorexia (par-ō-rek/-si-a): Morbid craving for certain foods or for substances that are not fit for food.

parosmia (par-os/-mi-a): Perverted sense of smell, usually of an hallucinatory nature.

parotid (pa-rot/-id): Situated near the ear. P. GLAND, the largest of the three salivary glands, located on either side of the face just in front of and below the ear; empties into the mouth via Stenson's duct which opens opposite the second upper molar tooth.

parotidectomy (par-ot-id-ek/-to-mi): Excision of the parotid salivary gland.

parotitis (par-ō-tī/-tis): Inflammation of one or both parotid glands. INFECTIOUS (SPECIFIC) P., mumps (*q.v.*). SEPTIC P. refers to ascending infection from the mouth via the parotid duct, when a parotid abscess may result.

parous (par/-us): Having borne a child or children.

paroxysm (par/-ok-sizm): 1. A sudden, temporary attack or convulsive seizure. 2. A sudden exacerbation or intensification of the symptoms of a disease.

paroxysmal (par-ok-siz/-mal): Coming on in attacks or paroxysms. P. DYSPNEA occurs mostly at night in patients with cardiac disease. P. FIBRILLATION occurs in the atrium of the heart and is associated with a ventricular tachycardia and total irregularity of the pulse rhythm. P. TACHYCARDIA may result from ectopic impulses arising in the atrium or in the ventricle itself.

parrot disease or fever: Psittacosis (*q.v.*).

partimute (par/-ti-mūt): A deaf-mute.

parturient (par-tū/-ri-ent): Pertaining to childbirth.

parturition (par-tū-rish/-un): The act of bearing a child; labor.

passive (pas/-iv): Not active. See **hyperemia, immunity.** P. CARRIER, one who harbors the causative organism of a disease without having had the disease. P. MOVEMENT OR EXERCISE, performed by the physiotherapist, the patient being relaxed.

passivism (pas/-i-vizm): Sexual perversion in which the individual submits to the will of another.

Pasteurella (pas-tūr-el/-la): A genus of bacteria. Short gram-negative rods, staining more deeply at the poles (bipolar staining). Pathogenic in man and animals. P. PESTIS is the causative organism of classical plague.

pasteurization (pas-tūr-īz-ā/-shun): A process whereby pathogenic organisms in fluid (especially milk) are killed by heat without affecting the food properties or flavor of the fluid. FLASH METHOD OF P. (H.T., S.T. —high temperature, short time), the fluid is heated to 161.5° to 162° F., maintained at this temperature for 15 seconds, then rapidly cooled. HOLDER METHOD OF P., the fluid is heated to 145° to 150° F., maintained at this temperature for 30 minutes, then rapidly cooled.

Pasteur's method, treatment: The method devised by Pasteur for preventing the development of rabies by injecting repeated doses of attenuated virus of the disease, gradually increasing the strength of the virus. [Louis Pasteur, French chemist and bacteriologist. 1822-1895.]

pastille (pas-tēl/): A medicated disk or lozenge intended to be held in the mouth until dissolved; used for local action on mucous membrane of mouth and throat.

patch: An area that differs in appearance from the surrounding surface. PEYER'S P's., small oval masses of lymphoid tissue found on the mucous membrane of the small intestine. P. TEST, a test for hypersensitiveness to certain foods, pollens, or other substances; a small amount of the suspected substance is applied to the skin.

patella (pa-tel/-a): The kneecap; a triangular, sesamoid bone.—patellar, adj., patellae, pl.

patellectomy (pa-tel-ek/-to-mi): Excision of the patella.

patent (pā/-tent): Open; not closed or occluded.—patency, n. P. DUCTUS ARTERIOSUS, failure of ductus arteriosus to close soon after birth, so that the abnormal shunt between the pulmonary artery and the aorta is preserved. P. INTERVENTRICULAR SEPTUM, a congenital defect in the dividing wall between the right and left ventricle of the heart.

patent medicine: A medicine that has been patented and can be sold without a prescription; must be labeled as to content and dosage.

paternity (pa-ter/-ni-ti): The state of being a father. P. TEST, a blood test in which the blood groups of the child, its mother and a certain man are compared to determine whether the man could be the father of the child; it does not prove paternity.

Paterson-Kelly syndrome: Plummer-Vinson syndrome (*q.v.*).

path-, patho-: Denotes: (1) disease; (2) pathology; (3) emotion.

-path: Denotes: (1) one suffering from a specific ailment; (2) a physician who practices a specific kind of medicine, *e.g.,* homeopath.

pathogen (path'-ō-jen): A disease producing agent, usually restricted to a living agent. —pathogenic, adj.; pathogenicity, n.

pathogenesis (path-ō-jen'-e-sis): The origin and development of disease.—pathogenetic, adj.

pathogenicity (path-ō-jen-is'-i-ti): The capacity to produce disease.

pathognomonic   (path-og-nō-mon'-ik): Characteristic of or peculiar to a disease or pathologic condition.

pathologist (path-ol'-ō-jist): A physician who is specially trained in pathology (*q.v.*).

pathology (path-ol'-ō-ji): The branch of medical science that deals with the cause and nature of disease and the changes in structure and function that result from disease processes.—pathological, adj.; pathologically, adv.

pathomimesis (path-ō-mim-ē'-sis): Intentional or unconscious mimicry of disease; malingering.

pathophobia (path-ō-fō'-bi-a): A morbid dread of disease.

pathway: In neurology, usually refers to a structure that carries an impulse to or from the central nervous system; an afferent or efferent neuron.

-pathy: Denotes: (1) disease of a specified part; (2) a system of therapy; (3) a feeling, *e.g.,* empathy.

patient (pā'-shent): A person who is physically or mentally ill or who is undergoing treatment for physical or mental illness.

patulous (pat'-ū-lus): Opened out; expanded.

Paul-Bunnell test: A serological test used in the diagnosis of infective mononucleosis. Antibodies to the virus of this disease agglutinate sheep's erythrocytes. [J. R. Paul, American physician. 1893- . W. W. Bunnell, American physician. 1902- .]

pavor (pā'-vor): Dread; terror. P. NOCTURNUS, night terrors during sleep.

PBI: Abbreviation for protein-bound iodine (*q.v.*).

p.c.: Abbreviation for *post cibum,* meaning after meals.

pearl: Perle (*q.v.*).

peccant (pek'-ant): Unhealthy; causing disease.

pectoral (pek'-tor-al): Pertaining to the breast or chest.

pectoralgia (pek-to-ral'-ji-a): Pain in the chest or breast.

pectoralis (pek-to-rā'-lis): 1. Pertaining to the breast or chest. 2.Any one of the four muscles of the chest. P. MAJOR, the large, fan-shaped muscle that covers the upper anterior chest. P. MINOR, the thin, triangular muscle underlying the P. MAJOR.

pectus (pek'-tus): The chest. P. CARINATUM, pigeon chest. P. EXCAVATUM, funnel chest.

ped-, pedi-, pedio-, pedo-: Denotes: (1) the foot; (2) having foot-like projections.

ped-, pedo-. Also **paed-, paedo-:** Denotes child, children.

pedal (ped'-al): Pertaining to the foot.

pedatrophia (ped-a-trō'-fi-a): Marasmus (*q.v.*); any wasting condition in children.

pederasty (ped'-er-as-ti): Homosexual intercourse by anus.

pederosis (ped-er-ō'-sis): A sexual interest in children; sexual abuse of children by adults.

pediatrician (pē-di-a-trish'-un): A physician who specializes in the health supervision and treatment of children.

pediatrics (pē-di-at'-riks): The branch of medicine that deals with the development and care of the child and with the diseases of children and their treatment

pedicle (ped'-ik-l): 1. A stalk, *e.g.,* the narrow part by which a tumor is attached to the surrounding structures. 2. The two processes that extend backward from the body of a vertebra and connect the laminae with the body of the vertebra.

pedicterus (ped-ik'-ter-us): Jaundice of the newborn; icterus neonatorum.

pediculicide (ped-ik'-ū-li-sīd): An agent that destroys lice (pediculi).

pediculosis (ped-ik-ū-lō'-sis): Infestation with lice (pediculi).

pediculous (ped-ik'-ū-lus): Infested with pediculi; lousy.

Pediculus (ped-ik'-ū-lus): A genus of wingless, blood-sucking insects (lice) important

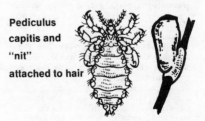

Pediculus capitis and "nit" attached to hair

pedodontics

as vectors of disease. P. CAPITIS, the head louse. P. CORPORIS, the body louse. P. PUBIS (more correctly, Phthirus), the pubic louse; also called the crab louse.

pedodontics (pē-dō-don'-tiks): The branch of dentistry that deals with the diagnosis and treatment of conditions of the teeth and surrounding tissues in children.

pedojet (ped-ō-jet'): Apparatus for introducing vaccine under pressure into the skin. Avoids use of the needle with consequent danger of spreading serum hepatitis.

pedophilia (pēd-ō-fil'-i-a): Abnormal fondness for children. P. EROTICA, sexual perversion in which children are the preferred objects.

peduncle (pēd-ungk'-l): A stalk-like structure, often acting as a support.—peduncular, pedunculated, adj.

pedunculus (pē-dung'-kū-lus): Peduncle (*q.v.*).

peeling: Desquamation (*q.v.*).

pejorative (pē'-jō-ra-tiv): Changing for the worse; unfavorable.

Pel-Ebstein's fever: Recurring bouts of pyrexia in regular sequence found in lymphadenoma (Hodgkin's disease). [Pieter Klazes Pel, Dutch physician. 1852-1919. Wilhelm Ebstein, German physician. 1836-1912.]

Pelizaeus-Merzbacher disease: Genetically determined degenerative disease associated with mental subnormality. [Friedrich Pelizaeus, German neurologist. 1850- . Ludwig Merzbacher, German physician in Argentina. 1875- .]

pellagra (pel-ag'-ra): A deficiency disease caused by lack of vitamin B complex (nicotinic acid) and protein. Syndrome includes glossitis, dermatitis, peripheral neuritis and spinal cord changes (even producing ataxia), anemia and mental confusion.

pellet (pel'-et): A small pill; may contain medication and be taken by mouth, or may contain pure steroid hormones and be implanted under the skin from which location it is slowly absorbed by the body.

pelmatogram (pel-mat'-o-gram): A footprint; an imprint of the sole of the foot made by pressing the inked sole on a piece of paper.

pelotherapy (pē-lō-ther'-a-pi): The use of mud in the treatment of disease.

pelvic (pel'-vik): Pertaining to the pelvis. P. GIRDLE, the bony framework of the pelvis; consists of the two innominate bones and the sacrum. P. FLOOR, the muscular lower part of the pelvis; includes the levator ani and coccygeus muscles, and fascia.

pelvimeter (pel-vim'-e-ter): An instrument especially devised to measure the pelvic diameters.

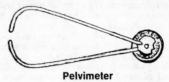

Pelvimeter

pelvimetry (pel-vim'-e-tri): The measurement of the dimensions of the pelvis by means of a pelvimeter. Four measurements are taken: the distances between (1) the anterior superior spines of the ilia; (2) between the crests of the ilia; (3) between the greater trochanters of the femurs; (4) between the spinous process of the 5th lumbar vertebra and the anterior surface of the symphysis pubis.

pelvis (pel'-vis): 1. A basin-shaped cavity, *e.g.*, pelvis of the kidney. 2. The large bony basin-shaped cavity formed by the innominate bones and sacrum, containing and protecting the bladder, rectum, and organs of generation.—pelvic, adj. CONTRACTED P., one in which one or more diameters are smaller than normal and this may result in difficulties in childbirth. FALSE P., the wide expanded part of the pelvis above the brim. TRUE P., that part of the pelvis below the brim.

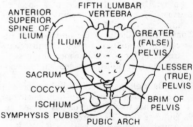

The bony pelvis

pemphigoid (pem'-fi-goid): 1. Allied to pemphigus. 2. A bullous eruption in the latter half of life. Of unknown cause. Histological examination of the base of a blister differentiates it from pemphigus.

pemphigus (pem'-fi-gus): Name applied to a group of skin conditions with bullous (blister) eruptions that absorb and leave pigmented spots, but more correctly used of a group of dangerous diseases called 'P. vulgaris,' 'P. vegetans' and 'P. erythematosus.' The latter two are rare. P. NEONATO-RUM: (1) a dangerous form of impetigo occurring as an epidemic in the hospital nursery; (2) bullous eruption in congenital syphilis of the newborn. P. VULGARIS is a bullous disease of middle age and later, of unknown etiology. Edema of the skin results in blister formation in the epidermis, with resulting secondary infection and rupture, so that large raw areas develop. Bullae develop also on mucous membranes. Death is from malnutrition or intercurrent disease.

pen-, pent-, penta-: Denotes: (1) five; (2) containing five atoms.

pendulous (pen'-dū-lus): Hanging down.

-penia: Denotes a deficiency of.

penicillin (pen-i-sil'-in): The first antibiotic; derived from cultures of certain molds of the genus Penicillium; widely used to treat infections due to gram-positive bacteria, some cocci and spirochetes. Many different preparations are available.

penicillinase (pen-i-sil'-in-āse): An enzyme that inactivates penicillin.

Penicillium (pen-i-sil'-i-um): A genus of fungi comprising the blue molds the hyphae of which bear spores characteristically arranged like a brush. Common contaminant of food. Found chiefly on decaying nonliving organic matter such as fruit. P. CHRYSOGENUM, is now used for the commercial production of penicillin.

penis (pē'-nis): The male organ of copulation.—penile, adj.

penitis (pē-nī'-tis): Inflammation of the penis. Also phallitis, priapitis.

Penrose drain: A 'cigarette' type of drain consisting of a piece of rubber tubing containing a length of absorbent gauze. [Charles B. Penrose, American gynecologist. 1862-1925.]

pentose (pen'-tōs): A class of monosaccharides with five carbon atoms in their molecule; abundant in some fruits.

pentosuria (pen-tō-sū'-ri-a): The occurrence of pentose in the urine. The alimentary type is temporary and due to ingestion of large amounts of certain foods, e.g., plums, cherries, or grapes. May be caused by a hereditary error of metabolism. Not significant except that it may be mistaken for diabetes.

peotomy (pe-ot'-o-mi): Surgical amputation of the penis.

pepsin (pep'-sin): A proteolytic enzyme of the gastric juice; converts the native proteins of foods into proteoses and peptones. Along with dilute hydrochloric acid, it is the chief active ingredient of gastric juice.

pepsinogen (pep-sin'-ō-jen): A pre-enzyme secreted by the peptic cells in the gastric mucosa and coverted into pepsin by contact with hydrochloric acid.

peptase (pep'-tās): An enzyme that splits peptides into amino acid.

peptic (pep'-tik): Pertaining to the stomach, to pepsin or to digestion generally. P. ULCER, a nonmalignant ulcer in those parts of the digestive tract which are exposed to the gastric secretions; hence usually in stomach or duodenum.

peptide (pep'-tīd): A chemical combination of two or more amino acids; e.g., dipeptide, tripeptide, polypeptide.

peptone (pep'-tōn): Substance produced when the enzyme pepsin acts upon the acid metaproteins produced in the first stage of digestion of proteins.

peptonuria (pep-tō-nū'-ri-a): The excretion of peptones in the urine.

per-: Denotes: (1) by, by means of, through; (2) completely, throughout, extremely. In chemistry, it denotes the highest member of a series.

peracidity (per-a-sid'-i-ti): Excessive acidity.

peracute (per-a-kūt'): extremely acute.

per anum (per ā'-num): By way of or through the anus.

percept (per'-sept): 1. An object perceived; the impression of an object obtained through the senses. 2. The mental product of a sensation; a sensation plus memories of similar sensations and their relationships.

perception (per-sep'-shun): The reception of a conscious impression through the senses by which we distinguish objects one from another and recognize their qualities according to the different sensations they produce. Intelligent discernment; insight.

percolation (per-kō-lā'-shun): The process by which fluid slowly passes through a hard but porous substance.

percussion (per-kush'-un): 1. A diagnostic procedure consisting of tapping or striking the surface of the body to determine the condition of the organs or tissues underneath by the resulting sound. Normally a finger of the left hand is laid on the patient's skin and the middle finger of the right hand is used to strike the left finger. Useful in detecting consolidation, fluid, or pus in a cavity, change in the size of an organ, etc.; used especially over the chest and abdomen. 2. A movement in massage consisting of taps of varying force.—percuss, v.t.

percussor (per-kus′-er): An instrument used in percussion, usually a hammer with a rubber or metal head.

percutaneous (per-kū-tā′-nē-us): Through unbroken skin.

perflation (per-flā′-shun): The blowing of air into a cavity or canal to force its walls apart or to force out any secretions or other substances.

perforating ulcer: One that erodes through the wall of an organ such as the stomach or intestine; a serious development requiring immediate surgery.

perforation (per-fo-rā′-shun): A hole in an intact sheet of tissue, or the act of making such a hole; may be pathogenic or intentional. Used especially in reference to the tympanic membrane or the wall of the stomach or intestine.

perfuse (per-fūz′): To spread or pour over or through.

perfusion (per-fū′-zhun): 1. The act of spreading or pouring over or through, specifically the artificial passage of fluid through an organ or tissue by way of the blood vessels. 2. The process whereby oxygen is carried from the lungs to body tissues and carbon dioxide is carried from tissues to the lungs.

peri-: Denotes: (1) all around, about; (2) near; (3) enclosing, surrounding.

periadenitis (per-i-ad-en-ī′-tis): Inflammation in soft tissues surrounding glands.

perianal (per-i-ān′-al): Around or surrounding the anus.

periapical (per-i-ap′-i-kal): Relating to the tissues that enclose the apex of a tooth. P. ABSCESS, one that forms at or near the apex of a tooth.

periarterial (per-i-art-ē′-ri-al): Around or surrounding an artery.

periarteritis (per-i-art-er-ī′-tis): Inflammation of the outer sheath of an artery and the periarterial tissue. P. NODOSA, a widespread disease of the arteries; frequently produces renal damage and hypertension; see **collagen, polyarteritis.**

periarthritis (per-i-arth-rī′-tis): Inflammation of the structures surrounding a joint. Sometimes applied to frozen shoulder (*q.v.*).

periarticular (per-i-art-ik′-ū-lar): Around or surrounding a joint.

periblepsis (per-i-blep′-sis): The characteristic staring expression of an insane or emotionally disturbed person.

pericardectomy (per-i-kard-ek′-to-mi): Surgical removal of a portion of the pericardium, thickened from chronic inflam-

mation and embarrassing the heart's action.

pericardiocentesis (per-i-kar-di-ō-sen-tē′-sis): The withdrawal of fluid from the pericardial sac by insertion of a hollow needle or cannula.

pericarditis (per-i-kar-dī′-tis): Inflammation of the outer, serous covering of the heart. It may or may not be accompanied by an effusion and formation of adhesions between the two layers. See **Broadbent's sign** and **pericardectomy.**

pericardium (per-i-kard′-i-um): The double fibroserous membranous sac which envelops the heart. The layer in contact with the heart is called 'visceral'; that reflected to form the sac is called 'parietal.' Between the two is the pericardial cavity, which normally contains a small amount of serous fluid.—pericardial, adj.

pericholangitis (per-i-kō-lan-jī′-tis): Inflammation of the tissues around the bile ducts.

perichondrium (pe-ri-kond′-ri-um): The membranous covering of cartilage.—perichondrial, adj.

pericolic (per-i-kō′-lik): Around the colon.

pericolitis (per-i-kō-lī′-tis): Inflammation of the tissues around the colon, especially of the peritoneal coat.

pericolpitis (per-i-kōl-pī′-tis): Inflammation of the tissues around the vagina.

pericranium (per-i-krān′-i-um): The periosteal covering of the cranium.—pericranial, adj.

perifollicular (per-i-fol-ik′-ū-lar): Around a follicle.

perikaryon (per-i-kar′-i-on): The protoplasmic part of the cell body, exclusive of the nucleus and processes.

perilymph (per′-i-limf): The fluid contained in the internal ear, between the bony and membranous labyrinth.

perimeningitis (per-i-men-in-jī′-tis): Inflammation of the dura mater. Syn., pachymeningitis.

perimetritis (per-i-mē-trī′-tis): Inflammation of the perimetrium (*q.v.*).

perimetrium (per-i-mēt′-ri-um): The peritoneal (serous) covering of the uterus.—perimetrial, adj.

perimetry (per-im′-e-tri): The determination of the extent of an individual's peripheral visual field.

perimysium (per-i-mis′-i-um): The delicate connective tissue sheath that envelops and separates the bundles of voluntary muscle fibers.

perinatal (per-i-nā′-tal): Occurring at, or pertaining to, the time of birth.

perineoplasty per-i-nē′-ō-plas-ti): Reparative or plastic surgery of the perineum.

perineorrhaphy (per-i-ne-or′-a-fi): The operation for the repair of a torn perineum.

perineotomy: Episiotomy (*q.v.*).

perinephric (per-i-nef′-rik): Around or surrounding the kidney.

perinephritis (per-i-nef-rī′-tis): Inflammation of the peritoneal covering of the kidney and of the surrounding tissues.

perineum (per-i-nē′-um): The area that lies between the vulva and the anus in the female and between the scrotum and the anus in the male. Often referred to as the pelvic floor (*q.v.*).

perineurium (per-i-nū′-ri-um): The connective tissue sheath that surrounds the separate bundles of fibers of peripheral nerves.

period: An interval or extent of time. GESTATION P., the period of pregnancy; in the human it is approximately 270 days. INCUBATION P., the time between the entrance of a pathogenic organism into the body and appearance of first symptoms of disease.

periodontal (per-i-ō-don′-tal): Around a tooth.

periomphalic (per-i-om-fal′-ik): Around the umbilicus.

perionychia (per-i-ō-nik′-i-a): Inflammation around a nail.

perioral (pe-ri-or′-al): Around or surrounding the mouth.

periosteitis (per-i-os-tē-ī′-tis): Periostitis (*q.v.*).

periosteoma (per-i-os-tē-ō′-ma): A neoplasm on the surface of a bone.

periosteomyelitis(per-i-os-tē-ō-mī-e-lī′-tis): Inflammation of the bone including the marrow and the periosteum.

periosteum (per-i-os′-tē-um): The thick, fibrous membrane that covers bones except at their articulations; it is protective and essential for regeneration of bone. Consists of two layers, the inner one being concerned with formation of bone tissue and the outer one serving to convey nerves and blood vessels to the bone.

periostitis (per-i-os-tī′-tis): Inflammation of the periosteum. P. DIFFUSE, that involving the periosteum of long bones. P. HEMORRHAGIC, that accompanied by bleeding between the periosteum and the bone.

periotic (per-i-ō′-tik): Around the ear.

peripatetic (per-i-pa-tet′-ik): Walking around. Descriptive of certain illnesses, particularly cases of typhoid fever in which the patient does not take to his bed.

peripheral (pe-rif′-er-al): Pertaining to or situated near the periphery (*q.v.*).

periphery (pe-rif′-er-i): The outward part or surface of the body; the parts away from the center or midline.

periproctitis (per-i-prok-tī′-tis): Inflammation of the tissues around the rectum and anus.

perirenal (per-i-rēn′-al): Around the kidney.

perisalpingitis (per-i-sal-pin-jī′-tis): Inflammation of the peritoneum and tissues around the fallopian tubes.

perisplentitis (per-i-splen-ī′-tis): Inflammation of the peritoneal coat of the spleen and of the adjacent structures.

perispondylitis (per-i-spon-di-lī′-tis): Inflammation of tissues around a vertebra.

peristalsis (per-i-stal′-sis): The characteristic wavelike movement of the intestine and certain other tubular structures in the body by which the contents of the lumen are moved forward toward its terminus. It consists of a wave of contraction preceded by a wave of relaxation.—peristaltic, adj. MASS P., strong peristaltic waves that occur in the large intestine several times a day and which move the contents from one division of the intestine to the next. REVERSED P., P. in which the wave is in a direction opposite to normal and the contents of the lumen are forced backward.

peritectomy (per-i-tek′-to-mi): Excision of a strip of conjunctiva at the edge of the cornea, a surgical treatment for pannus (*q.v.*).

peritendinitis (per-i-ten-di-nī′-tis): Inflammation of the sheath enclosing a tendon. Peritenonitis.

peritomy (per-it′-o-mi): 1. Surgical incision of the conjunctiva around the entire circumference of the cornea; peritectomy. 2. Circumcision.

peritoneocentesis (per-i-tō-nē-ō-sen-tē′-sis): Paracentesis of the abdominal cavity.

peritoneoscopy (per-i-tō-nē-os′-ko-pi): Inspection of the peritoneal cavity by means of an electrically lighted, tubular optical instrument (peritoneoscope) introduced through the abdominal wall.—peritoneoscopic, adj.; peritoneoscopically, adv.

peritoneum (per-i-tō-nē′-um): The delicate, smooth, transparent, serous membrane that lines the abdominal and pelvic cavities and also covers the organs contained in them, thus forming a sac.—peritoneal, adj.

peritonitis (per-i-tōn-ī′-tis): Inflammation of the peritoneum, usually secondary to disease of one of the abdominal organs.

peritonsillar (per-i-ton′-si-lar): Around the tonsil or tonsils. P.ABSCESS, quinsy (*q.v.*).

Peritricha (pe-rit′-ri-ka): A group of bacteria that have flagella over the entire surface of the cell.—peritrichous, adj.

perityphlitis (per-i-tif-li′-tis): Inflammation of the peritoneum around the cecum and the appendix; appendicitis.

periumbilical (per-i-um-bil′-ik-al): Around or surrounding the umbilicus.

periurethral (per-i-ū-rē′-thral): Surrounding the urethra, as a P. abscess.

periuterine (per-i-ū′-ter-in): Around the uterus.

perivascular (per-i-vas′-kū-lar): Around a blood vessel.

perivesical (per-i-ves′-i-kal): Around the bladder.

perkinism (per′-kin-izm): A formerly popular type of quackery in which the patient was treated by the application of certain metals that were supposed to have magic power to cure or alleviate a disease. [Elisha Perkins, New England physician. 1741–1799.]

perle (purl): A very small, thin glass ampule containing one dose of a volatile drug; it is to be crushed in a handkerchief and the contents inhaled.

perlèche (per-lesh′): An inflammation at the angles of the mouth with maceration, fissuring, or crust formation; causes lip licking and results in thickening and desquamation of the skin. Occurs mostly in malnourished children as a result of vitamin deficiency, thrush, bacterial infection, drooling or thumbsucking. In adults may result from poorly fitted dentures.

permeability (per-mē-a-bil′-it-i): In physiology, the ability of cell membranes to allow salts, glucose, urea and other soluble substances to pass into and out of the cells from the body fluids.

permit (per-mit′, per′-mit): 1. Permission. 2. To allow. OPERATIVE P., a statement signed by the patient, or his parent or guardian, permitting an operation to be performed on his body.

pernicious (per-nish′-us): Deadly, noxious, destructive. In medicine, usually denotes a disease of severe character and tending to a fatal outcome. P.ANEMIA, see **anemia**. P. VOMITING, see **vomiting**.

perniosis (per-ni-ō′-sis): Chronic chilblains. The smaller arterioles go into spasm readily from exposure to cold.

pero-: Denotes deformed.

peromelia (per-ō-mē′-li-a): Severe congenital deformity of the limbs, including absence of hand or foot.

perone (per-ō′-nē): Fibula.—peroneal, adj.

peroneal (per-o-nē′-al): Pertaining to the fibula or to the outer side of the leg, or to the muscles or tissues on the outer side of the leg.

peroneotibial (per-o-nē-ō-tib′-i-al): Pertaining to both the fibula and the tibia.

peroral (per-ō′-ral): By or through the mouth.

per os: By or through the mouth.

peroxide: See **hydrogen**.

perseveration (per-sev-er-ā′-shun): The continuation of an activity after the causative stimulus has been removed. In psychiatry, a mental symptom consisting of an apparent inability of the patient's mind to detach itself from one idea to another with normal speed. Thus shown a picture of a cow, the patient repeats 'cow' when shown further pictures of different objects. Common in senile dementia, schizophrenia.

persona (per-sō′na): In psychiatry, the outer or assumed personality that a person takes on to hide his true personality, as opposed to the anima (*q.v.*) which is his inner personality or actual character.

personality (per-so-nal′-i-ti): The total complex of individual mental attitudes, characteristics, and ways of behaving and reacting to the environment that distinguish a person. DISORDERED P., a condition in which a person thinks he is someone other than himself. DUAL P., a condition in which a person leads two lives, each independent of and not fully aware of the other. P. INVENTORY, an inventory for self-appraisal, containing statements about personal characteristics; the person judges whether they do or do not apply to him; it tests for neurotic tendencies, self-sufficiency, introversion, extroversion, sociability, etc. PSYCHOPATHIC P., descriptive of a person who has a persistent disorder of personality leading to aggressive, antisocial, or irresponsible behavior such as lying, cheating, criminalism, or sexual perversion; usually there is little evidence of guilt or concern about the effects of such behavior on others. SPLIT P., one composed of two or more groups of behavior tendencies, each acting independently and apparently dissociated from the other.

perspiration (per-spi-rā′-shun): 1. The excretion of sweat through the skin pores. INSENSIBLE P., invisible P.; the P. is evaporated immediately upon reaching the skin surface. SENSIBLE P., visible drops of sweat on the skin. 2. Sweat; the fluid secreted by the sweat glands.

perspire (per-spīr'): To sweat.

Perthes' disease (Legg-Perthes-Calvé's disease): Syn., pseudocoxalgia. A vascular degeneration of the upper femoral epiphysis; revascularization occurs, but residual deformity of the femoral head may subsequently lead to arthritic changes. [Georg Clemens Perthes, German surgeon. 1869-1927.]

pertussis (per-tus'-is): Whooping cough. An infectious disease of children with paroxysms of coughing that reach a peak of violence ending in a long-drawn inspiration that produces a characteristic 'whoop.' The basis of the condition is respiratory catarrh and the organism responsible is *Hemophilus pertussis.* Prophylactic vaccination is responsible for the decrease in case incidence.

perversion (per-vur'-shun): A turning away from what is normal or right. In medicine, a pathological alteration of function. SEXUAL P., indulgence in unnatural sexual practices.

pervert (per-vurt', per'-vurt): 1. To turn aside, or cause to be turned aside from what is considered right or normal; to lead astray. 2. A person who has turned aside from what is considered proper and normal behavior; applied especially to one who practices any unnatural sexual behavior.

pes: A foot or foot-like structure. P. CAVUS, 'hollow' foot when the longitudinal arch of the foot is accentuated. Clawfoot. P. PLANUS, flatfoot.

Pes cavus

Pes planus

pessary (pes'-a-ri): 1. An instrument inserted into the vagina to support the uterus or to correct uterine displacements. 2. A medicated suppository used to treat vaginal infections, or as a contraceptive.

pest: 1. An epidemic disease usually associated with high mortality, specifically the plague. 2. A destructive or annoying plant or animal.

pesthouse: A shelter, retreat. or hospital where persons with epidemic or communicable diseases are cared for.

pesticide (pes'-ti-sīd): A poisonous agent used to destroy a pest, *e.g.,* insect, rodent, fungus.

pestilence (pes'-ti-lens): 1. A virulent, communicable, devastating disease, specifically the plague. 2. Something that is pernicious or extremely destructive.—pestilential, adj.

pestis (pes'-tis): Plague.

petechia (pē-tē'-ki-a): A pinpoint hemorrhage into the skin.—petechiae, pl.; petechial, adj.

petit mal (pet'-ē mal): Minor epilepsy (*q.v.*). The convulsions are mild and the seizures transient; may be clouding or momentary loss of consciousness.

Petri dish: A round glass dish with a cover; used in the laboratory for growing bacterial cultures.

petrifaction (pet-ri-fak'-shun): Fossilization; calcification.

pétrissage (pā-tri-shazh'): A movement in massage that resembles kneading.

petrolatum (pet-rō-lā'-tum): A yellowish, semisolid substance obtained from petroleum; used as an emollient and as a base for many ointments. Petroleum jelly.

petroleum jelly: Petrolatum (*q.v.*).

petrosa (pē-trō'-sa): The hardened cone-shaped part of the temporal bone; it contains the structures of the inner ear.

petrous (pē'-trus): 1. Resembling stone. 2. Pertaining to the petrosa.

pexis (pek'-sis): The surgical fixation of a tissue or a part.

-pexy: Denotes fixation, a making fast.

Peyer's patches (pi'-ers): Flat patches of lymphatic tissue situated in the small intestine but mainly in the ileum; they are the seat of infection in typhoid fever; also known as 'aggregated lymph nodules.' [Johann Conrad Peyer, Swiss anatomist. 1653-1712.]

peyote (pā-ō'-tā): Mescaline (*q.v.*).

***p*H:** The concentration of hydrogen ions expressed as a logarithm. A neutral solution has a *p*H 7.0. With increasing acidity the *p*H falls and with increasing alkalinity it rises.

phac-, phaco-: Denotes: (1) a lentil or a thing shaped like a lentil; (2) a lens; (3) the crystalline lens of the eye.

phacolysis (fa-kol'-i-sis): 1. The operation of breaking down and then removing the crystalline lens of the eye. 2.The dissolution of the crystalline lens of the eye by means other than surgery.

phacomalacia (fak-ō-ma-lā′-shi-a): A soft cataract, or a softening of the crystalline lens.

phacosclerosis (fak-ō-skler-ō′-sis): A hard cataract, or a hardening of the crystalline lens.

phag-, phago-: Denotes: (1) eating, feeding, ingesting; (2) engulfing.

-phagia: Denotes a desire to eat a certain substance or food.

phagocyte (fag′-ō-sīt): A cell capable of engulfing, sometimes digesting, bacteria, foreign particles, cells, and other debris in the tissues.—phagocytic, adj.

phagocytose (fag-ō-sī′-tōs): To engulf and possibly destroy bacteria or other foreign material.

phagocytosis (fag-ō-sī-tō′-sis): The engulfment, and usually the isolation or destruction by phagocytes of foreign or other particles or cells harmful to the body.

phagomania (fag-ō-mā′-ni-a): Abnormal craving for or obsession with food. Morbid desire to eat continually.

phak-, phako-: See **phac-, phaco-**.

phalangectomy (fal-an-jek′-to-mi): Removal of one or more of the phalanges.

phalanges (fal-an′-jēz): Plural of phalanx (*q.v.*).

phalanx (fā′-lanks): Any one of the small bones of the fingers or toes; 14 in each appendage, two in the thumb and great toe and three in each of the other digits.—phalanges, pl.; phalangeal, adj.

phall-, phallo-: Denotes the penis.

phallectomy (fal-ek′-to-mi): Amputation of the penis.

phallitis (fal-ī′-tis): Inflammation of the penis.

phallodynia (fal-ō-din′-i-a): Pain in the penis. Phallalgia.

phalloncus (fal-ong′-kus): An abnormal swelling or tumor of the penis.

phallorrhea (fal-o-rē′-a): 1. A discharge from the penis. 2.Gonorrhea in the male.

phallus (fal′-us): The penis.—phallic, adj.

phantasm (fan′-tazm): A delusion or illusion. An impression not caused by an actual physical stimulus. Phantom.

phantasmatomoria (fan-taz-mat-ō-mō′-ri-a): Silly phantasies, delusions, or childishness; seen in demented persons.

phantasy: See **fantasy**.

phantom (fan′-tom): 1. A model of a part

of the body, *e.g.*, a model of the pelvis, used in teaching obstetrics. 2.An apparition; something that a person sees but which does not actually exist. P. LIMB, term applied to a sensation that a patient has of a limb although the limb has been amputated. P. PAIN, pain felt as though it were in an amputated limb.

pharmaceutic (far-ma-sū′-tik): Related to or pertaining to drugs.

pharmaceutical (far-ma-sū′-tik-al). 1. Relating to drugs. 2. A medicinal drug.

pharmacist (far′-ma-sist): One who is qualified and licensed to prepare and dispense drugs; a druggist.

pharmaco-: Denotes drug(s), medicine(s)

pharmacogenic (far-ma-kō-jen′-ik): Produced by drugs, usually referring to side-effects.

pharmacologist (far-ma-kol′-o-jist): One who studies drugs, their sources, uses, and actions.

pharmacology (far-ma-kol′-o-ji): The science that deals with drugs in all their aspects and relations.

pharmacomania (far-ma-kō-mā′-ni-a): A morbid desire to give or take medicines.

pharmacopeia (far-ma-kō-pē′-a): A book in which accepted drugs and their preparations are listed and described, including dosages and other pertinent information. Prepared by an official authority of the government or of a medical group and accepted as a legal standard. UNITED STATES P., the legally recognized P. for the U.S.; revised every ten years by a committee of physicians and pharmacists, and kept up-to-date by interim supplements. Abbreviated USP. Also pharmacopoeia.

pharmacopsychosis (far-ma-kō-sī-kō′-sis): Psychosis due to addiction to alcohol, a drug, or a poison.

pharmacotherapy (far-ma-kō-ther′-a-pi): Treatment of disease with drugs.

pharmacy (far′-ma-si): 1. The practice of preparing and dispensing medications. 2. A place where medications are prepared and dispensed; a drugstore.

pharyng-, pharyngo-: Denotes the pharynx.

pharyngectomy (far-in-jek′-to-mi): Removal of part of the pharynx.

pharyngismus (far-in-jis′-mus): Spasm of the muscles of the pharynx.

pharyngitis (far-in-jī′-tis): Inflammation of the pharynx.

pharyngolaryngeal (far-ing′-gō-la-rin′-jē-al): Pertaining to the pharynx and larynx.

pharyngolaryngectomy (far-ing′-gō-lar-in-jek′-to-mi): Surgical removal of the pharynx and larynx.

pharyngolaryngitis (far-ing-gō-lar-in-jī′-tis): Inflammation of both the pharynx and larynx.

pharyngoplasty (far-ing′-gō-plas-ti): Any plastic operation on the pharynx.

pharyngoplegia (far-ing-gō-plē′-ji-a): Paralysis of the muscles of the wall of the pharynx.

pharyngospasm (far-ing′-gō-spazm): Pharyngismus (*q.v.*).

pharyngotomy (far-ing-got′-o-mi): The operation of opening into the pharynx, done from either the outside or the inside.

pharynx (far′-ingks): The upper expanded portion of the digestive tube that forms the cavity at the back of the mouth. It is cone-shaped, 3 to 4 in. long, and is lined with mucous membrane; at the lower end it opens into the esophagus. The eustachian tubes pierce its lateral walls and the posterior nares pierce its anterior wall. The larynx lies immediately below it and in front of the esophagus. For descriptive purposes it is divided into the nasopharynx, that part above the level of the soft palate; the oropharynx, that part between the soft palate and the epiglottis; and the laryngopharynx, that part between the upper edge of the epiglottis and the larynx.—pharyngeal, adj.

-phasia, -phasy (pl., -phasias, -phasies): Denotes a speech disorder, especially as related to the symbolic use of language.

phen-, pheno-: Denotes: (1) appearance, showing; (2) derivation from benzene.

phenol (fē′-nol): Carbolic acid. Formerly widely used as a disinfecting agent. Strong solutions are caustic.—phenolic, adj. P. COEFFICIENT, the disinfecting power of a chemical as compared with phenol.

phenomenon (fe-nom′-e-non): 1. Any unusual occurrence or fact. 2. In medicine, a symptom or any occurrence in relation to disease, whether or not it is unusual or extraordinary.—phenomena, pl.

phenylketonuria (fe-nil-kē-tōn-ūr′-i-a): A rare genetic anomaly marked by the presence of phenylpyruvic acid in the urine; a metabolic disorder that results in severe mental deficiency, often seizures, other neurological symptoms. Syn., phenylpyruvic oligophrenia.

phenylpyruvic oligophrenia (fe-nil-pī-rū′-vik ol-ig-ō-frē′-ni-a): See **phenylketonuria**.

phial (fi′-al): A small glass bottle for medicine; a vial.

-phil, -phile: Denotes: (1) loving, having a fondness or affinity for; (2) one who loves or has an affinity for.

-philia: Denotes: (1) love or craving for; (2) tendency toward.

philtrum (fil′-trum): Anatomical term for the groove in the midline of the upper lip.

phimosis (fī-mō′-sis): Tightness of the prepuce so that it cannot be retracted over the glans penis.

phleb-, phlebo-: Denotes a vein(s).

phlebectomy (flē-bek′-to-mi): Excision of a portion of a vein, sometimes done to relieve varicose veins. MULTIPLE COSMETIC P., removal of varicose veins through little stab incisions that heal without scarring.

phlebitis (flē-bī′-tis): Inflammation of a vein.

phleboclysis (flē-bok′-li-sis): The injection of a solution into a vein.

phlebogram (fleb′-ō-gram): See **venogram.**

phlebolith (fleb′-ō-lith): A concretion which forms in a vein.

phleborrhagia (fleb-ō-rā′-ji-a): Hemorrhage from a vein.

phleborrhexis (fleb-ō-rek′-sis): Rupture of a vein.

phlebosclerosis (fleb-ō-skler-ō′-sis): Loss of elasticity of the walls of a vein.

phlebostenosis (fleb-ō-ste-nō′-sis): Narrowing of the caliber of a vein.

phlebothrombosis (fleb-ō-throm-bō′-sis): Thrombosis in a vein due to sluggish flow of blood rather than to inflammation in the vein wall, occurring chiefly in bedridden patients and affecting the deep veins of the lower limbs or pelvis. The loosely attached thrombus is liable to break off and lodge in the lungs as an embolus.

phlebotomy (flē-bot′-o-mi): Venesection (*q.v.*).

phlegm (flem): The secretion of mucus expectorated from the bronchi.

phlegmasia (fleg-mā′-zi-a): Inflammation. P. ALBA DOLENS, inflammation of the femoral vein; sometimes follows childbirth; marked by swelling of the leg, usually without redness. Milk leg.

phlegmatic (fleg-mat′-ik): Emotionally stable. Not easily excited.

phlyctenule (flik-ten′-ūl): A minute blister (vesicle) usually occurring on the conjunctiva or cornea.—phlyctenular, adj.

phob-, phobo-: Denotes fear, avoidance of.

-phobe: Denotes a person with a phobia.

phobia (fō´-bi-a): A persistent, unreasonable, exaggerated, often disabling, morbid fear or dread. The term is often used as the termination of a word in which the main stem indicates the object of the person's fear.—phobic, adj.

phocomelia (fō-kō-mē´-li-a): A developmental anomaly in which the hands and feet are attached directly to the trunk giving a seal-like appearance. Congenital absence of a part of a limb.

phon-, phono-: Denotes sound, voice, speech, tone.

phonal (fō´-nal): Pertaining to speech or the voice.

phonasthenia (fō-nas-thē´-ni-a): Weakness or hoarseness of the voice due to fatigue.

phonation (fō-nā´-shun): The act of uttering sounds.

phonetic (fō-net´-ik): Relating to the voice or to speech. Phonic.

phonetics (fō-net´-iks): The science of speech and of pronunciation. Syn., phonology.

phonocardiogram (fō-nō-kar´-di-ō-gram): A graphic record of heart sounds.

phonocardiography (fō-nō-kar-di-og´-ra-fi): The graphic recording of heart sounds and murmurs by electric reproduction.—phonocardiographical, adj.; phonocardiographically, adv.

phonopsia (fō-nop´-si-a): A sensation of seeing certain colors when one hears certain sounds.

phosphatemia (fos-fa-tē´-mi-a): The presence of a higher than normal concentration of phosphates in the blood.

phosphaturia (fos-fa-tū´-ri-a): Excess of phosphates in the urine.—phosphaturic, adj.

phosphonecrosis (fos-fō-nē-krō´-sis): 'Fossy-jaw' occurring in workers engaged in the manufacture of products made with white phosphorus, e.g., matches; necrosis of the jaw with loosening of the teeth.

phosphorus (fos´-fo-rus): A non-metallic element forming an important constituent of bone and nerve tissue. RADIOACTIVE P. (P^{32}) is used in treating certain pathologic conditions, e.g., various forms of leukemia, and as a tracer substance in certain physiological studies.

phot-, photo-: Denotes: (1) light; (2) photograph.

photalgia (fō-tal´-ji-a): Pain in the eyes from exposure to intense light.

photic (fō´-tik): Of, related to, or caused by light.

photochemical (fō-tō-kem´-ik-al): Related to or produced by the chemical properties of light.

photocoagulation (fō-tō-kō-ag-ū-lā´-shun): See **laser.**

photoerythema (fō-tō-er-i-thē´-ma): Erythema (q.v.) caused by exposure to light.

photomania (fō-tō-mā´-ni-a): 1. A morbid desire for light. 2. Insanity or maniacal symptoms induced by prolonged exposure to bright light.

photomicrograph (fō-tō-mī´-krō-graf): An enlarged photograph of an object seen under the microscope. Microphotograph.

photophobia (fō-tō-fō´-bi-a): 1. Inability to expose the eyes to light. 2. Dread or avoidance of light places.—photophobic, adj.

photoreceptor (fō-tō-rē-sep´-tor): A sensory end organ capable of receiving stimuli caused by light. Syn., photoceptor.

photosensitive (fō-tō-sen´-si-tiv): Sensitive to light as the pigments in the eye.

photosynthesis (fō-tō-sin´-the-sis): The formation, by sunlight, of carbohydrate (glucose) from carbon dioxide and water in the presence of chlorophyll.

phototherapy (fō-tō-ther´-a-pi): Exposure to artificial blue light. In hyperbilirubinemia it appears to dehydrogenate the bilirubin to biliverdin. Used for mild neonatal jaundice and to prevent jaundice in premature infants.

phren (fren): 1 The diaphragm. 2. The mind.—phrenic, adj.

phren-, phreni-, phreno-: Denotes: (1) the mind; (2) the diaphragm; (3) the phrenic nerve.

phrenasthenia (fren-as-thē´-ni-a): 1. Loss of muscle tone of the diaphragm. 2. Feeblemindedness; mental deficiency.

phrenetic (fren-et´-ik): 1. Frenzied. 2. A person who is maniacal or frenzied.

-phrenia: Denotes a disordered condition of mental functioning.

phrenic (fren´-ik): 1. Pertaining to the diaphragm. 2. Relating to the mind. P AVULSION, see **avulsion.**

phrenicectomy (fren-i-sek´-to-mi): Resection of all or part of the phrenic nerve.

phrenicotomy (fren-i-kot´-o-mi): Division of the phrenic nerve to paralyze one half of the diaphragm, done to produce compression of a diseased lung.

phrenitis (fren-ī´-tis): 1. Inflammation of the diaphragm. 2. Inflammation of the brain 3. Frenzy; delirium.

phrenology (fre-nol´-o-ji): The doctrine that

the external configurations of the skull indicate areas of development in the brain of certain mental faculties, and that therefore one's mental characteristics can be determined by examination of the various prominences of the skull.

phrenoplegia (fren-ō-plē′-ji-a): 1. Paralysis of the diaphragm. 2. Paralysis or sudden loss of mental faculties.

phrenotropic (fren-ō-trō′-pik): Having an effect upon the mind.

phthisis (tī′-sis): 1. Progressive, general, or local atrophy or wasting. 2. Old term for pulmonary tuberculosis.—phthisic, adj.

phylaxis (fī-laks′-is): The body's protection or defense against infection.

phylogenic (fī-lō-jen′-ik): Pertaining to the evolutionary development of a plant or animal species rather than of an individual of the species.

physiatrics (fiz-i-at′-riks): The use of physical agents in the diagnosis and treatment of disease. Physical therapy. Physical medicine.

physic (fiz′-ik): 1. Old term for the art and science of medicine. 2. A purgative or laxative drug.

physical (fiz′-i-kal): Pertaining to the body, nature, or the science of physics (q.v.).

physician (fi-zish′-un): A person fitted by knowledge and training and licensed by the proper authorities to care for the sick; a doctor. ATTENDING P., one who visits his patients in the hospital and gives orders for their care. HOUSE P., one who lives in the hospital and is responsible for the patients' care during the absence of attending physicians.

physicochemical (fiz-i-kō-kem′-ik-al): Pertaining to physics and chemistry.

physics (fiz′-iks): A fundamental science that deals with the phenomena and laws of nature; it treats particularly of the properties of matter and energy.

physiognomy (fiz-i-og′-nō-mi): The appearance; facial features and expression.

physiologic (fiz-i-ō-loj′-ik), **physiological** (fiz-i-ō-loj′-i-kal): 1. Of or related to physiology. 2. Denoting the action of a drug in a healthy person as distinguished from its therapeutic action. 3. Normal as opposed to pathologic; in accordance with natural processes of the body. Adjective often used to describe a normal process or structure, to distinguish it from an abnormal or pathological feature (e.g., the P. level of glucose in the blood is from 60 to 180 mg per 100 ml; higher and lower levels are

pathological and indicative of disease). P. SALINE (normal or isotonic), a 0.9 percent solution of sodium chloride in water. P. SOLUTION, a fluid isotonic with the body fluids and containing similar salts.

physiology (fiz-i-ol′-o-ji): The branch of biology that deals with the normal vital processes, activities, and functions of living organisms.

physiopsychic (fiz-i-ō-sī′-kik): Pertinent to or involving both the body and the mind.

physiotherapy (fiz-i-ō-ther′-a-pi): Treatment of disease by physical means, e.g., light, heat, electricity, water, massage, regulated exercises. Physical therapy. Physiatrics.

physique (fi-zēk′): The general bodily structure or type. Syn., build.

pia (pī′-a): P. MATER, the innermost of the three meninges (q.v.); the vascular membrane that lies in close contact with the substance of the brain and spinal cord. See **mater, meninges.**

pia-arachnitis (pī-a-ar-ak-nī′-tis): Leptomeningitis (q.v.).

pia-arachnoid (pī-a-ar-ak′-noid): Pertaining to the pia mater and the arachnoid membrane.

pial (pī′-al): Of or relating to the pia mater.

pica (pī′-ka): Desire for extraordinary articles of food and also substances not fit for food, e.g., plaster, chalk, ashes, clay. Often indicates a nutritional deficiency. See **geophagia.**

Pick's disease: 1. Syndrome of ascites, hepatic enlargement, edema, and pleural effusion occurring in constrictive pericarditis. [Friedel Pick, German physician. 1867-1926.] 2. A type of cerebral atrophy which produces mental changes similar to senescence (q.v.). [Arnold Pick, Czechoslovakian physician. 1851-1924.]

picorna virus: Term sometimes used for any one of a large group of viruses including enterovirus and Coxsackie groups, ECHO, and many rhinovirus types.

Pierre Robin syndrome: A condition in which micrognathia (q.v.) accompanies cleft palate and glossoptosis (q.v.).

piesesthesia (pī-es-es-thē′-zi-a): Sensivity to pressure.

pigeon breast: A deformity in which the chest is narrow and there is an anterior bulging of the sternum; occurs especially in rickets. Pectus carinatum.

pigeon toe: A condition in which the toes permanently turn inward toward the median line.—pigeon-toed, adj.

pigment (pig′-ment): In anatomy, any coloring matter in the body.

pigmentation (pig-men-tā′-shun): The deposit of pigment in any of the body tissues, especially when abnormal or excessive.

pigmentum nigrum (pig-men′-tum nī′-grum): The black pigment that lines the choroid coat of the eye.

piitis (pī-ī′-tis): Inflammation of the pia mater.

pil-, pili-, pilo-: Denotes hair(s).

pilar (pil′ar): Related to hair. Covered with hair.

piles: See **hemorrhoids.**

pili (pī′-li): Plural of pilus (*q.v.*).

pill: A small, usually rounded mass of some cohesive substance containing a medication; may or may not be coated; to be swallowed|whole. BREAD P., one made of bread crumbs pressed into a ball; usually a placebo. ENTERIC COATED P., one coated with a substance that will not dissolve until the pill reaches the intestine. PEP P., one|that contains a drug with a stimulating effect, especially benzedrine.

pillar: In anatomy, a supporting structure or part that resembles a column, usually in pairs, *e.g.,* the pillars of the fauces.

pilocystic (pī-lō-sis′-tik): Denoting a cyst that contains hair.

pilomotor (pī-lō-mō′-tor): Causing the hair to move. P. MUSCLES, the arrectores pili of the skin. P. NERVES, tiny nerves attached to the hair follicle; innervation causes the hair to stand upright and give the appearance of 'goose flesh.'

pilonidal (pī-lō-ni′-dal): Hair-containing. P. CYST, a sacrococcygeal dermoid cyst that contains hairs. P. SINUS, a sinus containing hairs and which usually occurs in hirsute people in the cleft between the buttocks; it is a congenital anomaly.

pilose (pī′-los): Covered with hair, especially that of a soft texture; hairy.

pilosebaceous (pī-lō-sē-bā′-shus): Pertaining to the hair follicle and the sebaceous gland opening into it.

pilosis (pī-lō′-sis): An abnormal growth of hair.

pilus (pī′-lus): A hair.—pili, pl.

pimple: A small, usually pointed protuberance on the skin, often suppurated. See **papule, pustule.**

pin: A slender metal rod used in the surgical fixation of the ends of fractured bones.

pineal (pin′-ē-al): 1. Having a shape like a pine cone. 2. Pertaining to the pineal body (*q.v.*).

pineal body (pin′-ē-al): A small reddish-gray conical structure on the dorsal surface of the midbrain. Its functions are not fully understood but there is some evidence that it is an endocrine gland concerned with growth.

pinealoma (pin-ē-a-lō′-ma): A tumor of the pineal gland; usually occurs in young people. Causes obesity and early puberty.

pinguecula (pin-gwek′-ū-la): A yellowish, slightly elevated thickening of the bulbar conjunctiva near the lid aperture. Associated with the aging eye.

pink disease: Erythredema polyneuritis (*q.v.*).

pinkeye: Popular name for acute contagious conjunctivitis.

pinna (pin′-a): That part of the ear which is external to the head; the auricle.

pint: A unit of capacity in the apothecaries' system; 16 fluid ounces, $^1/_2$ quart. Equivalent to 473.167 ml in the metric system.

pinta (pin′-ta): A chronic, nonvenereal disease caused by a spirochete; characterized by the eruption of patches of varying color that finally become white. Occurs mostly in children. Is endemic among dark-skinned peoples of the tropics and sub-tropics.

pinworm: Enterobius vermicularis (*q.v.*).

pipette (pī-pet′): A glass tube with a small lumen used in the laboratory for transferring and measuring small amounts of fluid.

piriform (pir′-i-form): Having the shape of a pear.

Pirquet's reaction (pir′-kāz): A local inflammatory reaction in response to the application of tuberculin to scarified skin to determine the presence of tuberculosis; used especially in children. [Baron Clemens von Pirquet, Austrian pediatrician. 1874-1929.]

pisiform (pī′-si-form): 1. Having the shape or size of a pea. 2. One of the bones of the carpus.

pit: 1. Any hollow or depression on the surface of the body or of an organ. 2. A dimple or pockmark. 3. A depression in the enamel of a tooth. 4. To make an indentation, as occurs when a finger is pressed against edematous tissue.

pith: 1. The spinal cord and medulla oblongata. 2. The center of a hair shaft. 3. To destroy the spinal cord or the entire central nervous system of an animal by introducing a sharp pointed instrument at the base of the skull or passing it down the spinal canal; done to destroy sensibility in animals to be used for experimental or teaching purposes.

pitting: (pit′-ting): 1. Making an indentation in dropsical tissues. 2. Depressed scars left on the skin, especially after smallpox.

pituitarism (pi-tū′-i-tar-izm): Any dysfunction of the pituitary gland.

pituitary gland: A small oval endocrine gland lying in the P. fossa of the sphenoid bone; the hypophysis cerebri. The anterior lobe secretes several hormones, having an effect upon other endocrine glands. Their general overall function is to regulate growth and metabolism. The posterior lobe secretes pituitrin, which has an effect on the fluid and electrolyte balance of the body; because it lessens the volume of urine formed it is called the antidiuretic hormone (ADH); also acts to regulate and stimulate smooth muscle tissue thus affecting blood pressure and the activity of uterine muscles.

pituitectomy (pi-tū-i-tek′-to-mi): Surgical removal of the pituitary gland.

pituitrin (pi-tū′-i-trin): 1. The secretion of the posterior lobe of the pituitary gland (*q. v.*). 2. Trademark for a preparation of pituitary extract made from the pituitary gland of an animal.

pityriasis (pit-i-rī′-a-sis): Name given to a group of skin diseases characterized by scaly (branny) eruption of the skin. P. CAPITIS, dandruff. P.ROSEA, a slightly scaly eruption of ovoid erythematous lesions which are widespread over the trunk and proximal parts of the limbs. There may be mild itching. It is a self-limiting condition. P. RUBRA, a form of exfoliative dermatitis. P. RUBRA PILARIS, a chronic skin disease characterized by tiny red papules of perifollicular distribution. P. VERSICOLOR, called also 'tinea versicolor,' is a fungus infection which causes the appearance of buff-colored patches on the chest.

Pityrosporum (pit-i-ros′-pŏr-um): A fungus associated with dandruff and seborrheic dermatitis.

PKU: Abbreviation for phenylketonuria (*q. v.*).

placebo (pla-sē′-bō): A harmless substance given for its psychologic or suggestive effect. In experimental research an inert substance, identical in appearance with the material being tested. Neither the physician nor the patient knows which is which.

placenta (pla-sen′-ta): Afterbirth. A flat, oval, spongy, vascular structure that develops about the third month of pregnancy and attaches to the inner wall of the uterus. Through it the fetus is supplied with oxygen and gets rid of its waste products.

Usually attaches to the upper part of the uterus and is expelled within an hour after the child is born. P. PREVIA, a P. that is attached to the lower part of the uterus so that it covers all or part of the internal os; usually causes antepartal hemorrhage. RETAINED P., one that is not expelled within the normal time after childbirth.—placental, adj.

placental insufficiency: Insufficiency of the placenta. Can be due to maternal disease or postmaturity of the fetus giving rise to a 'small for dates' baby.

placentography (pla-sen-tog′-ra-fi): X-ray examination of the placenta after injection of opaque substance.

plague (plāg): Any disease of wide prevalence and high mortality, but particularly the very contagious epidemic disease caused by *Pasteurella pestis,* and spread by infected rats who transfer the infection to man through the agency of fleas. It is characterized by high fever, prostration, a petechial eruption, glandular swellings. The main clinical types are bubonic, pneumonic, and septicemic. Also called pest, black death, oriental plague. See **bubo, bubonic plague.**

planta (plan′-ta): The sole of the foot.—plantae, pl.

plantar (plan′-tar): Pertaining to the sole of the foot. P. ARCH, the union of the P. and dorsalis pedis arteries in the sole of the foot. P. FLEXION, downward movement of the big toe. P. WART, one that occurs on the sole of the foot; usually very painful and difficult to cure; thought to be caused by a specific virus that attacks irritated tissue.

plaque (plak): 1. A blood platelet. 2. A small, flat, localized, abnormal area or patch on some body surface or part. 3. A deposit of fatty or fibrous consistency in the wall of a blood vessel, as occurs in atheroma (*q. v.*).

-plasia: Denotes formation, development.

plasm: 1. Plasma. 2. That part of the germ cell that contains the substance by which individual characteristics are transmitted from generation to generation.

plasm-, plasmo-: Denotes: (1) the blood plasma; (2) the substance of a cell.

plasma: 1. Cytoplasm or protoplasm. 2. The liquid fraction of lymph. 3. The liquid fraction of the circulating blood; to be differentiated from serum (*q. v.*). It is clear, straw-colored and 90 percent water; blood corpuscles and other formed substances, including fibrinogen, are suspended in it.

plasmapheresis (plaz-ma-fer′-e-sis): A technique whereby blood is removed from the body; the cells are separated from the plasma by centrifugation and are then added to a non-protein fluid and reinjected into the body; done for both experimental and therapeutic reasons.

plasmin (plaz′-min): A fibrinolysin (*q.v.*); a proteolytic enzyme found in the plasma and having an ability to dissolve fibrin clots.

plasminogen (plaz-min′-ō-jen): Precursor of plasmin. Release of activators from damaged tissue promotes the conversion of plasminogen into plasmin.

Plasmodium (plaz-mō′-di-um): A genus of protozoa, parasitic in the red blood cells of warm-blooded animals and which complete their sexual cycle in blood-sucking arthropods. Four species cause malaria in man.—plasmodial, adj.

plasmolysis (plaz-mol′-i-sis): Contraction or shrinking of a cell due to loss of water by osmosis; occurs when the cell is suspended in a hypertonic solution.

plasmoptysis (plaz-mop′-ti-sis): The swelling of a cell and bursting of its wall with the escape of protoplasm; occurs when the cell is suspended in a hypotonic solution.

plaster: A fabric or similar material, spread with a mixture or substance that may or may not contain a medication, to be applied externally. ADHESIVE P., fabric coated with a gummy substance; used to hold dressings in place, to protect wounds, sometimes for immobilization of a part. COURT P., P. made of isinglass spread on fine fabric; used for covering small lesions. MUSTARD P., made of mustard and flour mixed with water and spread on a cloth; a counterirritant. P. OF PARIS, calcium sulfate mixed with water and applied wet; hardens rapidly; used for casts and to immobilize a part.

plastic (plas′-tik): 1. Tending to build up or regenerate tissue. 2. Capable of taking the form of a mold. 3. A substance that has been produced chemically. P. SURGERY, a surgical procedure in which healthy tissue is transferred, or tissues are reconstructed or repaired in order to correct deformities or abnormalities present at birth or caused by injuries, burns, etc.

plastocyte (plas′-tō-sit): A blood platelet.

-plasty: Denotes: (1) molding or shaping; (2) repair, reconstruction, plastic surgery.

plate: 1. In anatomy, a thin, flat, differentiated structure, especially a bone. 2. A narrow, flat piece of metal that is screwed to the ends of fractured bones to keep them in alignment. 3. Common term for a denture.

platelet (plāt′-let): Small, oval, disk-like cell found in the blood plasma; does not contain hemoglobin; is essential for clotting. A thrombocyte.

platy-: Denotes broad, flat.

platycephalic (plat-i-se-fal′-ik): Having a skull that is flattened on top. Also platycephalous.

Platyhelminthes (plat-i-hel-min′-thēz): Flatworm; fluke. See **schistosomiasis**.

platymorphic (plat-i-mor′-fik): Having a flattened shape; used especially in reference to the eyeball.

platyopic (plat-i-ō′-pik): Having a broad face.

platypodia (plat-i-pō′-di-a): Flatfootedness.

platysma (pla-tiz′-ma): The broad, thin sheet of muscle on each side of the neck; it acts to depress the lower jaw and draw down the corners of the mouth.

pledget (plej′-et): A small compress of gauze or a tuft of wool or cotton.

-plegia, -plegy: Denotes paralysis.

pleio-, pleo-, plio-: Denotes more.

pleocytosis (plē-ō-sī-tō′-sis): 1. An increase of cells any place in the body. 2. An increase in the number of lymphocytes in the cerebrospinal fluid.

pleomastia (plē-ō-mas′-ti-a): The condition of having supernumerary breasts or nipples.

pleomorphism (plē-ō-mor′-fizm): Denotes a wide range in shape and size of individuals within a species or group of organisms.—pleomorphic, pleomorphous, adj.

pleonexia (plē-ō-nek′-si-a): Greediness.

plethora (pleth′-o-ra): Fullness; overloading. Used especially to describe a condition of overfullness of the blood vessels accompanied by congestion of tissues, a feeling of tension in the head, flushed complexion, bounding pulse.—plethoric, adj.

pleura (ploor′-a): A thin serous membrane covering the surface of the lung and reflecting, at the root of the lung, on to the chest wall. That portion lining the chest wall is termed 'parietal P.'; that closely adherent to lung tissue is 'visceral P.'—pleural, adj.

pleuracentesis (ploor-a-sen-tē′-sis): Surgical puncture of the chest wall for drainage of fluid. Pleurocentesis. Thoracocentesis.

pleuralgia (ploor-al′-ji-a): Pain in the pleura or in the side of the chest.—pleuralgic, adj,

pleurisy (ploo′-ri-si): Inflammation of the pleura. Pleuritis. May be fibrinous (dry), associated with an effusion (wet), or complicated by empyema.—pleuritic, adj.

pleuritis (ploo-rī′-tis): Pleurisy (*q.v.*).

pleurodynia (ploo-rō-din′-i-a): Intercostal myalgia or muscular rheumatism (f i-brositis). Is a feature of Bornholm disease (*q.v.*).

pleuropericarditis (ploo-rō-per-i-kar-dī′-tis): Inflammation of the pleura and the pericardium.

pleuropulmonary (ploo-rō-pul′-mon-a-ri): Pertaining to the pleura and lungs.

pleurothotonos (ploo-rō-thot′-o-nos): A bending of the body to one side, due to tetany of the muscles.

pleurotomy (ploo-rot′-o-mi): An incision into the pleural cavity to allow escape of effused fluid.

plexus (pleks′-us): A network of vessels or nerves.

-plexy: Denotes seizure or stroke.

plica (plī′-ka): A fold.—plicate, adj.; plication, n.

-ploid: Denotes: (1) multiple in form; (2) number of chromosomes.

plombage (plom-bazh′): The use of an inert material to produce compression of a tuberculous lung cavity.

plumbism: Chronic lead poisoning (*q.v.*).

plumbum (plum′-bum): Lead.

Plummer-Vinson syndrome: Also Kelly-Paterson syndrome. Combination of severe glossitis with dysphagia caused by degeneration of the muscle of the esophagus, atrophy of the papillae of the tongue, and secondary (nutritional) anemia. [Henry Stanley Plummer, American physician. 1874-1937. Porter Paisley Vinson, American surgeon. 1890- .]

pluri-: Denotes several, more.

pluriglandular (ploo-ri-gland′-ū-lar): Pertaining to or affecting several glands, as mucoviscidosis (*q.v.*).

pluripara (ploo-rip′-a-ra): Multipara.

P.M.: Abbreviation for *post meridian*, meaning after noon.

-pnea, -pnoea: Denotes: (1) breath; (2) breathing.

pneum-, pneumo-: Denotes: (1) lung(s); (2) respiration; (3) air or gas.

pneumat-, pneumato-: Denotes: (1) air or gas; (2) breathing.

pneumathemia (nū-ma-thē′-mi-a): Air embolism (*q.v.*); the presence of bubbles of air or gas in the blood.

pneumatosis (nū-ma-tō′-sis): An abnormal accumulation of air or gas in any part or tissue of the body.

pneumaturia (nū-ma-tū′-ri-a): The passage of flatus during or after urination; usually the result of a bladder-bowel fistula but may also be due to decomposition of bladder urine. Pneumatinuria.

pneumobacillus (nū-mō-ba-sil′-us): Friedländer's bacillus (*q.v.*).

pneumocentesis (nū-mō-sen-tē′-sis): Surgical puncture of a lung to allow drainage of accumulated fluid or pus; pneumonocentesis.

pneumococcus (nū-mō-kok′-us): *Diplococcus pneumoniae*. A gram-positive, encapsulated coccal bacterium, characteristically arranged in pairs; the common cause of lobar pneumonia; also causal agent for otitis media, mastoiditis, and leptomeningitis as well as many other infections.—pneumococcal, adj.

pneumoconiosis (nū-mō-kō-ni-ō′-sis): Dust disease. Fibrosis of the lung caused by long continued inhalation of dust in industrial occupations, such as coal mining, stone cutting, etc. The most important complication is the occasional superinfection with tuberculosis. Examples are silicosis, coal worker's P., asbestosis, siderosis, grinder's lung and byssinosis, described elsewhere.—pneumoconioses, pl.

pneumoencephalogram (nū-mō-en-sef′-a-lō-gram): X-ray picture of the brain after replacement of the cerebrospinal fluid with gas or air.

pneumoencephalography (nū-mō-en-sef-a-log′-ra-fi):The making of x-ray films of the head after the injection of air or gas into the subarachnoid space.—pneumoencephalogram, n.

pneumogastric (nū-mō-gas′-trik): Pertaining to the lungs and stomach. See **vagus.**

pneumohydrothorax (nū-mō-hī-drō-thō′-raks): The presence of both gas or air and fluid in the pleural cavity.

pneumokoniosis: See **pneumoconiosis.**

pneumolysis (nū-mol′-i-sis): Separation of the two pleural layers, or the outer pleural layer from the chest wall to collapse the lung. Also pneumonolysis.

pneumomediastinogram (nū-mō-mēd-i-as-tī′-nō-gram): X-ray of the mediastinum after rendering it opaque with air.

pneumomelanosis (nū-mō-mel-a-nō′-sis):A condition in which lung tissue becomes black due to inhalation of coal dust.

pneumomycosis(nū-mō-mi-kō′-sis):Fungus infection of the lung such as aspergillosis, actinomycosis, moniliasis.—pneumomycotic, adj.

pneumon-, pneumono-: Denotes lung(s).

pneumonectomy (nū-mo-nek′-to-mi): Excision of a lung or lung tissue.

pneumonia (nū-mō′-ni-a): Inflammation of the lung with production of alveolar exudate. Traditionally, two main types were recognized, on an anatomical or radiological basis, viz., lobar P. and broncho-P. The tendency these days is to classify according to the specific bacterium or virus causing the infection (specific pneumonias) on the one hand, and the aspiration or secondary pneumonias (nonspecific) on the other. ASPIRATION P., P. caused by inhalation of foreign particles such as vomitus inhaled by unconscious patients. HYPOSTATIC P. is the result of stasis and occurs in the case of debilitated patients from lack of movement in the dependent part of the lung. UNRESOLVED P., P. wherein the alveolar exudate does not liquefy but consolidation persists.—pneumonic, adj.

pneumonitis (nū-mō-nī′-tis): Inflammation of lung tissue.

pneumoperitoneum (nū-mō-per-it-o-nē′-um): Air or gas in the peritoneal cavity. May follow perforated gastric ulcer, peritonitis, other pathologic conditions, or may be introduced for diagnostic or therapeutic reasons.

pneumoradiography (nū-mō-rā-di-og′-ra-fi): Radiographic examination of a region after injection of air.

pneumoresection (nū-mō-rē-sek′-shun): Surgical removal of part of a lung.

pneumorrhagia (nū-mō-rā′-ji-a): Hemorrhage from the lungs.

pneumothorax (nū-mō-thō′-raks): Air or gas in the pleural cavity. ARTIFICIAL P., induced in the treatment of pulmonary tuberculosis. SPONTANEOUS P. occurs when an over-dilated pulmonary air sac ruptures, permitting communication of respiratory passages and pleural cavity. TENSION or VALVULAR P. occurs when a valve-like wound allows air to enter the pleural cavity at each inspiration but not to escape on expiration, thus progressively increasing intrathoracic pressure and constituting an acute medical emergency.—pneumothoraces, pl.

pneumotoxin (nū-mō-tok′-sin): An endotoxin produced by the pneumococcus and believed to be responsible for the systemic symptoms of lobar pneumonia.

pneumoventriculography (nū-mō-ven-trik-ū-log′-ra-fi): Examination of cerebral ventricles by x-ray after injection of air directly.

p.o.: Abbreviation for *per os*, meaning by mouth.

pock: A pustule, specifically the pustular lesion characteristic of smallpox.

pockmark: The small, depressed mark, scar, or pit left after the pustular lesion of smallpox heals.

pod-, podo-: Denotes foot or foot-like.

podagra (pō-dag′-ra): Gout in the foot, especially that in the great toe.

podalgia (pō-dal′-ji-a): Pain in the foot.

podiatrist (pō-dī′-a-trist): One who specializes in the diagnosis and treatment of diseases and defects of the feet. Syn., chiropodist.—podiatry, n.

podobromidrosis (pōd-ō-brō-mid-rō′-sis): Offensive perspiration of the feet.

pododynia (pōd-ō-din′-i-a): Pain in the foot. Syn., podalgia.

podogeriatric (pōd-ō-jer-i-at′-ric): Refers to foot care for the elderly.

podopompholyx (pōd-ō-pom′-fo-liks): See **cheiropompholyx.**

-poiesis: Denotes production or formation of.

poikilocytosis(poi-kil-ō-sī-tō′-sis):Variation in the shape of red blood corpuscles, *e.g.,* the pear-shaped cells found in pernicious anemia.

poison (poy′-z'n): Any substance that is harmful or lethal when applied to or taken into the body. P. IVY, see **ivy poisoning.**

poison control center: A facility equipped with personnel and reference works adequate to answer questions of the public about poisons and treatments for poisoning. Often associated with hospitals, medical schools or health departments. There are over 400 such centers in the U.S.; most of them are open 24 hours a day.

poli-, polio-: Denotes the gray matter of the nervous system.

polio: Colloquial term for poliomyelitis (*q.v.*).

polioencephalitis (pōl-i-ō-en-sef-a-lī′-tis): Inflammation of the gray matter of the brain; may or may not include the central nuclei. Caused by poliomyelitis virus; marked by fever, headache, anxiety, confusion, trembling, twitching of facial muscles, insomnia, sometimes convulsions, lethargy; often fatal.—polioencephalitic, adj.

poliomyelitis (pōl-i-ō-mī-e-lī′-tis): An acute

epidemic virus disease affecting children especially; marked by fever, headache, sore throat, stiff neck, gastrointestinal symptoms. May lead to paralysis and atrophy of one or more groups of skeletal muscles with resulting permanent deformity and disability. ACUTE ANTERIOR P., P. in which the virus attacks the anterior horns of the gray matter of the spinal cord. BULBAR P., a serious form in which the virus attacks the medulla oblongata; there may be inability to swallow, paralysis, respiratory distress leading to respiratory failure.

polio vaccine: Vaccine given for the purpose of conferring immunity to poliomyelitis.

poliovirus (pōl-i-ō-vī′-rus): The causative agent of poliomyelitis. Three types are recognized serologically, of which Type One is the most frequent cause of paralytic poliomyelitis.

Politzer's bag: A soft, rubber, pear-shaped bag for inflating the middle ear. [Adam Politzer, Austrian otologist. 1835-1920.]

pollex (pol′-eks): The thumb.

pollinosis (pol-i-nō′-sis): Allergic condition characterized by catarrhal condition of mucous membranes of eyes, nose, and respiratory tract; caused by sensitivity to pollen and recurs annually, usually in the spring or late summer. Hay fever and rose fever are examples of P. Also pollenosis.

pollution (po-lū′-shun): 1. Defilement; uncleanness; impurity. 2. Emission of semen at times other than during coitus, e.g., nocturnal emission.

poly: Abbreviation and colloquial term often used to designate polymorphonuclear leukocyte.

poly-: Denotes many, several, diverse, excessive, multiple.

polyadenitis (pol-i-ad-e-nī′-tis): Inflammation of several lymph nodes at the same time; refers especially to the cervical nodes.

polyarteritis (pol-i-ar-ter-i′-tis): Simultaneous inflammation of several arteries. P. NODOSA, inflammation of the coats of the arteries in multiple circumscribed areas resulting in the formation of nodules; see **periarteritis nodosa.**

polyarthritis (pol-i-ar-thrī′-tis): Inflammation of several joints at the same time. See **Still's disease.**

polyarticular (pol-i-ar-tik′-ū-lar): Pertaining to or affecting several joints simultaneously.

polyavitaminosis (pol-i-ā-vī-ta-min-ō′-sis): A pathological condition in which there is a deficiency of more than one vitamin in the diet.

polyblennia (pol-i-blen′-i-a): Excess production of mucus.

polycholia (pol-i-kō′-li-a): Excessive secretion of bile.

polychromia (pol-i-krō′-mi-a): Increased pigmentation or coloration in any part of the body.

polyclinic (pol-i-klin′-ik): Pertaining to a hospital that cares for several types of diseases and injuries.

polycrotic (pol-i-krot′-ik): Descriptive of a pulse that has several secondary waves following each pulse beat.

polycyesis (pol-i-sī-ē′-sis): Multiple pregnancy.

polycystic (pol-i-sis′-tik): Containing or composed of many cysts. P. kidney disease is congenital, and slowly fatal.

polycystoma (pol-i-sis-tō′-ma): A condition in which a part of the body has many cysts; said especially of the breast.

polycythemia (pol-i-sī-thē′-mi-a): Excess in the number of circulating red blood cells. This may result from dehydration or be a compensatory phenomenon to increase the oxygen carrying capacity, as in congenital heart disease. P. VERA, an idiopathic condition in which the red cell count is very high. The white cell count, platelets, volume and viscosity of the blood are also increased; there is hyperemia of all organs and enlargement of the spleen. The patient complains of headache and lassitude and there is danger of thrombosis and hemorrhage. RELATIVE P., a relative increase in red blood cell count, due to loss of fluid from the blood.

polycytosis (pol-i-sī-tō′-sis): An increase in the red and white cells of the blood with a reduction in blood volume.

polydactyly (pol-i-dak′-til-i): Having more than the normal number of fingers or toes. Also polydactylism.

polydipsia (pol-i-dip′-si-a): Frequent drinking because of excessive thirst.

polyemia (pol-i-ēm′-i-a): Excess amount of blood in the body.

polyethylene (pol-i-eth′-i-lēn): A synthetic plastic material, highly resistant to chemicals; frequently used to make tubing.

polygalactia (pol-i-ga-lak′-shi-a): Excess secretion of milk.

polygraph (pol′-i-graf): An instrument that records several impulses or pulsations simultaneously; e.g., pulse beat, blood pressure, and respiratory movements.

polyhidrosis (pol-i-hīd-rō′-sis): Excessive secretion of sweat.

polyhydramnios (pol-i-hī-dram′-ni-ōs): The

presence of more than the normal amount of amniotic fluid in the uterus at term.

polyhydruria (pol-i-hĭ-drŭ´-ri-a): Abnormal amount of water in the urine.

polyhypermenorrhea (pol-i-hĭ-per-men-ō-rē´-a): Frequent profuse menstruation.

polyhypomenorrhea (pol-i-hĭ-pō-men-ō-rē´-a): Frequent scanty menstruation.

polyinfection (pol-i-in-fek´-shun): Infection with several organisms at the same time.

polyleptic (pol-i-lep´-tik): Descriptive of diseases that have many remissions and exacerbations, *e.g.,* malaria.

polymastia (pol-i-mas´-ti-a): The condition of having more than two breasts.

polymer (pol´-i-mer): A natural or synthetic chemical compound that results when two or more molecules of the same substance are combined to form a larger molecule.

polymorphic (pol-i-mor´-fik): Multiform; existing or occurring in several forms.

polymorphonuclear (pol-i-mor-fō-nū´-klē-ar): Having a many-shaped or lobulated nucleus, usually applied to the neutrophil leukocytes (phagocytes) which constitute 70 per cent of the total white blood cells.

polymyositis (pol-i-mĭ-ō-sī´-tis): Inflammation of several muscles at the same time.

polyneuritis (pol-i-nū-rī´-tis): Inflammation of many peripheral nerves at the same time. Some of the causes are alcoholism; poisoning, particularly from metals; vitamin deficiency, especially of thiamine.—polyneuritic, adj.

polyopia (pol-i-ōp´-i-a): Seeing many images of a single object simultaneously; multiple vision.

polyorchidism (pol-i-or´-ki-dizm): The condition of having more than two testes.

polyp or **polypus** (pol´-ip (-us)): A small, smooth, finger-like growth arising from a mucous surface (cervical, uterine, nasal, etc.), usually attached by a stem. Usually benign but may become malignant.—polypi, pl.; polypous, adj.

polypectomy (pol-i-pek´-to-mi): Surgical removal of a polyp.

polypeptides (pol-i-pep´-tīdz): Proteins with long chains of amino acids linked together.

polyphagia (pol-i-fā´-ji-a): Pathological overeating; excessive appetite.

polyphobia (pol-i-fō´-bi-a): Morbid fear of many things.

polyphrasia (pol-i-frā´-zi-a): Excessive or insane talkativeness.

polyplegia (pol-i-plē´-ji-a): Paralysis of sev-eral muscles at the same time.

polypnea (pol-ip-nē´-a): Very rapid breathing; panting.

polypoid (pol´-i-poid): Resembling a polyp.

polyposis (pol-i-pō´-sis): A condition in which there are numerous polypi in an organ. P. COLI, a hereditary condition in which polypi occur throughout the large bowel and which leads eventually to carcinoma of the colon.

polysaccharide (pol-i-sak´-a-rīd): Carbohydrates containing a large number of monosaccharide groups. Starch, inulin, glycogen, dextrin and cellulose are examples.

polyserositis (pol-i-sē-rō-sī´-tis): Inflammation of several serous membranes.

polysinusitis (pol-i-sī-nus-ī´-tis): Inflammation of several sinuses at the same time.

polythelia (pol-i-thē´-li-a): The condition of having supernumerary nipples; may be on the breast or elsewhere on the body.

polytrichia (pol-i-trik´-i-a): Excessive hairiness.

polyuria (pol-i-ūr´-i-a): Excretion of an excessive amount of urine.—polyuric, adj.

polyvalent (pol-i-vāl´-ent): Refers usually to a serum or vaccine that is effective against several strains of a particular organism.

pompholyx (pom´-fol-iks): Vesicular skin eruption on the palms of the hands or soles of the feet. See **cheiropompholyx.**

pomphus (pom´-fus): A blister or wheal on the skin.—pomphoid, adj.

pons: A bridge; a process of tissue joining two sections of an organ.—pontine, adj. PONS VAROLII, the white convex mass of nerve tissue at the base of the brain which serves to connect the cerebrum, cerebellum, and medulla oblongata. [Constantio Varolius, Italian anatomist. 1543-1575.]

popliteal (pop-li-tē´-al): Pertaining to the posterior surface of the knee. P. SPACE, the diamond-shaped depression at the back of the knee joint, bounded by the muscles and containing the popliteal nerve and vessels.

poradenitis (por-ad-en-ī´-tis): Painful mass of iliac glands, characterized by abscess formation. Occurs in lymphogranuloma inguinale (*q.v.*).

pore: A small opening. One of the minute openings of the ducts that lead from the sweat glands to the surface of the skin; they are controlled by fine papillary muscles, contracting and closing in the cold, and dilating in the presence of heat.

porencephalia (pō-ren-se-fā´-li-a): A condition in which there is inflammation of the brain in early infancy with the formation of cavities in the brain substance; may be congenital, or due to imperfect development, infection, or injury following birth.

porosis (pō-rō′-sis): The formation of cavities or holes in tissue, *e.g.*, osteoporosis (*q.v.*).

porphyria (por′-fi-ri-a): A pathological state, due to an inborn error of metabolism of blood pigments, resulting in the production of excess porphyrins (*q.v.*) which are present in the blood and urine. Symptoms include pathological changes in nervous and muscular tissue and, in some cases, splenomegaly, anemia, sensitivity to light, and a variety of mental symptoms.

porphyrin (por′-fi-rin): Any one of a group of organic pigments that are widely distributed in nature and also exist in small amounts in the human body. Chlorophyll and hemoglobin are examples.

porphyrinuria (por-fi-rin-ūr′-i-a): Excretion of porphyrins in the urine. Such pigments are produced as a result of an inborn error of metabolism. The urine becomes red or dark brown in color. See **porphyria**.

porrigo (po-rī′-go): Any disease condition of the scalp in which there is scaling or loss of hair.

porta: The depression (hilum) of an organ at which the vessels and nerves enter and, in some organs, excretory ducts leave.—portal, adj. P.HEPATIS, the transverse fissure through which the portal vein, hepatic artery and bile ducts pass on the under surface of the liver.

portacaval (por-ta-kā′-val): Pertaining to the portal vein and inferior vena cava. P. ANASTOMOSIS, a fistula made between the portal vein and the inferior vena cava with the object of reducing the pressure within the portal vein in cases of cirrhosis of the liver. P SHUNT, P. anastomosis.

portahepatitis (por-ta-hep-a-tī′-tis): Inflammation around the transverse fissure of the liver.

portal: 1. Pertaining to any porta or hilum, especially to the porta hepatis (*q.v.*). 2. The point of entrance of a pathogenic organism into the body. P.VEIN, that conveying blood into the liver; it is about 3 in. long and is formed by the union of the superior mesenteric and splenic veins.

portogram (por′-tō-gram): X-ray of portal vein after splenic puncture and injection of radiopaque liquid, or after injection of ra-

diopaque liquid into the portal vein at operation.

port-wine stain or mark: A purplish-red superficial hemangioma of the skin occurring as a birthmark; a nevus (*q.v.*).

position: Posture; attitude. An arrangement of the parts of the body considered desirable or necessary for some medical or surgical procedure or for an examination. In obstetrics, the situation of the fetus in the pelvis as determined by the relation of an arbitrary point (occiput, chin, sacrum) to the right or left side of the mother.

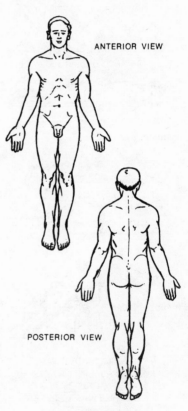

ANTERIOR VIEW

POSTERIOR VIEW

Anatomical position

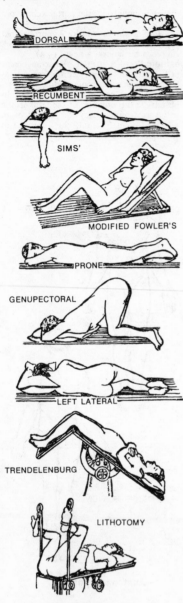

DORSAL

RECUMBENT

SIMS'

MODIFIED FOWLER'S

PRONE

GENUPECTORAL

LEFT LATERAL

TRENDELENBURG

LITHOTOMY

Positions

positive: Indicates that a substance or microorganism tested for is present in the material examined.

positive pressure breathing (PPB): Inflation of the lungs with air (or oxygen) under pressure to produce inspiration. Exhaled air, hand bellows or more sophisticated apparatus can be used. Elastic recoil of lungs produces expiration.

posology (pō-sol′-o-jē): That branch of materia medica that is concerned with dosage.

post-: Denotes: (1) behind, after, posterior; (2) subsequent to, later.

postanal (pōst-ān′-al): Behind the anus.

postanesthetic (pōst-an-es-thet′-ik): After anesthesia.

postcibal (pōst-sī′-bal): After a meal or after taking food. Abbreviated p.c.

postclimacteric (pōst-klī-mak′-ter-ik): Occurring after the menopause.

postconcussional syndrome (pōst-konkush′-on-al sin′-drōm): The association of headaches, giddiness and a feeling of faintness, which may persist for a considerable time after a head injury.

postdiphtheritic (pōst-dif-ther-it′-ik): Following an attack of diphtheria. Refers especially to paralysis of the limbs and palate.

postencephalitic (pōst-en-sef-al-it′-ik): Following encephalitis lethargica. The adjective is commonly used to describe the syndrome of parkinsonism, which so often results from an attack of this kind of encephalitis.

postepileptic (pōst-ep-i-lep′-tik): Following or occurring as a consequence of an epileptic seizure. P. AUTOMATISM, a fugue state, following a fit, when the patient may undertake a course of action, even involving violence, without having any memory of this.

posterior (pos-tē′-ri-or): Situated at the back.—posteriorly, adv. P. CHAMBER OF THE EYE, space between the anterior surface of lens and P. surface of iris. See **aqueous.**

postero-: Denotes posterior, behind, at the back part of.

posteroanterior (post-er-ō-an-tē′-ri-or): From back to front.

posterolateral (post-er-ō-lat′-er-al): Situated behind and to one side of the body, specifically the outer side.

posteromedian (post-er-ō-mēd′-i-an): Situated at the back and at or near the midline.

postganglionic (pōst-gang-gli-on′-ik): Situated distal to a collection of nerve cells (ganglion) as a P. nerve fiber.

posthepatic (pŏst-hep-at′-ik): Behind the liver.

postherpetic (pŏst-her-pet′-ik): Occurring after an attack of shingles or as a sequel.

posthetomy (pos-thet′-o-mi): Circumcision (*q. v.*).

posthitis (pos-thĭ′-tis): Inflammation of the prepuce.

posthumous (pos′-tū-mus): 1. After death. 2. Born after the father's death. 3. In obstetrics, born by cesarean section after the mother's death.

posthypnotic (pŏst-hip-not′-ik): After hypnotism. P. SUGGESTION, one made while the person is under hypnosis but carried out after he has returned to his normal state, usually without his awareness of the origin of the suggestion.

posthypophysis (pŏst-hī-pof′-i-sis): The posterior part of the pituitary body.

postictal (pŏst-ik′-tal): Following a sudden attack or seizure such as an epileptic seizure.

postmature (pŏst-ma-tūr′): 1. Overly developed. 2. Past the expected date of delivery. A baby is postmature when labor is delayed beyond 40 weeks.—postmaturity, n.

postmenopausal (pŏst-men-ō-pawz′-al): Occurring after the menopause has been established.

postmortal (pŏst-mor′-tal): Occurring after death.

post mortem: After death.

postmortem (pŏst-mor′-tem): 1. Related or pertaining to the period after death. 2. Pertaining to an examination of the body after death. P. EXAMINATION, an examination of the dead body to determine the cause of death or the pathological changes produced by the disease; autopsy.

post myocardial infarction syndrome: Pyrexia and chest pain associated with inflammation of the pleura, lung, or pericardium. Due to sensitivity to released products from dead muscle.

postnasal (pŏst-nā′-zal): Situated behind the nose and in the nasopharynx.—postnasally, adv. P. DRIP, the continual dripping of nasal mucus down the back of the throat instead of out of the nostrils; often more annoying than significant. Causes include allergies, low-grade infections, cold or foggy climate, polluted air, excessive smoking.

postnatal (pŏst-nā′-tal): Occurring after birth.

postocular (pŏst-ok′-ū-lar): Situated behind the eyeball.

postoperative (pŏst-op′-er-at-iv): After a surgical operation.—postoperatively, adv.

postoral (pŏst-or′-al): Situated behind or in the back part of the mouth.

postpartum (pŏst-par′-tum): Occurring after childbirth. P. HEMORRHAGE, H. that occurs soon after childbirth and is a result of it. P. PSYCHOSIS, a P. arising soon after childbirth; often schizophrenic in nature; cause may be organic or emotional.

postprandial (pŏst-pran′-di-al): Following a meal.

postsplenic (pŏst-splen′-ik): Behind the spleen.

postulate (pos′-tū-lat): A claim, demand, requirement, or basic principle. KOCH'S P'S., a list of four experimental conditions that an organism must meet before it can be declared to be the cause of a disease.

postural (pos′-tū-ral): Pertaining to or affected by posture. P. DRAINAGE, usually infers drainage from the respiratory tract, by elevation of the foot of the bed or using a special frame. P. HYPOTENSION, see **hypotension.**

posture (pos′-tùr): Active or passive arrangement of the whole body, or a part, in a definite manner.

postvaccinal (pŏst-vak′-sin-al): After vaccination.

postvagotomy diarrhea: Three types: 1. Transient D. shortly after operation, lasting from a few hours to a day or so. These episodes disappear in 3 to 6 months. 2. If they recur later than this and the attacks last longer, the term recurrent episodic diarrhea is used. 3. An increased daily bowel frequency—may be of disabling severity, but often acceptable in contrast to preoperative constipation. See **vagotomy.**

potable (pō′-ta-b'l): Drinkable; suitable for drinking.

potassemia (pot-a-sē′-mi-a): The presence of more than the normal amount of potassium in the blood.

potassium (pō-tas′-i-um): A soft, silverwhite metallic element occurring widely in nature but always in combination. Present in all animal cells and thought to be important for normal growth and muscle function. Because potassium is present in many foods the daily requirement is easily met. Its salts have long been used in medicine.

potassium deficiency: Disturbed electrolyte balance; can occur after excessive vomiting, and/or diarrhea; after prolonged use of diuretics, steroids, etc. Signs and symptoms variable, but nausea and muscle weakness often present. Heart failure can quickly supervene.

potbelly: A large, protruding belly; a fairly common condition in middle-aged males, due to a collection of fat in the omentum (*q.v.*). In children, often a symptom of a disease condition or the result of improper or inadequate diet.

potency (pō′-ten-si): Strength, force, power.

potent (pō′-tent): 1. Possessing strength, force. 2. Describing a medicinal preparation that is highly effective. 3. The ability of a male to engage in sexual intercourse.

potential (pō-ten′-shal): Latent; existing in possibility and having the power to eventually become an actuality. P. ENERGY, energy that is stored in the body but not in actual use.

potion (pō′-shun): A large draught of liquid medicine or other liquid mixture.

potomania (pō-tō-mā′-ni-a): 1. An abnormal desire to drink, said especially of alcoholics. 2. Delirium tremens.

Pott's disease: Spondylitis; spinal caries; tuberculosis of one or more of the vertebrae causing necrosis of the bone and resulting in kyphosis (*q.v.*). [Percival Pott, English surgeon. 1714-1788.]

Pott's fracture: A fracture at the lower end of the fibula and of the medial malleolus of the tibia with an outward displacement of the foot.

Potts' operation: A direct side-to-side anastomosis between the aorta and the pulmonary artery; used in cases of tetralogy of Fallot. [Willis J. Potts, American surgeon. 1895- .]

Potts-Smith-Gibson operation: Potts' operation (*q.v.*).

pouch: A pocket, recess, or cul-de-sac. P. OF DOUGLAS, see **Douglas' pouch.**

poultice (pōl′-tis): A soft, moist, pulpy mass spread between two layers of material and applied, usually hot, to an external surface to relieve pain and congestion and improve circulation in the area, or to hasten suppuration. Materials used include bread, mustard, flaxseed, linseed.

pound: A unit of weight; in the avoirdupois system the pound contains 16 ounces; in the apothecaries' system it contains 12 ounces.

Poupart's ligament (poo′-pars): The inguinal ligament; between the anterior superior iliac and the pubic spines. [Francois Poupart, surgeon of Paris. 1616-1708.]

powder: 1. A mass of dry substance separated into minute particles. 2. A single dose of a drug in powdered form. 3. To reduce a solid mass of a substance to fine particles.

pox: 1. Any disease characterized by an eruption, especially a pustular eruption. 2. An eruption. 3. Colloquial term for syphilis. See **smallpox, chickenpox.**

PPD: Purified Protein Derivative (*q.v.*).

PPLO: Abbreviation for pleuropneumonia-like organisms, including Eaton agent (*q.v.*).

practical nurse: See **nurse.**

practitioner (prak-tish′-on-er): 1. A person who practices medicine. 2. A person engaged in practice in any profession.

prae-: See **pre-.**

pragmatic (prag-mat′-ik): Practical; matter-of-fact; concerned with the practical aspects.

pre-: Denotes: (1) anterior, before, in front of; (2) preparatory, beforehand.

preanesthesia (prē-an-es-thē′-zi-a): Preliminary or light anesthesia; usually produced by medication and induced prior to general anesthesia.

preanesthetic (prē-an-es-thet′-ik): Pertaining to preanesthesia or to the period preceding anesthesia.

preauricular (prē-aw-rik′-ū-lar): Situated in front of the auricle of the ear; used especially with reference to the lymphatic nodes in this area.

precancer (prē′-kan-ser): A condition that is expected to eventually become malignant.

precancerous (prē-kan′-ser-us): 1. Occurring before cancer with special reference to nonmalignant pathological changes which are believed to lead on to, or to be followed by, cancer. 2. Tending to become malignant.

precipitate (pre-sip′-i-tāt): 1. To separate out or cause a substance in a solution or suspension to separate out. 2. A solid that is separated out from a solution or suspension. 3. Hasty or unduly rapid, as labor.— precipitation, n.

precipitin (prē-sip′-i-tin): An antibody which forms a specific complex with precipitinogen (antigen), and under certain physiochemical conditions this results in the formation of a precipitate. This reaction forms the basis of many delicate diagnostic serological tests for the identification of minute traces of material and bacteria. See **antibodies.**

preclinical (prē-klin′-i-kal): 1. Referring to the period before symptoms of a disease are recognizable. 2 The period in the education of a physician or nurse before there is contact with patients.

precocious (prē-kō′-shus): Unusually early development.

preconscious (prē-kon′-shus): In psycho-analysis, thoughts that are not present in the consciousness but which one can recall easily when one wishes to do so.

precordialgia (prē-kōr-di-al′-ji-a): Pain in the precordium (*q.v.*).

precordium (prē-kōr′-di-um): The area on the ventral surface of the body that lies immediately over the heart and stomach; comprises the epigastrium and lower, middle part of the thorax.—precordial, adj.

precursor (prē-kurs′-or): Forerunner.

prediabetes (prē-dī-a-bē′-tēz): Potential predisposition to diabetes mellitus. Urine testing can detect the condition and it can sometimes be controlled by diet alone.—prediabetic, adj.; n.

predigestion (prē-di-jest′-chun): Partial artificial digestion of foods before they are ingested.

predisposing (prē-dis-pōz′-ing): Rendering one more vulnerable or susceptible to a disease condition.

predisposition (prē-dis-pō-zi′-shun): A latent or increased susceptibility to develop or contract certain diseases.

preeclampsia (prē-ē-klamp′-si-a): A condition characterized by albuminuria, edema, hypertension, headache, and visual disturbances; arising usually in latter part of pregnancy.—preeclamptic, adj.

prefrontal (prē-front′-al): Situated in the anterior portion of the frontal lobe of the cerebrum. See **leukotomy.**

preganglionic (prē-gang-gli-on′-ik): Preceding or in front of a collection of nerve cells (ganglion) as a P. nerve fiber.

pregnancy (preg′-nan-si): Being with child, *i.e.*, from conception to parturition, normally 40 weeks or 280 days. ABDOMINAL P., development of the ovum in the peritoneal cavity; usually follows rupture of tubal P., primary abdominal implantation seldom occurs. EXTRAUTERINE P., see **ectopic p.** MULTIPLE P., more than one fetus in the uterus. PHANTOM P., see **pseudocyesis.**

pregnant: Gravid; being with child; containing unborn young within the body.

prehensile (prē-hen′-sil): Equipped or adapted for grasping or seizing.

prehension (prē-hen′-shun): The act of grasping or taking hold of.

prehypophysis (prē-hī-pof′-i-sis): The anterior lobe of the pituitary body.

preictal (prē-ik′-tal): Occurring before a stroke or a seizure, such as an epileptic seizure.

premature (prē-ma-tūr′): Occurring before the usual or proper time. P. BABY, one whose weight at birth is less than 5.5 pounds (2.5 kg) and therefore special treatment is needed. Current synonyms are low-weight or dysmature baby. Not all low birth weight babies are premature, but are included in a new category 'small for dates.' See **placental insufficiency.** P. BEAT, extrasystole (*q.v.*). P. LABOR, expulsion of the fetus before the 280th day of pregnancy.

premedication (prē-med-i-kā′-shun): Drugs given before the administration of another drug, *e.g.*, those given before an anesthetic for the purposes of allaying apprehension, producing sedation, inhibiting secretion of saliva and mucus from the upper respiratory tract, or to facilitate the administration of the anesthetic.

premenstrual (prē-men′-stroo-al): Preceding menstruation. The term cyclical syndrome (*q.v.*) now preferred for P. syndrome-complex. P. TENSION, the nervousness, irritation, and physical discomfort experienced by some women during the days immediately preceding appearance of the menses.

premolar (prē-mōl′-ar): One of 8 bicuspid teeth. There are two on each side of each jaw, between the canine and first molar.

premonitory (prē-mon′-i-tō-ri): Giving advance warning or notice, *e.g.*, P. SYMPTOMS may warn of a disease condition before it is fully developed.

prenaris (prē-nar′-is): One of the anterior nares; nostril.—prenares, pl.

prenatal (prē-nā′-tal): Occurring or existing before birth. Antenatal.—prenatally, adv.

preoperative (prē-op′-er-at-iv): Before operation.—preoperatively, adv.

prep: Colloquial term meaning the preparation of an area (cleansing, shaving, etc.) for surgery, delivery, or other procedure.

preparalytic (prē-par-a-lit′-ik): Before the onset of paralysis, often referring to the early stage of poliomyelitis.

prepartal (prē-par′-tal): Before labor.

prepatellar (prē-pa-tel′-ar): In front of the kneecap. P. BURSITIS, inflammation of the large bursa in front of the patella; housemaid's knee.

prepuce (prē′-pūs): The foreskin; the free fold of skin that covers most of the glans penis.

preputium (prē-pū′-shi-um): The prepuce (*q.v.*).—preputial, adj.

prerectal (prē-rek′-tal): In front of the rectum.

presacral air insufflation: Injection of air into retroperitoneal interstitial tissues, mainly used to demonstrate renal and adrenal outlines.

presby-, presbyo-: Denotes: (1) old; (2) old age.

presbycusis (pres-bi-kū′-sis): Loss of ability of older people to perceive or discriminate sounds; usually progressive and bilateral. Also presbyacusia, presbyacousia, presbycusia.

presbyope (pres′-bi-ōp): A farsighted person.

presbyophrenia (pres-bi-ō-frē′-ni-a): A mental disorder most often seen in the elderly; characterized by memory loss; disorientation, and confabulation. Often judgment remains relatively unimpaired. Wernicke's syndrome.

presbyopia (pres-bi-ōp′-i-a): Farsightedness due to loss of elasticity of the crystalline lens of the eye with consequent failure of accommodation; seen mostly in persons 45 and more years of age.—presbyopic, adj.; presbyope, n.

prescribe (prē-skrīb′): To give directions orally or in writing for the administration of a remedy in the treatment of any disease condition.

prescription (prē-skrip′-shun): A written formula, signed by a physician, directing the preparation and administration of a remedy. Also refers to instructions for grinding corrective lenses for eyeglasses.

presenility (prē-sē-nil′-i-ti): 1. Before senility is established. 2. Premature old age.—presenile, adj.

present (prē-sent′): 1. To precede or appear first, as the part of the fetus that appears first at the os uteri. 2. To come forward as a patient.

presentation: The part of the fetus which first enters the pelvic brim and will be felt by the examining finger through the cervix in labor. May be vertex, face, brow, shoulder or breech.

pressor (pres′-or): 1. A substance that tends to raise blood pressure. 2. Involving or stimulating the vasomotor center in the brain.

pressure: 1. A force or compression exerted against an area of the body. 2. The sensation of touch aroused by compression against the skin. BLOOD P., see **blood**. DIASTOLIC P., arterial blood pressure during the period of dilatation of the chambers of the heart. INTRACRANIAL P., the pressure of the cerebrospinal fluid in the space between the brain and the skull. INTRAOCULAR P., see **intraocular**. NEGATIVE P., pressure that is less than

that of the atmosphere. OSMOTIC P., the pressure with which a fluid passes through a semipermeable membrane. PULSE P., the difference between the systolic and diastolic blood pressures. SYSTOLIC P., arterial pressure during the period of contraction of the ventricles. P. AREAS, bony prominences of the body, over which the flesh of bedridden patients is denuded of its blood supply as it is compressed between the bone and an external source of pressure; the latter is usually the bed, but may be a splint, plaster, upper bedclothes, etc. P. BANDAGE, see **compression bandage**. P. DRESSING, one applied firmly enough over a wound to exert compression. P. POINT, a place at which an artery passes over a bone, against which it can be compressed, to stop bleeding. Term also used synonymously with pressure area. P. SORE, decubitus ulcer (*q.v.*).

presystole (prē-sis′-to-li): The interval just preceding the systole or contraction of the heart muscle.—presystolic, adj.

preventive (prē-ven′-tiv): Acting to prevent the occurrence of. P. MEDICINE, that branch of medicine that deals with preventing the occurrence of disease in individuals or in the community at large.

preventorium (prē-ven-tō′-ri-um): An institution for the care of persons (usually children) who are believed to be in danger of contracting some disease (usually tuberculosis), either because they have been exposed to it or are in poor physical condition.

prevesical (prē-ves′-ik-al): Anterior to a bladder, especially the urinary bladder.

priapism (prī′-a-pizm): [*Priapus*, the god of procreation.] Prolonged penile erection in the absence of sexual stimulation.

prickly heat: A noncontagious eruption that often occurs in hot humid weather; consists of small red pimples that itch, burn and tingle. See **miliaria**.

primary (prī′-ma-ri): 1. First or most important in order of time or development. 2. First in rank or importance. P. COMPLEX or GHON'S FOCUS, the initial tuberculous infection in a person, usually in the lung, and manifest as a small focus of infection in the lung tissue and enlarged, caseous, hilar glands. It usually heals spontaneously. [Anton Ghon, Austrian pathologist. 1866-1936.]

primigravida (prim-i-grav′-i-da): A woman who is pregnant for the first time.—primigravidae, pl.

primipara (prī-mip′-a-ra): A woman who

287 prognosis

is giving birth to her first child.—primiparous, adj.

primordial (prī-mor′-di-al): Primitive, original; applied to the ovarian follicles present at birth.

principle (prin′-si-p'l): In pharmacology, the constituent of a drug or compound that is chiefly responsible for its action.

privates: The external organs of generation.

p.r.n.: Abbreviation for *pro re nata*, meaning whenever necessary.

pro-: Denotes: (1) earlier than, prior to, before; (2) anterior to, located in front of; (3) projecting.

proband (prō′-band): Propositus (*q.v.*).

probe (prōb): 1. A slender, somewhat flexible rod-like metal instrument with a blunt tip, used typically for exploring body cavities or wounds. 2. To use a probe for exploration purposes.

procedure (prō-sē′-dūr): A series of orderly steps followed in carrying out a treatment or operation.

procephalic (prō-se-fal′-ik): Related to or situated on or near the anterior part of the head.

process (pros′-es): 1. A projection or outgrowth from the mass of an organism or part, especially from a bone. 2. A method, system, or mode of action utilized in doing something.

procidentia (prō-si-den′-shi-a): Complete prolapse of an organ or part, especially the uterus so that it lies within the vaginal sac but outside the contour of the body.

procreate (prō′-krē-āt): To beget; produce offspring. Term applied usually to the male parent.

proct-, procti-, procto-: Denotes anus or rectum, or both.

proctalgia (prok-tal′-ji-a): The presence of pain in the rectal region.

proctatresia (prok-ta-trē′-zi-a): Imperforation of the anus.

proctectomy (prok-tek′-to-mi): Surgical removal of the rectum, usually because of the presence of a malignancy.

proctitis (prok-tī′-tis): Inflammation of the mucous membrane of the rectum.

proctocele (prok′-tō-sēl): Rectocele (*q.v.*).

proctoclysis (prok-tok′-li-sis): The slow continuous injection of large quantities of fluid into the rectum. Murphy drip (*q.v.*).

proctocolectomy (prok-tō-kol-ek′-to-mi): Surgical excision of the rectum and colon.

proctocolitis (prok-tō-kō-lī′-tis): Inflammation of the rectum and colon; usually a type of ulcerative colitis.

proctology (prok-tol′-o-ji): That branch of medicine that deals with the study of the anus, rectum, and sigmoid and the treatment of their diseases.

proctoperineoplasty (prok-tō-per-i-nē′-ō-plas-ti): An operation for repair of the anus and perineum. Also proctoperineorrhaphy.

proctopexy (prok′-to-pek-si): Operation for fixation of the rectum to some other part.

proctoplasty (prok′-to-plast-ti): Plastic surgery of the anus and rectum.

proctoptosis (prok-top-tō′-sis): Prolapse of the anus and rectum.

proctorrhagia (prok-to-rā′-ji-a): Bleeding from the anus.

proctorrhea (prok-to-rē′-a): Discharge of mucus from the rectum.

proctoscope (prok′-tō-skōp): An instrument for dilating and visually examining the rectum. See **endoscope.**—proctoscopic, adj.; proctoscopy, n.

proctosigmoidectomy (prok-tō-sig-moid-ek′-to-mi): Surgical removal of the sigmoid colon and the rectum.

proctosigmoiditis (prok-tō-sig-moid-ī′-tis): Inflammation of the rectum and sigmoid colon.

proctosigmoidoscopy (prok-tō-sig-moi-dos′-kop-i): Direct inspection of the rectum and the sigmoid colon with a sigmoidoscope.

proctostasis (prok-tos′-ta-sis): Constipation with retention of feces in the colon due to the inability of the rectum to respond to the stimulus for defecation.

proctostenosis (prok-tō-ste-nō′-sis): Narrowing or stricture of the rectum or anus.

prodromal (prō-drō′-mal): Preceding, as the transitory rash before the true rash of an infectious disease.

prodrome (prō′-drōm): An early or premonitory symptom or sign of disease.—prodromata, pl.; prodromal, adj.

proenzyme (prō-en′-zīm): A precursor of an enzyme which requires some change to render it active, *e.g.*, pepsinogen. Zymogen.

progestational (prō-jes-tā′-shun-al): 1. Before pregnancy; favoring pregnancy. 2. Term applied to the phase of the menstrual cycle that immediately precedes menstruation.—progestation, n.

progesterone (prō-jes′-ter-ōn): A hormone produced by the corpus luteum; plays an important part in regulation of the menstrual cycle and in pregnancy.

proglottis (prō-glot′-is): Sexually mature segment of tapeworm.—proglottides, pl.

prognathic (prog-nā′-thik): Having projecting jaws.

prognosis (prog-nō′-sis): A forecast of the

probable course, duration, and termination of a disease.—prognostic, adj.

programmed instruction: Medium for self-instruction that is individualized so that the student can progress at his own speed by a technique that enables him to pace himself. The unit of instruction is an individual frame in which a question is asked, a response is requested, and knowledge of the correct response is available through feedback. May be presented on paper or by a teaching machine, film, recording or flip chart. Sometimes used in teaching certain subjects in nursing school curriculums.

progressive patient care: A system of caring for patients whereby the facilities are adapted to the needs of various types of patients. Acutely ill patients are cared for in an intensive care unit; those who are moderately ill are cared for in an intermediate care unit; those who need very little assistance with their physical care but who must remain in the hospital, are cared for in a self-care unit. The objective is to allow patients to live as nearly normal lives as possible and to make the best use of the available nursing staff.

projectile vomiting: Sudden vomiting, usually without preceding nausea, so forcibly that the vomitus is projected for some distance.

projection (pro-jek'-shun): A prominence or extending process of a bone. In psychology, a mental mechanism occurring in normal people unconsciously, and in an exaggerated form in mental illnesses, especially paranoia, whereby the person fails to recognize certain motives and feelings in himself but attributes them to others.

prolactin (prō-lak'-tin): A hormone produced in the hypophysis cerebri; stimulates the production of milk.

prolapse (prō-laps'): Descent; downward displacement of an organ or body structure from its usual position. P. OF THE CORD, premature expulsion of the cord during labor. P. OF THE IRIS, part of the iris bulges forward through a corneal wound. P. OF THE RECTUM, the lower part of the intestinal tract extends downward in varying degrees, sometimes protruding through the external anal sphincter. P. OF THE UTERUS, the uterus descends into the vagina and may be visible at the vaginal orifice. See **procidentia.** P. OF AN INTERVERTEBRAL DISK (PID), nucleus pulposis; see **nucleus.**

proliferate (prō-lif'-er-āt): Increase by cell division.—proliferation, n.; proliferative, adj.

prolific (prō-lif'-ik): Fruitful, multiplying abundantly.

promontory (prom'-on-to-ri): A projection; a prominent part.

pronate (prō'-nāt): To turn the ventral surface downward, e.g., to lie on the face; to turn the palm of the hand downward.—pronation, n. Opp., supinate.

pronator (prō-nā'-tor): That which pronates, usually applied to a muscle. Opp., supinator.

prone (prōn): Lying with the face downward. Opp., supine.

prophylaxis (prō-fi-lak'-sis): Prevention.—prophylactic, adj.; prophylactically, adv.

propositus (prō-poz'-i-tus): In studies in human genetics, the person whose particular mental or physical characteristics served as a stimulus for the study. Also called proband.

proprietary (prō-prī'-e-ta-ri): Refers to any medicine that is protected from competition by secrecy as to its composition or manufacture, or by trademark, copyright, or patent.

proprioceptor (prō-pri-ō-sep'-tor): One of the sensory nerve terminals of the afferent nerves in the deeper structures of the body, e.g., muscles, tendons, joints. They are responsible for the sensation of the position of the body and its parts and of changes in position.

proptosis (prop-tō'-sis): Forward protrusion of any organ, especially of the eyeball. OCULAR P., exophthalmos (q.v.).

pro re nata: Whenever necessary; as the occasion arises. Sometimes used in prescription writing to indicate that the medicine is to be given according to the patient's need for it. Abbreviated p.r.n.

prosop-, prosopo-: Denotes: (1) the face; (2) a person.

prosopoplegia (prōs-ō-pō-plē'-ji-a): Facial paralysis.

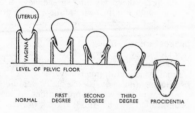

Degrees of prolapse of uterus

UTERUS

VAGINA

LEVEL OF PELVIC FLOOR

NORMAL FIRST DEGREE SECOND DEGREE THIRD DEGREE PROCIDENTIA

prostate (pros'-tāt): A small conical gland at the base of the male bladder and surrounding the first part of the urethra. It secretes a milky fluid that is discharged into the urethra and mixes with the semen at the time of emission.

prostatectomy (pros-ta-tek'-to-mi): Surgical removal of part or all of the prostate gland.

prostaticovesical (pros-tat-i-kō-ves'-i-kal): Pertaining to both the prostate gland and the bladder.

prostatitis (pros-ta-tī'-tis): Inflammation of the prostate gland.

prostatocystitis (pros-ta-tō-sis-tī'-tis): Inflammation of the prostatic urethra and the male urinary bladder.

prostatomegaly (pros-ta-tō-meg'-a-li): Enlargement or hypertrophy of the prostate gland.

prostatorrhea (pros-ta-tō-rē'-a): A thin catarrhal discharge from the prostate gland; often occurs in prostatitis.

prosthesis (pros-thē'-sis): An artificial substitute for a missing part, *e.g.*, eye, tooth, limb, breast.—prostheses, pl.; prosthetic, adj.

prosthetics (pros-thet'-iks): The art and science of making and adjusting artificial parts of the body (prostheses).

prosthetist (pros'-the-tist): One skilled in making and adjusting prostheses.

prosthokeratoplasty (pros-thō-ker'-a-tō-plas-ti): Keratoplasty (*q.v.*) in which the corneal implant is of some material other than human or animal tissue.

prostration (pros-trā'-shun): Complete exhaustion; extreme loss of strength. NERVOUS P., neurasthenia (*q.v.*). See **heat exhaustion.**

prot-, proto-: Denotes: (1) first in time, formation, rank, status, or importance; (2) giving rise to.

protanopia (prō-ta-nō'-pi-a): Red-green color blindness.

protease (prō'-tē-ās): Any protein-splitting enzyme. GASTRIC P., pepsin.

protein (pro'-tē-in): A highly complex, nitrogenous compound, found in all animal and vegetable tissues. Proteins are built up of amino acids and are essential for growth and repair of body. Those from animal sources are of high biological value since they contain the essential amino acids. Those from vegetable sources do not contain all, but some of the essential amino acids. P. are hydrolyzed in the body to produce amino acids which are then used to build up new body proteins.

proteinemia (prō-tē-in-ē'-mi-a): More than the normal amount of protein in the blood.

protein-bound iodine: Iodine combined with protein as part of the thyroid hormone. It is low in thyroid deficiency.

proteinuria (prō-tē-in-ūr'-i-a): Protein in the urine. Syn., albuminuria.

proteolysis (prō-tē-ol'-i-sis): The breaking down of proteins into simpler substances. —proteolytic, adj.

proteose (prō'-tē-ōs): The first cleavage product in the breakdown of proteins, intermediate between protein and peptone.

Proteus (prō'-tē-us): A genus of gram-negative, flagellated, motile, rod-shaped microorganisms; found in damp surroundings, fecal and other putrefying material. May be pathogenic, especially in wound or urinary tract infections as a secondary invader.

prothrombin (prō-throm'-bin): A factor in the plasma of the blood; a precursor of thrombin. It is synthesized in the liver when the supply of vitamin K is adequate. In the presence of thromboplastin and calcium it is converted into thrombin. P. TIME is a measure of its production and concentration in the blood; it is increased in certain hemorrhagic conditions.

prothymia (prō-thīm'-i-a): Mental alertness.

proton (prō'-ton): One of the basic parts of the nucleus of the atom, around which the electrons revolve; it carries a positive charge.

protopathic (prō-tō-path'-ik): Primary; primitive. P. SENSIBILITY, term applied to peripheral sensory fibers that are of low sensibility for degree and location of the sensations of pain and heat. Opp. to epicritic (*q.v.*).

protoplasm (prō'-tō-plazm): The complex chemical compound constituting the main part of the tissue cells; it may be clear or granulated.—protoplasmic, adj.

protopsis (prō-top'-sis): Protrusion of the eyeball; exophthalmos.

protosyphilis (prō-tō-sif'-i-lis): Primary syphilis.

prototype (prō'-tō-tīp): 1. The primitive or original member of a class or species on which subsequent members are modeled. 2. An individual or quality that exemplifies the standard for members of a particular class or species.

protozoa (prō-tō-zō'-a): The smallest type of animal life; single-celled organisms, capable of asexual reproduction. Diseases produced by them include malaria, amebic dysentery, leishmaniasis.—protozoon, sing.; protozoal, adj. See **ameba.**

protozoology (prō-tō-zō-ol′-o-ji): The science that treats of protozoa.

protuberance (prō-tū′-ber-ans): A projecting part, outgrowth, swelling, knob.

proud flesh: Excessive growth of granulation tissue in a wound or ulcer with little tendency toward scar formation.

provitamin (prō-vī′-ta-min): A principle in certain foods which the body is able to convert into a vitamin, *e.g.*, carotene is converted into vitamin A.

proximal (prok′-si-mal): Nearest the head or source. In anatomy, the part of an extremity, nerve, vessel, etc. that is nearest the trunk or point of origin of the part.—proximally, adv.

prurigo (proo-rī′-gō): A chronic skin disease marked by formation of papules that itch intensely, occurring most frequently in children. P. ESTIVALE, hydroa aestivale (*q.v.*). P. FEROX, a severe form. P. MITIS, a mild form. P. NODULARIS, a rare disease of the adult female in which intensely pruritic pea-sized nodules occur on the arms and legs.

pruritus (proo-rī′-tus): Itching. May be caused by drugs, bites, or disease, including allergy. P. ani and P. vulvae are considered to be psychosomatic conditions (neurodermatitis) except in the few cases where a local cause can be found, *e.g.*, worm infestation, vaginitis. Generalized P. may be a symptom of systemic disease as in diabetes, icterus, Hodgkin's disease, carcinoma, etc. It may be psychogenic, *e.g.*, widow's itch which occurs shortly after bereavement.—pruritic, adj.

prussic acid (prus′-ik as′-id): A 4 percent solution of hydrogen cyanide; hydrocyanic acid. Both the solution and its vapor are poisonous, with death occurring very rapidly from respiratory paralysis.

psellism (sel′-izm): Stammering; stuttering; mispronunciation or substitution of letter sounds.

pseud-, pseudo-: Denotes: (1) false, counterfeit, feigned, fake, or illusory; (2) a deceptive resemblance; (3) abnormal, aberrant.

pseudacousis (sū-da-koo′-sis): A defect in hearing in which sounds are heard as altered in pitch or quality.

pseudaphia (sū-daf′-i-a): A defect in the perception of touch.

pseudarthrosis (sū-dar-thrō′-sis): A false joint, *e.g.*, due to ununited fracture; also congenital. Occurs primarily in the long bones. Also pseudoarthrosis.

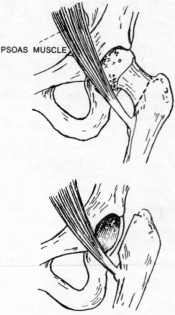

PSOAS MUSCLE

Pseudarthrosis of hip

pseudoangina (sū-dō-an-jī′-na): False angina. Sometimes referred to as 'left mammary pain,' it occurs in anxious individuals. Usually there is no cardiac disease present. May be part of effort syndrome (*q.v.*).

pseudoblepsis (sū-dō-blep′-sis): A condition in which a person sees objects as different from what they really are.

pseudocide (sū′-dō-sīd): Consciously acting to harm oneself in such a way as to attract attention or gain sympathy without intending to take one's life.

pseudocoxalgia (sū-dō-kok·sal′-ji-a): See **Perthes' disease.**

pseudocrisis (sū-dō-krī′-sis): A rapid reduction of body temperature resembling a crisis, followed by further fever.

pseudocroup (sū-dō-kroop′): Laryngismus stridulus (*q.v.*).

pseudocyesis (sū-dō-sī-ē′-sis): The existence of the signs and symptoms of pregnancy in a woman who believes that she is pregnant, when, in fact, this is not so.

pseudodementia (sū-dō-dē-men′-shi-a): Extreme apathy and indifference to environment and general behavior simulating dementia but without impairment of the mental faculties.

pseudogeusia (sū-dō-gū′-si-a): A sensation of taste arising without any external stimulus to produce it.

pseudohemophilia (sū-dō-hē-mō-fil′-i-a): A non-hereditary disease of both men and women in which the clotting time is normal but the bleeding time is prolonged. False hemophilia.

pseudohermaphrodite (sū-dō-her-maf′-rō-dīt): A person in whom the gonads of one sex are present, whilst the external genitalia resemble those of both sexes.

pseudohypertrophic muscular dystrophy: A type of muscular dystrophy, occurring most often in young boys; probably hereditary. Marked by hypertrophy of the muscles, especially those of the calf and shoulder, difficulty in walking, and later dystrophy of the muscles.

pseudologia fantastica (sū-dō-lō′-ji-a fantas′-ti-ka): A constitutional tendency to tell, and defend, fantastic lies plausibly, found in some hysterics.

pseudomembrane (sū-dō-mem′-brān): A false membrane such as that which forms on the mucous membrane of the throat in diphtheria.

pseudomnesia (sū-dom-nē′-zi-a): False memory. Memory of events that have never occurred.

Pseudomonas (sū-dō-mōn′-as): A bacterial genus. Gram-negative motile rods, found commonly in water, soil and decomposing vegetable matter. Some are pathogenic to plants and animals and occasionally to man, *e.g.*, *P. pyocyanea (Bacillus pyocyaneus)*, found commonly in intestinal dejecta, sinuses and suppurating wounds; a secondary invader in some urinary tract infections and wound infections; produces a blue or blue-green pigment which colors the exudate or pus.

pseudonystagmus (sū-dō-nis-tag′-mus): Rhythmic jerking movements of the eyeball occurring as a symptom in various diseases of the central nervous system.

pseudoparalysis (sū-dō-pa-ral′-i-sis): See **pseudoplegia**.

pseudo-parkinsonism (sū-dō-park′-in-sonizm): Signs and symptoms of paralysis agitans (*q.v.*) when they are not postencaphilitic.

pseudoplegia (sū-dō-plē′-ji-a): Paralysis mimicking that of organic nervous disorder but usually hysterical in origin.

pseudopodia (sū-dō-pō′-di-a): False legs. The temporary projection of protoplasmic processes of an ameba or of ameboid cells (leukocytes) for the purposes of locomotion or for the ingestion of food or other particles.—pseudopodium, sing.

pseudopolyposis (sū-dō-pol-i-pō′-sis): Widely scattered polypi, usually result of previous inflammation—sometimes ulcerative colitis.

pseudopsia (sū-dop′-si-a): False vision; visual hallucinations. See **pseudoblepsia**.

pseudosmia (sū-doz′-mi-a): The subjective sensation of smelling something that is not present.

psilosis (sī-lō′-sis): 1. Sprue (*q.v.*). 2. Falling of the hair.

psittacosis (sit-a-kō′-sis): Virus disease of parrots, pigeons and budgerigars which is occasionally responsible for a form of pneumonia in man.

psoas (sō′-as): One of two muscles of the loins.

psoriasis (so-rī′-a-sis): A chronic skin condition characterized by bright red, slightly elevated, round or oval areas that are covered with dry adherent scales that leave bleeding points when removed; when scales are scraped they produce a shiny, silver sheen that is diagnostic. Non-infectious; cause unknown. May occur on any part of the body but characteristic sites are extensor surfaces, especially over the knees and elbows.—psoriatic, adj.

PSP: Abbreviation, used in laboratory reports, for phenolsulfonphthalein (tests).

psych-, psycho-: Denotes: (1) the mind, mental processes; (2) spirit, soul.

psychalgia (sī-kal′-ji-a): Mental pain or distress; sometimes caused by mental effort; seen especially in states of melancholia.

psychanopsia (sī-kan-op′-si-a): Psychic blindness.

psychasthenia (sī-kas-thē′-ni-a): A form of psychoneurosis marked by mental fatigue, unreasonable fears, obsessions and compulsion, feelings of inadequacy, lack of self-control, a sensation of unreality of self and surroundings, preoccupation with minor details to the extent that nothing worthwhile is accomplished.

psyche (sī′-ke): The mind. The intellect, including both conscious and unconscious mental processes.

psychedelic (sī-ke-del′-ik): 1. Mind-manifesting or mind-expanding. 2. Pertaining to drugs that have the immediate action of producing highly creative and imaginative thought patterns, enlarging the vision, and producing freedom from anxiety, *e.g.,* peyote, LSD-25. Also psychodelic.

psychiatrist (sī-kī′-a-trist): One who specializes in psychiatry (*q. v.*).

psychiatry (sī-kī′-at-ri): That branch of medical science that is devoted to the origin, diagnosis, and treatment of mental, emotional or behavioral disorders; by extension includes problems of personal adjustment and such special fields as mental retardation.—psychiatric, adj.

psychic (sī′-kik): 1. Pertaining to the psyche; of the mind; mental. 2. A person who is thought to have unusual sensitivity to non-physical forces; a spiritualistic medium. P. ENERGIZER, popular term for a drug that elevates or stimulates the mood of a depressed person.

psychoanalysis (sī-kō-a-nal′-i-sis): A specialized branch of psychiatry founded by Freud. Briefly, the method is to recall and analyze a person's past emotional experiences and dreams with the purpose of understanding the origin of the patient's symptoms and furnishing hints as to the kind of psychotherapy that may eventually alleviate the symptoms.—psychoanalytic, adj.

psychoanalyst (sī-kō-an′-al-ist): One who specializes in psychoanalysis (*q. v.*).

psychobiology (sī-kō-bī-ol′-o-ji): The branch of biology that deals with the interactions of the mind and the body in relation to the development and functioning of the personality.

psychochemotherapy (sī-kō-kĕm-ō-ther′-a-pi): The use of drugs to improve or cure pathological changes in the emotional state.—psychochemotherapeutic, adj.; psychochemotherapeutically, adv.

psychodrama (sī-kō-dra′-ma): A method of psychotherapy whereby patients act out their personal problems by taking roles in spontaneous dramatic performances.

psychodynamics (sī-kō-dī-nam′-iks): The science of the mental processes, especially of the causative factors in mental activity.

psychogenesis (sī-kō-jen′-e-sis): The development of mental and emotional traits.

psychogenic (sī-kō-jen′-ik): Arising from or originating in the psyche or mind as opposed to having a physical basis. P. SYMPTOM, a neurotic symptom.

psychogeriatrics (sī-kō-jer-i-at′-riks): Psychology applied to geriatrics.

psychokinesia (sī-kō-kī-nē′-zi-a): Impulsive behavior; a burst of violent behavior, often maniacal, resulting from lack of inhibition.

psychokinesis (sī-kō-ki-nē′-sis): The production or alteration of movement by the direct influence of the mind without any somatic influence.

psychologist (sī-kol′-o-jist): One who specializes in the study of the mind, especially as it affects behavior.

psychology (sī-kol′-o-ji): The science that deals with the emotions, mental processes, and behavior of an organism in its environment. Medically, the study of human behavior.—psychologic, adj.; psychologically, adv.

psychometric (sī-kō-met′-rik): Related to or being a measurement of the duration and force of mental processes.

psychometry (sī-kom′-e-tri): 1. The science of measuring the duration and force of mental processes. 2. The measurement of mental potential, ability, and functioning by means of psychometric tests (sometimes called intelligence tests); *e.g.,* the Binet-Simon test.

psychomotor (sī-kō-mō′-ter): Pertaining to the motor effect of psychic or cerebral activity. P. EPILEPSY, recurrent, periodic disturbances of behavior in which the person carries out certain repetitive movements semiautomatically. P. RETARDATION, general retardation in both physical and emotional development.

psychoneurosis (sī-kō-nū-rō′-sis): A functional disorder of the mind, usually mild in character, based on psychogenic factors. Neurosis.—psychoneurotic, adj.

psychopath (sī′-kō-path): An eccentric, unstable or mentally ill person with a poorly balanced personality that leads to egocentric, impulsive, immoral, or antisocial behavior. See **personality.**—psychopathic, adj.

psychopathology (sī-kō-path-ol′-o-ji): The study of pathology of the mind, personality or social adjustment.—psychopathological, adj.; psychopathologically, adv.

psychopathy (sī-kop′-a-thi): Any disease of the mind.—psychopathic, adj.

psychopharmacology (sī-kō-far-ma-kol′-o-ji): The study of the action of drugs on the affective or emotional state, or the use of such drugs.

psychophysics (sī-kō-fiz′-iks): A branch of experimental psychology dealing with the study of stimuli and sensations.—psychophysical, adj.

psychoprophylactic (sī-kō-prō-fi-lak′-tik): That which aims at preventing mental disease.

psychosexual (sī-kō-seks′-ū-al): Pertaining to the emotional factors of sex. P. DEVELOPMENT, that which takes place in the libido from infancy to adulthood; influences a person's basic personality; includes phases described as oral, anal, phallic, latent, and genital.

psychosis (sī-kō′-sis): Insanity. A severe mental disorder arising in the mind itself, as opposed to a neurosis in which the mind is affected by factors in the environment. Marked by such abnormal mental function or behavior as loss of contact with reality, distortions of perception, diminished control of elementary desires and impulses, delusions, hallucinations. The deterioration of personality may be so great as to be incompatible with self-sustained social adjustment.—psychoses, pl.; psychotic, adj.

psychosocial (sī-kō-sō′-shul): Involving both the psychological and social aspects (of a person's environment, personality, or health care services).

psychosomatic (sī-kō-sō-mat′-ik): Pertaining to the intimate relationship of mental and bodily functions and their effects upon each other. Most commonly used to describe symptoms or illnesses that are at least partly psychic or emotional in origin.

psychosomimetic (sī-kō-sō-mī-met′-ik): 1. Pertaining to symptoms that resemble those of psychosis or to drugs that produce psychosis-like symptoms. 2. A hallucinogen. Also psychotomimetic.

psychosurgery (sī-kō-ser′-jer-i): Surgery on the brain for the treatment of an emotional disorder; e.g., frontal lobotomy.

psychotherapy (sī-kō-ther′-a-pi): A form of therapy that may be used either in the treatment of organic diseases or in neuroses and psychoses; it is based on psychological methods, e.g., psychoanalysis, hypnosis, suggestion, or persuasion rather than medical, pharmaceutical, or surgical methods. GROUP P., see **therapy, group.**

psychotic (sī-kot′-ik): 1. Related to or characterized by psychosis (q.v.). 2. A person suffering from psychosis.

psychotomimetic (sī-kō-tō-mī-met′-ik): Psychosomimetic (q.v.).

psychotropic (sī-kō-trō′-pik): That which exerts its specific influence upon the psyche or mind. Term often used to describe the action of such drugs as LSD (q.v.).

psychro-: Denotes cold, freezing.

psychrotherapy (sī-krō-ther′-a-pi): Treatment of disease by the application of cold.

psyllium (si′-li-um): The seeds of an African plant. They contain mucilage, which swells on contact with water; useful as a bulk-forming laxative.

pt: Abbreviation for: (1) patient; (2) pint.

PT: Abbreviation for physical therapy.

pterygium (te-rij′-i-um): A triangular mass of conjunctiva and blood vessels extending from the inner canthus of the eye toward the pupil; encroaches on the cornea causing disturbance of vision. Occurs mostly in people habitually exposed to wind and dust. Removable.—pterygial, adj.

pterygoid (te′-ri-goid): Resembling a wing. P. MUSCLES, four muscles that originate on the pterygoid process and insert into the mandible; they open and close the jaw and move it forward and from side to side. P. PROCESS, one of two processes that extend downward from either side of the sphenoid bone at the junctions of the wings with the body of the sphenoid.

ptilosis (ti-lō′-sis): Falling out of the eyelashes.

ptomaine (tō′-mān): A chemical substance formed by the putrefactive action of bacteria on protein. P. POISONING, term formerly applied to food poisoning.

ptosed (tōsd): Prolapsed.

ptosis (tō′-sis): A drooping, falling or sinking down of an organ or part, particularly the drooping of an upper eyelid. See **visceroptosis.**—ptotic, adj.

-ptosis: Denotes: (1) sagging, falling; (2) prolapse of an organ or part.

ptyal-, ptyalo-: Denotes: (1) saliva; (2) salivary gland(s).

ptyalagogue (ti-al′-a-gog): An agent that increases the flow of saliva. Also ptyalogogue. Syn., sialagogue.

ptyalin (tī′-a-lin): Salivary amylase, an enzyme which in an alkaline medium converts starch into dextrin and maltose.

ptyalism (tī′-a-lizm): Excessive flow of saliva; salivation.

ptyalolith (tī′-a-lō-lith): A salivary calculus.

ptyalorrhea (ti-a-lō-rē′-a): Abnormally heavy flow of saliva.

pubertas (pū′-ber-tas): Puberty (q.v.). P. PRAECOX, premature (precocious) sexual development.

puberty (pū′-ber-ti): The age at which the reproductive organs become functionally active. It is accompanied by secondary sex

pubes 294

characteristics. Occurs typically between 13 and 16 years of age in boys and between 11 and 14 in girls.

pubes (pū'-bēz): 1. The hairy region covering the pubic bone. 2. Plural of pubis.

pubescence (pū-bes'-ens): Approaching or being at the age of puberty.—pubescent, adj.

pubic (pū'-bik): Related to or concerning the os pubis. P. ARCH, that formed by the union of the inferior rami of the two pubic bones at the symphysis. P. BONE, the os pubis; the lower anterior part of the innominate bone. P. SYMPHYSIS, the rather rigid joint at the center of the front of the bony pelvis formed by the union of the two pubic bones by a thick pad of fibrocartilaginous tissue.

pubiotomy (pū-bi-ot'-o-mi): A rather rare surgical operation involving the separation of the pubic bone to facilitate delivery of a live child.

pubis (pū'-bis): The pubic bone or os pubis; it is the center bone of the front of the pelvis.—pubes, pl.; pubic, adj.

public health: Descriptive of all phases of health promotion and preventive medicine carried on in a community under federal, state, county, or local agencies for the benefit of the public in general.

public health nurse: One who is engaged in caring for the sick in their homes and in guiding both them and their families in health matters at home, in school, at work or health centers, and who works with other paramedical and medical groups as well as citizens' groups in planning and carrying out community programs concerned with physical and mental health.

pudendal block: The rendering insensitive of the pudendum by the injection of local anesthetic. Used mainly for episiotomy and forceps delivery. See **transvaginal.**

pudendum (pū-den'-dum): The external reproductive organs, especially of the female.—pudenda, pl.; pudendal, adj.

puerile (pū'-er-il): Pertaining to children or the period of childhood. Childlike.

puerilism (pū'-er-il-izm): Childishness; second childhood.

puerpera (pū-er'-per-a): A woman who has just delivered a child.

puerperal (pū-er'-pe-ral): Pertaining to the puerperium (q.v.). P. ECLAMPSIA, convulsions that occur during the puerperium. See **eclampsia.** P. FEVER, that which occurs after delivery and usually relates to P.

infection. P INFECTION, a general term for infection of the genital tract after delivery or abortion. Also called childbed fever, lying-in fever, puerperal sepsis. P. PSYCHOSIS or INSANITY, a psychotic state that occurs during the puerperium.

puerperium (pū-er-pē'-ri-um): The period immediately following childbirth to the time when involution is completed, usually 6 to 8 weeks.—puerperia, pl.

pulmo-: Denotes lung (s).

pulmonary (pul'-mon-ar-i): Pertaining to the lungs. P. DISTRESS SYNDROME, see **respiratory distress syndrome.** P. EMBOLISM, the blocking or closing of the pulmonary artery by an embolus; a not uncommon cause of death.

pulmonectomy (pul-mō-nek'-to-mi): Pneumonectomy (q.v.).

pulmonic (pul-mon'-ik): 1. Pertaining to or affecting the lungs. 2. A person suffering from a pulmonary disease.

pulmonitis (pul-mo-nī'-tis): Inflammation of the lung; pneumonia; pneumonitis.

pulmotor (pul'-mō-tor): A portable apparatus for forcing oxygen or air or both, into and out of the lungs; used to induce artificial respiration in emergencies such as drowning, asphyxiation by gas, smoke inhalation, etc. Most local police and fire departments have at least one.

pulp: The soft, interior part of some organs and structures. DENTAL P., found in the P. cavity of teeth; carries blood, nerve and lymph vessels. DIGITAL P., the tissue pad of the finger tip.

pulsate (pul'-sāt): To throb, move, or beat rhythmically; to vibrate.

pulsatile (pul'-sa-tīl): Beating, throbbing.

pulsating mattress: Syn., alternating pressure mattress. A mattress made of plastic and consisting of separate cells that are inflated alternately with air about every 3 minutes. Useful for patients who are long confined to bed, debilitated, or subject to decubitus ulcers.

pulsation (pul-sā'-shun): Beating or throbbing, as of the heart or arteries.

pulse: The impulse transmitted to arteries by contraction of the left ventricle, and customarily palpated in the radial artery at the wrist. The P. rate is the number of beats or impulses per minute and is about 130 in the newborn infant, 70 to 80 in the adult and 60 to 70 in old age. The P. rhythm is its regularity—can be regular or irregular; the P. volume is the amplitude of expansion of the arterial wall during the passage of the wave; the P. force or tension is its strength, estimated by the force needed to obliterate it by pressure of the finger. ALTERNATING P., a regular P. with alternate beats of weak and strong amplitude. BIGEMINAL P., one in which the beats occur in pairs each pair being followed by a prolonged pause. BOUNDING P., one of large volume and force. CORRIGAN'S P., the water-hammer P. of aortic incompetence, with high initial upthrust that rapidly falls away; also called collapsing P. P. DEFICIT, the difference in rate of the heart (counted by stethoscope) and the pulse (counted at the wrist). It occurs when some of the ventricular contractions are too weak to open the aortic valve and hence produce a beat at the heart but not at the wrist. DICROTIC P., a double pulse beat with the second beat being weaker. P. PRESSURE is the difference between the systolic and diastolic pressures. SOFT P., one of low tension. THREADY P., a weak, usually rapid and scarcely perceptible P. See **beat.**

'pulseless' disease: Progressive obliterative arteritis of the vessels arising from the aortic arch resulting in diminished or absent pulse in the neck and arms. Thrombo-endarterectomy or a by-pass procedure may prevent blindness by improving the carotid blood flow at its commencement in the aortic arch.

pulv.: Abbreviation for *pulvis,* meaning powder.

pulvis (pul'-vis): A powder.

pump: An apparatus for forcing or drawing fluid or gas to or from a part. BREAST P., one for withdrawing milk from the breast. STOMACH P., one for withdrawing the contents of the stomach.

pump-oxygenator: An apparatus used during open heart surgery; it substitutes for both the heart and lungs in that it pumps the blood through the body and also oxygenates it.

punctate (pungk'-tăt): Dotted or spotted, *e.g.,* punctate basophilia describes the immature red cells in which there are droplets of blue-staining material in the cytoplasm.

punctum (pungk'-tum): An extremely small point or spot. P. LACRIMALE, the minute opening on either the upper or lower eyelid near the canthus through which excess tears enter the lacrimal duct and are carried to the nasal cavity.—puncta, pl.

puncture (pungk'-tūr): 1. A stab wound, hole or other perforation made with a sharp pointed hollow instrument for the withdrawal or injection of fluid or other substance. 2. To make such a wound or perforation. CISTERNAL P., insertion of a special hollow needle with stylet through the atlantooccipital ligament between the occiput and atlas, into the cisterna magna. One method of obtaining cerebrospinal fluid. LUMBAR P., insertion of a special hollow needle with stylet either through the space between the third and fourth lumbar vertebrae or lower, or into the subarachnoid space to obtain cerebrospinal fluid for examination, to remove excess fluid, or to inject a drug; *e.g.,* an anesthetic. STERNAL P., insertion of a special guarded hollow needle with stylet into the body of the sternum for aspiration of a bone marrow sam-

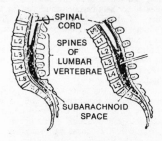

Site of lumbar puncture

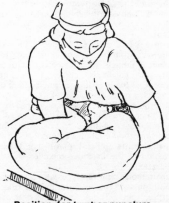

Position for lumbar puncture

ple. VENTRICULAR P., a highly skilled
method of puncturing a cerebral ventricle
for a sample of cerebrospinal fluid. P.
WOUND, see **wound.**

pungent (pun'-jent): Sharp, bitter, biting,
acrid as to taste or odor.

PUO: Abbreviation for pyrexia of unknown
origin. Term often used in reference to a
fever that occurs before the diagnosis of the
condition causing it has been made.

pupil (pū'-pil): The contractile circular
opening in the center of the iris which allows the passage of light rays to the retina.
—pupilary, pupillary, adj. ARGYLL ROB-
ERTSON P., one that responds to accommodation but not to light. PINHOLE or PIN-
POINT P., extremely contracted pupil sometimes caused by miotics or certain brain
disorders.

Pure Food and Drug Act: A federal law, originally enacted in 1906 and amended many
times since. Sets certain standards for the
purity of drugs and manufactured food
products, with the intention of protecting
the consuming public.

purgation (pur-gā'-shun): Catharsis; vigorous evacuation of the bowels effected by a
cathartic drug.

purgative (pur'-ga-tiv): 1. Causing copious
evacuation of the bowels. 2. A drug that
causes copious evacuation of the bowels.
DRASTIC P., one which causes an unusually copious evacuation of watery feces.

purge (purj): 1. To cause a thorough evacuation of the bowels. 2. A drug that causes
such an evacuation.

Purified Protein Derivative: A purified protein derivative of tuberculin, used in intradermal test for tuberculosis. See **Mantoux
test.**

purin(e)s (pū'-rinz): Constituents of nucleoproteins from which uric acid is derived.
Gout is thought to be associated with the
disturbed metabolism and excretion of uric
acid; thus foods of high purine content are
excluded in its treatment.

Purkinje's cells: Large flask-shaped cells
with many branching dendrites, located in
middle layer of the cerebral cortex; they
are important efferent neurons.

purohepatitis (pū-rō-hep-a-tī'-tis): Inflammation of the liver accompanied by suppuration.

puromucous (pū-rō-mū'-kus): Containing
both pus and mucus. Syn., mucopurulent.

purple (pur'-p'l): A color between red
and blue. VISUAL P., a photosensitive pigment in the rods of the retina; rhodopsin
(*q.v.*).

purpura (pur'-pū-ra): A disorder characterized by spontaneous extravasation of blood
from the capillaries into the skin, or into or
from the mucous membranes. Manifest
either by small red spots (petechiae) or
large plaques (ecchymoses) or by oozing,
the latter, in the absence of trauma, being
confined to the mucous membranes. It is
believed that the disorder can be due to
impaired function of the capillary walls, or
to defective quality or quantity of the blood
platelets, and can be caused by many different conditions, *e.g.,* infective, toxic, allergic, etc. See **Schönlein's disease.** P.
HEMORRHAGICA, (thrombocytopenic P.),
of unknown cause, is characterized by a
greatly diminished platelet count. The clotting time is normal but the bleeding time is
prolonged. HENOCH'S P., a disorder mainly affecting children; characterized by pur-
puric bleeding into and from the wall of the
gut, resulting in abdominal colic, vomiting,
diarrhea, distension of the abdomen, renal
colic, and melena. Skin purpura and fleeting joint pains may or may not be present.
Recurrences are common. [Edward Henoch, German pediatrician. 1820-1910.]

purulence (pūr'-ū-lens): The state of being
purulent, or of containing pus.

purulent (pūr'-ū-lent): Pertaining to, resembling, containing, or producing pus; suppurative (*q.v.*). Term is often combined
with the part affected, *e.g.,* purulent meningitis.

pus: A thick, opaque fluid or semifluid substance; the product of inflammation;
formed in certain infections, and composed
of serum, leukocytes, tissue and dead cell
debris, living and dead bacteria, fibrin, and
various foreign elements; varying in color,
odor, and consistency with the particular
causative organism.

pustule (pus'-tūl): A small, circumscribed
inflammatory elevation on the skin containing pus, *e.g.,* the lesions of acne, eczema, smallpox, chickenpox, impetigo.—
pustular, adj. MALIGNANT P., cutaneous
anthrax (*q.v.*).

putrefaction (pūt-re-fak'-shun): The process
of rotting; the destruction of organic material by bacteria.—putrefactive, adj.

putrescible (pu-tres'-ib-l): Capable of undergoing putrefaction.

putrid (pū'-trid): Decayed, rotten.

py-, pyo-: Denotes: (1) suppuration; (2)
pus; (3) pus-producing infection.

pyarthrosis (pī-ar-thrō'-sis): Pus or suppuration in a joint cavity.

pycn-, pycon-: See **pykn-, pykno-.**

pyel-, pyelo-: Denotes the renal pelvis.

pyelitis (pī-e-lī′-tis): Inflammation of the pelvis of the kidney. A mild form of pyelonephritis (*q.v.*) with pyuria but minimal involvement of renal tissue. P. on the right side is a common complication of pregnancy.

pyelocystitis (pī-e-lō-sis-tī′-tis): Inflammation of the renal pelvis and the urinary bladder.

pyelography (pī-e-log′-raf-i): Radiographic visualization of the renal pelvis and ureter after injection of a radiopaque liquid. The liquid may be injected into the blood stream whence it is excreted by the kidney (intravenous P.) or it may be injected directly into the renal pelvis or ureter by way of a fine catheter introduced through a cystoscope (retrograde or ascending P.).—pyelogram, n.; pyelographic, adj.

pyelolithotomy (pī-el-ō-lith-ot′-om-i): The operation for removal of a stone from the renal pelvis.

pyelonephritis (pī-e-lō-ne-frī′-tis): A form of renal infection which spreads outwards from the pelvis to the cortex of the kidney. The origin of the infection is usually from the ureter and below, or from the bloodstream.—pyelonephritic, adj.

pyelonephrosis (pī-e-lō-ne-frō′-sis): A pathological condition of the kidney and its pelvis.

pyeloplasty (pī′-el-ō-plas-ti): A plastic operation on the kidney pelvis.

pyeloscopy (pī-e-los′-ko-pi): Fluoroscopic examination of the pelvis of the kidney after introduction of radiopaque material.

pyelostomy (pī-e-los′-to-mi): The operation of making an incision into the pelvis of the kidney and inserting a tube to divert the flow of urine from the ureter. The tube is connected with drainage apparatus in which the urine is collected.

pyelotomy (pī-e-lot′-o-mi): An incision into the pelvis of the kidney, usually for the removal of a calculus.

pyemesis (pī-em′-e-sis): The vomiting of material containing pus.

pyemia (pī-ē′-mi-a): A grave form of general septicemia (*q.v.*) in which blood-borne bacteria from an acute primary focus of infection lodge and grow in distant organs, *e.g.,* brain, kidneys, lungs, or heart, and form multiple abscesses.—pyemic, adj.

pyencephalus (pī-en-sef′-a-lus): Abscess of the brain.

pyesis (pī-ē′-sis): Pyosis (*q.v.*).

pykn-, pykno-: Denotes compact, dense, bulk.

pyknic (pik′-nik): A type of body structure; the P. individual has a large head and chest, broad shoulders, large body cavities, generally stocky body with considerable subcutaneous fat. See **Kretschmer's personality types.**

pyknolepsy (pik′-nō-lep-si): A familial condition marked by epileptiform seizures resembling petit mal, occurring primarily in female children. Attacks may number a hundred or more in a day. Also pyknoepilepsy.

pyknosis (pik-nō′-sis): Thickening, inspissation. Refers especially to the degenerative changes in cell nuclei whereby they shrink and condense into a mass of chromatin with no specific structure or form. Also pycnosis.

pyl-, pyle- Denotes the portal vein.

pylephlebitis (pī-lē-fle-bī′-tis): Inflammation of the veins of the portal system, usually secondary to intra-abdominal sepsis.

pylethrombosis (pī-lē-throm-bō′-sis): Intravascular blood clot in portal vein or any of its branches.

pylic (pī′-lik): Of or pertaining to the portal vein.

pyloroduodenal (pī-lor-ō-dū-ō-dēn′-al): Pertaining to the pyloric sphincter and the duodenum.

pyloromyotomy (pī-lor-ō-mī-ot′-o-mi): Incision of the pyloric sphincter muscle, as in pyloroplasty.

pyloroplasty (pī-lor′-ō-plas-ti): A plastic operation on the pylorus, designed to widen the passage.

pylorospasm (pī-lor′-ō-spazm): Spasm of the pyloric sphincter muscle or of the pyloric portion of the stomach; usually due to the presence of a duodenal ulcer, but is also frequently of emotional origin.

pylorus (pī-lō′-rus): The opening of the stomach into the duodenum, encircled by a sphincter muscle.—pyloric, adj.

pyochezia (pī-ō-kē′-zi-a): The presence of pus in the feces. Also pyofecia.

pyococcus (pī-ō-kok′-us): Any one of the coccal organisms that cause suppuration, *e.g., Streptococcus pyogenes.*

pyocolpocele (pī-ō-kol′-pō-sēl): An accumulation of pus in the vagina or a vaginal tumor containing pus. Also pyocolpos.

pyoderma (pī-ō-der′-ma): Any inflammatory disease of the skin that is marked by formation of pus-containing lesions, *e.g.,* impetigo contagiosa, ecthyma. Also pyodermia.

pyogen (pī′-ō-jen): An agent that causes the formation of pus.—pyogenic, pyogen-ous, adj.; pyogenesis, n.

pyogenic (pī-ō-jen′-ik): 1. Pertaining to or characterized by the formation of pus. 2. Pus-forming.

pyometra (pī-ō-mē′-tra): Pus retained in the uterus and unable to escape through the cervix; may be due to malignancy or atresia.—pyometric, adj.

pyometritis (pī-ō-mē-trī′-tis): Purulent inflammation of the uterus.

pyonephritis (pī-ō-ne-frī′-tis): Suppurative inflammation of the kidney.

pyonephrosis (pī-ō-ne-frō′-sis): Distension of the pelvis of the kidney with pus; there is suppurative destruction of the functional structures of the kidney with severe loss of renal function.—pyonephrotic, adj.

pyopericarditis (pī-ō-pe-ri-kar-dī′-tis): Pericarditis with purulent effusion.

pyoperitonitis (pī-ō-per-i-to-nī′-tis): Inflammation of the peritoneum, with suppuration.

pyopneumothorax (pī-ō-nū-mō-thō′-raks): Pus and gas or air within the pleural sac.

pyopoiesis (pī-ō-poi-ē′-sis): Formation of pus.

pyoptysis (pī-op′-ti-sis): The spitting of material containing pus.

pyorrhea (pī-or-rē′-a): A flow of pus. P. ALVEOLARIS, an inflammatory condition involving the gums and the peridontal membrane, often with a discharge of pus from the alveoli; the breath has a foul odor and the teeth often become loose.

pyosalpingitis (pī-ō-sal-pin-jī′-tis): Suppurative inflammation of a fallopian tube.

pyosalpinx (pī-ō-sal′-pingks): A fallopian tube containing pus.

pyosis (pī-ō′-sis): Pus formation. Also pyesis.

pyothorax (pī-ō-thō′-raks): Pus in the pleural cavity; empyema (*q.v.*).

pyr-, pyro-: Denotes: (1) fire, heat; (2) fever, fever production.

pyramid (pir′-a-mid): Descriptive of anatomical structures that are shaped like a wide-based, pointed cone. PETROUS P., the pyramid-like part of the temporal bone that contains the inner ear structures. RENAL P., one of the cone-shaped structures in the medulla of the kidney; contains the collecting tubules.

pyramidal(pi-ram′-id-al): Applied to some conical-shaped eminences in the body. P. CELLS, nerve cells in the pre-rolandic area of the cerebral cortex, from which originate impulses to voluntary muscles. P. TRACTS in the brain and spinal cord transmit the fibers arising from the P. cells.

pyrectic (pī-rek′-tik): 1. An agent that induces fever. 2. Pertaining to fever. 3. Feverish; febrile.

pyretherapy (pī-re-ther′-a-pi): Treatment of disease by artificially inducing fever; may involve the use of diathermy or the injection of malarial organisms. Also called fever therapy, pyrotherapy, pyretotherapy. See **malariotherapy.**

Pyrex (pī′-reks): Trade name for a kind of glass that is extremely resistant to heat, chemicals and electricity; much used in laboratories and for cooking utensils.

pyrexia (pī-rek′-si-a): Fever; elevation of the body temperature above normal.—pyrexial, adj.

pyridoxin (e): A member of the vitamin B complex; vitamin B_6. May be connected with the utilization of unsaturated fatty acids or the synthesis of fats from proteins. Found in wheat germ, fish liver, meat; an ordinary mixed diet provides an adequate amount. Deficiency may result in symptoms of nervous irritability and convulsions (in infants), dermatitis and neuritic pains.

pyrogen (pī′-rō-jen): A substance capable of producing pyrexia (*q.v.*). DISTILLED WATER P., a substance of unknown nature, found sometimes in distilled water and which causes a rise in the patient's temperature when used in solutions that are injected into the body.—pyrogenic, adj.

pyrolysis (pī-rol′-i-sis): Decomposition of an organic substance by the application of heat.

pyromania (pī-rō-mā′-ni-a): Excessive preoccupation with fires. Insane desire to start fires, in psychoanalysis thought to be due to desire to obtain erotic gratification. —pyromaniac, n.

pyrosis (pī-rō′-sis): Heartburn; water-brash. Eructation of acid gastric contents into the mouth, accompanied by a burning sensation.

pyruvic acid (pī-roo′-vik): An important intermediate compound produced during carbohydrate metabolism and dependent upon an adequate supply of thiamine for its proper oxidation.

pyuria (pī-ū′-ri-a): Pus in the urine (more than 3 leukocytes per high-power field). —pyuric, adj.

Q

q: Abbreviation for *quaque,* meaning every.

q.d.: Abbreviation for every day (*quaque die*).

Q fever: A mild rickettsial infection somewhat like Rocky Mountain spotted fever, characterized by fever, chills, muscle pain; transmitted by raw milk, contact with infected animals, or by ticks which serve as vectors. The name is derived from the fact that the disease was first described in Queensland, Australia.

q.h.; q.2 h.; q.3 h., etc.: Abbreviations for every hour (*quaque hora*); every two hours; every three hours; etc.

q.i.d.: Abbreviation for *quater in die,* meaning four times a day.

q.s.: Abbreviation for *quantum satis,* meaning as much as is needed.

q-sort: A personality assessment technique in which a person sorts cards carrying representations of certain objects according to his interpretation of their meaning to him.

qt: Abbreviation for quart.

quack (kwak): One who fraudulently represents himself as having medical skill and knowledge; a medical charlatan; a fraud.

quackery (kwak′-er-i): The pretensions and methods employed by a quack (*q.v.*).

quadr-, quadri-, quadro-: Denotes four, fourth.

quadrant (kwod′-rant): A quarter of a circle. In anatomy, an area that is roughly circular may be divided into quadrants for descriptive purposes, *e.g.,* the surface of the abdomen.

quadratus (kwod-rā′-tus): Square. In anatomy, descriptive of skeletal muscles that are more or less four-sided, *e.g.,* the quadratus lumborum.

quadriceps (kwod′-ri-seps): Having four heads; denoting the great extensor muscle of the front of the thigh which has four heads.

quadripara (kwod-rip′-a-ra): A woman who has had four full term pregnancies.

quadriplegia (kwod-ri-plē′-ji-a): Paralysis of both arms and both legs.

quadriplegic (kwod-ri-plē′-jik): 1. Pertaining to quadriplegia. 2. A person with quadriplegia.

quadruplet (kwod-rup′-let): One of four children born at a single birth.

qualitative analysis: Laboratory analysis of a material or compound to determine what kind of substance(s) it is composed of. See **quantitative analysis.**

quantitative analysis: Laboratory analysis of a material or compound to determine how much of a certain kind (or kinds) of substance it contains. See **qualitative analysis.**

quarantine (kwar′-an-tēn): 1. To detain or isolate a person who has been exposed to a communicable disease for a period of time equal to the longest incubation period. 2. To restrict persons from an area or premises where a case of communicable disease exists. 3. To detain a ship coming from an infected port or carrying passengers who are suspected of having or of having been exposed to a communicable disease. 4. A place where persons under quarantine are kept, *e.g.,* an isolation hospital.

quart: A unit of capacity. Liquid quart is equal to one-fourth of a gallon; 0.9463 of a liter. Dry quart is slightly larger than a liquid quart.

quartan (kwar′-tan): Recurring every fourth day, reckoning inclusively. Malaria in which the paroxysms occur every 72 hours.

quasi (kwa′-si): Having some resemblance to a given thing; seemingly; in some sense or degree. Often joined by a hyphen to another word element naming the thing or condition that is resembled.

quickening: The first movements of the fetus that are perceptible to the mother; usually occur at 16 to 18 weeks gestation.

quicklime: Calcium oxide; unslacked lime. Formerly much used as a deodorant and mild disinfectant, particularly for excreta.

quicksilver: Mercury (*q.v.*).

quiescent (kwī-es′-ent): Arrested; not active; causing no symptoms. Said especially of a skin disease which is settling under treatment.

Quincke's disease: Angioneurotic edema (*q.v.*).

quinine (kwī′-nīn): The chief alkaloid of cinchona, once the standard treatment for malaria. Now largely replaced by more modern drugs.

quininism (kwin′-in-izm): Headache, noises in the ears and partial deafness, disturbed vision and nausea arising from an idiosyncrasy to, or long-continued use of quinine or cinchona.

quinsy (kwin'-zi): Acute inflammation of the tonsil and surrounding loose tissue, with abscess formation. Peritonsillar abscess.

quint-, quinti-: Denotes five, fifth.

quintan (kwin'-tan): Recurring every fifth day.

quintipara (kwin-tip'-a-ra): A woman who has had five full term pregnancies.

quintuplet (kwin'-tup-let): One of five children born at a single birth.

quotidian (kwō-tid'-i-an): Recurring daily. A form of malaria in which paroxysms er-cur daily. DOUBLE Q., recurring twice daily.

quotient (kwō'-shent): A number obtained by division. ACHIEVEMENT Q., a percentage statement of the amount a child has learned in relation to his inherent intellectual ability. INTELLIGENCE Q., the estimate of intelligence; obtained by dividing the mental age, as determined by standard tests, by the chronological age, and multiplying the result by 100. Expressed as IQ. RESPIRATORY Q., the ratio between the CO_2 expired and the O_2 inspired during a specified time.

q.v.: Abbreviation for: (1) *quod vide,* meaning which see; (2) *quantum vis,* meaning as much as you wish.

R

R: Abbreviation for right, rectal, respiration.

Ra: Chemical symbol for radium.

rabbit fever: Tularemia (*q.v.*).

rabid (rab′-id): 1. Pertaining to rabies. 2. Affected with rabies. 3. Extremely violent, furious.

rabies (rā′-bēz): An acute infectious disease of warmblooded animals, especially the dog, cat, wolf, fox; caused by a filterable virus; attacks chiefly the nervous system; fatal if untreated. May be transmitted to man through the infected saliva of a rabid animal, usually through a bite, primarily dog-bite. Hydrophobia (*q.v.*).—rabid, rabic, adj.

racemose (ras′-e-mōs): Resembling a bunch of grapes, as a gland that is divided and subdivided, *e.g.,* a salivary gland.

rachi-, rachio-: Denotes the spine.

rachiocampsis (rā-ki-ō-camp′-sis): Curvature of the spine.

rachis (rā′-kis): The spinal column.

rachitic (ra-kit′-ik): Pertaining to or affected with rickets. R. ROSARY or BEADS, a row of bead-like nodules that form on the ribs at their junctions with the cartilage, sometimes seen in children with rickets.

radial (rā′-di-al): 1. Pertinent to the radius. R. ARTERY, the artery at the wrist. 2. Radiating or expanding outward from a common point, as the rays of the sun.

radiant (rā′-di-ant): Emitting rays or beams of light. R. ENERGY, E. that is transmitted in the form of waves, including radiowaves, infrared and ultraviolet rays, visible light, x- and gamma rays.

radiation (rā-di-ā′-shun): 1. Divergence in all directions from a common center. 2. In anatomy, a structure made up of divergent elements, particularly a group of nerve fibers which diverge from a common origin. 3. A general term for any form of radiant energy such as that emitted from a luminous body, x-ray tube or radioactive substance such as radium. R. SICKNESS, that which follows therapeutic use of radium or x-rays; term also applied to effects of exposure to radioactivity released in atomic bomb explosions.

radical (rad′-ik-al): 1. A group of atoms that act as a single atom in chemical processes, *e.g.,* the sulfate radical, SO_4. 2. Pertaining to or going to the root of a thing; in medicine, going to the root of a disease process. R. OPERATION, one that is extensive and thorough so that it is curative, not palliative.

radicle (rad′-i-k'l): The smallest branch of a vessel or nerve; a rootlet.—radicular, adj.

radiculitis (ra-dik-ū-lī′-tis): Inflammation of the root of a nerve, particularly a spinal nerve.

radio-: Denotes: (1) radiation; (2) radiant energy; (3) the radius; (4) radium.

radioactive (rā-di-ō-ak′-tiv): Giving off penetrating rays due to spontaneous breaking up of atoms. R. GOLD, used for investigation of liver disease. R. IODINE, see **iodine.** R. MERCURY, used for investigation of brain lesions. R. TECHNETIUM, used for investigation of visceral lesions.

radioactivity (rā-di-ō-ak-tiv′-i-ti): The quality or property of emitting radiant energy; possessed naturally by certain elements such as radium and uranium; certain other elements become radioactive after bombardment with neutrons or other particles. The three major forms of radioactivity are designated as alpha, beta, and gamma.

radiobiology (rā-di-ō-bī-ol′-ō-ji): The study of the effects of radiation on living tissue. —radiobiological, adj.; radiobiologically, adv.

radiocarbon (rā-di-ō-kar′-bon): A radioactive form of the element carbon used for research into metabolism, diagnostic procedures, etc.

radiocarpal (rā-di-ō-kar′-pal): Pertaining to the radius and the carpus.

radiocobalt (rā-di-ō-kō′-balt): Any radioactive isotope of cobalt; medical uses include treatment of malignancies.

radiodermatitis (rā-di-ō-der-ma-tī′-tis): Irritation of the skin due to overexposure to x-rays or radium.

radiodiagnosis (rā-di-ō-dī-ag-nō′-sis): Diagnosis made by use of x-ray pictures.

radioepidermitis (rā-di-ō-ep-i-der-mī′-tis): Destructive changes in the skin resulting from overexposure to radiation.

radiographer (rā-di-og′-ra-fer): X-ray technician.

radiography (rā-di-og′-ra-fi): The making of a photograph or record by the action of certain rays on a sensitized surface such as a film. Roentgenography.

radio-iodinated human serum albumin: Used for detection and localization of brain lesions, determination of blood and plasma volumes, circulation time, and cardiac output.

radioiodine (rā-di-ō-ī'-ō-dēn): A radioactive isotope of iodine, I^{130} and I^{131} being most frequently used in medicine for the diagnosis and treatment of disorders of the thyroid gland. R. UPTAKE TEST, the person is given a small dose of radioactive iodine and the radioactivity of the thyroid gland is subsequently measured. If the gland is overactive, more than 45 percent of the iodine will be taken up by the gland within four hours. If the gland is underactive, less than 20 percent will be taken up after 48 hours.

radioisotope (rā-di-ō-ī'-sō-tōp): A radioactive isotope (*q.v.*) of an element; an element that has the same atomic number as another but a different atomic weight, exhibiting the property of spontaneous decomposition. When fed or injected can be traced with a Geiger-Muller counter. R. SCAN, pictorial representation of the distribution and amount of radioactive isotope present.

radiologist (rā-di-ol'-ō-jist): One skilled in the use of x-rays and other forms of radiant energy for the diagnosis and treatment of disease.

radiology (rā-di-ol'-ō-ji): The science that deals with radioactive substances, particularly that branch of medicine that is concerned with the use of the sources of radiant energy in the diagnosis and treatment of disease.—radiologic. radiological, adj.

radiometer (rād-i-om'-e-ter): An instrument used for detecting and measuring radiant energy, particularly small amounts of such energy.

radiomimetic (rā-di-ō-mĭ-met'-ik): Producing effects similar to those of radiotherapy. See **cytotoxic.**

radiopaque (rā-di-ō-pāk'): Referring to a substance that does not permit the passage of x-rays or other forms of radiation. Areas or organs treated with a R. substance prior to taking x-ray pictures appear light or white on the film.

radiosensitivity(rā-di-ō-sen -si-tiv'-i-ti):The condition of being sensitive to the effects of radiant energy; term often used to describe cells that can be destroyed by radiation.—radiosensitive, adj.

radiotherapist (rā-di-ō-ther'-a-pist): One who specializes in radiotherapy (*q.v.*).

radiotherapy (rā-di-ō-ther'-a-pi): Treatment of disease by x-rays, radium, radon seeds, sunlight, or other forms of radioactive substances or radiant energy.

radioulnar (rā-di-ō-ul'-nar): Pertaining to both the radius and ulna, bones of the forearm.

radium (rā'-di-um): One of the earliest known naturally radioactive elements. More radioactive than uranium and found in the same ores. Used in radiotherapy, particularly in the treatment of malignancies.

radius (rā'-di-us): 1. The bone on the outer side of the forearm. 2. A line radiating from the center to the periphery of a circle or sphere.—radial, adj.

radon (rā'-don): A radioactive gas that is an intermediary product of the disintegration of radium. It is used therapeutically for the same purposes as radium. R. SEEDS, capsules containing radon gas, designed to be placed where it would not be convenient to place or remove radium from; the rays lose their effect in a few days and the capsule remains harmlessly in the tissues.

ragweed: A common weed the pollen of which is the most frequent cause of asthma and hay fever.

rale (ral): Abnormal sound heard on auscultation of lungs, when fluid is present in bronchi.

Ramstedt's operation: An operation to relieve pyloric stenosis in infants by dividing the pyloric muscle, leaving the mucous lining intact. [Conrad Ramstedt, Emeritus Chief Surgeon, Rafael Clinic, Münster. 1867- .] Fredet-Ramstedt operation.

ramus (rā'-mus): 1. An elongated process of a bone. 2 A branch. Term used to describe the smaller structure formed when a larger one divides or forks; applied to bones, nerves, blood vessels.—rami, pl.

rancid (ran'-sid): Having a rank, disagreeable smell or taste; said of fatty substances that are undergoing or have undergone decomposition.—rancidity, n.

ranula (ran'-ū-la): A retention cyst that forms underneath the tongue on either side of the frenum due to obstruction in the duct of a sublingual or mucous gland.

Ranvier's nodes (ron-vē-āz'): Regularly spaced constrictions in myelinated nerve fibers; at these points the myelin sheath is absent.

rape (rāp): Unlawful sexual use of another, usually of a female by a male, without her consent, and chiefly by force or deception.

raphe (rā'-fē): A seam, suture, ridge, or crease marking the line of fusion of two similar parts, *e.g.,* the median furrow on the dorsal surface of the tongue.

rapport (ra-pōr'): A relation characterized by harmony and accord. In psychiatry, a

303 recessive

conscious feeling of accord, trust, confidence and responsiveness to another, particularly the therapist, with willingness to cooperate. Cf., **transference.**

rarefaction (rar-e-fak'-shun): Becoming less dense or thinning, but not being reduced in volume, as occurs in some bone diseases.

rash: A localized or general temporary skin eruption, often a characteristic of certain infectious diseases. NETTLE R., urticaria (*q.v.*). SERUM R., one following injection of a serum, *e.g.,* antitoxin; due to hypersensitivity.

rat-bite fever: A relapsing fever caused by the *Streptobacillus moniliformis* or the *Spirillum minus;* the result of a bite by an infected rat, sometimes an experimental animal. The wound often ulcerates and becomes abscessed. In the spirillary infection the blood Wassermann test is positive.

rational (rash'-un-al): 1. Of sound mind; not delirious. 2. Reasonable. 3. In medicine, treatment that is based on reason or general principles rather than empiricism. See **empirical.**

rationalization (rash-un-al-ī-zā'-shun): A mental process whereby a person explains an emotionally motivated occurrence by substituting an unconscious excuse that is more acceptable than the truth, both to himself and to others. The excuse must be acceptable enough for self-deception and he feels completely justified.

Rauwolfia (rau-wol'-fi-a): A genus of trees and shrubs found in South America, Africa, and Asia and formerly much used in those areas as the source of drugs for tranquilizing, nervous system depressant, and hypotensive actions. Now also popular in the U.S. for the treatment of such conditions as require the use of drugs with these actions.

raw: 1. Uncooked. 2. Not pasteurized (*q.v.*), as applied to milk.

ray: A beam of light or other radiant energy. A stream of particles from a radioactive substance (alpha, beta, gamma rays). ROENTGEN R., x-ray (*q.v.*).

Raynaud's disease (rā'-nōz): Idiopathic trophoneurosis. Paroxysmal spasm of the digital arteries producing numbness, tingling, and pallor or cyanosis of fingers or toes and occasionally resulting in gangrene. Primarily a disease of young and nervous women; is brought on by emotion, shock or exposure to cold. [Maurice Raynaud, French physician. 1834-1881.]

RBC: Abbreviation for red blood cells; also for red blood cell count.

RDS: Abbreviation for respiratory distress syndrome. See **respiratory.**

re-: Denotes: (1) again; (2) back, backward.

react (rē-akt'): 1. To respond to a stimulus in a particular way. 2. To undergo a chemical reaction. 3. To tend to move toward a prior condition. 4. To exert a counteracting or reciprocal influence.

reaction (rē-ak'-shun): 1. Response to stimulation. 2. Result of a test to determine acidity or alkalinity of a solution; usually expressed as pH. 3. The interaction of two or more different types of molecules with the production of a new type of molecule. ALLERGIC R., (see **sensitization**) is a hypersensitivity disorder to certain proteins with which the patient is brought into contact through the medium of his skin, his digestive or respiratory tract, resulting in eczema, urticaria, hay fever, etc. Inheritance and emotion contribute to the allergic tendency. The basis of the condition is probably a local antigen-antibody R.

reagent (rē-ā'-jent): An agent capable of producing a chemical change; when added to a complex solution it may determine the presence or absence of certain substances.

reagin (rē'-a-jin): An antibody associated with allergic reactions. Present in the serum of naturally hypersensitive people.

rebore: Disobliteration (*q.v.*).

recalcitrant (rē-kal'-si-trant): Refractory. Describes medical conditions which are resistant to treatment.

recall (rē-kawl'): The revival of a past mental image or event; to remember. R. is one phase of memory, the other two being memorization and retention.

recannulation (rē-kan-ū-lā'-shun): Reestablishment of patency of a vessel.

receptaculum (rē-sep-tak'-ū-lum): Receptacle, often acting as a reservoir. R. CHYLI, the pear-shaped sac at the lower end of the thoracic duct, in front of the first lumbar vertebra. It receives the digested fat from the intestine.

receptor (rē-sep'-tor): Sensory afferent nerve ending capable of receiving and transmitting stimuli.

recessive (rē-ses'-iv): Receding; having a tendency to disappear. R. GENE, one of a gene pair that determines the character trait in an individual only if the other member of the pair is also recessive. R. TRAIT, an inherited characteristic that remains latent when paired with a dominant trait in selective mating. See **Mendel's law.** Opp. to dominant.

recidivation(rē-sid-i-vā′-shun): Relapse of a disease or recurrence of a symptom.

recipe (res′-i-pi): 1. A prescription. 2. A word at the head of a written prescription meaning *take*; usually represented by R_x.

recipient (rē-sip′-i-ent): One who receives; usually refers to the person who receives blood in a transfusion. UNIVERSAL R., one who can receive any type of blood in a transfusion without harmful effects.

Recklinghausen's disease (rek-ling-howz′-enz): Name given to two conditions: (1) osteitis fibrosa cystica—the result of over-activity of the parathyroid glands (hyperparathyroidism) resulting in decalcification of bones and formation of cysts; (2) multiple neurofibromatosis—an hereditary skin disease in which tumors of all sizes appear on the skin along the course of the cutaneous nerves all over the body; the skin is pigmented in various areas; there is mental retardation and skeletal deformity. [Friedrich Daniel von Recklinghausen, German pathologist. 1833-1910.]

recovery room: A special room where patients are kept until they recover from anesthesia. It is usually located near the operating suite so that if emergency care is needed it can be given quickly by the anesthesiologist or surgeon. Specially prepared nurses are present at all times to observe the patients and care for them.

recrudescence (rē-kroo-des′-ens): The return of symptoms or of a pathological state after a period of apparent improvement.

rectalgia (rek-tal′-ji-a): Proctalgia (*q.v.*).

rectocele (rek′-tō-sēl): Hernial protrusion of the rectum or part of it through the vagina caused by injury to the posterior vaginal wall; may occur during childbirth. Repaired by posterior colporrhaphy.

rectoclysis (rek-tok′-li-sis): Proctoclysis (*q.v.*).

rectopexy (rek′-tō-pek-si): Surgical fixation of a prolapsed rectum.

rectoscope(rek′-tō-skōp): An instrument for examining the rectum. See **endoscope.** —rectoscopic, adj.

rectosigmoid (rek-tō-sig′-moid):The rectum and sigmoid portions of the colon. Also descriptive of the place where the rectum and sigmoid join.

rectosigmoidectomy (rek-tō-sig-moid-ek′-to-mi): Surgical removal of the rectum and sigmoid colon.

rectouterine (rek-tō-ū′-ter-in): Pertaining to the rectum and uterus.

rectovaginal (rek-tō-vaj′-in-al): Pertaining to rectum and vagina. R. FISTULA, one between the rectum and vagina.

rectovesical (rek-tō-ves′-ik-al): Pertaining to the rectum and bladder. R. FISTULA, one between the rectum and the bladder.

rectum (rek′-tum): The lower part of the large intestine between the sigmoid flexure and anal canal.—rectal, adj.; rectally, adv.

rectus (rek′-tus): Straight; in anatomy a straight muscle. R. ABDOMINIS MUSCLE, the straight muscle that extends from the pubis to the xiphoid process; it compresses the abdomen and assists to flex the trunk. R. FEMORIS MUSCLE, the large muscle on the front of the thigh; it flexes the thigh and extends the leg. The R. MUSCLES OF THE EYE include the superior, inferior, lateral and medial; they control the movements of the eyeball.

recumbent (rē-kum′-bent): Lying or reclining.—recumbency, n.

recuperate (rē-kū′-per-āt): To regain health or strength.

recurrent (re-kur′-ent): Occurring again after a period of quiescence or abatement, *e.g.*, fever, hemorrhage. R. BANDAGE, see **bandage.**

red blood cell: Erythrocyte (*q.v.*).

red bone marrow: See **marrow.**

Red Cross: 1. Abbreviation for a local, national, or the International Red Cross Society. 2. The insignia adopted by the various Red Cross Societies; consists of a red Geneva cross on a white ground. 3. A sign of neutrality used for protection of the sick and wounded and those caring for them in time of war. See **International Red Cross.**

reduce (rē-dūs′): 1. To restore something to its normal place or position, as in hernia, fracture or dislocation. 2. In chemistry, to remove oxygen from a chemical substance. 3. To decrease in volume or size.—reduction, n.

reduction (rē-duk′-shun): In chemistry, the removal of oxygen or addition of hydrogen to a compound. In medicine, the replacement of a part to its normal position in the body. CLOSED R., refers to reduction of a fracture by manipulation without making an incision. OPEN R., refers to reduction of a fracture after incision of the tissues over the site of the fracture.

referred pain: Pain which is felt as occurring at a place which is distant from its origin, *e.g.*, the pain felt in the arm during an attack of angina pectoris.

reflex (rē′-fleks): Reflected or thrown back. An involuntary activity. R. ACTION, an

305

rehabilitation

involuntary response by the body or any of its parts to a stimulus; the testing of various reflexes provides valuable information in the localization and diagnosis of disorders involving the nervous system. R. ARC, a sensory neuron, a connective neuron and a motor neuron which, acting together, carry out a reflex action. ACHILLES R., contraction of the calf muscles causing flexion of the foot when the Achilles tendon is struck. ACCOMMODATION R., constriction of the pupils and convergence of the eyes for near vision. BABINSKI'S REFLEX, see under **Babinski.** CONDITIONED R., one that is not inborn but developed through training and repeated association with a definite stimulus. CORNEAL R., the reaction of blinking when the cornea is touched. PATELLAR R., the forward jerk of the leg when the tendon immediately below the patella is struck; also called knee-jerk R. PLANTAR R., the involuntary movement of the toes when the sole of the foot is stroked. PUPILLARY R., change in the size of the pupil in response to a stimulus such as light. STARTLE R., the contraction of leg and neck muscles of an infant when dropped a short distance or in response to a sudden loud sound or a jerk.

reflux (rē′-fluks): Backward flow or return of a fluid; regurgitation.

refraction (rē-frak′-shun): 1. The bending of light rays as they pass through media of different densities. In normal vision, the light rays are so bent that they meet on the retina. 2. The process of measuring errors of refraction in the eyes and correcting them by eyeglass lenses.—refractive, adj.

refractory (rē-frak′-tor-i): Resistant to treatment; stubborn, unmanageable; rebellious. R. PERIOD, the time immediately after a nerve has received a stimulus and during which it cannot respond to another stimulus, regardless of its strength.

refracture (rē-frak′-chur): The operation of rebreaking a bone that has united improperly after fracture.

refrigeration (rē-frij-er-ā′-shun): Cooling of the body or any part of it, to reduce basal metabolism or to render a part insensitive as is needed for minor surgery. See **hibernation, hypothermia.**

regeneration (rē-jen-er-ā′-shun): The natural renewal or repair of tissue after injury.

regimen (rej′-i-men): A systematic plan of diet, medication, and activities designed to restore or maintain a certain state of health or keep a certain condition under control.

region: In anatomy, a limited area of the surface of the body. ABDOMINAL REGIONS: epigastric, umbilical, pubic, and the right and left hypochondriac, lateral, and inguinal.

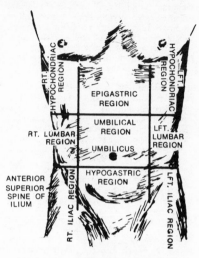

Abdominal regions

registered nurse: See **nurse.**

registry (rej′-is-tri): A placement bureau or office where a nurse may list her name as available for nursing duty.

regression (rē-gresh′-un): 1. A return to a former state or condition. 2. The subsidence or abatement of symptoms or of a disease condition. 3. In psychiatry, a turning back to an earlier stage of development in order to escape a frustrating or unbearable situation; occurs in dementia, especially senile dementia.

regurgitation (rē-gur-ji-tā′-shun): Backward flow, as of stomach contents into or through the mouth, or of blood into the heart or between the chambers of the heart when the valves do not function properly.

rehabilitation (rē-ha-bil-i-tā′-shun): The restoration of an individual's ability to function as efficiently and normally as his condition will permit following injury, illness, or accident. It involves re-education and retraining of those who have become partially or wholly incapacitated by such conditions as blindness, deafness, heart disease, amputation, paralysis, etc.—rehabilitate, v.t.

rehabilitee (rē-ha-bil′-i-tē): One who is undergoing or has undergone rehabilitation (*q.v.*).

Rehfuss' tube (rā′-fus): Consists of a graduated syringe attached to a fine-caliber stomach tube that has a bulbous perforated metal tip. Used in obtaining gastric juice for study and for gastric feeding.

rehydration (rē-hī-drā′-shun): The restoration of water to the body after dehydration (*q.v.*).

Reil's island (rīls): See **insula.**

reimplantation (rē-im-plan-tā′-shun): The replacement into its former position of a part that has been removed, *e.g.*, a tooth.

reinfection (rē-in-fek′-shun): A second infection during convalescence or after recovery from a previous infection caused by the same or a very similar organism.

reinnervation (rē-in-er-vā′-shun): The operation of restoring the nerve supply of an organ or muscle by grafting in a living nerve when the motor nerve supply has been lost.

relapse (rē-laps′): The return of a disease or of serious symptoms after the disease has apparently been overcome.

relapsing fever: Louse-borne or tick-borne infection caused by spirochetes of genus Borrelia. Prevalent in many parts of the world. Characterized by a febrile period of a week or so, with apparent recovery, followed by a further bout of fever.

relaxant (rē-laks′-ant): An agent or drug that reduces tension or activity.

REM: Abbreviation for rapid eye movements. Term is used by scientists in their studies of sleep. REM sleep is the deep sleep during which there are coordinated eye movements. This is also the period of sleep during which one dreams, and this has been suggested as a possible reason for the movements. See **NREM.**

remedial (re-mē′-di-al): Having curative properties.

remedy (rem′-e-di): Any agent that prevents, cures, or alleviates a disease or its symptoms.

remission (rē-mish′-un): 1. Lessening or abatement of the symptoms of a disease. 2. A period of temporary abatement of the symptoms of a disease, *e.g.*, a fever.

remittent (rē-mit′-ent): Increasing and decreasing at periodic intervals.

ren (ren): The kidney.—renal, adj.

ren-, reni, reno-: Denotes the kidney.

renal (rē′-nal): Pertaining to the kidney. R. ASTHMA, hyperventilation of lung occurring in uremia as a result of acidosis. R. CALCULUS, stone in the kidney. R. COLIC, severe pain in the lower back, radiating down the groin and sometimes down the leg, caused by presence of a renal calculus in the kidney or ureter. R. GLYCOSURIA occurs in patients with normal blood sugar and a lowered R. threshold for sugar. R. INSUFFICIENCY, inability of the kidney to properly perform its functions. R UREMIA, is uremia (*q.v.*) following kidney disease itself, in contrast to uremia from failure of the circulation of the blood.

renin (rē′-nin): A protein substance, found only in the kidney cortex; it acts like an enzyme. Is a powerful vasodilator.

rennet (ren′-et): An extract made of calf's stomach. Used in preparing certain foods and in cheese making.

rennin: A coagulating enzyme occurring in the gastric juice of the calf; the active principle in rennet; able to curdle milk. Prepared commercially from the mucous lining of the calf's stomach.

renography (re-nog′-ra-fī): See **nephrogram.**

reovirus (rē′-ō-vī-rus): Respiratory enteric orphan virus (*q.v.*). Has an indefinite relationship to ECHO virus (*q.v.*). R. TYPE 3 has been isolated from Burkitt's tumors and from the lesions of herpes simplex.

Rep.: Abbreviation for the expression, let it be repeated.

reportable disease: Communicable or other disease of humans or animals that the physician or other responsible person is required by law to report to the appropriate authority. The list of such diseases is made up by each health jurisdiction.

repression (rē-presh′-un): The refusal to recognize the existence of urges and feelings which are painful, or are in conflict with the individual's accepted moral principles. Freud called this refusal 'repression,' because the painful idea was repressed into the unconscious mind.

reproduction (rē-prō-duk′-shun): The production of offspring, usually by sexual means.

resection (rē-sek′-shun): Surgical removal of a section or segment of an organ or structure. SUBMUCOUS R., incision of nasal mucosa, removal of deflected nasal septum, replacement of mucosa.—resect, v.t.

resectoscope (rē-sek′-tō-skōp): An instrument passed along the urethra; it permits resection of tissue from the base of the bladder and prostate under direct vision. See **prostatectomy.**

resident (rez'-i-dent): A graduate licensed physician who serves as a house officer in a hospital following his internship in order to gain additional clinical training. So called because formerly he lived in the hospital.

residual (rē-zid'-ū-al): Remaining. In physiology, refers to something remaining in a body cavity after normal expulsion has occurred. Also refers to a disability or deformity that remains after recovery from disease or operation, as a limp or a scar. R. AIR, the air remaining in the lung after forced expiration. R. URINE, urine remaining in the bladder after micturition.

resilient (rē-zil'-yent): Elastic. Having a tendency to return to previous shape, position, or condition.

resistance (rē-zis'-tens): 1. Opposition to the passage of an electrical current. 2. Power of opposing an active force. 3. In psychology, the name given to the force that prevents repressed thoughts from reentering the consciousness. R. TO INFECTION, the power of the body to withstand infection. See **immunity.** PERIPHERAL R., that offered by the capillaries to the blood passing through them.

resolution (rez-ō-loo'-shun): The subsidence or spontaneous arrest of an inflammatory process without suppuration; the breaking down and removal or absorption of the products of inflammation, as seen, *e.g.,* in lobar pneumonia when the consolidation begins to liquefy.

resonance (rez'-o-nans): The sound elicited when percussing a part that can vibrate freely, as for example, a hollow organ or a cavity containing air. VOCAL R., is the reverberating note heard through the stethoscope on auscultation of the chest while the patient is speaking.

resorption (rē-sorp'-shun): The loss or removal of a body substance by a physiological or pathological process, *e.g.,* callus following a bone fracture, the root of a tooth, or blood from a hematoma.

respiration (res-pi-rā'-shun): 1. The physical and chemical process by which the cells and tissues of an organism receive the oxygen needed for carrying on their physiological processes and are relieved of the carbon dioxide resulting from these activities. 2. The act or function of breathing.—respiratory, adj. ABDOMINAL R., the use of the diaphragm and abdominal muscles in

breathing. CHEYNE-STOKES R., a type of breathing in which the respirations gradually increase in depth until they reach a maximum and then decrease in depth finally ceasing for a period of time; then the cycle is repeated; it generally has an ominous prognosis. EXTERNAL R., the exchange of oxygen and carbon dioxide in the lungs. INTERNAL R., the exchange of gases in the tissues. PARADOXICAL R., inward movement of the chest wall during inspiration, outward movement during expiration. PERIODIC R., Cheyne-Stokes R. STERTOROUS R., noisy breathing due to breathing with the mouth open; often occurs in comatose patients.

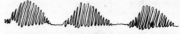

Pattern of Cheyne-Stokes respiration

respirator (res'-pi-rā-tor): 1. An appliance worn over the nose and mouth and designed to filter out irritating or poisonous substances such as gases, fumes, smoke or dust, or to warm the air before it enters the respiratory tract. 2. An apparatus which artificially and rhythmically inflates and deflates the lungs as in normal breathing, when for any reason the natural nervous or muscular control of respiration is impaired. The apparatus may work on either positive or negative pressure or on electrical stimulation. DRINKER R., used when it is necessary to supply artificial respiration for a long period of time. Consists of a metal tank that encloses the entire body except the head; commonly called 'iron lung.'

respiratory (res-pir'-a-to-ri): Related or pertaining to respiration. R. CENTER, the area in the medulla oblongata that regulates respiratory movements; it is stimulated by the carbon dioxide in the blood. R. DISTRESS SYNDROME, dyspnea in the newly born. Due to failure of formation of special protein-lipid complex in the tiny air spaces of the lung on first entry of air, causing atelectasis. Also called hyaline membrane disease. Clinical features include severe retraction of chest wall with every breath, cyanosis, an increased respiratory rate and an expiratory grunt. R. FUNCTION TESTS; numerous tests are available including tests for vital capacity, forced vital capacity, forced expiratory volume, and maximal breathing capacity. R. SYNCYTIAL VIRUS, many strains; responsible for both upper and lower respiratory infections.

respirometer (res-pi- rom′-e-ter): An instrument used for studying and measuring the extent and character of the respiratory movements.

responaut (res′-po-nawt): A person with permanent respiratory paralysis and need- ing a mechanical breathing device.

restorative (re-stor′-a-tiv): 1. An agent that serves to restore health, strength or consciousness. 2. Promoting or tending to restore health, strength or consciousness.

restraint (re-strănt′): 1. Forcible restriction of the movements of an excessively restless, irrational or psychotic patient in order to prevent him from injuring himself or others. 2. The means used to restrain a patient who is delirious, irrational, or psychotic; may be a drug or a mechanical appliance. May consist simply of a sheet applied firmly over the thighs and fastened to the bed frame, or cuffs, straps, splints, restraining jacket, etc.

resuscitation (re-sus-i-tā′-shun): The restoration to life of one who is apparently dead (collapsed or shocked).—resuscitate, v.t.; resuscitative, adj. MOUTH-TO-MOUTH R., a method of giving artificial respiration in which the rescuer forces his own expired air directly into the mouth of the victim; also called oral resuscitation.

retardate (re-tard′-āt): A mentally retarded person.

retardation (re-tar-dā′-shun): Delay; hindrance; slowing down; backwardness. MENTAL R., the lack of normal mental development; falling behind the norm for one's age. PSYCHOMOTOR R., abnormal slowness or lack of progress in mental and physical development.

retching: Straining at vomiting.

rete (re′-te): A mesh or network; in anatomy, a network or plexus of nerve fibers or blood vessels.—retia, pl.

retention: 1. Retaining information and facts in the mind; memory. 2. Accumulation of that which is normally excreted. R. CYST, one caused by the retention of secretion in a gland. 3. Keeping within the body that which normally belongs there, particularly food and liquid in the stomach. 4. Keeping in the body that which should normally be discharged. R. OF URINE, accumulation of urine within the bladder. R. ENEMA, one given with the intent that it be retained in order to provide nourishment, medication, or anesthesia. See **catheter, indwelling.**

reticular (re-tik′-ū-lar): Resembling a net.

reticulocyte (re-tik′-ū-lō-sīt): A young circulating red blood cell, which still contains traces of the nucleus which was present in the cell when developing in the bone marrow. Increased numbers of reticulocytes in the blood is evidence of active blood regeneration. Reticulocytes normally constitute about 1% of the circulating red blood cells.

reticulocytopenia (re-tik-ū-lō-sī-tō-pē′-ni-a): A decrease in the normal number of reticulocytes in the circulating blood.

reticulocytosis (re-tik-ū-lō-sī-tō′-sis): A condition in which there is more than the normal number of reticulocytes in the peripheral blood, due either to irritation of the bone marrow or to excessive formation; may occur after hemorrhage, in high altitude, and in some types of anemia.

reticuloendothelial (re-tik-ū-lō-end-ō-the′-li-al): Related to or pertaining to the reticuloendothelium (q.v.).

reticuloendothelium (re-tik-ū-lō-end-ō-the′-li-um): A series of cells, diffusely scattered throughout the body, that have the property of taking up and removing bacteria, foreign particles, and cellular debris from the blood. They are found mainly in the bone marrow, liver, spleen, lymph glands, connective tissue, and some of the formed elements of the blood. Play an important part in immunity.

reticulosis (re-tik-ū-lō′-sis): Proliferative disease of the reticuloendothelial system. An ill-defined group of fatal conditions of unknown etiology in which glandular and splenic enlargement is commonly found, and of which the three commonest members are Hodgkin's disease (lymphadenoma), lymphosarcoma, and reticulum cell sarcoma. See **mycosis.**—reticuloses, pl.

retina (ret′-i-na): The delicate, light-sensitive innermost of the three coats of the eyeball. The optic nerve enters the posterior of the eyeball and then expands. to form the retina which extends forward to the margin of the pupil. Thus it is composed of nervous tissue which receives stimuli from light and transmits them to the visual center in the brain. It is soft in consistency, translucent, and of a pinkish color. It is made up of layers, the outer one being pigmented and the 7 inner ones being nervous tissue the innermost of which contains the rods and cones which are the receptors for light. In the center of the posterior of the retina is the *macula lutea* or yellow spot, and in the center of it is the *fovea centralis*, the area of most acute vision. DETACHED R., see **retinal**.

retinal (ret′-i-nal): Related to the retina. R. DETACHMENT, occurs when the retina becomes partially detached from the choroid; a serious condition as it may lead to blindness unless treated.

retinitis (ret-i-nī′-tis): Inflammation of the retina. R. PIGMENTOSA, a familial, degenerative condition which progresses to blindness.

retinoblastoma (ret-i-nō′-blas-tō′-ma): A malignant tumor of the neuroglial element of the retina, occurring exclusively in children; usually bilateral. Often several in a family are affected.

retinopathy (ret-i-nop′-ath-i): Any noninflammatory disease of the retina.

retinoscope (ret-i-nō′-skōp): Instrument for detection of refractive errors by illumination of retina using a mirror.

retractile (rĕ-trak′-til): 1. Capable of being drawn back. 2. The state of being drawn back.

retraction (rē-trak′-shun): A drawing back or backward. R. OF NIPPLE, frequently a sign of breast cancer.

retractor (rē-trak′-tor): 1. An instrument for drawing apart the edges of a wound during surgery so as to expose the deeper structures or make them more accessible. 2. A muscle that draws a part backward.

retrad (rē′-trad): Toward the back or posterior.

retro-: Denotes: (1) backward; (2) located behind; (3) contrary to a natural or ordinary course.

retrobulbar (ret-rō-bul′-bar): 1. Behind the medulla oblongata. 2. Pertaining to or located at the back of the eyeball or behind it. R. NEURITIS, inflammation of that portion of the optic nerve behind the eyeball.

retrocecal (ret-rō-sē′-kal): Behind the cecum, *e.g.*, a retrocecal appendix.

retrocession (ret-rō-sesh′-un): 1. Going backward; a relapse. 2. A backward displacement, particularly of the uterus as a whole.

retrocolic (ret-rō-kol′-ik): Behind the colon.

retrocollic (ret-rō-kol′-lik): Relating to the back of the neck. R. SPASM, spasm of the muscles of the back of the neck.

retroflexion (ret-rō-flek′-shun): The state of being bent backward, specifically the bending backward of the body of the uterus at an acute angle, the cervix remaining in its normal position. Opp. to anteflexion.

retrograde (ret′-rō-grād): Going backward.

R. PYELOGRAPHY (*q.v.*). R. AMNESIA, loss of memory for events that occurred just before trauma, illness, or emotional shock.

retrography (ret-rog′-ra-fi): Mirror writing.

retrogression (ret-rō-gresh′-un): 1. Reversal in a condition or development. 2. Degeneration; catabolism.

retrolental (ret-rō-len′-tal): Behind the crystalline lens. R. FIBROPLASIA, the presence of fibrous tissue in the vitreous, from the retina to the lens, causing blindness. Noticed shortly after birth, more commonly in premature babies who have had continous oxygen therapy.

retroocular (ret-rō-ok′-ū-lar): Behind the eye.

retroperitoneal (ret-rō-per-i-tō-nē′-al): Behind the peritoneum.

retropharyngeal (ret-rō-fa-rin′-jē-al): Behind the pharynx. R. ABSCESS, one between the pharynx and the spine.

retroplacental (ret-rō-pla-sen′-tal): Behind the placenta.

retroplasia (ret-rō-plā′-zi-a): Degeneration of a cell or tissue in which it reverts to an earlier or more primitive form.

retropleural (ret-rō-ploo′-ral): Behind the pleura.

retropubic (ret-rō-pū′-bik): Behind the pubis.

retropulsion (ret-rō-pul′-shun): 1. Forcing back of any part, *e.g.*, forcing back the fetal head during labor. 2. The involuntary tendency to walk backward as sometimes occurs in tabes dorsalis or Parkinson's disease.

retrosternal (ret-rō-ster′-nal): Behind the breastbone.

retrosymphysial (ret-rō-sim-fiz′-i-al): Behind the symphysis pubis.

retrotracheal (ret-rō-trā′-kĕ-al): Behind the trachea.

retroversion (ret-rō-ver′-shun): Turning backward. R. OF THE UTERUS, tilting of the whole of the uterus backward with the cervix pointing forward.—retroverted, adj.

revascularization(rē-vas-kū-lar-ī-zā′-shun): 1. The regrowth of blood vessels in a tissue or organ after deprivation of the normal blood supply. 2. The reestablishment of the blood supply to a part by the operation of grafting a blood vessel.

reversion (rē-ver′-zhun): 1. The appearance of an inherited characteristic in an individual after several generations in which it has not appeared. 2. A return to a previous state or condition.

rhachi-, rhachio-: See **rachi-, rachio-**.

rhagades (rag′-a-dēz): Cracks or fissures in

the skin, especially around a body orifice, seen in vitamin deficiencies and syphilis. When they occur around the nares and mouth in cases of congenital syphilis, they leave superficial elongated scars that are pathognomic for the disease.

-rhage, -rrhage, -rrhagia: Denotes hemorrhage, a bursting forth, or profuse flow.

-rhaphy, -rrhaphy: Denotes a joining together in a seam; suturing.

-rhea, -rrhea, -rrhoea: Denotes flow, discharge.

Rhesus factor: See **blood groups.**

rheum (room): A watery discharge from a mucous membrane.

rheumatic (roo-mat′-ik): Pertaining to or affected with rheumatism. R. FEVER, see **acute rheumatism.** R. HEART DISEASE, a serious clinical form of rheumatic fever that may occur as an accompaniment or sequela of that disease. Usually involves the endocardium, including the mitral valve, the myocardium and the pericardium. The heart may be seriously and permanently damaged. A not infrequent cause of death in children and young adults.

rheumatism (roo′-ma-tizm): A non-specific term embracing a diverse group of diseases and syndromes which have in common, disorder or disease of connective tissue and hence usually present with pain, or stiffness, or swelling of muscles and joints. The main groups are rheumatic fever, rheumatoid arthritis, ankylosing spondylitis, nonarticular rheumatism, osteoarthritis and gout. ACUTE R. (rheumatic fever), a disorder tending to recur but initially commonest in childhood, classically presenting as fleeting polyarthritis of the larger joints, pyrexia and carditis within 3 weeks following a streptococcal throat infection. Atypically, but not infrequently, the symptoms are trivial and ignored, but carditis may be severe and result in permanent cardiac damage; the most common cause of mitral stenosis in later life because of scar tissue resulting from inflammation of the valve. GONORRHEAL R., that which results from a systemic infection with the gonococcus. INFLAMMATORY R., an acute form (R. fever) that tends to affect the heart. LUMBAR R., lumbago. MUSCULAR R., term for a number of muscle conditions characterized by pain, tenderness and local spasm; includes myalgia, myositis, fibromyositis, torticollis. NONARTICULAR R., involves the soft tissues; includes fibrositis. OSSEOUS R., arthritis deformans. TUBERCULOUS R.,

inflammation of joints due to the toxins of the tubercle bacillus.

rheumatoid (roo′-mat-oid): Resembling rheumatism. R. ARTHRITIS, a chronic disease of unknown etiology, characterized by polyarthritis mainly affecting the smaller peripheral joints, accompanied by general ill health and resulting eventually in varying degrees of ankylosis, crippling joint deformities, and associated muscle wasting. See **Still′s disease.**

rhexis (rek′-sis): Rupture or bursting of an organ, blood vessel, or tissue.

Rh factor: Rhesus factor. See **blood groups.**

Rh hemolytic disease: Erythroblastosis fetalis. See **erythroblastosis.**

rhin-, rhine-, rhino-, -rrhine: Denotes the nose.

rhinal (rī′-nal): Pertaining to the nose.

rhinalgia (rī-nal′-ji-a): Pain in the nose.

rhinedema (rī-ne-dē′-ma): Swelling of the nose or of the nasal mucosa.

rhinencephalon (rī-nen-sef′-a-lon): The part of the cerebral cortex concerned with the reception and interpretation of olfactory stimuli.

rhinesthesia (rī-nes-thē′-zi-a): The sense of smell.

rhinitis (rī-nī′-tis): Inflammation of the nasal mucous membrane. ACUTE R., coryza; the common cold.

rhinochiloplasty (rī-nō-kī′-lō-plas-ti): Plastic surgery of the nose and upper lip. Also rhinocheiloplasty.

rhinokyphectomy (rī-nō-kī-fek′-to-mi): A plastic operation to remove an abnormal hump on the nose.

rhinokyphosis (rī-nō-kī-fō′-sis): The presence of an excessively prominent hump on the bridge of the nose.

rhinolalia (rī-nō-lā′-li-a): Having a voice of nasal quality due to some defect of structure or pathology of the nose.

rhinolaryngitis (rī-nō-lar-in-jī′-tis): Inflammation of the mucous membrane of the nose and of the larynx occurring at the same time.

rhinology (rī-nol′-o-ji): That branch of medical science that has to do with the nose and pathological conditions of the nose.

rhinomiosis (rī-nō-mī-ō′-sis): A plastic operation for reducing the size of the nose.

rhinomycosis (rī-nō-mī-kō′-sis): A fungal infection of the mucous membrane of the nose.

rhinonecrosis (rī-nō-ne-krō′-sis): Necrosis of the bones of the nose.

rhinopharyngitis (rī-nō-far-in-jī′-tis): Inflammation of the mucous membrane of the nose and pharynx at the same time.

rhinophonia (rī-nō-fō′-ni-a): Having a voice of nasal quality. Rhinolalia (*q.v.*).

rhinophyma (rī-nō-fī′-ma): A form of rosacea (*q.v.*) characterized by nodular swellings or tumors of the skin of the nose, red coloration, and congestion.

rhinoplasty (rī′-nō-plas-ti): Plastic surgery of the nose.

rhinopolypus (rī-nō-pol′-i-pus): A polyp on the mucous membrane of the nose.

rhinorrhagia (rī-nō-rā′-ji-a): Nosebleed.

rhinorrhea (rī-nō-rē′-a): Free discharge of thin watery mucus from the nose.

rhinoscopy (rī-nos′-ko-pi): Examination of the nose by means of an instrument called a rhinoscope.

rhinosporidiosis (rī-nō-spō-rid′-i-ō sis): Fungal condition caused by the Rhinosporidium, affecting the mucosa of the nose, eyes, ears, larynx and occasionally the genitalia; characterized by persistent polypi.

rhinostenosis (rī-nō-ste-nō′-sis): Narrowing or constriction of the nasal passages.

rhinovirus (rī-nō-vī′-rus): Any one of a large group of viruses considered to be the cause of common colds.

rhizoid (rī′-zoid): Resembling a root.

rhizotomy (rī-zot′-o-mi): Surgical division of a root, especially that of a nerve. ANTERIOR R., sectioning of the anterior root of a spinal nerve for the relief of essential hypertension. POSTERIOR R., sectioning of the posterior root of a spinal nerve for the relief of intractable pain. CHEMICAL R., accomplished by injection of a chemical, often phenol.

rhodopsin (rō-dop′-sin): The visual purple contained in the retinal rods. Its color is preserved in darkness; bleached by daylight. Its formation is dependent on vitamin A.

rhomboid (rom′-boid): Diamond-shaped.

rhomboideus (rom-boi′-dē-us): One of the two diamond-shaped muscles of the back. They lie under the trapezii and act to draw the scapula upward and toward the median line and to rotate it.

rhonchus (rong′-kus): 1. A whistling or sonorous sound heard on auscultation when there is exudate or fluid in the bronchi. 2. A rattling in the throat. See **sibilus.**

Rh sensitivity: The state of being or becoming sensitized to the Rh factor, *e.g.*, as happens when an Rh-negative woman is pregnant with an Rh-positive fetus. See **blood groups.**

Rhus: A genus of shrubs that contain an oil that causes dermatitis on contact with the skin; includes poison ivy, poison oak, and poison sumac.

rhythm (rith′-em): The regular recurrence of a similar feature, action, or situation, *e.g.*, the pulse beat. R. METHOD, a method of contraception that involves abstinence from sexual intercourse during the period of the menstrual cycle when ovulation is most likely to occur.

rhytidectomy (rit-i-dek′-to-mi): The surgical removal of wrinkles. Face-lifting. Also called rhytidoplasty.

rib: Any one of the paired bones, 12 on either side, which articulate with the twelve dorsal vertebrae posteriorly and form the walls of the thorax. The upper seven pairs are TRUE R. and are attached to the sternum anteriorly by costal cartilage. The remaining five pairs are the FALSE R. The first three pairs of these do not have an attachment to the sternum but are bound to each other by costal cartilage. The lower two pairs are the FLOATING R. which have no anterior articulation. CERVICAL R. are formed by an extension of the transverse process of the seventh cervical vertebra in the form of bone or a fibrous tissue band; this causes an upward displacement of the subclavian artery; a congenital abnormality.

riboflavin (rī-bō-flā′-vin): A member of the vitamin B complex. Essential for growth, good vision; aids in digestion and carbohydrate metabolism. Found in liver, milk, eggs, kidney, lean meats, malt, yeast, green leafy vegetables, whole grain and enriched flour and cereals; also synthesized. Deficiency may result in lowered resistance and vitality, cracks at corners of mouth and lesions on lips.

ribonucleic acid (RNA) (rī-bō-nū-klē′-ik): A nucleic acid substance found chiefly in the cytoplasm of cells; an intermediate of DNA (deoxyribonucleic acid) (*q.v.*).

rice-water stool: The stool of cholera. The 'rice grains' are small pieces of desquamated epithelium from the intestine.

ricin (rī′-sin): A poisonous substance found in the seeds of the castor bean plant from which castor oil is derived.

rickets (rik′-ets): A disorder of calcium and phosphorus metabolism associated with a deficiency of vitamin D, and beginning most often in infancy and early childhood between the ages of 6 months and 2 years. There is proliferation and deficient ossification of the growing epiphyses of bones, producing 'bossing,' softening and bending of the long weight-bearing bones, muscular hypotonia, head sweating, delayed closure of the fontanelles, degeneration of the liver and spleen and, if the blood calcium falls sufficiently, tetany. FETAL R., see **achondroplasia.** RENAL R., condition of decalcification (osteoporosis) of bones associated with chronic kidney disease and clinically simulating R. It occurs in later age groups than R. and is characterized by excessive urinary calcium loss.

Rickettsia (ri-ket′-si-a): A group of small parasitic gram-negative, non-filterable microorganisms that are like bacteria in some ways and like viruses in others. Their natural habitat is the gut of arthropods such as lice, mites, ticks, fleas. They are the vectors of many diseases, transmitting the organisms to man through their bites. Rickettsial diseases include Q fever, Rocky Mountain spotted fever, and the typhus group of fevers. [Howard Taylor Ricketts, American pathologist. 1871-1910.]

rickettsial (ri-ket′-si-al): Caused by or pertaining to a Rickettsia. R. DISEASES, see **Rickettsia.**

rickety rosary: See **rachitic.**

rigidity (ri-jid′-i-ti): Stiffness, inflexibility or rigor, particularly that which is abnormal or pathological.

rigor (ri′-gor): 1. Stiffness, rigidity. 2. A sudden chill, accompanied by severe shivering. The body temperature rises rapidly and remains high until perspiration ensues and causes a gradual fall in temperature. R. MORTIS, the stiffening of the body after death.

rima (ri′-ma): A slit, cleft, or fissure between two like parts. R. GLOTTIDIS, the slit between the vocal cords. R. PALPEBRARUM, the slit between the eyelids when the eye is closed.

ring: In chemistry, a closed chain of atoms in a cyclic compound, *e.g.*, the benzene R. In anatomy, a more or less circular structure that surrounds an opening or an area. EXTERNAL INGUINAL R., the opening in the fascia of the transversalis muscle through which the vas deferens or the round ligament passes into the inguinal canal. INTERNAL INGUINAL R., the opening in the aponeurosis of the external oblique muscle through which the spermatic cord or round ligament passes. WALDEYER'S R., the ring of lymphoid tissue in the throat; made up of the lingual, faucial, and pharyngeal tonsils.

Ringer's solution: An isotonic solution containing a mixture of sodium, potassium and calcium chlorides. [Sydney Ringer, English physiologist. 1835-1910.]

ringworm: A broad general term used to describe a group of diseases of the skin and its appendages; caused by a fungus. So called because the common manifestations are circular, scaly patches. See **tinea** and **mycosis.**

Rinne's test: Testing of air conduction and bone conduction hearing, by tuning fork. [Friedrich Heinrich Rinne, German otologist. 1819-1868.]

risus sardonicus (ri′-sus sar-don′-i-kus): An expression resembling a grin, caused by spasm of facial muscles; seen in tetanus and in strychnine poisoning.

ritual (rit′-ū-al): In psychiatry, any psychomotor activity that a person persists in performing when there is no need for it; a means of relieving anxiety. See **obsessional neurosis.**

R.N.: Abbreviation for Registered Nurse. See **nurse.**

RNA: Abbreviation for ribonucleic acid (*q.v.*).

Robertson's pupil: See **Argyll Robertson pupil.**

Rocky Mountain spotted fever: An infectious rickettsial disease formerly thought to be confined to the Rocky Mountain area, but now known to occur in many parts of the Western hemisphere. It is transmitted by the bite of an infected tick or by contamination of the skin with the crushed tissues or feces of an infected tick. It is characterized by fever, headache, conjunctivitis, and a maculopapular rash.

rod: In anatomy, a slender mass of substance, specifically the rodlike bodies found in the retina.

rodent (rō′-dent): A gnawing animal.

roentgen (rent′-gen): The international unit used in measuring dosage of x- or gamma rays. R. RAYS, x-rays. [Wilhelm Konrad von Röntgen, German physicist. 1845-1923.]

roentgenography (rent-gen-og′-ra-fi): Examination of a part of the body by means of a photograph made by exposure of the part to roentgen rays. See **radiography.**

rolandic (rō-lan′-dik): Pertaining to structures first described by Rolando. R. AREA, the area in the cortex of the cerebrum that is concerned with control of motor activities. R. FISSURE, the boundary between the frontal and parietal lobes of the cerebrum. [Luigi Rolando, Italian anatomist. 1773-1831.]

Rolando (rō-lan′-dō): See **rolandic.**

role: The kind of behavior expected of a person because of his particular place in social arrangements, *e.g.,* the mother's role, nurse's role, etc. Every person assumes or fulfills more than one role on various occasions as demanded by his situation, *e.g.,* the mother role and the nurse role may be enacted simultaneously.

Romberg's sign: A sign of ataxia (*q.v.*). Inability to stand erect (without swaying) when the eyes are closed and the feet together. Also called 'rombergism.' [Moritz Romberg, German neurologist. 1795-1873.]

rooming-in: The practice in maternity units or hospitals of keeping the baby in a crib in the mother's room instead of in a nursery.

Rorschach test (ror′-shahk): A psychologic test which also measures the elements of personality; consists of a series of ink blots which the patient is told to look at and then simply tell what he sees. [Herman Rorschach, Swiss psychiatrist. 1884-1922.]

rosacea (rō-zā′-sē-a): A chronic skin disease affecting the nose particularly; marked by flushing due to chronic dilatation of the capillaries, often complicated by the appearance of papules and acne-like pustules. Called also acne roseacea, acne erythematosa, brandy face, rum nose, rum blossom.

rosary: RACHIṬIC R., rachitic bead; see **bead.**

rose cold, rose fever: Seasonal allergy that occurs in the spring or early summer, due to pollens. Symptoms are those of a common cold.

roseola (rō-zē-ō′-la): A rose- or scarlet-colored rash. EPIDEMIC R., rubella (*q.v.*). SYPHILITIC R., the rose-colored eruption of early secondary syphilis; usually appears 6-12 weeks after the initial lesion of the disease; spreads over most of the body except for the skin of the hands and face.

rose spots: The rose-colored papular eruption that appears on the abdomen and loins during the first week of typhoid fever; the spots disappear on pressure.

Rose-Waaler test: A serological test used in the diagnosis of rheumatoid arthritis. The presence of rheumatoid factor is detected in the serum by the agglutination of sheep's red blood cells sensitized with rabbit gamma globulin.

rotating tourniquet: See **tourniquet.**

rotator (rō′-tā-tor): A muscle having the action of turning a part.

roughage (ruf′-ij): Coarse food containing much indigestible vegetable fiber com-

posed of cellulose. It provides bulk in the diet and by this means helps to stimulate peristalsis and eliminate waste products. Lack of R. may cause atonic constipation. Too much R. may cause spastic constipation.

rouleau (roo′-lō): A row of red blood cells, resembling a roll of coins.—rouleaux, pl.

roundworm: One of the more prevalent intestinal worms parasitic to man. See **Ascarides.**

Rous sarcoma: A type of fibrosarcoma that arose spontaneously in fowl and which furnished the basis for study and experimental work important to the concept of a viral causation of sarcoma.

Roux-en-Y operation: Originally the distal end of divided jejunum was anastomosed to the stomach and the proximal jejunum containing the duodenal and pancreatic juices was anastomosed to the jejunum about 3 inches below the first anastomosis. The term is now used to include joining of the distal jejunum to a divided bile duct, esophagus or pancreas, in major surgery of these structures. [Cesar Roux, Swiss surgeon. 1857-1926.]

Rovsing's sign: Pressure in the left iliac fossa causes pain in the right iliac fossa in appendicitis. [Niels Thorkild Rovsing, Danish surgeon. 1862-1927.]

-rrhacis: Denotes the spine.

-rrhexis: Denotes rupture; splitting.

RSV: Abbreviation for respiratory syncytial virus (see under **respiration**); or Rous sarcoma virus (see **Rous sarcoma**).

rubedo (roo-bē′-do): Blushing or other temporary reddening of the skin.

rubefacient (roo-be-fā′-shent): 1. Producing redness of the skin. 2. An agent that acts as a counterirritant and produces a reddening when applied to the skin.

rubella (roo-bel′-a): Syn., German measles. An acute, infectious, eruptive fever (exanthema) caused by a virus and spread by droplet infection. There is pyrexia, coryza, conjunctivitis, a pink rash, enlarged occipital and posterior cervical glands. Complications are rare, except when contracted in the first 3 months of pregnancy when it may produce fetal deformities. Referred to as the rubella syndrome.

rubor (roo′-bor): Redness; one of the four classic signs of inflammation, the other three being pain, heat, and swelling.

rudimentary (roo-di-men′-ta-ri): Imperfectly or incompletely developed.

Ruffini's corpuscles (roo-fē′-nēz): Specialized encapsulated sensory nerve endings in the subcutaneous connective tissue of the finger; they are sensitive to warmth. [Angelo Ruffini, Italian anatomist. 1864-1929.]

rugae (roo'-jē): Wrinkles, corrugations, folds, often of an impermanent nature and allowing for distension, *e.g.,* the wrinkles and folds seen on the inner surface of the stomach and vagina.—ruga, sing.; rugose, rugous, adj.

rupia (roo'-pē-a): A skin eruption in which vesicles or ulcers form and become scabby with yellowish or brown crusts; almost always indicative of tertiary syphilis.—rupial, adj.

rupture (rup'-chur): Tearing, splitting, bursting of a part. A popular name for hernia (*q.v.*).

℞: Recipe (*q.v.*). Term used at the head of a prescription. It is a symbol that stands for the word 'recipe.'

S

S: Abbreviation for (1) *sinister,* meaning left; (2) *semis,* meaning one half. In the latter case it is usually written ss.

s̄: Abbreviation for *sans,* meaning without.

Sabin: SABIN'S VACCINE, an orally administered vaccine used to produce immunity against poliomyelitis; contains three types of live, attenuated polioviruses that have been cultured on monkey tissue culture. See **Salk.** [Albert B. Sabin, American virologist. 1906- .]

sac (sak): A small pouch or bag-like cavity. —saccular, sacculated, adj. AIR S., an air vesicle of the lung; an alveolus. AMNIOTIC S., the membrane that holds the fetus and amniotic fluid when in utero. CONJUNCTIVAL S., the potential space between the eyeball and the conjunctiva. HERNIAL S., the pouch of peritoneum that contains a hernia. LACRIMAL S., the expanded portion of the upper part of the lacrimal duct.

saccate (sak'-āt): Shaped like a sac; pouched.

sacchar-, sacchari-, saccharo-: Denotes sugar.

saccharic (sak'-ar-ik): Pertaining to sugar.

saccharide (sak'-a-rīd): 1. A simple sugar such as glucose. 2. A compound made up of sugar and another substance. 3. The carbohydrate grouping contained in each of the three types of carbohydrates (*q.v.*).

saccharin (sak'-a-rin): A well-known sugar substitute.

saccharine (sak'-a-rin): Sweet.

saccharogalactorrhea (sak-ar-ō-gal-ak-tō-rē'-a): The secretion of milk that has a higher than normal amount of lactose.

saccharolytic (sak-ar-ō-lit'-ik): Having the capacity to ferment or otherwise disintegrate carbohydrate molecules.

Saccharomyces (sak-a-rō-mī'-sēz): A genus of yeasts which includes baker's and brewer's yeast.

saccharose (sak'-ar-ōs): Cane sugar; sucrose.

saccharum (sak'-ar-um): Sugar.

saccharuria (sak-a-rū'-ri-a): Glycosuria (*q.v.*).

sacculation (sak-ū-lā'-shun): The formation of a saccule (*q.v.*).

saccule (sak'-ūl): 1. A minute sac. 2. The lower portion of the vestibule of the inner ear. —saccular, sacculated, adj.

sacculus (sak'-ū-lus): Saccule (*q.v.*).

sacr-, sacro-: Denotes the sacrum.

sacral (sā'-kral): Involving, pertaining to, or in the area of the sacrum.

sacralgia (sā-kral'-ji-a): Pain in the sacral region.

sacroanterior (sā-krō-an-tē'-ri-er): Used to describe a breech presentation in midwifery. The fetal sacrum is directed to one or the other acetabulum of the mother.— sacroanteriorly, adj.

sacrococcygeal (sā-krō-kok-sij'-ē-al): Pertaining to the sacrum and the coccyx.

sacrocoxalgia (sā-krō-koks-al'-ji-a): Pain in the sacroiliac joint or region.

sacrocoxitis (sā-krō-kok-sī'-tis): Inflammation of the sacroiliac joint.

sacroiliac (sā-krō-il'-i-ak): Pertaining to the sacrum and the ilium; or denoting the articulation between the two bones.

sacroiliitis (sā-krō-il-ē-ī'-tis): Inflammation of the sacroiliac joint.

sacrolumbar (sā-krō-lum'-bar): Pertaining to the sacrum and the loins.

sacroposterior (sā-krō-pos-tē'-ri-er): Used to describe a breech presentation in midwifery. The fetal sacrum is directed to one or other sacroiliac joint of the mother.— sacroposteriorly, adj.

sacrosciatic (sā-krō-si-at'-ik): Pertaining to both the sacrum and the ischium.

sacrospinalis (sā-krō-spī-nal'-is): The long large muscle that passes up on either side of the vertebral column from the sacrum to the head. Extends the trunk, bends the head and vertebral column to the side.

sacrum (sā'-krum): The triangular bone lying between the fifth lumbar vertebra and the coccyx; forms the back of the pelvis. It consists of five vertebrae fused together, and it articulates on each side with the innominate bones of the pelvis, forming the sacroiliac joints.—sacral, adj.

saddle: TURK'S or TURKISH SADDLE, sella turcica (*q.v.*).

saddlenose: One with a flattened bridge; often a sign of congenital syphilis.

sadism (sā'-dizm): The obtaining of pleasure from inflicting pain, violence or degradation on another person, or the sexual partner. Opp. to **masochism.**

sadist (sā'-dist): One who practices sadism.

sadistic (sā-dis'-tik): Pertaining to or marked by sadism.

316

safflower oil (saf'-flow-er): Oil obtained from an herb; contains unsaturated fats; used in the diets of those in whom it is desirable to keep the blood cholesterol low.

sagittal (saj'-it-al): 1. Shaped like an arrow; straight. 2. A lengthwise plane of the body, running from front to back; divides the body into right and left halves. s. SUTURE, the immovable joint formed by the union of the two parietal bones.

Saint Anthony's fire: An old term for certain inflammatory conditions of the skin resulting from ergotism.

Saint Vitus's dance: Chorea (*q.v.*).

salicylates (sal-is'-i-lāts): A large group of drugs commonly used for their analgesic effects in the treatment of such conditions as rheumatism, dysmenorrhea, arthritis, and a variety of other aches and pains.

saline (sā'-lēn, sā'-lĭn): 1. Salty, containing salt, or resembling a salt. 2. A solution containing salt. NORMAL or PHYSIOLOGICAL s., a 0.9% solution of salts in water that is of the same osmotic pressure as the blood; see **hypertonic, hypotonic, isotonic**.

saliva (sa-lī'-va): The secretion of the salivary glands; spittle. It contains water, mucus and ptyalin. Its function is to keep the inside of the mouth moist, to moisten and dissolve foods, and to start the digestion of carbohydrates.

salivary (sal'-i-var-i): Pertaining to saliva. s. AMYLASE, ptyalin (*q.v.*). s. CALCULUS, a stone formed in a salivary duct. s. GLANDS, those which secrete saliva, *e.g.*, parotid, submaxillary, and sublingual.

salivate (sal'-i-vāt): To produce an excessive amount of saliva.

salivation (sal-i-vā'-shun): An increased secretion of saliva. Ptyalism.

Salk: SALK VACCINE, a vaccine used to confer active artificial immunity to poliomyelitis; consists of three types of killed polioviruses; given by injection. [Jonas E. Salk, American bacteriologist. 1914- .]

sallow: Having a skin that is pale yellow or unhealthy looking.

Salmonella (sal-mō-nel'-a): A genus of bacteria. Gram-negative rods. Parasitic in many animals and man in whom they are often pathogenic. Some species, such as *S. typhi*, are host-specific, infecting only man, in whom they cause typhoid fever. Others, such as *S. typhimurium*, may infect a wide range of host species, usually through contaminated foods. Some species cause mild gastroenteritis, others a severe and sometimes fatal food poisoning.

salmonellosis (sal-mō-nel-lō'-sis): Infection with a Salmonella organism.

salping-, salpingo-: Denotes: (1) the fallopian tube(s); (2) less often, the eustachian tube(s).

salpingectomy (sal-pin-jek'-to-mi): Excision of a fallopian tube.

salpingitis (sal-pin-jī'-tis): Acute or chronic inflammation of one or both of the fallopian tubes. The term is also sometimes applied to inflammation of the eustachian tube.

salpingocyesis (sal-ping-gō-sī-ē'-sis): Ectopic pregnancy (*q.v.*).

salpingogram (sal-ping'-gō-gram): Radiological examination of tubal patency after injecting an opaque substance into the uterus and along the tubes.—salpingography, n.; salpingographic, adj.; salpingographically, adv.

salpingo-oophorectomy (sal-ping-gō-ō-of-ō-rek'-to-mi): Excision of a fallopian tube and ovary.

salpingoperitonitis (sal-ping-gō-per-i-tō-nī'-tis): Inflammation of the fallopian tube(s) and the peritoneum.

salpingostomy (sal-ping-gos'-to-mi): The operation performed to restore tubal patency.

salpinx (sal'-pingks): A tube, especially the fallopian tube or the eustachian tube.

salt: 1. Sodium chloride; common salt; table salt. 2. A compound formed by the chemical interaction of an acid and a base. 3. A saline purgative. s. SOLUTION, see **saline solution**.

salt rheum (room): An old term for any one of a variety of skin conditions resembling eczema.

salubrious (sa-lū'-bri-us): Wholesome; healthful. Usually in reference to climate or environment.

salve (sav): An ointment.

sanatorium (san-a-tō'-ri-um): An institution, usually private, for the treatment of patients with such chronic disorders as tuberculosis, nervous disease, etc., and who are not extremely ill.

sandfly (*Phlebotomus*): Responsible for short, sharp, pyrexial fever called 'sandfly fever' of the tropics, and for various types of leishmaniasis (*q.v.*).

sane: Of sound mind.

sangui-: Denotes blood.

sanguineous (sang-gwin'-ē-us): Pertaining to or containing blood.

sanguinopurulent (sang-win-ō-pūr'-ū-lent): Pertaining to an exudate that contains both blood and pus.

sanitarian (san-i-tar′-i-an): A person who specializes in matters of sanitation, particularly as they relate to public health. Sanitary engineer.

sanitary (san′-i-ta-ri): Healthful; promoting health.

sanitation (san-i-tā′-shun): The science of using measures that prevent diseases and that promote either individual or community health, or both.

sanitize (san′-i-tiz): To clean or sterilize something so as to make it sanitary (q.v.), e.g., eating utensils.

sanity (san′-i-ti): Soundness, particularly of the mind.

San Joaquin Valley fever (san wa-kĕn′): Coccidioidomycosis (q.v.).

S-A node: Sinoatrial node. See **node**. Also sinus node, sinuatrial node.

saphenous (sa-fē′-nus): Apparent; manifest. The name given to the two main veins in the leg, the internal and the external, and to the nerves accompanying them.

saponaceous (sa-pō-nā′-shus): Soapy.

saponification (sa-pon-i-fi-kā′-shun): Conversion into soap or a soapy substance.

sapphism (saf′-izm): Lesbianism (q.v.).

sapr-, sapro-: Denotes: (1) rotten, putrid, decayed; (2) dead or decaying organic matter.

sapremia (sa-prē′-mi-a): A pathological condition caused by the absorption and circulation in the blood stream of toxins and breakdown products resulting from the action of saprophytic organisms on dead tissue.

saprogen (sap′-rō-jen): Any microorganism that causes putrefaction (q.v.).

saprogenic (sap-rō-jen′-ik): Causing putrefaction or resulting from it.

saprophyte (sap′-rō-fīt): Free-living microorganisms obtaining food from dead and decaying animal or plant tissue.—saprophytic, adj.

sarc-, sarco-, -sarc: Denotes muscle or flesh.

sarcoblast (sar′-kō-blast): An embryonic cell that becomes a muscle cell.

sarcoid (sar′-koid): 1. Resembling flesh. 2. Sarcoidosis (q.v.).

sarcoidosis (sar-koi-dō′-sis): A chronic granulomatous disease of unknown etiology characterized by the presence of tubercles that histologically resemble those of tuberculosis and range in size from that of a pinhead to that of a bean. May affect any organ of the body but most commonly presents as a condition of the skin, lymph nodes, lungs, liver, spleen, or the small bones of the hands and feet. See **lupus**.

sarcolemma (sar-kō-lem′-ma): The delicate outer elastic membranous covering of the striated muscle fibers.

sarcoma (sar-kō′-ma): A tumor arising in the connective tissue; often highly malignant; tends to grow rapidly and to metastasize. Seen most frequently in children or young adults. The most common type is OSTEOSARCOMA, usually of the tibia, femur, or humerus. CHONDROSARCOMA arises in cartilage; FIBROSARCOMA contains much fibrous tissue. MELANOTIC S., a very malignant type containing melanin. ROUND CELL S. and GIANT CELL S. are named for the type of cell they contain. OAT CELL S. contains cells that are long and blunted at the ends.—sarcomatous, adj.; sarcomata, pl.

sarcoplasm (sar′-kō-plazm): The cytoplasmic substance of muscle in which the muscle fibers are imbedded.

Sarcoptes scabiei (sar-kop′-tēz skā′-bē-ī): The itch mite which causes scabies (q.v.).

sardonic grin (sar-don′-ik): See **risus sardonicus**.

sartorious (sar-tōr′-i-us): A long muscle of the thigh; originates on the anterior superior spine of the ilium and inserts on the medial surface of the upper end of the tibia. It adducts the leg and enables one to sit with one leg crossed over the other; so called because tailors formerly sat in this cross-legged position while at work.

saturated solution: A liquid that contains as much of a solute as it is capable of holding in solution.

satyriasis (sat-i-rī′-a-sis): Excessive sexual craving in a male. Same as nymphomania in a female.

sauna (saw′-na): Steam bath followed by plunge in the snow; originated in Finland and adapted for use in other countries using cold shower as a substitute for snow.

s.c.: Abbreviation for subcutaneous(ly).

scab: A dried crust forming over an open wound.

scabies (skā′-bi-ēz):A parasitic skin disease caused by the itch mite which bores beneath the skin; highly contagious. Characterized by intense itching and eczematous lesions caused by scratching. Sites most affected are the skin between fingers and toes, axillae, genital region, around the breasts. Syn., itch, 7-year itch.—scabious, adj.

scald: 1. A burn caused by moist heat, either steam or a hot liquid. 2.To burn the skin with moist heat.

scalp: The skin that covers the top of the head.

scalpel (skal'-pel): A small pointed knife, used in surgery.

scan: Usually used with another, designating word; *e.g.*, brain scan, thyroid scan. See **scanning.**

scanning (skan'-ing): 1. Visually examining a small area or several different isolated areas in great detail. In radioisotope s., a two-dimensional picture is made showing the gamma rays that are emitted by the isotope which is concentrated in the particular tissue, *e.g.*, brain, thyroid. 2. Scanning speech is a form of dysarthria that occurs in disseminated sclerosis; the speech is slow, or jumpy or stacatto.

scaphoid (skaf'-oid): Boat-shaped as a bone of the tarsus and carpus.

scapula (skap'-u-la): The shoulder blade—a large, flat, triangular bone.—scapular, adj.

scar: The dense, avascular white fibrous tissue, formed as the end result of healing, especially in the skin. Cicatrix. See **keloid.**

scarification (skar-i-fi-kā'-shun): The making of a series of small superficial incisions or punctures in the skin.

scarf skin: A popular name for the epidermis.

scarlatina (skar-la-tē'-na): Scarlet fever. Acute infection by hemolytic streptococcus producing a scarlet rash. Occurs mainly in children. Begins commonly with a throat infection, leading to pyrexia and the outbreak of a punctate erythematous eruption of the skin followed by desquamation. Characteristically, the area around the mouth escapes (circumoral pallor).—scarlatinal, adj.

scarlet fever: Scarlatina (*q. v.*).

Scarpa's triangle: An anatomical area just below the groin. The base of the triangle is uppermost and is formed by the inguinal ligament. The vessels and nerves passing to and from the thigh are superficial here. [Antonio Scarpa, Italian anatomist and surgeon. 1747-1832.]

SCAT: Abbreviation for sheep cell agglutination test; a test for the presence of rheumatoid factors in the blood.

scat-, scato-: Denotes feces, dung.

scatophagy (ska-tof'-a-ji): The eating of excrement.

Schaefer's method: A method of performing manual (prone pressure) artificial respiration. [Albert Edward Sharpey-Schaefer, English physiologist. 1850-1935.]

Scheuermann's disease: Osteochondritis of the vertebral bodies. Occurs chiefly in adolescents. [Holger Werfel Scheuermann, Danish orthopedic surgeon. 1877-1960.]

Shick test: A test used to determine a person's susceptibility or immunity to diphtheria. It consists in the injection of 2 or 3 minims of freshly prepared toxin beneath the skin of the left arm. A similar test is made into the right arm, but in this the serum is heated to 75° C for 10 minutes, in order to destroy the toxin but not the protein. A positive reaction is recognized by the appearance of a round red area on the left arm within 24 to 48 hours, reaching its maximum intensity on the fourth day, then gradually fading with slight pigmentation and desquamation. This reaction indicates susceptibility or absence of immunity. No reaction indicates that the subject is immune to diphtheria. Occasionally a pseudo-reaction occurs, caused by the protein of the toxin; in this case the redness appears on both arms, hence the value of the control. [Bela Schick, Austrian pediatrician. 1877-1967.]

Schilder's disease: Genetically determined degenerative disease associated with mental subnormality. [Paul Schilder, German-American psychiatrist. 1886-1940.]

Schilling test: A test for the detection of malabsorption or deficiency of Vitamin B_{12}. Following the oral administration of a small dose of radioactive B_{12}, urine for the test is collected for 24 hours.

schisto-: Denotes split, cleft.

schistocephalus (skis-tō-sef'-al-us): A fetus with an unclosed cranium.

schistoglossia (skis-tō-glos'-i-a): A congenitally cleft tongue.

Schistosoma (skis-tō-sō'-ma): A genus of trematode worms or flukes which infest man. See **schistosomiasis.**

schistosomiasis (skis-tō-sō-mī'-a-sis): Infestation of the human body by Schistosoma. The worm, often present in contaminated water, penetrates the skin, enters the bloodstream and is carried to other parts of the body, giving rise to dysentery, hematuria, anemia. Bilharziasis.

schiz-, schizo-: Denotes split or divided.

schizoid (skiz'-oid): 1. Resembling schizophrenia; having an unsocial, introspective personality. 2. A person exhibiting such traits.

Schizomycetes (skiz-ō-mī-sē'-tēz): Unicellular vegetable microorganisms that multiply by fission. May be saprophytic, parasitic, or pathogenic to man.

schizonychia (skiz-ō-nik'-i-a): Splitting of the nails.

schizophrenia (skiz-ō-frē'-ni-a): A group of mental illnesses characterized by disorganization of the patient's personality, often resulting in chronic life-long ill health and hospitalization. The onset, commonly in youth or early adult life, is either sudden or insidious. Bleuler described four main types: (1) S. SIMPLEX, the patient is dull, withdrawn, solitary and inactive; (2) CATATONIC S. (catatonia), characterized by stages of excitement alternating with phases of stupor (*q.v.*) and a peculiar rigidity; (3) PARANOID S., characterized by persecutory ideas; (4) HEBEPHRENIC S. (hebephrenia), characterized by confusion of thought; silly, purposeless behavior, mannerisms and speech. All types of s. may exhibit delusions, usually of a bizarre type, and hallucinations.

schizophrenic (skiz-ō-fren/-ik): Pertaining to schizophrenia. S. SYNDROME, in childhood considered a better label than autism or psychosis.

Schlatter's disease: Also Osgood-Schlatter's disease. Osteochondritis of the tibial tuberosity. [Carl Schlatter, Swiss surgeon. 1864-1934. Robert Bayley Osgood, American orthopedic surgeon. 1873-.]

Schlemm's canal: A lymphaticovenous canal in the inner part of the sclera, close to its junction with the cornea which it encircles. It receives the aqueous humor from the anterior chamber; obstruction leads to increased intraocular pressure. [Friedrich Schlemm, German anatomist. 1795-1858.]

Schölz's disease: Genetically determined degenerative disease associated with subnormality; the familial form of juvenile demyelinating encephalopathy.

Schönlein's disease: A form of anaphylactoid purpura occurring in young adults, without apparent cause; associated with damage to the capillary walls and accompanied by swollen, tender joints and mild fever. See **purpura**. [Johann Lukas Schönlein, German physican. 1793-1864.]

school nurse: See **nurse**.

school phobia: Term used to describe a child's irrational fear of attending school; thought to result from an intense separation anxiety caused by dependency on the mother.

Schultz-Charlton reaction: A blanching produced in the skin of a patient showing scarlatinal rash, around an injection of serum from a convalescent case, indicating neutralization of toxin by antitoxin. [Werner Schultz, German physician. 1878-1947.]

Schwann, sheath of: The neurilemma. [Theodor Schwann, German anatomist. 1810-1882.]

sciatic (sī-at/-ik): Pertaining to the ischium or the region of the hip. S. NERVE, the largest nerve in the body; it extends from the hip down the back of the leg after passing under the buttock; at the level of the knee it divides into the tibial and common peroneal nerves.

sciatica (sī-at/-i-ka): Pain along the line of distribution of the sciatic nerve (buttock, back of thigh, calf and foot).

science (sī/-ens): Any branch of systematized knowledge that is a specific object of study or practice.

scintillation (sin-ti-lā/-shun): 1. A sensation as of seeing sparks or flashing lights. 2. A flashing or sparkling. 3. A particle emitted when radioactive substances disintegrate.

scintiscan (sin/-ti-scan): 1. To use a scintiscanner, *i.e.*, to count by automation the gamma rays emitted by a radioisotope, revealing their concentration and location. 2. The record made on a scintigram.

scintiscanner (sin-ti-skan/-er): A device that scans a part of the body, measures the amount of and distribution of radioactive tracer substances, and records this information on a grid called a scintigram.

scirrho-: Denotes hard.

scirrhous (skir/-us): Hard; resembling a scirrhus.

scirrhus (skir/-us): A carcinoma which provokes a considerable growth of hard, connective tissue; a hard carcinoma of the breast.—scirrhoid, adj.

scissor leg: Abnormal crossing of the legs as a result of double hip joint disease or as a manifestation of Little's disease (*q.v.*). S. L. GAIT, crossing the legs in walking.

scler-, sclera-, sclero-: Denotes: (1) hard or dry; (2) the sclera.

sclera (sklēr/-a): The 'white' of the eye; the opaque bluish-white fibrous outer coat of the eyeball covering the posterior five sixths; it merges into the cornea at the front.—scleral, adj.; sclerae, pl.

scleradenitis (sklē-rad/-en-ī-tis): Inflammation and induration of a gland.

sclerectomy (sklē-rek/-to-mi): 1. Surgical removal of a portion of the sclera of the eye. 2. Operation for the removal of sclerosed parts of the middle ear after otitis media.

scleredema (sklē-rē-dē/-ma): A condition of edema and induration of the skin; often follows an acute infection; more common in females than males. Frequently confused with scleroderma (*q.v.*).

sclerema (sklē-rē'-ma): Hardening of the skin; scleroderma. S. OF THE NEWBORN, a usually fatal disease of premature or undernourished children; excessive drying and hardening of the skin with limitation of movement.

scleritis (sklē-rī'-tis): Inflammation of the sclera.

scleroconjunctival (sklē-rō-kon-junk-tī'-val): Pertaining to both the sclera and the conjunctiva.

sclerocorneal (sklē-rō-kor'-nē-al): Pertaining to the sclera and the cornea, as the circular junction of these two structures.

scleroderma (sklē-rō-der'-ma): A disease in which localized edema of the skin is followed by hardening, atrophy, deformity and ulceration. Occasionally it becomes generalized, producing immobility of the face, contraction of the fingers; diffuse fibrosis of the myocardium, kidneys, digestive tract and lungs. The localized form is called morphea. See **collagen** and **dermatomyositis**.

sclerodermatitis (sklē-rō-der-ma-tī'-tis): Inflammation and hardening of the skin.

scleroid (sklē'-roid): Of unusually hard or firm texture.

sclerokeratitis (sklē-rō-ker-a-tī'-tis): Inflammation of both the sclera and cornea.

scleroma (sklē-rō'-ma): A circumscribed area or patch of hardened skin or mucous membrane.

scleromalacia (sklē-rō-ma-lā-shi-a): Softening or thinning of the sclera; sometimes seen in persons with rheumatoid arthritis.

scleronychia sklē-rō-nik'-i-a): Thickening and drying of the nails.

sclerose (sklē-rōs'): To become hardened.—sclerosed, sclerotic, adj.

sclerosis (sklē-rō'-sis): Term used in pathology to describe abnormal hardening or fibrosis of a tissue. AMYOTROPHIC LATERAL S., hardening of the motor tracts of the lateral columns of the spinal cord; results in progressive atrophy of muscles. DISSEMINATED S., multiple S. LATERAL S., S. of the pyramidal tracts in the spinal cord; results in slowly progressive weakness and disability of the legs; usually occurs after age 50. MULTIPLE S., a variably progressive disease of the nervous system, most commonly first affecting young adults, in which patchy, degenerative changes occur in nerve sheaths in the brain, spinal cord

and optic nerves, followed by sclerosis (glial scar). The presenting symptoms can be diverse, ranging from diplopia to weakness or unsteadiness of a limb; disturbances of micturition are common. TUBEROUS S., see **epiloia**.

sclerotherapy (sklē-rō-ther'-a-pi): The treatment of varicose veins, *e.g.*, hemorrhoids, by the injection of a sclerosing fluid which obliterates the lumen of the affected vessel.

sclerotic (sklē-rot'-ik): Relating to: (1) the sclera of the eye; (2) sclerosis or the hardening of tissue.

sclerotitis (sklē-rō-tī'-tis): Scleritis (*q.v.*).

sclerotomy (sklē-rot'-o-mi): Incision of the sclera. ANTERIOR S., incision into the anterior chamber of the eye for the relief of acute glaucoma. POSTERIOR S., incision into the vitreous chamber of the eye for treatment of detached retina or removal of a foreign object.

scolex (skō'-leks): The head of the tapeworm by which it embeds into the intestinal wall, and from which the segments proglottides) develop.

scolio-: Denotes twisted, crooked.

scoliokyphosis (skō-li-ō-kī-fō'-sis): Combined lateral and posterior curvature of the spine.

scoliosis (skō'-li-ō-sis): Lateral curvature of the spine.

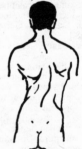

Scoliosis

-scope: Denotes an instrument for viewing or examining.

-scopy: Denotes the act of viewing, examining, observing.

scorbutic (skor-bū'-tik): Pertaining to scorbutus, the old name for scurvy.

scoto-: Denotes darkness.

scotoma (skō-tō'-ma): An area of darkness or blindness within the visual field; may be of varying size and shape. In psychiatry, refers to a 'blind spot' in a person's psychological awareness.

scotophilia (skō-tō-fil′-i-a): Fondness for the night or for being in the dark.

scotopic vision: The ability to see well in poor light. Dark-adaptation.

scratch test: A test for allergy. The superficial layer of skin is scratched and the suspected allergen rubbed in. If a redness or wheal appears at the site of the scratch the test is said to be negative. A safe test because so little of the allergen is used; as many as 30 may be done at one time.

screening: 1. Fluoroscopy (*q.v.*). 2.Mass examination of the population in a certain area for the detection of such diseases as diabetes, tuberculosis.

scrivener's palsy (skriv′-ner): Writer's cramp (*q.v.*).

scrofula (skrof′-ū-la): An old term for a constitutional state that predisposes the individual to tuberculosis; also descriptive of tuberculosis of the lymph glands and sometimes of the bones; seen mostly in the young.—scrofulous, adj.

scrofuloderma (skrof-ū-lō-der′-ma): A skin disease marked by exudative and crusted lesions, often with sinuses, resulting from a tuberculous lesion underneath, as in bone or lymph glands.

scrotitis (skrō-tī′-tis): Inflammation of the scrotum.

scrotocele (skrō′-to-sēl): A hernia into the scrotum.

scrotum (skrō′-tum): The pouch in the male which contains the testes and their accessory structures.—scrotal, adj.

scrubbing: The thorough cleansing of the hands and nails with soap, water and a brush before carrying out or assisting with a surgical or other procedure requiring aseptic technique (*q.v.*).

scrub nurse: A nurse who assists a surgeon by handing him things he needs during an operation, holding retractors, etc.; she scrubs hands and arms thoroughly and dons sterile gown, mask and gloves before the operation begins.

scrub typhus: A rickettsial disease occurring mostly in Asia and Australia; characterized by a primary lesion at the site of attachment of an infected mite, fever, headache, conjunctival injection and lymphadenopathy, followed by a red maculopapular eruption. Seen mostly in adults who frequent scrub terrain. Mites and various rodents are reservoirs of infection. Syn., tsutsugamushi disease. See **typhus fever.**

scruple (skroo′-p'l): A unit of weight in the apothecaries' system; the equivalent of 20 grains or 1.296 grams by weight, or one-third of a dram liquid measure.

scultetus (skul-tē′-tus): See **bandage.**

scurf (skurf): A flaky desquamation of the epidermis, especially of the scalp; dandruff.

scurvy (skur′-vi): A deficiency disease caused by lack of vitamin C (ascorbic acid). Clinical features include fatigue and hemorrhage. Latter may take the form of oozing at the gums or large ecchymoses. Tiny bleeding spots on the skin around hair follicles are characteristic. In children painful subperiosteal hemorrhage (rather than other types of bleeding) is pathognomonic.

scybala (sib′-a-la): Rounded hardened masses of fecal matter in the intestine.—scybalum, sing.; scybalous, adj.

seam: In anatomy, a line of union.

seasickness: See **motion sickness.**

seatworm: Pinworm; *Enterobius vermicularis* (*q.v.*).

sebaceous (sē-bā′-shus): Pertaining to fat or suet. S. CYST, one due to the retention of sebaceous material in a sebaceous follicle; a wen. S. GLANDS, the cutaneous glands which secrete an oily substance called 'sebum.' The ducts of these glands are short and straight and open into the hair follicles.

seborrhea (seb-ō-rē′-a): A functional disturbance of the sebaceous glands, marked by overactivity and resulting in a greasy condition of the skin of the face, scalp, sternal region, and elsewhere, usually accompanied by itching and burning. The seborrheic type of skin is especially liable to conditions such as alopecia, seborrheic dermatitis, acne, etc.—seborrheal, seborrheic, adj.

sebum (sē′-bum): The normal secretion of the sebaceous glands; it contains fatty acids, cholesterol and dead cells.

secondary: Second or inferior in either time, place, or importance. S. ANEMIA, see **anemia.** S. INFECTION, see **infection.** S. SEX CHARACTERISTICS, those that develop at puberty but are not directly associated with reproduction. S. SEX ORGANS, those that are characteristic of one's sex but are not directly associated with reproduction, *e.g.*, the breasts in the female. S. SYPHILIS, the second stage of syphilis; usually occurs 6 weeks to 3 months after infection.

second intention: See **healing.**

secretagogue (sē-krēt′-a-gog): An agent

secrete **322**

that stimulates secretion by a gland.

secrete (sē-krēt′): To produce or elaborate a new product from substances in the blood and to either pass it into the bloodstream, or transport it by a duct to the area where it is required or to the exterior of the body.

secretin (sē-krē′-tin): A hormone produced in the duodenal mucosa, which stimulates the secretion of pancreatic juice.

secretion (sē-krē′-shun): 1. A fluid or substance, formed or concentrated in a gland, and passed into the alimentary tract, the blood or to the exterior. 2. The process of formulating such a substance.

secretory (sē-krēt′-o-ri): Describes a gland which secretes.

section: 1. The act of cutting. 2. A cut surface. 3. A thin slice that has been prepared for microscopic examination. 4. A segment or division of an organ or structure. ABDOMINAL S., laparotomy (*q.v.*). CESAREAN S., incision through the abdominal and uterine walls for the delivery of a fetus. CORONAL S., a section of the skull that is parallel with the coronal suture. FROZEN S., a thin slice that has been cut from tissue that has been frozen; for microscopic study. SAGITTAL S., one that follows the sagittal suture and runs the entire length of the body dividing it into right and left halves.

secundigravida (se-kun-di-grav′-i-da): A woman pregnant for the second time.

secundipara (se-kun-dip′-a-ra): A woman who has borne two live children at different labors.

sedation (sē-dā′-shun): The production of a state of lessened functional activity.

sedative (sed′-a-tive): 1. Allaying physical activity and excitement. 2. An agent that lessens functional activity.

sedimentation (sed-i-men-tā′-shun): The settling of a solid substance in a fluid to the bottom of a container, or causing this to happen by the use of a centrifuge. ERYTHROCYTE S. RATE, the rate at which red blood cells settle to the bottom of a tube of drawn blood; the rate differs in different diseases and in different stages of a disease; determination of the S. rate assists the physician to follow the course of the disease; also called ESR and sed. rate.

sed. rate: Abbreviation for (erythrocyte) sedimentation rate.

segment (seg′-ment): A small section; a part of an organ or structure.—segmental, adj.; segmentation, n.

segregation (seg-rē-gā′-shun): A setting apart, usually for a particular reason,

e.g., to put those with the same or similar disease in a particular area.

seizure (sē′-zhur): 1. A sudden attack or sudden occurrence of symptoms, *e.g.,* convulsions. 2. An epileptic attack or fit.

selective action: The tendency of disease-producing agents to attack certain parts of the body.

self: The sum total of all that an individual can call his alone, including both mental and physical data. Term used to denote the feeling of self-awareness or personal identity. S.-ABUSE, common term for masturbation.

self-demand schedule: A plan of infant feeding based on the infant's behavior rather than following a set time schedule; feeding when the child indicates he is hungry.

self-limited: Descriptive of a pathological condition that runs a definite course regardless of external factors or influences.

sella turcica (sel′-a tur′-sik-a): Now called 'pituitary fossa.' A depression in the sphenoid bone which contains the pituitary gland; so named from its resemblance in shape to a Turkish saddle.

semeiologic, semiologic (sē-mi-ō-loj′-ik): Pertaining to the symptoms of a disease.

semeiology, semiology (sē-mi-ol′-o-ji): Symptomatology (*q.v.*).

semen (sē′-men): The secretion from the testicles and accessory male organs, *e.g.,* prostate. It contains the spermatozoa.

semi-: Denotes: (1) half, in quantity or value; (2) partial, to some extent, incompletely.

semicircular canals (se-mi-sir′-kū-lar ka-nalz′): Three membranous semicircular tubes contained within the bony labyrinth of the internal ear. They are concerned with appreciation of the body's position in space.

semicomatose (sem-i-kō′-ma-tōs): Condition bordering on the unconscious.

semilunar (sem-i-lūn′-ar): Shaped like a crescent or half-moon. S. CARTILAGES, the crescentic interarticular cartilages of the knee joint (menisci). S. VALVES, those guarding the opening between the right ventricle and the pulmonary artery and between the left ventricle and the aorta.

seminal (sem′-in-al): Pertaining to semen.

seminiferous (sem-i-nif′-er-us): Carrying or producing semen.

seminoma (sem-i-nō′-ma): A malignant tumor of the testis.—seminomata, pl.; seminomatous, adj.

semipermeable (sem-i-per′-mē-a-b'l): Used to describe a membrane which is permeable to some substances in solution, but not to others.

semiplegia (sem-i-plē′-ji-a): Hemiplegia (*q.v.*).

semis (sē′-mis): Half. Used in prescription writing; abbreviated s̄s̄.

senescence (se-nes′-ens): Normal changes of mind and body in increasing age.—senescent, adj.

Sengstaken-Blakemore tube: A tube with an attached inflatable balloon that is inserted into the esophagus and retained there to cause pressure on bleeding esophageal varices. [Robert Sengstaken, American neurosurgeon. 1923- . Arthur H. Blakemore, American Surgeon. 1897-1970.]

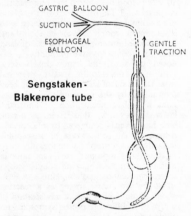

GASTRIC BALLOON
SUCTION
ESOPHAGEAL BALLOON
GENTLE TRACTION

Sengstaken-Blakemore tube

senile (sē′-nīl): Pertaining to or characteristic of old age. S. DEMENTIA, S. PSYCHOSIS, organic loss of intellectual function due to age, characterized by loss of memory, irritability, personality deterioration.

senility (sē-nil′-i-ti): 1. Feebleness or deterioration of mind and/or body when it occurs in the aged. 2. Old age.

sensation (sen-sā′-shun): The perception or mental image produced in the brain by a stimulus which has been carried there by a sensory nerve.

sense: 1. The property of perceiving. 2. Feeling or sensation. S. ORGAN, a specialized structure for receiving certain stimuli, *e.g.*, the eye, ear. SPECIAL S., any one of the five senses of feeling, hearing, seeing, tasting, smelling.

sensible (sen′-si-b'l): 1. Endowed with the sense of feeling. 2. Detectable by the senses. S. PERSPIRATION, see **perspiration.**

sensitive (sen′-si-tiv): 1. Capable of receiving and responding to a stimulus. 2. Responding to a stimulus. 3. Being unusually aware of factors in interpersonal relations. 4. Being abnormally susceptible to a substance such as a drug or foreign protein.

sensitivity (sen-si-tiv′-i-ti): The quality or state of being sensitive (*q.v.*) to certain agents.

sensitization (sen-si-ti-zā′-shun): Rendering sensitive. Persons may become sensitive to a variety of substances which may be food (*e.g.*, shellfish), bacteria, plants, chemical substances, drugs, sera, etc. Liability is much greater in some persons than others. Sensitizing agent acts as an antigen leading to development of antibodies in the blood. See **allergy, anaphylaxis.**

sensorimotor (sen-so-ri-mō′-tor): Both sensory and motor; descriptive of a nerve that has both afferent and efferent fibers.

sensorium (sen-sō′-ri-um): A term that implies the presence of memory and orientation to time, place and person; roughly the same as consciousness.

sensory (sen′-so-ri): Pertaining to sensation. S. NERVES, those which convey impulses to the brain and spinal cord.

sentient (sen′-shi-ent): Capable of feeling; sensitive.

sentiment: An attitude or thought arising from an emotional experience, *e.g.*, love, hatred, contempt or self-regard, with reference to some particular situation, person or object. Sentiments increase with experience of the environment.

separation anxiety: A state usually seen in infants from six to ten months of age, marked by fear and apprehension when the mother or mother surrogate is not present; may continue into later life when the person is separated from his normal environment or from persons who are significant to him.

sepsis (sep′-sis): The state of being infected with pus-forming or other pathogenic bacteria or their toxins.—septic, adj.

sept-, septi-: Denotes seven, seventh.

sept-, septo-: Denotes a septum.

septic (sep′-tik): Pertaining to or caused by the presence of pathogenic organisms or their poisonous products. S. SORE THROAT, streptococcic inflammation of the throat, accompanied usually by fever and prostration.

septic-: Denotes poison, sepsis.

septicemia (sep-ti-sē′-mi-a): A systemic condition resulting from the invasion of the body by living pathogenic organisms and their persistence and multiplication in the bloodstream. —septicemic, adj.

septum (sep′-tum): A thin partition between two cavities, e.g., between the nasal cavities.—septa, pl.; septal, septate, adj.

sequela (se-kwe′-la): Any morbid condition, lesion or affection that occurs consequent to a disease.—sequelae, pl.

sequestration (se-kwes-tra′-shun): 1. The formation of a sequestrum (q.v.). 2. The isolation of a person who has a communicable disease.

sequestrectomy (se-kwes-trek′-to-mi): Excision of a sequestrum (q.v.).

sequestrum (se-kwes′-trum): A piece of dead bone which separates from the healthy bone but remains within the tissues; occurs in certain diseases of the bone, particularly osteomyelitis.—sequestra, pl.

sero-: Denotes: (1) a watery consistency; (2) the blood serum.

serocolitis (se-ro-ko-li′-tis): Inflammation of the external serous coat of the colon; pericolitis.

serodiagnosis (se-ro-di-ag-no′-sis): Diagnosis that is based on the results of a test or tests on the serum of the blood.

serologist (se-rol′-o-jist): A person who specializes in serology (q.v.).

serology (se-rol′-oj-i): The branch of science dealing with the study of sera.—serological, adj.; serologically, adv.

seromucous (se-ro-mu′-kus): Pertaining to a gland which produces a watery mixture that contains both serum and mucus.

seropurulent (se-ro-pur′-u-lent): Containing serum and pus.

serosa (se-ro′-sa): A serous membrane, e.g., the peritoneal covering of the abdominal viscera.—serosal, adj.

serosanguineous (se-ro-sang-win′-e-us): Descriptive of a discharge or exudate that contains both serum and blood.

serositis (se-ro-si′-tis): Inflammation of a serous membrane.

serosynovitis (se-ro-sin-o-vi′-tis): Synovitis accompanied by copious serous effusion.

serotherapy (se-ro-ther′-a-pi): Treatment by injection of serum containing specific antibodies; may be either prophylactic or curative.

serotonin (se-ro-ton′-in): A potent vasoconstrictor found particularly in blood platelets, brain and intestinal tissue. During dissolution of blood platelets this substance is liberated, along with histamine and, since both are vasoconstrictors, this may aid in the physiological control of blood loss.

serous (se′-rus): Pertaining to, containing or producing serum. S. MEMBRANE, one lining a cavity which has no communication with the external air and covering the organs that lie in those cavities.

serpiginous (ser-pij′-in-us): Snake-like, coiled, irregular; term often used to describe the margins of skin lesions, especially ulcers and ringworm which sometimes heal at one side while spreading from the other.

serration (ser-a′-shun): A sawtooth-like notch.—serrated, adj.

serum (se′-rum): 1. Any thin watery fluid produced by serous membranes and which serves to keep serous surfaces moist. 2. The fluid part of the blood that remains after the blood has clotted and removed the corpuscles. 3. The fluid part of the blood of an animal that has been inoculated with a specific microorganism or its toxins and has become immunized against the disease; used to produce passive immunity in exposed or susceptible individuals.—sera, serums, pl. ANTITOXIC SERUM, prepared from the blood of an animal that has been immunized by the requisite toxin; it contains a high concentration of antitoxin. CONVALESCENT S., that from a person who has recently recovered from a specific disease; given to exposed or susceptible individuals as a prophylactic measure or to modify the symptoms; used especially in measles, mumps, whooping cough, scarlet fever, chickenpox, poliomyelitis. S. SICKNESS, the symptoms arising as a reaction about 10 days after the administration of serum of a different species; symptoms include urticarial rash, pyrexia, joint pains.

serum glutamic oxaloacetic transaminase: SGOT (q.v.).

serum gonadotropin (se-rum go-nad-o-tro′-pin): An ovarian-stimulating hormone obtained from the blood serum of pregnant mares. It is used in amenorrhea, often in association with estrogens (q.v.).

sesamoid (ses′-a-moid): Resembling a sesame seed. S. BONES, small bony masses formed in tendons, e.g., the patella, and the pisiform bones.

sesqui-: Denotes one and one-half.

sesquihora (see-kwi-ho′-ra): Every one and one-half hours.

sessile (ses′-il): Without a peduncle or stalk; having a broad base or attachment.

sex: 1. Either of the two divisions of organisms that are distinguished as male and female. 2. Sexual intercourse.—sexual, adj. S. DEVIANT, a person exhibiting paraphilia (*q.v.*). S. HORMONE, one having an effect on growth or functions of the reproductive organs or on the development of secondary sex characteristics. S.-LIMITED, descriptive of conditions that affect one sex only. S.-LINKED, descriptive of characteristics that are transmitted by genes that are located on the sex chromosomes.

sexology (seks-ol′-o-ji): That branch of science that deals with sex and relations between the sexes from a biological point of view.

SGOT: Serum glutamic oxaloacetic transaminase, an enzyme normally found in the blood and which increases when the heart muscle is damaged, *e.g.*, in infarction; the level may increase as much as 4 to 10 times normal during the first 24 hours after an infarction; determination of the serum level of SGOT is a diagnostic procedure.

shaft: An elongated structure, *e.g.*, the long part of a bone between its wider ends or extremities.

shaking palsy: Paralysis agitans (see **paralysis**).

shell shock: Term first used during World War I to designate a wide variety of psychotic or neurotic disturbances thought to be caused by the noise of bursting shells and other combat experiences. See **shock.**

sheltered workshop: An institution, usually operated by a nonprofit agency, that provides suitable employment for disabled individuals, some of whom are later able to enter competitive employment. Work is done on subcontracts from private industry and includes reclaiming and repairing salvage items or manufacturing items that the workshop itself has developed.

shield (shēld): A protecting tube or cover. BULLER'S S., a watch glass that is taped over one eye to protect it from infection from the other eye, *e.g.*, in gonorrheal ophthalmia. LEAD S., a lead plate that is placed between the operator and an x-ray machine to protect him from the x-rays. NIPPLE S., a device made of a glass dome and rubber teat that is placed over the nipple of a nursing mother to protect it when the infant is suckled.

Shiga's bacillus (*Shigella dysenteriae*): One of the bacteria that produce dysentery. Most common in the Middle and Far East. Infection often serious. [Kiyoshi Shiga, Japanese bacteriologist. 1870-1957.]

Shigella (shi-gel′-la): A genus of microorganisms; many of them are causative agents in various forms of dysentery.

shigellosis (shi-gel-ō′-sis): Bacillary dysentery caused by one of the Shigella organisms; tends to be endemic in certain lower social and economic areas.

shin: The front of the leg below the knee. S. BONE, the tibia.

shingles: See **herpes.**

shock: A state in which the vital processes of the body are profoundly depressed as the result of the circulatory disturbance produced by severe injury or illness and due in large part to reduction in blood volume. Its features include a fall in blood pressure, rapid pulse, pallor, restlessness, thirst and a cold clammy skin. ANAPHYLACTIC S., a violent attack of severe symptoms of shock produced when a sensitized individual receives a second injection of a serum or protein. ELECTRIC S., the sudden violent convulsive effect of the passage of an electric current through the body. INSULIN S., hypoglycemia produced by an overdose of insulin; also a therapeutic measure used in certain psychoses. PRIMARY S., that which occurs immediately after an injury. SECONDARY S., that which occurs several hours after an injury or after surgery. SHELL S., a type of psychoneurosis experienced by soldiers; a form of hysteria in which the symptoms often indicate functional disorder, *e.g.*, blindness, deafness, paralysis. S. THERAPY, use of convulsant drug or electric shock as a palliative or therapeutic measure in some psychoneurotic and psychotic conditions.

shortsightedness: Myopia (*q.v.*).

shoulder: The part of the body on each side of the base of the neck where the arm joins the trunk and where the clavicle, scapula and humerus meet. S. BLADE, the scapula. S. GIRDLE, formed by clavicle and scapula on either side. FROZEN S., inability to abduct or rotate the arm due to inflammation of subacromial bursa.

show: A popular name for the blood-stained vaginal discharge at the commencement of labor.

shunt: 1. To turn to one side; divert from a normal path or course. 2. In surgery, the anastomosis of blood vessels to change the course of blood flow. PORTACAVAL S., anastomosis of the portal vein with a vein of the general circulation, specifically the vena cava.

sial-, sialo-: Denotes: (1) saliva; (2) salivary gland(s).

sialadenitis (sī-al-ad-e-nī′-tis): Inflammation of a salivary gland.

sialagogue (sī-al′-a-gog): An agent which increases the flow of saliva.

sialic (sī-al′-ik): Pertaining to saliva.

sialism (sī′-al-izm): Salivation.

sialogram (sī-al′-ō-gram): Radiographic picture of the salivary glands and ducts, usually after injection of radiopaque medium.—sialography, n.; sialographic, adj.; sialographically, adv.

sialolith (sī-al′-ō-lith): A stone in a salivary gland or duct.

sialorrhea (sī-al-ō-rē′-a): Salivation; ptyalism.

sib: Sibling (*q.v.*).

sibilus (sib′-il-us): Rhonchus, or dry rale. Whistling sound heard on auscultation of the chest, *e.g.,* in cases of bronchitis, where the bronchi are narrowed by presence of edema or exudate.—sibilant, adj.

sibling (sib′-ling): One of a family of children having the same parents. S. RIVALRY, jealousy between brothers and sisters, often based on competition for parental affection.

sick bay: The infirmary or dispensary on a ship.

sickle cell anemia: See **anemia.**

sickness: A disordered, weakened or unsound mental or physical condition; disease. AIR S.,see **motion s.** ALTITUDE S., condition characterized by giddiness, nausea, dyspnea, thirst, prostration; caused by atmosphere that has less oxygen than one is accustomed to breathing. CAR S., see **motion s.** DECOMPRESSION S., see **caisson disease.** FALLING S.,epilepsy. RADIATION S., see **radiation.** SEASICKNESS, see **motion s.** SLEEPING S., see **African trypanosomiasis.**

sideboards, siderails: Protective devices attached to the sides of the bed to prevent restless, delirious or aged persons from falling out of bed.

side-effect: A result other than the one for which an agent or drug was administered; sometimes but not always an undesirable effect.

sider-, sidero-: Denotes iron.

sideropenia (sid-er-ō-pē′-ni-a): Iron deficiency.

sideropenic dysphagia (sid-er-ō-pē′-nik dis-fā′-ji-a): See **Plummer-Vinson syndrome.**

siderosis (sid-er-ō′-sis): 1. Excess of iron in the blood or tissues. 2. A form of pneumoconiosis caused by the inhalation of iron or other metallic particles.

SIDS: Sudden infant death syndrome. Unexplained crib death; occurs mostly during sleep; no warning cry; occurs most often in cold seasons and more often among nonwhite children from low income groups; most likely victims are children of low birth weight. The greatest single cause of death between one week and one year of age.

Sig: Abbreviation for *signetur,* meaning let it be labeled; used in prescription writing.

sigmatism (sig′-ma-tizm): A form of stammering in which the individual cannot properly articulate the letter S.

sigmoid (sig′-moid): Shaped like the letter S, or the Greek sigma. S. FLEXURE, an S-shaped curve of intestine joining the descending colon above to the rectum below.

sigmoidoscope (sig-moi′-do-skōp): An instrument for visualizing the rectum and sigmoid flexure of the colon. See **endoscope.**—sigmoidoscopic, adj.; sigmoidoscopy, n.

sigmoidostomy (sig-moid-os′-to-mi): The formation of a colostomy in the sigmoid colon.

sign (sīn): Any objective evidence of disease.

silica (sil′-i-ka): A substance that occurs naturally and abundantly in the earth in several forms; used in making glass and ceramic products and as an abrasive and adsorbent.

silicosis (sil-i-kō′-sis): Fibrosis of the lung from the inhalation of particles of silica. A form of pneumoconiosis or 'industrial dust disease,' found in miners, metal-grinders, stone-workers, etc.

Silvester's method: A manual performance of artificial respiration. [Henry Robert Silvester, English physician. 1829-1908.]

Simmonds' disease: Hypopituitary cachexia. Results from destruction of anterior pituitary lobe with consequent absence of secretions which normally stimulate other endocrine glands, especially the gonads, thyroid, and the adrenal glands. The BMR is very low, there is loss of pubic and axillary hair, loss of sexual desire, premature aging, progressive emaciation. Confirmation of diagnosis is by finding excretion of 17-ketosteroids (*q.v.*) and corticosteroids in the urine to be very low. [Morris Simmonds, physician in Germany. 1855-1925.]

Sims' position: The patient lies on the side with the under arm placed behind the back and with the thighs flexed, the upper being flexed more than the lower; facilitates vaginal examination.

sinew (sin′-ū): A ligament or tendon.

singultus (sing-gul′-tus): A hiccup.

sinistr- sinistro-: Denotes the left; toward or on the left side.

sinistral (sin′-is-tral): Pertaining to the left side.

sinistromanual (sin-is-trō-man′-ū-al): Left-handed.

sinoatrial (sī-nō-ā′-tri-al): Pertaining to the sinus venosus and the right atrium of the heart. See **S-A node.**

sinogram (sī′-nō-gram): Radiographic picture of a sinus after injection of radiopaque medium.

sinus (sī′-nus): 1. A hollow or cavity, especially one in a cranial bone. 2. A channel containing blood, especially venous blood, *e.g.,* the sinuses of the brain. 3. Any abnormal tract leading from a suppurating area; a fistula. CORONARY S., the dilated portion of the great cardiac vein; it is about one inch in length and opens into the lower part of the right atrium. PARANASAL SINUSES, air spaces in the bones around the nose; they are lined with mucous membrane and communicate with the nasal passages; include the ethmoid; sphenoid, frontal and maxillary sinuses. See **cavernous, pilonidal.**

sinusitis (sī-nus-ī′-tis): Inflammation of a sinus, particularly one or more of the paranasal sinuses.

sinusoid (sī′-nus-oid): 1. Resembling a sinus. 2. A dilated channel into which arterioles open in some organs and which take the place of capillaries; found in such organs as the heart, spleen, liver, pancreas, and the suprarenal, parathyroid, and carotid glands.

Sippy method: A regimen for the treatment of peptic ulcer. The objective is to neutralize the hydrochloric acid in the stomach by frequent feedings and the use of alkalinizing agents. [Bertram W. Sippy, American physician. 1866-1924.]

-sis: Denotes: (1) diseased state; (2) disease produced by the agent named in the stem; *e.g.,* amebiasis. Usually appears as aisis, esis, iasis, osis.

sito-: Denotes food, nutrition.

sitology (sī-tol′-o-ji): The science of nutrition; dietetics.

sitotherapy (sī-tō-ther′-a-pi): Treatment of disease through diet; dietotherapy.

sitz bath: Hip bath; immersion of the body from the waist down in hot water for therapeutic purposes.

Sjögren's syndrome (swā′-grens): A condition seen mostly in menopausal or post-menopausal women, characterized by deficient secretion from lacrimal, salivary and other glands, keratoconjunctivitis, dry tongue, hoarse voice, tenderness of joints, muscular weakness, and anemia. Thought to be due to an autoimmune process, possibly influenced by changes in the functioning of endocrine glands.

Sjögren-Larrson syndrome: Genetically determined congenital ectodermosis. Associated with mental subnormality.

skatole (skā′-tol): A strong-smelling crystalline compound in the human feces; the product of decomposition of proteins in the intestine.

skeleton (skel′-e-ton): The bony framework of the body, supporting and protecting the soft tissues and organs.—skeletal, adj. APPENDICULAR S., the bones forming the upper and lower extremities. AXIAL S., the bones forming the head and trunk.

Skene's glands: Two small glands at the entrance to the female urethra; the paraurethral glands. [Alexander Johnston Chalmers Skene, American gynecologist. 1838-1900.]

skia-: Denotes shadow, especially one produced by internal organs on x-ray film.

skiagram (skī′-a-gram): An x-ray photograph.

skiagraphy (ski-ag′-ra-fi): The making of x-ray pictures.

Skillern's fracture: A fracture in the lower one-third of the radius with a greenstick fracture of the ulna in the same region. [Penn G. Skillern, American surgeon. 1882- .]

skin: The tissue which forms the outer covering of the body; it consists of two main layers: (1) the epidermis, or cuticle, forming the outer coat; (2) the dermis, or cutis vera, the inner or true skin, lying beneath the epidermis. Also called the integument.

skull: The bony framework of the head. See **cranium.**

sleeping sickness: 1. A disease endemic in Africa, characterized by increasing somnolence; caused by protozoal parasites transmitted by the tsetse fly. 2. Any one of the viral encephalitides that is characterized by somnolence, especially equine encephalitis.

sleep walking: See **somnambulism.**

slide: A glass plate on which something to be viewed through the microscope is placed.

sling: A bandage that supports the whole

body or any part of it, particularly the arm.

slough (sluf): 1. A mass of necrotic tissue that separates from the healthy tissue and is eventually washed away by exudated serum. 2. To separate or cast off necrotic tissue from the healthy tissue underneath.

small for dates: Term used to describe an infant whose birth weight is below the normal average but whose gestational period may be of normal length.

smallpox: Variola. An acute infectious disease caused by a virus identical with that of vaccinia (cowpox). Endemic in many parts of the world. Headache, vomiting, and high fever precede the eruption of a widespread rash which is papular, vesicular and finally pustular. The eruption follows a set pattern of dissemination, commencing on the head and face. When the final stage of desiccation is passed, scars (pock-marks) are left to disfigure the skin. Prophylaxis against the disease is by vaccination. See **vaccinia.**

smear: A film of material spread out on a glass slide for microscopic examination.

smegma (smeg′-ma): An ill-smelling sebaceous secretion which accumulates under the prepuce and in the folds of the vagina.

smelling salts: A mixture of compounds usually containing some form of ammonia, which when inhaled acts as a stimulant or restorative, *e.g.*, to prevent or relieve fainting.

Smith-Petersen nail: A trifid, cannulated metal nail used to provide internal fixation of the head of the femur in fracture of the femoral neck. [Marius Nygaard Smith-Petersen, American surgeon. 1886-1953.]

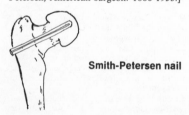

Smith-Petersen nail

snare (snâr): A surgical instrument with a wire loop at the end; used for removal of polypi, tumors or any soft fleshy projection such as a tonsil.

Snellen's test type   Block letters of varying sizes arranged on charts; used for testing visual acuity.

snow: Solid carbon dioxide; dry ice. Used for local freezing of the tissues in minor surgery. S. BLINDNESS, that caused by the glare of sun on snow.

snuffles (snuf′-lz): A snorting inspiration due to congestion of nasal mucous membranes when the nasal discharge may be mucopurulent or bloody; seen in newborn infants. Usually indicative of congenital syphilis.

soap: A cleansing agent formed by the action of an alkali on fatty acid. CASTILE S., hard soap made with olive oil. MEDICINAL SOFT S., made of vegetable oils; a soft soap used in treating certain skin conditions; also called green soap because of its color.

social sciences: The sciences that deal with social institutions, the functioning of human society, and the relationships between individuals in society.

social service: Organized activities designed to aid the sick and destitute by promoting their social welfare.

sociocultural: Pertaining to culture in its sociological setting.

sociology (sō-si-ol′-o-ji): The scientific study of interpersonal and intergroup social relationships.—sociological, adj.

sociomedical(sō-si-ō-med′-ik-al):Pertaining to the problems of medicine as they are related to society.

sociopath (sō′-si-ō-path): One who has a pathological attitude toward society; a person with a psychopathic personality (*q.v.*).

sociopathic (sō-si-ō-path′-ik): Pertaining to or characterized by asocial or antisocial behavior.

socket (sok′-et): 1. A hollow part or depression into which a part fits, as the eye socket. 2. The hollow part of a bone at a joint which receives part of another bone.

soda: A term often loosely used in reference to the salts of sodium, *e.g.*, sodium carbonate (washing soda), sodium bicarbonate (baking soda).

sodium (sō′-dē-um): A soft white metallic element many of the salts of which are used in medicine. S. BICARBONATE is an important constituent of the blood; it acts as a 'buffer' substance helping to maintain the correct *p*H of the blood. S. CHLORIDE is also an important constituent of blood and body tissues; it is an important factor in maintaining the water balance of the body.

sodomy (sod′-o-mi): Unnatural sexual relations between a human and an animal or between humans of the same sex. Bestiality.

soft sore: The primary ulcer of the genitalia occurring in the venereal disease, chancroid (*q. v.*).

solarium (sō-lar′-i-um): 1. A room or porch enclosed by glass; a sun room. 2. A room or place in a hospital where patients may expose their bodies to the sun for therapeutic purposes.

solar plexus: A large network of sympathetic nerve ganglia situated behind the stomach and in front of the aorta, and which sends nerve fibers to all of the abdominal organs; the pit of the stomach.

sole: The bottom of the foot.

solute (sol′-ūt): That which is dissolved in a fluid.

solution (sō-lū′-shun): A fluid that contains one or more dissolved substances that are evenly distributed throughout. The dissolving liquid is called the solvent and the dissolved substance is called the solute. SATURATED S., one in which as much of the solid is dissolved as will be held in solution without depositing or floating.

solvent (sol′-vent): An agent, usually liquid, which is capable of dissolving other substances.

soma (sō′-ma): 1. The body as distinguished from the psyche or the mind. 2. The walls of the body as distinguished from the viscera. 3. The trunk of the body as distinguished from the appendages.

somasthenia (sō-mas-the′-ni-a): General chronic weakness of the body.   Also somatasthenia.

somat-, somato-: Denotes the body.

somatesthesia (sō-ma-tes-the′-zi-a): Being conscious of having a body; being sensitive to bodily sensation. Also somesthesia.

somatic (sō-mat′-ik): 1. Pertaining to the body. 2. Pertaining to the trunk. 3. Pertaining to the wall of the body cavity rather than to the viscera. S. NERVES, nerves controlling the activity of striated, skeletal muscle.

somatomegaly (sō-ma-tō-meg′-a-li): The condition of having an unusually large body; gigantism.

somatopathy (sō-ma-top′-a-thi): Disorder of the body as distinguished from that of the mind.

somatopsychic (sō-ma-tō-sī′-kik): Pertaining or relating to both the body and the mind.

somatotrophin (sō-ma-tō-trō′-fin): The growth factor secreted by the anterior pituitary gland.

somnambulism (som-nam′-bū-lizm): Sleep walking; a state of dissociated consciousness in which sleeping and waking states are combined; the individual performs purposeful and often complex acts but has no memory of them upon awakening. Considered normal in children but as an illness having a physical or psychological basis in adults.

somnambulist (som-nam′-bū-list): An individual who habitually walks in his sleep.

somni-: Denotes sleep.

somnifacient (som-ni-fā′-shent): 1. Causing sleep; hypnotic, soporific. 2. An agent that causes sleep.

somnific (som-nif′-ik): Producing sleep.

somniloquism (som-nil′-ō-kwism): Talking in one's sleep.

somnolence (som-nō′-lens): Excessive or prolonged sleepiness or drowsiness.—somnolent, adj.

Sonne dysentery (son′-ne dis′-en-ter-i): Bacillary dysentery caused by infection with *Shigella sonnei.* [Carl Sonne, Danish bacteriologist. 1882-1948.]

sopor (sō′-por): Unnaturally deep or profound sleep; stupor.

soporific (sō-pō-rif′-ik): 1. An agent which induces profound sleep.   2. Producing sleep.

sorbefacient (sor-be-fā′-shent): 1. Causing absorption. 2. An agent that causes absorption.

sordes (sor′-dēz): Dried, fetid brown crusts that form on the teeth, tongue, lips, and around the mouth in illness especially fevers like typhoid; due to improper oral hygiene; consist of saliva, mucus, food particles, epithelial matter, and microorganisms.

sore: 1. Painful. 2. A general term for any ulcer or lesion on the skin or mucous membrane. BEDSORE, decubitus ulcer (*q.v.*). CANKER S., an ulcer on the mucous membrane of the mouth. COLD S., herpes simplex (*q.v.*). PRESSURE S., decubitus ulcer (*q.v.*). VENEREAL S., any lesion accompanying a venereal infection; usually refers to chancre (*q.v.*).

SOS: Abbreviation for *si opus sit,* meaning if it is necessary. Term used in written orders, usually for medication.

souffle (soo′-fl): Puffing or blowing sound heard on auscultation. FUNIC S., auscultatory murmur of pregnancy. Synchronizes with the fetal heartbeat and is caused by pressure on the umbilical cord.

UTERINE S., soft, blowing murmur that can be auscultated over the uterus after the fourth month of pregnancy.

sound: 1. Vibrations that stimulate the receptors and organs of the sense of hearing and result in a mental image. 2. Normal or abnormal noise produced in an organ of the body and audible on auscultation, *e.g.,* heart sound. 3. Sane or healthy. 4. A long, slender, cylindrical instrument to be inserted into a hollow organ for examination or exploration or to detect a foreign body, or into a duct to dilate it.

Southey's tubes: Small, perforated metal tubes used for draining away the fluid from dropsical tissues. [Reginald Southey, English physician. 1835-1899.]

soya bean: A highly nutritious legume that contains high-quality protein and little starch. Is useful in diabetic preparations. Also soybean.

space medicine: The branch of aeromedicine that deals with medical problems that develop in those who enter outer space.

spasm: Convulsive, involuntary muscular contraction. CLONIC S., s. in which fairly short periods of contraction alternate with periods of relaxation. HABIT S., an involuntary s. which occurs in a muscle that is ordinarily under voluntary control; a tic. TETANIC S., that which occurs in tetanus; tonic s. TONIC S., s. in which the rigidity persists for some time. WINKING S., involuntary contraction of muscles of the eyelid resulting in a wink; also nictitating s.

spasmodic (spaz-mod′-ik): 1. Recurring at intervals. 2. An agent that produces spasm. 3. Pertinent to or like a spasm.

spasmolytic (spaz-mō-lit′-ik): Current term for antispasmodic drugs.—spasmolysis, n.

spastic (spas′-tik): In a condition of muscular rigidity or spasm, *e.g.,* spastic diplegia (Little's disease (*q.v.*)).

spasticity (spas-tis′-it-i): Condition of rigidity or spasm of muscles.

spatula (spat′-ū-la): A flat flexible knife with blunt edges for making poultices and spreading ointment. TONGUE S. a rigid, blade-shaped instrument for depressing the tongue.

spay: To remove the ovaries by surgery. Term is usually used for animals rather than humans.

species (spē′-shēz): A subdivision of genus. A group of individuals having common characteristics and differing only in minor details.

specific (spē-sif′-ik): 1. Special; characteristic; peculiar to. 2. Pertaining to a spe-

cies. 3. A medication that has special curative properties for a particular disease, as quinine for malaria. S. DISEASE, one that is always caused by a specified organism. S. GRAVITY, the weight of a substance, as compared with that of an equal volume of water, the latter being represented by 1000.

specimen (spes′-i-men): 1. A sample or small part of a substance or a thing taken for the purpose of determining the character of the whole, *e.g.,* urine, sputum, blood, or a small portion of tissue. 2. A preparation of normal or abnormal tissue prepared for study or pathological examination.

speculum (spek′-ū-lum): An instrument used to hold the orifice or walls of a cavity apart, so that the interior of the cavity can be examined.—specula, pl.

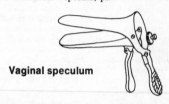

Vaginal speculum

sperm: Abbreviation for spermatozoon.

spermatic (sper-mat′-ik): Pertaining to or conveying semen. S. CORD, suspends the testis in the scrotum and contains the S. artery and vein and the vas deferens.

spermatogenesis (sper-mat-ō-jen′-e-sis): The formation and development of sperm. —spermatogenetic, adj.

spermatorrhea (sper-mat-ō-rē′-a): Involuntary discharge of semen without orgasm.

spermatozoon (sper-mat-ō-zō′-on): A mature, male reproductive cell produced in the testes; consisting of a head or nucleus, neck, and tail; about 1/500 of an inch in length.—spermatozoa, pl.

spermicide (sper′-mi-sid): An agent that kills spermatozoa. Also spermatocide.— spermicidal, adj.

sp gr: abbreviation for specific gravity. See **specific.**

sphacelate (sfas′-e-lāt): To slough or become gangrenous.—sphacelation, n.; sphacelous, adj.

sphen-, spheno-: Denotes: (1) wedge-shaped; (2) the sphenoid bone.

sphenoid (sfē′-noid): 1. Wedge-shaped. 2. A wedge-shaped bone at the base of the skull, articulating with the occipital bone at the back, the ethmoid in front and the parietal and temporal bones at the sides. —sphenoidal, adj.

spherocyte (sfĕ/-rŏ-sīt): Round red blood cells, as opposed to biconcave.–spherocyt-ic, adj.

sphincter (sfink/-ter): A circular muscle, contraction of which serves to constrict a natural passage or to close a natural orifice. ANAL S., that which surrounds the anus. CARDIAC S., surrounds the esophagus at its opening into the stomach. OCULAR S., surrounds the eye. PUPILLARY S., surrounds the pupil. PYLORIC S., located at the junction of the stomach and small intestine.

sphincterotomy (sfink-ter-ot/-o-mi): Surgical division of a sphincter.

sphygmic (sfig/-mik): Pertaining to or relating to the pulse.

sphygmo-: Denotes the pulse.

sphygmocardiograph (sfig-mŏ-kar/-di-ŏ-graf): An apparatus for simultaneous graphic recording of the radial pulse and heartbeats.—sphygmocardiographic, adj.; sphygmocardiographically, adv.

sphygmomanometer (sfig-mŏ-ma-nom/-e-ter): An instrument for measuring the force of the arterial blood pressure.

spica (spī/-ka): A bandage applied in a figure-of-eight pattern.

spicule (spi/-kūl): A small, spike-like fragment, especially of bone.—spicular, adj. Also spiculum.

spike: The pointed element in a graph or chart that is created by a rising and falling vertical line. The spikes on a fever chart represent the high temperatures that are recorded. The spike in an electroencephalogram represents a brief electrical discharge.

spiloma (spī-lō/-ma): A nevus (q.v.).

spina bifida (spī/-na bif/-i-da): A congenital defect in which the vertebral neural arches fail to close, so exposing the contents of the spinal canal posteriorly. The fissure usually occurs in the lumbosacral region. The contents of the canal may or may not protrude through the opening: this latter condition is called 'spina bifida occulta.'

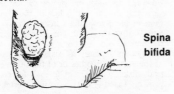

Spina bifida

spinal (spī/-nal): Pertaining to a spine or to

the vertebral column. S. ANESTHETIC, a local anesthetic solution is injected into the subarachnoid space so that it renders the area supplied by the selected s. nerves insensitive. S. BULB, the medulla oblongata. S. CANAL, the central hollow throughout the S. column. S. CARIES, disease of the vertebral bones. S. CAVITY, the S. canal. S. COLUMN, a bony structure formed by 33 separate bones; the lower ones fuse together; the rest are separated by pads of cartilage; the backbone. S. CORD, the continuation of the nervous tissue of the brain down the s. canal to the level of the first or second lumbar vertebra. S. CURVATURE, an exaggerated curve in the s. column; see **kyphosis, lordosis, scoliosis.** S. FLUID, cerebrospinal fluid (q.v.). S. FUSION, an operation in which the articulations of vertebrae are destroyed thus rendering a portion of the spine rigid (ankylosed). S. GANGLION, a group of sensory nerve cells on the posterior root of a spinal nerve. S. NERVES, 31 pairs leave the s. cord and pass out of the s. canal to supply the periphery. S. PUNCTURE, lumbar puncture (q.v.). S. TAP, s. puncture.

spine (spīn): 1. A popular term for the bony spinal or vertebral column. 2. A sharp process of bone.—spinous, spinal, adj.

spinifugal (spī-nif/-ŭ-gal): Moving away from the spinal cord, particularly the efferent fibers of the spinal nerves.

spinipetal (spī-nip/-e-tal): Conducting or moving in a direction toward the spinal cord, particularly the efferent fibers of the spinal nerves.

spinobulbar (spī-nŏ-bul/-bar): pertaining to the spinal cord and the medulla oblongata.

spinocerebellar (spī-nŏ-ser-e-bel/-lar): Pertaining to the spinal cord and cerebellum.

spinous (spī/-nus): Pertaining to or resembling a spine or a spinelike process. Also spinose.

Spirillum (spī-ril/-um): A bacterial genus. Cells are rigid screws or portions of a turn. Common in water and organic matter. *Sp. minus* is found in rodents and may infect man, in whom it causes one form of ratbite fever.—spirilla, pl.; spirillary, adj.

spirit: 1. An alcoholic solution. 2. A distilled solution.

spirochete (spī/-ro-kēt): A bacterium having a spiral shape. — spirochetal, adj.

Spirochetes

spirochetemia (spī-rō-kē-tē′-mi-a): Spirochetes in the bloodstream. This kind of bacteremia occurs in the secondary stage of syphilis and in the syphilitic fetus.—spirochetemic, adj.

spirocheticide (spī-rō-kĕt′-i-sīd): An agent that destroys spirochetes.—spirocheticidal, adj.

spirograph (spī′-rō-graf): An apparatus which records the depth and rapidity of movement of the lungs.—spirographic, adj.; spirographically, adv.; spirography, n.

spirometer (spī-rom′-e-ter): An instrument for measuring the air capacity of the lungs. See **bronchospirometer**.—spirometric, adj.; spirometry, n.

spissated (spis′-āt-ed): Inspissated (*q.v.*).

spittle (spit′l): Sputum or saliva that is expectorated.

splanchnic (splangk′-nik): Pertaining to or supplying the viscera, especially the abdominal viscera. S. NERVES, those of the sympathetic system that supply the abdominal viscera.

splanchnicectomy (splangk-ni-sek′-to-mi): Surgical removal of the splanchnic nerves, whereby the viscera are deprived of sympathetic impulses; occasionally performed in the treatment of essential hypertension or for the relief of certain kinds of visceral pain.

splanchno-: Denotes the viscera.

splanchnology (splangk-nol′-o-ji): The study of the structure and function of the viscera.

splanchnomegaly (splangk-nō-meg′-a-li): Abnormal enlargement of one or more of the viscera.

splayfoot (splā′-foot): Flatfoot.

spleen (splēn): An elongated, oval, lymphoid, vascular organ lying in the upper left quadrant of the abdominal cavity, immediately below the diaphragm at the tail of the pancreas and behind the stomach. It is one of the blood-forming organs, stores blood, and acts as a blood filter. Apparently not essential to life as it can be removed without endangering the patient's life.—splenic, adj.

splen-, spleno-: Denotes the spleen.

splenadenoma (splēn-ad-en-ō′-ma): Hyperplasia of the spleen.

splenectasia (splēn-ek-tā′-si-a): Enlargement of the spleen.

splenectomy (splēn-ek′-to-mi): Surgical removal of the spleen.

splenic (splen′-ik): Pertaining to the spleen. S. ANEMIA, Banti's disease (*q.v.*). S. FLEX-

URE, the bend in the colon just beneath the spleen where the transverse colon becomes the descending colon.

splenitis (splēn-ī′-tis): Inflammation of the spleen.

splenocaval (splēn-ō-kā′-val): Pertaining to the spleen and inferior vena cava, usually referring to anastomosis of the splenic vein to the inferior vena cava.

splenogram (splēn-ō-gram): Radiographic picture of the spleen after injection of radiopaque medium.—splenograph, splenography, n.; splenographical, adj.; splenographically, adv.

splenomegaly (splēn-ō-meg′-al-i): Enlargement of the spleen.

splenoportal (splēn-ō-por′-tal): Pertaining to the spleen and portal vein.

splenoportogram (splēn-ō-port′-ō-gram): Radiographic picture of the spleen and portal vein after injection of radiopaque medium.—splenoportograph, splenoportography, n.; splenoportographical, adj.; splenoportographically, adv.

splenorenal (splēn-ō-rē′-nal): Pertaining to the spleen and kidney, as anastomosis of the splenic vein to the renal vein; a procedure carried out in some cases of portal hypertension.

splenorrhagia (splēn-ō-rāj′-i-a): Hemorrhage from a ruptured spleen.

splint: An apparatus, usually rigid, used to prevent movement between the broken ends of a bone, to immobilize a joint or other part, or to restrict motion of a part of the body.—splint, v.t.

spondyl-, spondylo-: Denotes a vertebra.

spondyl(e) (spon′-dil): A vertebra.

spondylitis (spon-di-lī′-tis): Inflammation of one or more vertebrae. Pott's disease (*q.v.*). RHEUMATOID S., a condition of unknown etiology, characterized by pain, stiffness, and ankylosing of the sacroiliac, intervertebral, and costovertebral joints, rigidity of the spine and thorax. Occurs mostly in men between 20 and 40 years of age. Also called ankylosing S.

spondylolisthesis (spon-di-lō-lis-thē′-sis): Forward displacement of one of the lower vertebrae on the one below it; more common in men; resulting deformity makes it appear that the trunk has descended into the pelvis.

spondylosis (spon-di-lō′-sis): Degeneration of the vertebral bodies or of the intervertebral disks with an abnormal fusion or growing together of two or more vertebrae.

Often called osteoarthritis of the spine.

spondylosyndesis (spon-di-lō-sin′-de-sis): Spinal fusion; surgical immobilization or ankylosis of the vertebrae.

sponge: 1. The elastic, fibrous skeleton of a marine organism. 2. A folded piece of gauze or a piece of cotton used for mopping up fluids, for dressings, etc.

spontaneous (spon-tān′-ē-us): Occurring without apparent cause. S. ABORTION, unexpected premature delivery of the contents of a pregnant uterus. S. FRACTURE, one occurring without apparent injury; sometimes seen in certain diseases of the bone. S. GENERATION, an obsolete theory in microbiology that microorganisms arise spontaneously.

sporadic (spō-rad′-ik): Scattered; occurring in isolated cases; not epidemic.—sporadically, adv.

spore (spōr): A phase in the life cycle of a limited number of bacterial genera where the vegetative cell becomes encapsulated and metabolism almost ceases. These spores are highly resistant to environmental conditions such as heat and desiccation. The spores of important species such as *Clostridium tetani* and *Cl. botulinum* are ubiquitous so that sterilization procedures must ensure their removal or death.

sporicidal (spōr-i-sī′-dal): Lethal to spores.—sporicide, n.

sporotrichosis (spōr-ō-tri-kō-sis): A subacute or chronic disease caused by infection of a wound with a fungus (*Sporotrichum schenkii*). There results a primary sore with lymphangitis and subcutaneous painless granulomata which tend to break down and become ulcerous. Occurs among those working in the soil.

sport: An organism that varies entirely or partly from others of the same type and which may transmit this variation to its offspring; a mutation.

sporulation (spōr-ū-lā′-shun): The formation of spores.

spot: In medicine, a circumscribed area that differs from the surrounding area in color, texture, elevation or other characteristics; a macule. See **rose spots, liver spots, Koplik's spots.**

spotted fever: 1. A name given to several eruptive fevers that are characterized by the appearance of distinctive spots, including typhus and Rocky Mountain spotted fever. 2. Endemic cerebrospinal fever, caused by the meningococcus.

spotting: The loss of a slight amount of blood between menstrual periods, but enough to spot a napkin.

sprain: Injury to the soft tissues surrounding a joint caused by forcible wrenching or hyperextension of the joint; sometimes ligaments or tendons are ruptured but the bone is not fractured or dislocated; accompanied by pain, swelling, and discoloration.

Sprengel's shoulder deformity: Congenital high scapula, a permanent elevation of the shoulder, often associated with other congenital deformities, *e.g.,* the presence of a cervical rib or the absence of vertebrae. [Otto G. K. Sprengel, German surgeon. 1852-1915.]

sprue (sproo): A chronic disorder due to malabsorption in the intestinal tract, occurring mostly in the tropics and characterized by glossitis, indigestion, weakness, emaciation, anemia, diarrhea, steatorrhea.

spur: A projection as from a bone. CALCANEAL S., one on the lower surface of the heel bone; causes pain in walking.

sputum (spū′-tum): Excess of secretion from the respiratory passages expectorated through the mouth; consists mainly of mucus and saliva, but may also contain blood, pus, microorganisms.

SQ: One abbreviation for subcutaneous.

squama (skwā′-ma): 1. A scale from the outer layer of skin. 2. A thin plate of bone.—squamous, adj.; squamae, pl.

squamous (skwā′-mus): 1. Scaly. 2. Pertaining to a squama. S. EPITHELIUM, the nonglandular epithelial covering of the external body surfaces. S. CARCINOMA, arising in squamous epithelium; epithelioma.

squint (skwint): Syn., strabismus. Incoordinated action of the muscles of the eyeball, such that the visual axes of the two eyes fail to meet at the objective point. CONVERGENT S., when the eyes turn toward the medial line. DIVERGENT S., when the eyes turn outward.

SR: Abbreviation for sedimentation rate.

s̄s̄: Abbreviation for *semis,* meaning one-half.

s.s.: Abbreviation for soapsuds.

staccato speech (sta-ka′-tō): A jerky manner of speaking with interruptions between words or syllables; scanning speech (*q.v.*).

stage (stāj): 1. The platform-like part of a microscope upon which a slide is placed for viewing. 2. A phase or period in the course of a disease or in the life of an organism.

stain (stān): A dye or other pigment or coloring matter used to color microorganisms or tissue for microscopic examination.

stalk (stawk): In anatomy, a narrow connecting or supporting structure.

stamina (stam'-i-na): Endurance, vigor, strength.

stammer (stam'-er): A speech disorder characterized by halting, repeating, mispronouncing, or inability to pronounce certain sounds; most often seen in children; may be caused by excessive nervousness, agitation, being constantly scolded, emotional states such as fear, worry, insecurity.

standardization (stan-dard-ī-zā'-shun): The bringing of any drug or other substance into conformity with a set standard of purity, concentration, etc.

Stanford-Binet test: The Binet-Simon intelligence test as it has been revised and prepared at Stanford University; it is an individually administered test used to measure intelligence.

stapedectomy (stā-pe-dek'-to-mi): Surgical removal of stapes for otosclerosis.

stapes (stā'-pēz): The stirrup-shaped innermost bone of the middle ear.—stapedial, adj. S. MOBILIZATION, release of a stapes rendered immobile by otosclerosis.

Staph: Common abbreviation for Staphylococcus.

staphyl-, staphylo-: Denotes: (1) the uvula; (2) a structure or arrangement that resembles a bunch of grapes.

staphylectomy (staf-i-lek'-to-mi): Amputation of the uvula.

staphylitis (staf-i-lī'-tis): Inflammation of the uvula.

Staphylococcus (staf-i-lō-kok'-us): A genus of bacteria. Gram-positive cocci occurring in clusters. May be saprophytic or parasitic. Common commensals of man, in whom they are responsible for much minor pyogenic infection, and a lesser amount of more serious infection. A common cause of hospital cross-infection.—staphylococcal, staphylococcic, adj.; staphylococci, pl. S. AUREUS, produces a golden-yellow pigment on culture media; responsible for many diseases and infections in man.

staphyloma (staf-i-lō'-ma): A protrusion of the cornea or sclera of the eye.—staphylomata, pl.

staphylorrhaphy (staf-i-lor'-a-fi): The operation for closing or uniting a cleft uvula or a cleft palate.

starch: A complex carbohydrate, classed as a polysaccharide, found abundantly in nature in rice, corn and other cereals, in vegetables, and in unripe fruits.

stasis (stā'-sis): Stagnation, cessation or stoppage of flow of blood, urine or other body fluid, or of the motion of a part, *e.g.,* the intestines. INTESTINAL S., atony or sluggish bowel contractions resulting in constipation, auto-intoxication, neurasthenia and other symptoms.

Stat: Abbreviation for *statim,* meaning immediately.

state medicine: A method of managing medical treatment in which a governmental body supervises medical care and regulates financial aspects of care, the objective being to furnish medical care to all who need it.

static (stat'-ik): Not dynamic; not moving; resting.

status (stā'-tus): State. Condition. S. ASTHMATICUS is a prolonged and refractory attack of asthma. S. EPILEPTICUS describes epileptic attacks following each other almost continuously. S. LYMPHATICUS is a morbid condition found mostly in children, in which there is hypertrophy of lymphoid tissue, particularly of the thymus; sudden death is not unusual in these patients, especially when they are under the influence of an anesthetic.

steapsin (stē-ap'-sin): The lipase of the pancreatic juice which splits fat into fatty acids and glycerine.

steat-, steato-: Denotes fat.

steatolysis (stē-a-tol'-i-sis): The process by which fats are emulsified in the intestine.

steatoma (stē-a-tō'-ma): 1. A retention cyst of a sebaceous gland. 2. A lipoma. Also steatocystoma.

steatorrhea (stē-a-tō-rē'-a): A syndrome of varied etiology associated with multiple defects of absorption from the gut and characterized by the passage of pale, bulky, greasy stools.

Steinmann's pin: An alternative to the use of a Kirschner wire (*q.v.*) for applying skeletal traction to a limb. [Fritz Steinmann, Swiss surgeon. 1872-1932.]

stellate (stel'-āt): Star-shaped. S. GANGLION, a large collection of nerve cells (ganglion) on the sympathetic chain in the root of the neck.

Stellwag's sign: Occurs in exophthalmic goiter (Graves' disease). Patient does not blink so often as usual, and the eyelids close only imperfectly when he does so, also the upper eyelid is retracted so that the palpebral opening is widened. [Carl Stellwag von Carion, Austrian ophthalmologist. 1823-1904.]

stem: A supporting structure; a stalk. BRAIN S., all of the brain except the cerebrum and the cerebellum.

sten-, steno-: Denotes narrow; constricted.

stenocoriasis (sten-ō-ko-rī'-a-sis): Contraction of the pupil.

stenosed (sten-ōst'): Narrowed; constricted.

stenosis (sten-ō'-sis): Abnormal narrowing of any canal or orifice.—stenotic, stenosed, adj. AORTIC S., narrowing of the orifice between the heart and the aorta CARDIAC S., narrowing of any of the heart cavities or orifices. MITRAL S., narrowing of the bicuspid opening between the left atrium and ventricle. PULMONARY S., narrowing of the orifice between the right ventricle and pulmonary artery. PYLORIC S., narrowing of the orifice between the stomach and small intestine. TRICUSPID S., narrowing of the orifice between the right atrium and ventricle.

Stensen's duct (sten'-sen): The duct leading from the parotid gland and opening in the cheek opposite the upper second molar tooth. [Niels Stensen or Steno, Danish anatomist. 1638-1686.]

stercobilin (ster-kō-bī'-lin): The brown pigment of feces; it is derived from the bile pigments.

stercobilinogen: Urobilinogen (*q.v.*).

stercolith (ster'-kō-lith): A hard, dry mass of fecal matter in the intestine.

stercoraceous (ster-kō-rā'-shus): Consisting of, containing, or resembling feces. Also stercoral. S. VOMITING, the vomiting of material that contains feces.

stereognosis (ster-ē-og-nō'-sis): Recognition of objects by handling them; perception through the sense of touch.—stereognostic, adj.

stereoscope (ster'-ē-ō-skōp): An instrument that projects two images of the same object which when blended, give an impression of depth to a single picture of that object.

stereotactic surgery: Electrodes and cannulae are passed to a predetermined point in the brain for physiological observation or destruction of tissue in such diseases as paralysis agitans, epilepsy, multiple sclerosis. Used for the relief of intractable pain also.—stereotaxy, stereotaxis, n.

sterile (ster'-il): 1. Free from living microorganisms and their products. 2. Not fertile; barren.—sterilize, v.t.

sterility (ster-il'-i-ti): 1. Being free from microorganisms. 2. Being unable to conceive or bear offspring.

sterilization (ster-il-i-zā'-shun): 1. The process of completely ridding material or tissue of living microbes. 2. Rendering an individual incapable of reproduction.

sterilizer (ster'-i-līz-er): A mechanism, chemical, or method used for making any material or object free of living microorganisms.

stern-, sterno-: Denotes the sternum or breast.

sternal (ster'-nal): Pertaining to or related to the sternum. S. PUNCTURE, aspiration of bone marrow from the sternum for diagnosis of certain diseases of the blood or bone marrow.

sternoclavicular (ster-nō-kla-vik'-ū-lar): Pertaining to the sternum and the clavicle. Also sternocleidal.

sternocleidomastoid (ster-nō-klī-dō-mas'-toid): S. MUSCLE, a strap-like muscle arising from the sternum and clavicle, and inserting into the mastoid process of the temporal bone. It draws the head toward the shoulder and assists to flex the head and neck. See **torticollis.**

sternocostal (ster-nō-kos'-tal): Pertaining to the sternum and ribs.

sternotomy (ster-not'-om-i): Surgical division of the sternum.

sternum (ster'-num): The breastbone; a narrow, flat bone, shaped like a dagger, with a handle (manubrium), blade (body), and tip (xiphoid). The first seven costal cartilages are attached to it on either side; it articulates with the clavicles above.—sternal, adj.

sternutation (ster-nū-tā'-shun): Sneezing, or a sneeze.

steroids (stē'-roidz): A term embracing a naturally occurring group of chemicals allied to cholesterol and including sex hormones, adrenal cortical hormones, bile acids, etc. By custom it often now implies the natural adrenal glucocorticoids, viz., hydrocortisone and cortisone, or synthetic analogues such as prednisolone and prednisone.

sterol (stēr'-ol): Any one of a class of solid alcohols widely distributed in nature; they are waxy materials found in plant and animal tissues; cholesterol is the best known of the group.

stertor (ster'-tor): A snore. Noisy or laborious breathing as occurs in deep sleep or in coma.—stertorous, adj.

stertorus 336

stertorous (ster'-tor-us): Pertaining to or characterized by stertor or snoring.

steth-, stetho-: Denotes the chest.

stethoscope (steth'-ō-skōp): An instrument used for listening to the various body sounds, especially those of the heart and lungs —stethoscopic, adj.; stethoscopically, adv.

Stevens-Johnson syndrome: A severe type of erythema multiforme of unknown etiology which affects children and young adults. Sometimes attacks follow administration of sensitizing drugs. It is characterized by the abrupt onset of fever, malaise and ulcerative lesions of the mouth, pharynx, and anogenital region, conjunctivitis, keratitis; ulceration of the cornea may cause gradual loss of vision. Syn., ectodermosis erosiva pluriorificialis. [Albert Mason Stevens, American pediatrician. 1884-1945. Frank Chambliss Johnson, American pediatrician. 1894-1934.]

-sthen: Denotes strength, power.

sthenia (sthēn'-i-a): A condition of normal strength and activity. Opp., asthenia.

stiff neck: Torticollis; wryneck. Rigidity of neck muscles due to spasm.

stigma (stig'-ma): In medicine (1) a spot or mark on the skin; or (2) any physical or mental mark or characteristic that aids in diagnosis of a particular condition, e.g., facies of congenital syphilis.—stigmata, stigmas, pl.; stigmatic, adj.

stilette (stil-et'): 1. A thin wire or metal rod for maintaining patency of a hollow instrument or rigidity of a catheter. 2. A small, slender, sharp surgical probe. Also stylet.

stillborn: Born dead.

Still's disease: A form of rheumatoid polyarthritis, of unknown cause, character-

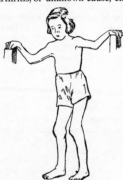

Still's disease

ized by high fever, skin rashes, abdominal discomfort, progressive pain and tenderness of joints, especially the larger joints; later by lymphadenectomy, splenomegaly, valvular heart disease, ankylosis, especially of the cervical spine, impaired growth and development. Occurs in young children. Also called 'arthritis deformans juvenilis.' [George Frederic Still, English physician. 1868-1941.]

stimulant (stim'-ū-lant): Stimulating or promoting functional activity. An agent which excites or increases function.

stimulate (stim'-ū-lāt): 1. To excite to functional activity or growth. 2. To elicit a response in a special organ or system.—stimulation, n.

stimulus (stim'-ū-lus): Anything that is capable of exciting functional activity in an organ or part.—stimuli, pl. ADEQUATE S., one that arouses a response in a particular receptor. INADEQUATE or SUBLIMINAL S., one that is too weak to arouse a response. THRESHOLD S., one that is just strong enough to arouse an appropriate response.

stirrup bone: The stapes (q.v.).

stitch: 1. A sudden, sharp, darting pain. 2. A suture. 3. To fix an organ or part in a certain position or to bring the edges of a wound together with a needle and some suture material used as thread. S. ABSCESS, one that forms at the site of a wound, made by a stitch, and due to nonsterile suture material or pus-forming bacteria on the skin.

stockinet, stockinette (stok-i-net'): A soft, circular-knit material, usually cotton, having elastic properties and used for bandages, under casts, etc.

Stokes-Adams syndrome: A fainting (syncopal) attack, commonly transient, which frequently accompanies heart block; characterized by slow and occasionally irregular pulse, vertigo, fainting, sometimes convulsions, Cheyne-Stokes respiration, and unconsciousness. Also Adams-Stokes syndrome. [William Stokes, Irish physician. 1804-1878. Robert Adams, Irish physician. 1791-1875.]

stom-, stoma-, stomo-, stomata-, -stoma: Denotes a mouth or opening.

stoma (stō'-ma): 1. Any minute pore, orifice or opening. 2. The mouth. 3. An artificial opening established surgically between an organ and the exterior or between two organs or parts.—stomal, adj.; stomata, pl.

stomach (stum'-ak): The most dilated part of the digestive tube, situated between the

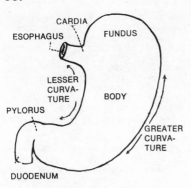

CARDIA
ESOPHAGUS
FUNDUS
LESSER CURVATURE
BODY
PYLORUS
GREATER CURVATURE
DUODENUM

The stomach when full

esophagus (cardiac orifice) and the beginning of the small intestine (pyloric orifice); it lies just under the diaphragm in the epigastric, umbilical and left hypochondriac regions of the abdomen. The wall is composed of four coats: serous, muscular, submucous, and mucous. HOURGLASS S., one partially divided into two halves by an equatorial constriction following scar formation. UPSIDE-DOWN S., common term for a S. that is wholly or partially situated above the diaphragm. S. TUBE., one inserted into the S. through the mouth and used for feeding or for washing out the S.

stomachic (stum-ak′-ik): 1. Pertaining to the stomach. 2. An agent that increases the appetite and improves digestion, especially one of the bitters.

stomatic (stŏm-at′-ik): Relating to the mouth.

stomatitis (stŏ-ma-tī′-tis) Inflammation of the mucous membrane of the mouth. ANGULAR S., fissuring in the corners of the mouth, usually due to riboflavin deficiency, pellagra or sensitivity to dental materials. APHTHOUS S., recurring crops of small ulcers in the mouth; relationship to herpes simplex suspected but not proven. See **aphthae.** GANGRENOUS S., see **cancrum oris.** ULCERATIVE S., characterized by chronically recurring painful shallow ulcers on cheeks, tongue, lips.

-stomy: Denotes a surgical opening into a hollow organ or a new opening between two structures.

stone (stŏn): Calculus; a hardened mass of mineral matter.

stool: The feces. An evacuation of the bowels.

strabismus (stra-biz′-mus): A condition in which the axis of one eye is not parallel with that of the other. It is called convergent s. when the eye turns toward the nose and divergent s. when it turns outward. See **squint.**

strain (strān): 1. To exert effort to the limit of one's ability. 2. An injury resulting from over-exercise, overuse or improper use. 3. To overstretch some part of the musculature of the body. 4. To filter. 5. A group of microorganisms within a species whose common properties are maintained through successive generations.

strait (strāt): A constricted or narrow space or passage, as of the pelvic canal.

strait jacket: Common name for a device used to restrain irrational or restless patients; consists of a shirt with long sleeves which are fastened so as to restrict movement of the arms.

strangle (strang′-g'l): 1. To suffocate, choke, or cause one to be choked by compression or obstruction of the trachea sufficiently to prevent breathing. 2. To deny an organism or a part of a vital substance such as blood, water, air.

strangulated (strang′-ū-lāt-ed): The condition of being compressed or constricted so as to cut off the supply of air, blood or other vital substance from a part. S. HERNIA, see **hernia.**

strangulation (strang-ū-lā′-shun): 1. Choking caused by compression, constriction or obstruction of air passages with consequent arrest of breathing. 2. Arrest of blood circulation to a part by compression or constriction of the blood vessels.

strangury (strang′-gŭ-ri): Frequent desire to urinate with slow and painful micturition; due to spasm of the urethral muscles.

strapping: The application of strips of adhesive tape that overlap; used to cover, support, exert pressure on, or immobilize a part in such condition as strain, sprain, dislocation or fracture.

Strassmann's operation: A plastic operation to make a bicornuate (*q.v.*) uterus a more normal shape. [Paul F. Strassmann, German gynecologist. 1866-1938.]

stratified (strat′-i-fīd): Arranged in layers.

stratum (strā′-tum): A lamina or layer of differentiated tissue, *e.g.*, one of the layers of the skin.—strata, pl.; stratified, adj.

streph-, strepho-, strepto-: Denotes twisted, a twisted chain.

strephosymbolia (stref-ō-sim-bō′-li-a): Reversal of letters, words, or phrases in reading or writing, *e.g.*, g-o-d for d-o-g; found mainly in children; may result from forcing a left-handed person to use the right hand for eating, writing, etc.

strepticemia (strep-ti-sē′-mi-a): Streptococcemia (*q.v.*).

streptococcal (strep-tō-kok′-al): Pertaining to or caused by a streptococcus.

streptococcemia (strep-tō-kok-sē′-mi-a): The presence of streptococcic organisms in the bloodstream.

Streptococcus (strep-tō-kok′-us): A genus of more or less round bacteria that do not form spores, are nonmotile, gram-positive, and occur in chains of varying lengths. Saprophytic and parasitic species. Pathogenic species produce powerful exotoxins. In man, they are responsible for septic sore throat, tonsillitis, urinary tract infections, puerperal infections, scarlatina, septicemia, erysipelas, endocarditis, rheumatic fever, pneumonia, mastoiditis, glomerulonephritis, wound infections in hospitals.—streptococcal, streptococcic, adj.

streptodornase (strep-tō-dor′-nās): An enzyme used with streptokinase (*q.v.*) in liquefying pus and blood clots. thus promoting healing.

streptokinase (strep-tō-kī′-nās): An enzyme derived from cultures of certain hemolytic streptococci. Because of its fibrinolytic effect, it is usually administered with streptodornase to dissolve and remove clotted blood, fibrinous or purulent accumulations.

streptolysins (strep-tol′-i-sinz): Hemolytic toxins produced by streptococci. Antibody produced in the tissues against streptolysin may be measured and taken as an indicator of recent streptococcal infection.

Streptomyces (strep-tō-mī′-sēz): A genus of microorganisms found mostly in the soil but also occasionally on plants and animals; the source of several antibiotics in common use.

streptosepticemia (strep-tō-sep-ti-sē′-mi-a): Septicemia (*q.v.*) that is caused by a streptococcal organism.

stress: 1. Intense effort; emphasis; pressure; a constraining force or influence. 2. A condition of strain resulting from inability to adjust to factors in the environment and causing physiological tensions; may even be a contributory cause of disease.

stria (strī′-a): A streak; stripe; narrow band. —striae, pl.; striated, adj. STRIAE GRAVIDARUM, lines which appear, especially on the abdomen, as a result of stretching of the skin in pregnancy; due to rupture of the lower layers of the dermis. They are red at first and then become silvery-white.

striated (strī′-āt-ed): Striped. In anatomy, term usually applies to skeletal muscles.

stricture (strik′-tūr): An abnormal congenital or acquired narrowing of a tube, canal or passage; may be temporary or permanent; usually due to inflammation, infection, injury, scar formation, muscle spasm, or growth of abnormal tissue.

stridor (strī′-dor): A harsh high-pitched sound in breathing, caused by air passing through constricted air passages,—stridulous, adj.

stroke (strōk): A sudden severe attack, particularly one resulting from cerebrovascular accident. APOPLECTIC S., one in which sudden unconsciousness occurs as a result of intracranial hemorrhage, thrombosis or embolism. HEAT S., one resulting from hyperpyrexia due to inhibition of the heat-regulating mechanism in conditions of high temperatures or high humidity or because sweating is interfered with; marked by dry skin, vertigo, headache, nausea, muscular cramps. PARALYTIC S., one in which injury to the brain or spinal cord causes paralysis of some part or parts of the body. S. VOLUME, the amount of blood ejected by the left ventricle at each heart beat.

stroma (strō′-ma): The interstitial substance or supporting framework of a structure as distinguished from its specific functional physiological element.—stromal, stromatic, adj.

strontium 90: Radioactive isotope with a relatively long half-life (28 years).

strophulus (strof′-ūl-us): Prickly heat; miliaria (*q.v.*).

struma (stroo′-ma): 1. Goiter. 2. Scrofula (*q.v.*).

Stryker frame (strī′-ker): An anterior and posterior frame mounted on a stand with a device by which they can be pivoted and the patient turned from his back to his face. He is placed on the posterior frame, the anterior frame is placed over him and he is securely fastened between the two frames before he is turned. Then the first frame is removed and he remains on his face until it is time to turn him again and the process is repeated. Used in cases where it is necessary to keep the spine immobile, for burn cases and other instances when the patient cannot be turned in the ordinary manner.

stump: The remaining distal end of a part that has been amputated.

stun: To knock unconscious by a blow or other force; to daze.

stupe (stoop): A piece of cloth, usually woolen, or a sponge, that has been placed in hot water and then wrung almost dry before being applied to a part of the body; a medicament with irritating properties or turpentine may be added to the water. See **fomentation.**

stupefacient (stū-pē-fā′-shent): 1. Inducing stupor. 2. An agent that causes stupor.

stupor (stū′-por): A state of marked impairment of, but not complete loss of consciousness. The victim shows gross lack of responsiveness, usually reacting only to noxious stimuli. In psychiatry there are three main varieties of s.: depressive, schizophrenic and hysterical.—stuporous, adj.

Sturge-Weber syndrome: A genetically determined congenital ectodermosis; associated with mental subnormality and buphthalmos (*q.v.*). [William A. Sturge, English physician. 1850-1919. Frederick Parkes Weber, English physician. 1863-1962.]

stutter (stut′-ter): To speak with hesitation and spasmodic repetition of the initial consonant of a word or syllable due to anxiety, nervousness, or an impediment.

St. Vitus's dance: Chorea (*q.v.*). Called after a 3rd century child martyr who was invoked by sufferers of chorea.

sty, stye (stī): Inflammation of one of the sebaceous glands at the edge of the eyelid. Syn., hordeolum.

styl-, styli- stylo-: Denotes: (1) pillar or pillar-like; (2) a projecting bony process.

styloid (stī′-loid): Long and pointed; resembling a pen or stylus. Used especially in reference to a bony process.

stylus (stī′-lus): In pharmacology, a pencil-shaped stick of some substance containing a medicament such as a caustic.

styptic (stip′-tik): 1. Astringent or hemostatic in action. 2. An astringent applied locally to stop bleeding.

sub-: Denotes: (1) under, below; (2) near, almost, moderately; (3) less than normal.

subacute (sub-a-kūt′): Moderately severe. Often the stage between the acute and chronic phases of a disease. S. BACTERIAL ENDOCARDITIS, see **endocarditis.**

subarachnoid (sub-a-rak′-noid): Beneath the arachnoid membrane. S. SPACE, the space between the arachnoid membrane and the pia mater; it contains cerebrospinal fluid.

subaural (sub-aw′-ral): Beneath the ear.

subclavian (sub-klā′-vi-an): Beneath the clavicle.

subclinical (sub-klin′-ik-al): 1. The period in the course of a disease before the symptoms are severe enough to make the disease identifiable. 2. A condition or infection not severe enough to cause the classic identifiable disease.

subconjunctival (sub-con-jungk-tī′-val): Under the conjunctiva.—subconjunctivally, adv.

subconscious: 1. That portion of the mind outside the range of clear consciousness, but capable of affecting conscious mental or physical reactions. 2. Partially but not wholly conscious.

subcostal (sub-kos′-tal): Beneath a rib or ribs.

subcutaneous (sub-kū-tā′-nē-us): Beneath the skin.—subcutaneously, adj.

subcuticular (sub-kū-tik′-ū-lar): Beneath the cuticle or epidermis as a s. abscess.

subdermal (sub-der′-mal): Subcutaneous (*q.v.*).

subdiaphragmatic (sub-dī-a-frag-mat′-ik): Beneath the diaphragm.

subdural (sub-dū′-ral): Beneath the dura mater; between the dura and arachnoid membranes.

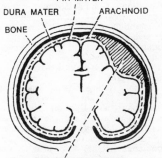

Subdural hematoma

subendocardial (sub-end-ō-kar′-di-al): Immediately beneath the endocardium.

subhepatic (sub-hep-at′-ik): Beneath the liver.

subinvolution (sub-in-vō-lū′-shun): The failure of an organ to return to its normal size and condition after enlargement; said especially of the uterus that fails to return to its normal size after childbirth. See **involution.**

subjacent (sub-jā′-sent): Lying below or under.

subjective (sub-jek′-tiv): Internal; personal; arising from the senses and not influenced by the environment or perceptible to others. Opp., objective. S. SYMPTOMS, those perceived only by the patient and not perceptible to the observer.

sublatio (sub-lā′-shi-ō): The removal or detachment of a part; sublation (q.v.). S. RETINAE, detachment of the retina.

sublation (sub-lā′-shun): Detachment, removal or elevation of an organ or part.

sublethal (sub-lē′-thal): Almost fatal. S. DOSE, one that contains not quite enough of a toxic substance to cause death.

sublimate (sub′li-māt): A solid deposit resulting from the condensation of a vapor. In psychiatry, to redirect a drive or primitive desire into some more socially acceptable channel, e.g., a strong tendency to aggressiveness sublimated into athletic activity.—sublimation, n.

subliminal (sub-lim′-in-al): Inadequate for perceptible response. Below the threshold of consciousness. See liminal, stimulus.

sublingual (sub-ling′-gwal): Beneath the tongue.

sublobular (sub-lob′-ū-lar): Beneath a lobule. S. VEINS, those below the liver that receive the blood from the intralobular veins.

subluxation (sub-luk-sā′-shun): Incomplete or partial dislocation of a joint.

submandibular (sub-man-dib′-ū-lar): Below the mandible.

submaxilla (sub-mak-′sil-a): The lower jawbone; the mandible.

submaxillary (sub-mak-′sil-a-ri): Beneath the lower jaw.

submental (sub-men′-tal): Beneath the chin.

submucosa (sub-mū-kō′-za): The layer of areolar connective tissue beneath a mucous membrane which attaches it to the underlying tissues.—submucous, submucosal, adj.

submucous (sub-mū′-kus): Beneath a mucous membrane. S. RESECTION, an operation for the correction of a deviated septum in the nose.

subnormal (sub-nor′-mal): Having less of something than is normal; said especially of intelligence. Being inferior to an accepted standard.

subnormality: A state of arrested or incomplete development of mind which includes s. of intelligence and is of a nature or degree which requires or is susceptible to medical treatment or other special care or training of the patient. SEVERE S., a state of arrested or incomplete development of mind which includes s. of intelligence and is of such a nature or degree that the patient is incapable of living an independent life or of guarding himself against exploitation, or will be so incapable when of a normal age to do so.

suboccipital (sub-ok-sip′-it-al): Beneath the occiput; in the nape of the neck.

subperiosteal (sub-per-i-os′-ti-al): Beneath the periosteum of bone.

subperitoneal (sub-per-i-to-nē′-al): Beneath the peritoneum.

subphrenic (sub-fren′-ik): Beneath the diaphragm.

subpituitarism (sub-pi-tū′-i-tar-izm): Hypopituitarism (q.v.).

subpubic (sub-pū′-bik): Situated or performed below the pubic arch. See **suprapubic.**

subscapular (sub-skap′-ū-lar): Beneath the scapula.

substance (sub′-stans): The material of which something is made; in the body it refers to the materials that make up the organs and tissues and to which they owe their characteristic qualities.

substandard (sub stan′-dard): Descriptive of something that falls short of the usual or accepted standard of quality.

substantia (sub-stan′-shi-a): In anatomy, substance or tissue.

substernal (sub-ster′-nal): Beneath the breastbone (sternum).

substitution (sub-sti-tū′-shun): 1. In chemistry, the replacement of one substance in a compound by another substance. 2. Something that is used in place of another substance; may be cheaper or inferior, or not. 3. An artificial product used in place of a natural one; usually to correct a deficiency of the natural product, e.g., a hormone. 4. In psychology and psychotherapy, the person who takes the place of or acts for another person in relation to the patient. 5. The unconscious acceptance of a suitable goal or emotion for one that is unacceptable or unattainable.

substratum (sub-strā′-tum): A lower stratum or layer; an underlying structure or part.

subsultus (sub-sul′-tus): Muscular twitching, jerking or tremor. S. TENDINUM, twitching of tendons and muscles particularly around the wrist in severe fever, such as typhoid.

subtotal (sub′-tō-tal): Somewhat less than total or complete. S. HYSTERECTOMY, see **hysterectomy.**

subungual (sub-ung′-gwal): Beneath a finger or toe nail.

Sucaryl sodium (soo′-ka-ril): Trademark for

a calorie-free liquid sweetener; a preparation of cyclamate.

succagogue (suk′-a-gog): Stimulating a glandular secretion or the flow of a juice, or an agent that does this.

succorrhea (suk-ō-rē′-a): An abnormal increase in the flow of a secretion or a juice, *e.g.*, saliva, intestinal juice.

succus (suk′-us): A juice, especially that secreted by glands in the small intestine and which functions in the digestive process; it is called succus entericus.

succussion (su-kush′-on): Splashing sound produced by fluid in a hollow cavity on shaking the patient, *e.g.*, liquid content of dilated stomach in pyloric stenosis. HIPPOCRATIC S., the splashing sound, on shaking, when fluid accompanies a pneumothorax.

suckle (suk′-l): 1. To suck or draw nourishment from the breast. 2. To feed an infant at the breast.

sucrase (sū′-krās): An intestinal enzyme that acts to split sucrose; invertase.

sucrose (sū′-krōs): Cane, beet or maple sugar. A disaccharide. It is normally converted into dextrose and levulose in the body.

sucrosemia (sū-krō-sē′-mi-a): The presence of sucrose in the blood.

sucrosuria (sū-krō-sū′-ri-a): The presence of sucrose in the urine.

suction (suk′-shun): The act or process of sucking up or aspirating.

sudamina (sū-dam′-i-na): Minute, transient, whitish vesicles caused by the retention of sweat in the ducts or the corneum of the skin occurring after profuse perspiration; sweat rash.—sudamen, sing.

sudden infant death syndrome: See SIDS.

sudor (sū′-dor): Sweat.—sudoriferous, adj.

sudoresis (sū-dō-rē′-sis): Profuse sweating.

sudorific (sū-dor-if′-ik): An agent which induces sweating. Diaphoretic.

sudorrhea (sū-dō-rē′-a): Excessive sweating; hyperhidrosis.

suffocation (suf-ō-kā′-shun): Asphyxia (*q.v.*).

suffusion (su-fū′-zhun): 1. Extravasation or spreading of blood or other body fluid into surrounding parts. 2. A sudden reddening of the surface as in blushing. 3. The act of pouring a fluid over the body or wetting it.

sugar: A sweet carbohydrate of animal or vegetable origin. See **carbohydrate.**

suggestibility (sug-jes-ti-bil′-i-ti): Susceptibility to suggestion (*q.v.*); is heightened in hospital patients, in the dependence on others that illness brings, in children, some mental defectives, and those with a tendency to hysteria.

suggestion (sug-jest′-shun): The implanting in a person's mind of an idea which he accepts fully without logical reason. In psychiatric practice, s. is used as a therapeutic measure sometimes under hypnosis or narcoanalysis (*q.v.*).

sulcus (sul′-kus): A furrow or groove, particularly one separating gyri or convolutions of the cortex of the brain.—sulci, pl.

sulf-, sulfo-: Denotes sulfur, or derivation from sulfur or sulfuric acid.

sulf-, sulfa-, sulph-, sulpha-: Denotes derivation from sulfanilic acid.

sulfa drugs: Sulfonamides (*q.v.*).

sulfanilamide(sul-fa-nil′-a-mīd): The first sulfonamide (*q.v.*), and parent of the other sulfa drugs.

sulfate (sul′-fāt): Any salt of sulfuric acid. See **salt.**

sulfide (sul′-fīd): A compound of sulfur and an element or base.

sulfite (sul′-fīt): Any salt of sulfurous acid.

sulfonamides (sul-fon′-a-mīds): A group of synthetic drugs derived from sulfonic acid. Their action is bacteriostatic,thus they prevent multiplication of bacteria and allow the body to build its defenses against the organisms.

sulfones (sul′-fōns): A group of synthetic drugs related to the sulfonamides, useful in treatment of leprosy; also sometimes used in tuberculosis.

sulfur (sul′-fur): A non-metallic element, frequently used in various combinations in medicine.

sulfuric acid (sul-fū′-rik): Heavy, colorless, odorless, oily liquid; extremely corrosive and caustic.

sulph-: For words beginning thus, and not found here, see words beginning sulf-.

sum: Abbreviation for *sumat*, meaning let him take. Used in prescription writing.

sunburn: Reddening of the skin and dermatitis caused by direct exposure to the rays of the sun. The reaction varies with the individual and the degree of exposure.

sunstroke: A condition produced by overexposure to the direct rays of the sun; marked by convulsions, coma, and high temperature of the skin. See **stroke.**

super-: Denotes: (1) situated above, over; (2) extra, in addition; (3) in excess; (4) higher in degree, quantity or quality.

supercilium (sū-per-sil′-i-um): The eyebrow. —supercilia, pl.; superciliary, adj.

superego (sū-per-ē′-gō): That part of the personality that is concerned with moral standards and ideals, derived mainly from parents, teachers, and others in the environment. The theoretical part of the mind; popularly referred to as the conscience.

superficial (sū-per-fish′-al): At or near the surface.

supergenual (sū-per-jen′-ū-al): Above the knee.

superinfection (sū-per-in-fek′-shun): A second infection developing in a person who has not recovered from another one.

superior (sū-pē′-ri-or): Situated above. In anatomy, the upper of two parts.

supernatant (sū-per-nā′-tant): 1. Above or on the top of something. 2. The upper layer of material, liquid or solid, that remains after the precipitation of a solid part of a mixture.

supernumerary (sū-per-nū′-mer-ar-i): In excess of the normal number; additional.

supersaturate (sū-per-sat′-ū-rāt): To add more of an ingredient than can be held in solution permanently, the excess being precipitated when the physical conditions are changed.

supinate (sū′-pin-āt): To turn face or palm upward. Opp., pronate.—supination, n.

supinator (sū-pin-ā′-tor): That which supinates (q.v.), usually applied to a muscle. Opp., pronator.

supine (sū-pīn′): Lying on the back with the face and palms of the hands turned upward. Having the palm of the hand turned upward or outward. Opp., prone.

supplemental air: That air that remains in the lung after an ordinary expiration but which can be exhaled when one makes a forcible effort to do so.

suppository (su-poz′-i-tō-ri): Medicament in a semi-solid base that remains solid at room temperature but melts at body temperature, for insertion into a body orifice other than the mouth, e.g., rectum, vagina, urethra. Usually shaped like a cone or cylinder.

suppression (su-presh′-un): 1. Holding back; repressing; arresting. 2. Cessation or arrest of a secretion (e.g., urine) or a normal process (e.g., menstruation), as distinguished from retention (q.v.). In psychology, the conscious, intentional forcing out of the mind of painful thoughts or feelings; may result in the precipitation of a neurosis (q.v.).

suppuration (sup-ū-rā′-shun): The formation or discharge of pus.—suppurative, adj.; suppurate, v.i.

supra-: Denotes: (1) a situation above, over or higher; (2) beyond; (3) the same as super-, and often used interchangeably with it.

supraclavicular (soop-ra-kla-vik′-ū-lar): Above the collar bone (clavicle).

supracondylar (soop-ra-kon′-dil-ar): Above a condyle.

supradiaphragmatic (soop-ra-dī-a-fragmat′-ik): Above the diaphragm.

supralethal (soop-ra-lē′-thal): More than enough to kill.

supraliminal (soop-ra-lim′-i-nal): Above the threshold of consciousness.

supraorbital (soop-ra-or′-bit-al): Above the orbits. S. RIDGE, the ridge formed by the prominence of the frontal bone, covered by the eyebrows.

suprapubic (soop-ra-pū′-bik): Above the pubic arch. S. CYSTOTOMY, surgical opening of the bladder just above the pubis.

suprarenal (soop-ra-rē′-nal): 1. Above the kidney. 2. Tiny endocrine gland just above each kidney. Syn., adrenal (q.v.).

suprasternal (soop-ra-ster′-nal): Above the breast bone (sternum).

supravergence (soop-ra-ver′-jens): The upward movement of one eye while the other eye remains stationary.

sura (sū′-rah): The calf of the leg.—sural, adj.

surdity (sur′-di-tē): Deafness.

surfactant (sur-fak′-tant): A phospholipid that is manufactured in the alveoli of the lungs, lines them, and prevents them from collapsing during exhalation. In the newborn, it reduces the adhesion between the unexpanded walls of the alveoli.

surgeon (sur′-jun): A medical practitioner who treats diseases, disorders or deformities by operative procedures.

surgery (sur′-jer-i): That branch of medicine that treats diseases, deformities and injuries, wholly or in part, by manual or operative procedures. ASEPTIC S., that performed in a field kept free of pathogenic bacteria. CLOSED S., that done without making an incision, e.g., reduction of a dislocation. CONSERVATIVE S., that in which diseased or injured parts are repaired but removal is avoided if possible. MAJOR S., important and serious operations that may involve risk to life. MINOR S., simpler, less serious operations that do not usually involve risk to life. OPEN-HEART S., corrective operation on heart valves after they have been exposed to direct vision. ORAL S., that done to treat disorders of the mouth and teeth; a branch of dentistry. ORTHOPEDIC S., that which treats diseases or deformities of the skeletal system. PLASTIC S., that which repairs or reconstructs a tissue or part by such methods as skin grafting or transplanting of other tissue. RADICAL S., see **radical.**

surrogate (sur'-ō-gāt): A substitute or replacement for something or someone.

susceptibility (sus-sep-ti-bil'-i-ti): The opposite of resistance. Usually refers to a disposition to infection.

suspension (sus-pen'-shun): 1. Temporary cessation, as of a vital process. 2. A mixture in which finely divided particles are dispersed throughout a liquid but are not dissolved in it. 3. A method of treatment whereby a part or the whole of a patient's body is suspended in a desired position. 4. The fixation of an organ or part in correct position by suturing it to other tissues, *e.g.,* suspension of the uterus.

suspensory (sus-pen'-so-ri): 1. Descriptive of a structure, often a ligament, that functions to hold an organ or part in correct position. 2. A bandage or other material used to support a dependent part or organ, *e.g.,* the scrotum.

suture (sū'-tūr): 1. The jagged line of union of cranial bones. 2. A stitch or series of stitches used to close a wound. 3. The act of stitching to close a wound. 4. The material used to close a wound by stitching; see **ligature.** ABSORBABLE S., one made with a material that is liquefied in the body and absorbed. CONTINUOUS S., one of a series of sutures made with one length of

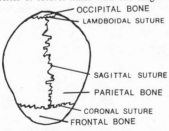

OCCIPITAL BONE
LAMDBOIDAL SUTURE
SAGITTAL SUTURE
PARIETAL BONE
CORONAL SUTURE
FRONTAL BONE

Sutures of the skull

material. INTERRUPTED S., one of a series of sutures each one being made with a separate piece of material. NON-ABSORBABLE S., one that is not liquefied and absorbed by the body. PURSE-STRING S., a stitching around the edge of a circular opening that is then drawn up tightly to close the opening.

swab (swob): 1. To use a small tuft of cotton or similar material to cleanse an area or a cavity or absorb an exudate. 2. A small piece of cotton or similar material wound firmly around one or both ends of a shaft of wire or wood; used to cleanse a cavity, apply a medication or collect a specimen for laboratory examination; in the latter case it is sterilized within a protective tube.

swathe (swath): To envelop, cover, wrap or bind tightly as with a bandage.

sweat: 1. Sudor; a clear, watery, slightly salty fluid secreted by the sweat glands in the skin. 2. To perspire or sweat. S. TEST, a diagnostic procedure used in fibrocystic disease of the pancreas; it is a meaurement of sodium in the sweat; see **cystic fibrosis.** NIGHT S., profuse sweating while asleep, often a symptom of pulmonary tuberculosis.

sweetbread: The pancreas of an animal, usually the calf, used as a food.

swelling (swel'-ling): A transient, abnormal elevation or enlargement of a body part or area, usually on the surface, that is not caused by new growth or proliferation of cells; may be due to injury, inflammation or edema.

swoon: Syncope (*q.v.*).

sycoma (sī-kō'-ma): A large soft wart-like growth.

sycosis (sī-kō'-sis): A skin disease in which inflammation of the hair follicles, usually by a staphylococcal organism, results in papules or pustules and scab formation. S. BARBAE, pustular folliculitis of the beard area in men; barber's itch. S. NUCHAE is a similar folliculitis at the nape of the neck which leads to keloid thickening (acne keloid).

Sydenham's chorea: Chorea with comparatively moderate convulsive muscular movements; chorea minor. [Thomas Sydenham, famous English physician. 1624-1689.]

sylvian (sil'-vi-an): Referring to the fissure of Sylvius (*q.v.*).

Sylvius (sil'-vi-us): FISSURE OF S., a deep fissure at the side of each cerebral hemisphere; the temporal lobe lies below it. [Franciscus de le Boë Sylvius, Dutch physician. 1614-1672.]

sym-, syn-: Denotes: (1) together, union of, association, similar; (2) at the same time.

symbiosis (sim-bĭ-ō'-sis): The living together or association of two or more organisms of different species in which the participants may or may not mutually aid and benefit one another.—symbiotic, adj.

symblepharon (sim-blef'-a-ron): Adhesion of one or both of the lids to the eyeball.

symbol (sim'-bol): A letter or mark that represents an idea or word (s) or, in chemistry, an atom or group of atoms of a substance.

symbolism (sim'-bol-izm): In psychiatry, the unconscious substitution of a symbol to express thoughts or ideas that the individual had previously been unable or unwilling to accept or express.

Syme's amputation: Amputation at the ankle joint with removal of both malleoli. Provides an end-bearing stump. Especially useful in primitive conditions where elaborate artificial limbs are not available. [James Syme, Scottish surgeon. 1799-1870.]

symmetry (sim'-e-tri): Correspondence or equality of size, shape and general characteristics of two similar parts of the body.

sympathectomy (sim-pa-thek'-to-mi): Surgical excision of a sympathetic nerve or surgical interruption of sympathetic nerve pathways.—sympathectomize, v.t.

sympathetic (sim-pa-thet'-ik): 1. Exhibiting sympathy. 2. Influenced by or produced by disease in another part of the body. s. NERVOUS SYSTEM, a portion of the autonomic nervous system; composed of a chain of ganglia on either side of the vertebral column in the thoracolumbar region; sends fibers to all involuntary muscle tissue and glands.

sympathin (sim'-pa-thin): An old name for chemical substances liberated by sympathetic nerve endings; now known to be epinephrine and norepinephrine.

sympathomimetic (sim-path-ō-mĭ-met'-ik): Capable of producing changes similar to those produced by stimulation of the sympathetic nerves.

symphysiotomy (sim-fiz-i-ot'-o-mi): The surgical separation of the pubic bone, at its symphysis, to facilitate the birth of a living child.

symphysis (sim'-fi-sis): A very slightly movable joint in which there is a fibrocartilaginous union of bones, as occurs between the two parts of the pubic bone, the vertebrae, and the sacrum and ilium.—symphysiac, symphyseal, symphysial, adj.; symphyses, pl.

symptom (simp'-tom): Any morbid phenomenon, condition, or evidence of disease. CARDINAL S., a major s., especially one that pertains to temperature, pulse, or respiration. DEFICIENCY S., one that indicates reduction in or lack of secretion of an endocrine gland, or lack of a vital element in the patient's diet. OBJECTIVE S., one apparent to the observer. PRESENTING S., the s. or group of s's. the patient complains of most. PRODROMAL S., one that precedes the diagnostic s's. of a disease. SUBJECTIVE S., one that is apparent only to the patient. SYMPTOM COMPLEX, a group of symptoms which, occurring together, typify a particular disease or syndrome.—symptomatic, adj.

symptomatology (sim-tom-a-tol'-o-ji): 1. The branch of medicine concerned with symptoms. 2. The combined symptoms typical of a particular disease.

Synanon (sin'-a-non): A social movement, begun in 1958, that is concerned with the reeducation of persons affected with drug addiction, alienation, or any other type of antisocial behavior. This is accomplished through a drug-free, crime-free, totally integrated community. S. HOUSES are maintained in 6 U.S. cities for the 1300 resident members; the 6000 nonresident members go to these houses for various activities connected with their reeducation. Partly self-supporting, it also receives some community support.

synapse (sin'-aps): The point of communication between two neurons. The place where the axon of one neuron comes into contact with the dendrites of another and an impulse is chemically transmitted from one neuron to the other.

synarthrosis (sin-ar-thrō'-sis): An immovable articulation of bones, as the cranial sutures.—synarthroses, pl.

synchondrosis (sin-kon-drō'-sis): The joining of bones by cartilage, as occurs, *e.g.,* between the diaphysis and shaft of long bones in immature individuals.

synchronous (sin'-kro-nus): Occurring at the same time.

synchysis (sin'-ki-sis): A degenerative condition of the vitreous body of the eye which renders it fluid. S. SCINTILLANS, the appearance of flashes of reflected light caused by the presence of fine crystals in the vitreous; they are usually cholesterol or fatty acid crystals.

syncope (sin′-ko-pi): A faint; caused by cerebral anemia. May be a symptom of disease or may result from an emotional experience such as fright when the peripheral blood vessels dilate and drain the blood from the brain. The loss of consciousness is usually temporary.—syncopal, adj.

syndactyly (sin-dak′-ti-li): A congenital anomaly in which the fingers and/or toes are webbed. Also syndactylism, syndactylia.—syndactylous, adj.

syndesmosis (sin-des-mō′-sis): A fixed joint (synarthrosis) in which the surfaces of the bones are joined to each other by fibrous connective tissue, e.g., the joint at the distal ends of the tibia and fibula.

syndrome (sin′-drōm): A group of symptoms and/or signs that, occurring together, produce a pattern or symptom complex that is typical of a particular disease, disturbance, disorder or lesion.

synechia (sin-ek′-i-a): Abnormal union of parts, especially adhesion of the iris to the cornea in front, or the lens capsule behind. —synechiae, pl.

synergism (sin′-er-jizm), **synergy** (sin′-er-ji): The harmonious working together of two agents, such as drugs, microoganisms, muscles, etc., so that their combined efforts produce an effect that could not be obtained by their separate actions.—synergic, adj.

synergist (sin′-er-jist): An agent cooperating with another. One partner in a synergic action. See **synergism**.

synesthesia (sin-es-thē′-zi-a): A secondary or concomitant sensation accompanying a sensory response, or one perceived by a sense organ other than the one stimulated as happens, e.g., when a certain sound produces a sensation of color.

synovectomy (si-nov-ek′-to-mi): Excision of synovial membrane. Current early treatment for rheumatoid arthritis, especially of the hands and of the knees.

synovia (si-nō′-vi-a): The transparent, alkaline, viscous fluid secreted by the membrane lining a joint cavity; its function is to lubricate and thus minimize friction during joint movement. Also synovial fluid.

synovial membrane (si-nō′-vi-al mem′-brān): That lining a joint capsule; it does not cover the articular surfaces. It secretes a lubricating fluid, synovia. See **bursa**.

synovioma (si-nō-vi-ō′-ma): A tumor of synovial membrane origin, benign or malignant.

synovitis (sin-ō-vī′-tis): Inflammation of a synovial membrane.

synthesis (sin′-the-sis): The chemical building up of complex substances from simpler substances.—synthetic, adj.; synthesize, v.t.

syphilid(e) (sif′-i-lid): General term for any syphilitic skin lesion.

syphilis (sif′-il-is): [Syphilis, syphilitic shepherd in poem by Fracastorius (1530), in which the term first appears.] A severe contagious venereal disease, caused by the *Treponema pallidum*. Infection is acquired, commonly by sexual intercourse, or the fetus may acquire it from the mother while in utero. CONGENITAL S., marked by coryza, skin eruptions, malformed teeth, wasting of the tissues, and craniotabes (*q.v.*). ACQUIRED S., manifests in: (1) The primary stage; appears 4 to 5 weeks (or later) after infection when a primary chancre associated with swelling or local lymph glands appears. (2) The secondary stage in which the skin eruption appears. (3) The third (tertiary) stage occurs 15 to 30 years after initial infection. Gummata appear, or neurosyphilis and cardiovascular S. intervene. The commonest types of nervous system involvement are general paralysis of the insane and tabes dorsalis (locomotor ataxia). Cardiovascular involvement produces cerebrovascular disasters, aortic aneurism, or destruction of the aortic valve.—syphilitic, syphilous, adj.

syphiloma (sif-i-lō′-ma): A tumor of syphilitic origin; a gumma.

syrigmus (si-rig′-mus): Ringing in the ears.

syringe (si-rinj′): An instrument for injecting or withdrawing liquids; of differing sizes and designs depending upon the specific purpose for which it is used.

syringomyelia (si-ring-gō-mī-ē′-li-a): An uncommon, progressive disease of the nervous system of unknown cause, beginning mainly in early adult life. Cavitation and surrounding fibrous tissue reaction, in the upper spinal cord and brain stem, interfere with sensations of pain and temperature, and sometimes with the motor pathways. The characteristic symptom is painless injury, particularly of the exposed hands. Touch sensation is intact.

syringomyelocele (si-ring-gō-mī′-e-lō-sēl): Most severe form of meningeal hernia (spina bifida). The central canal is dilated

syrup

and the thinned-out posterior part of the spinal cord is in the hernia.

syrup: A concentrated solution of sugar and water usually containing a drug.

system (sis′-tem): 1. A collection of parts that unite in the performance of a particular duty. In anatomy, a group of organs that work together to perform a particular function. 2. The entire (physical) body organism.—systemic, adj.

systemic (sis-tem′-ik): 1. Related to a particular system of the body. 2. Related to the body as a whole.

systole (sis′-to-li): The contraction phase of the cardiac cycle.—systolic, adj. EXTRA S., a premature contraction of an atrium or ventricle, or both, which does not alter the fundamental rhythm of contractions.

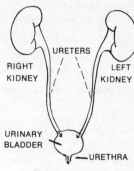

Urinary system

T

T: Abbreviation for (1) temperature; (2) tension.

TA: Abbreviation for toxin-antitoxin.

TAB: A mixed vaccine containing killed *Salmonella typhi, Paratyphi A* and *B*; used to produce immunity to typhoid and paratyphoid fever; usually given in 3 ascending doses a week apart; confers immunity for varying lengths of time, usually one to three years.

Tab: Abbreviation for tablet.

tabes (tā′-bēz): Progressive emaciation; wasting away. Term usually used in connection with tabes dorsalis. T. DOR-SALIS (locomotor ataxia), is a variety of neurosyphilis in which there is progressive sclerosis of the posterior (sensory) columns of the spinal cord, the sensory nerve roots and the peripheral nerves. It is marked by muscular incoordination, ataxia (*q.v.*), anesthesia, joint disorders, neuralgia, sometimes paralysis. Usually occurs after middle life. T. MESENTERICA, tuberculous enlargement of the peritoneal lymph nodes; seen in children.

tabetic (ta-bet′-ik): 1. Pertaining to tabes. 2. Affected with tabes.

table: In anatomy, the external or internal layer of compact bone separated by a layer of cancellous bony tissue called the diploë, that make up the bones of the cranium.

tablespoon: A large spoon used in household measurements; holds approximately 4 fluidrams or 15 milliliters.

tablet: In pharmacology, a small disk of varying size and thickness, containing a dose of a medication, in either pure or diluted form.

taboo, tabu (ta-bu′): A prohibition imposed by social usage or for the protection of the group; in primitive groups often related to the supernatural.

taboparesis (tā-bō-par-ē′-sis): A condition of general paralysis of the insane in which the spinal cord shows the same lesions as in tabes dorsalis (*q.v.*).

tache (tahsh): A macule, blemish or spot, *e.g.*, a freckle.—tachetic, adj.

tachy-: Denotes rapid, swift.

tachycardia (tak-i-kar′-di-a): Excessively rapid action of the heart with resulting increase in the pulse rate; some of the causes are heart disease, hyperthyroidism, high fever, toxemia. PAROXYSMAL T., sudden marked increase in the pulse rate, lasting for variable lengths of time and then suddenly disappearing; sometimes accompanies failing heart muscle action but in some people it is of nervous origin.—tachycardiac, tachycardic, adj.

tachylalia (tak-i-lā′-li-a): Rapidity of speech.

tachyphagia (tak-i-fā′-ji-a): Abnormally rapid eating; bolting of food.

tachyphrasia (tak-i-frā′-zi-a): Volubility; extremely rapid flow of speech; may be seen in certain nervous disorders. Also tachyphasia.

tachypnea (tak-ip-nē′-a): Abnormal frequency of respiration, frequently seen in hysteria, neurasthenia, high fevers, respiratory infections; sometimes but not always accompanied by dyspnea (*q.v.*).

tactile (tak′-til): 1. Pertaining to the sense of touch. 2. Perceptible through the sense of touch. 3. Real; tangible. T. CORPUSCLES, see **Meissner's corpuscles.**

tactual (tak′-tū-al): Pertaining to or caused by touch.

Taenia (tē′-ni-a): A genus of flat, parasitic worms; cestodes or tapeworms. T. ECHIN-OCOCCUS, the adult worm lives in the dog's intestine (the definitive host) and man (the intermediate host) is infested by swallowing eggs from the dog's excrement. These become embryos in the human small intestine, pass via the bloodstream to organs, particularly the liver, and develop into hydatid cysts. T. SAGINATA, larvae present in infested, undercooked beef. In man's (the definitive host) intestinal lumen they develop into the adult tapeworm, which, by its four suckers attaches itself to the gut wall. It grows to 12-25 feet in length and is the most common tapeworm of man in the U.S. Consists of a head and numerous segments, each one being capable of independent existence, therefore in treatment it is necessary for the head to be expelled. T. SOLIUM resembles T. SAGINATA, but has hooklets as well as suckers. The larvae are ingested in infested, undercooked pork; man can also be the intermediate host for this worm by ingesting eggs which, developing into larvae in his stomach, pass via the bowel wall to reach organs, and there develop into cysts. In the brain these may give rise to epilepsy.

talc, talcum: A naturally occurring soft white powder consisting of magnesium silicate.

taliped (tal'-i-ped), **talipedic** (tal-i-pēd'-ik): Clubfooted.

talipes (tal'-i-pēz): Descriptive of several types of congenital foot deformities, especially clubfootedness of which there are four main types. T. CALCANEUS, dorsal flexion of the foot results in walking with only the heel touching the ground. T. EQUINUS, hyperflexion of the foot results in walking with only the toes touching the ground. T. VALGUS, eversion of the foot results in walking on the inner edge of the foot only. T. VARUS, inversion of the foot results in walking on the outer edge of the foot only; the opp. of valgus.

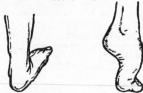

talipes calcaneus   talipes equinus

talipes valgus   talipes varus

talus (tā'-lus): The astragalus; situated between the tibia proximally and the calcaneus distally, thus directly bearing the weight of the body. It is the second largest bone of the ankle.

tampon: A ball of absorbent cotton, gauze, sponge or similar substance used to pack or plug a canal or cavity to restrain hemorrhage, absorb secretions, or apply medication.

tamponade: 1. The insertion of a tampon. See **cardiac.** 2. A device for checking internal hemorrhage.

tantalum (tan'-ta-lum): A rare, noncorrosive, malleable metal, used sometimes in the form of wire sutures, flat plates to re-pair skull injuries, or wire mesh to reinforce weak areas in the body, as in the repair of a large hernia.

tantrum: An unreasoning fit of anger accompanied usually by violent physical gestures, seen in children and sometimes in mentally disturbed patients.

tapeworm: Taenia (*q.v.*).

tapotement (ta-pōt'-mon): A percussive or tapping movement in massage, usually performed with the side of the hand.

tapping: Aspiration. Paracentesis (*q.v.*).

tarsal: 1. Relating to the eyelid or the plates of cartilage in the eyelid. 2. Relating to the bones of the tarsus (*q.v.*).

tarsalgia (tar-sal'-ji-a): Pain in the foot or ankle.

tarsometatarsal (tar-sō-met'-a-tar-sal): Pertaining to the tarsal and metatarsal regions.

tarsoplasty (tar'-sō-plas-ti): Any plastic operation to the eyelid.

tarsoptosia (tar-sop-tō'-si-a): Flatfootedness; falling of the tarsus.

tarsorrhaphy (tar-sor'-ra-fi): Suturing together of the eyelids, partially or entirely, to shorten the palpebral fissure or to protect the cornea when there is paralysis of the obicularis muscle or to allow healing in case of chronic ulcer. Also blepharorrhaphy.

tarsus (tar'-sus): 1. The part of the foot that is behind the metatarsals; made up of seven bones: the calcaneus or heel bone, the talus or ankle bone, and the cuboid, navicular, and first, second and third cuneiform bones. 2. The thin elongated plates of dense connective tissue found in each eyelid, contributing to its form and support.—tarsal, adj.

tartar: A hard yellowish deposit that forms on the teeth.

taste: 1. The power to perceive and distinguish flavors. 2. The sensation produced when the specialized nerve endings in the taste buds are stimulated. T. BUDS, small clusters of specialized cells located in the epithelium of the tongue and the inside of the mouth; they connect with the surface by small pores through which substances in solution enter and stimulate the nerve endings contained in the buds thus giving rise to the sensation of taste. They are classified according to the composition of the substance to which they are sensitive: sweet, acid, salty, bitter.

TAT: 1. Abbreviation for toxin-antitoxin. 2. Abbreviation for thematic apperception test; used in psychiatry; the patient is shown a series of drawings that depict life scenes and situations and his interpretations of these pictures are thought to be indicative of his mood and personality.

taut (tawt): Tightly drawn or tensely stretched; not loose or flabby.

-taxia, -taxis, -taxy: Denotes order, arrangement.

taxis (tak′-sis): 1. The restoration of a displaced part to its normal position by manual manipulation; term often used in relation to the reduction of a hernia by manipulation. 2. The reflex movement that occurs in response to a stimulus; term is usually attached to a word that designates the kind of stimulus, *e.g.,* chemotaxis, thermotaxis.

taxonomy (taks-on′-o-mi): The scientific and orderly classification of plants and animals, or the principles and laws upon which such classification is made.

Tay-Sachs disease: Amaurotic familial idiocy (*q.v.*). Thought to be an error of fat metabolism resulting in cerebral lipoidosis. [Warren Tay, English physician. 1843-1927. Bernard Sachs, New York neurologist. 1858-1944.]

TB: Abbreviation for (1) tubercle bacillus; (2) tuberculosis.

T-bandage: See **bandage**. Also called T-binder.

tbsp: Abbreviation for tablespoon.

TD: Abbreviation for tetanus and diphtheria toxoids.

tears (tērz): The clear, slightly alkaline secretion formed by the lacrimal gland; function is to keep the conjunctiva moist. Contain the enzyme lysosome which acts as an antiseptic. See **lacrimal**.

tease: To draw or pull out or separate into fine threads or minute shreds; refers especially to preparation of tissue for microscopic examination.

teaspoon: A spoon of small size used in household measurements; contains approximately 1 fluidram or 4 milliliters.

teat (tēt): A nipple.

technic, technique (tek-nēk′): The detailed systematic manner in which a specific procedure, such as a mechanical or surgical operation or a test, is performed. ISOLATION T., the methods used to prevent the spread of pathogenic organisms or infection from one patient to other individuals.

technician (tek-nish′-un): One who has had training in and uses the techniques required

for carrying out the specific procedures of a profession.

technologist (tek-nol′-o-jist): Technician (*q.v.*).

teeth: Any of the small bone-like structures that are set in the jaws and used for chewing; they also assist in articulation. Each tooth is made up of a pulp cavity which contains a soft pulpy substance that supports blood vessels and nerves, and a solid part consisting of dentin or ivory which is covered above the gum with enamel—the hardest substance in the body—and below the gum with cementum. The part above the gum is called the crown and the part below is the root. In man, the deciduous, baby or milk teeth erupt between the 6th and 24th months of life and are shed by the age of approximately 7 years. The permanent set, 32 in number, is usually complete in the late teens and consists of 4 incisors, 2 canines, 4 premolars, and 6 molars in each jaw. CANINE or EYE T. have a sharp fang-like edge for tearing food. IMPACTED T., T. so placed that they cannot erupt into their normal position. INCISOR T. have a knife-like edge for biting food. PEG or PEGGED T., Hutchinson's T. (*q.v.*). PREMOLAR and MOLAR T., have a squarish termination for chewing and grinding food. STOMACH T., the lower canine T. WISDOM T., the last molar T., one at either side of each jaw.

teething (tēth′-ing): Dentition; the eruption of teeth. Term is usually applied to eruption of the first or deciduous set.

tegmentum (teg-men′-tum): 1. A covering. 2. That part of the brain stem that lies behind the peduncles that connect the cerebrum with the pons.—tegmental, adj.

tegument (teg′-ū-ment): The skin or covering of the animal body; the integument.—tegumental, tegumentary, adj.

tel-, tele-, telo-: Denotes far off, at a distance, over a distance.

tela (tē′-la): In anatomy any web-like structure; a thin, delicate tissue.—telae, pl.

telangiectasia (tel-an-ji-ek-tā′-si-a): Abnormal dilatation of the terminal capillaries on a body surface; seen frequently on the face in certain disorders of the circulation. When the condition is congenital it results in a discoloration commonly called a 'birthmark.'

telangioma (tel-an-ji-ō′-ma): An angioma made up of dilated terminal capillaries.

telepathy (te-lep′-a-thi): Mental communication, without any obvious means, between people who are at a distance from

each other. Thought transference. Also
called extrasensory perception.

teleradium (tel-e-rā/-di-um): Radium whose
radiation is directed into the body from an
external source; radium beam.

teletherapy (tel-e-ther/-ap-i): 1. By custom
refers to treatment with teleradium (*q.v.*).
2. Absent treatment, as that used by
mental healers.—teletherapeutic, adj.; tele-
therapeutically, adv.

temp: An abbreviation for temperature.

temperament (tem/-per-a-ment): The habitual mental and emotional attitude of an
individual as distinct from mood, which is
temporary. Four types originally described
were sanguine, phlegmatic, bilious or choleric, and melancholic.

temperature (tem/-per-a-tūr): The degree of
heat or coldness of an object or substance
as measured by a thermometer. AXILLARY
T., that registered on a thermometer placed
in the axilla or armpit. INVERSE T., body
temperature that is lower in the evening
than in the morning. MEAN T., the average
temperature of the atmosphere in an area
over a period of time. NORMAL T., usually
refers to that considered normal for the
human body; 36.9° C or 98.4° F. ORAL T.,
that registered on a thermometer placed in
the mouth. RECTAL T., that registered on a
thermometer placed in the rectum. ROOM
T., the ordinary temperature of the atmosphere in a room. SUBNORMAL T., usually
refers to temperature of the body that is
below that considered normal. See **fever,
pyrexia.**

temple: 1. The flattened area on either side
of the head lying between the outer angle of
the eye and the top of the ear flap. 2. One
of the side supports for a pair of spectacles.

temporal (tem/-por-al): 1. Limited in time
or pertinent to time. 2. Relating to the
temple (*q.v.*). T. BONES, one on either side
of the head below the parietal bone; contain the middle ear. T. LOBE, one of the
five lobes of each hemisphere of the cerebrum; lies under the T. bone and contains
the auditory center.

temporofrontal (tem-por-ō-fron/-tal): Pertaining to the temporal and frontal regions
or bones.

temporomandibular (tem-por-ō-man-dib/-
ū-lar): Pertaining to the temporal region
or bone, and the lower jaw.

temporo-occipital (tem-por-ō-ok-sip/-it-al):
Pertaining to the temporal and occipital
regions or bones.

temporoparietal (tem-por-ō-par-ī/-et-al):

Pertaining to the temporal and parietal
regions or bones.

tenacious (te-nā/-shus): 1. Sticky, adhesive,
holding fast. 2. Thick and viscid, usually
said of sputum or other body fluid.

tenaculum (te-nak/-ū-lum): 1. A hook-like
instrument with a sharp point. 2. In anatomy, a fibrous band that helps to hold a
part in its proper position and place.

tendinitis (ten-di-nī/-tis): Inflammation of
a tendon. Also tenonitis, tenontitis, tenosi-
tis.

tendon: A band or cord of firm, white, in-
elastic tissue that forms the termination of
a muscle and attaches it to a bone or other
structure. Syn., sinew.—tendinous, adj. T.
OF ACHILLES, that which connects the gastrocnemius and soleus muscles to the heel
bone. KANGAROO T., T. from the tail of a
kangaroo, used for sutures when delay of
absorption of sutures is desired, *e.g.*, in
orthopedic surgery.

tendovaginitis (ten-dō-vaj-i-nī/-tis): See
tenosynovitis.

tenesmus (ten-ez/-mus): Painful, ineffectual
straining to empty the bowel or bladder.

tenia (tē/-ni-a): 1. An organism of the genus
Taenia (*q.v.*). 2. A flat band or strip of
soft tissue. T. COLI, three flat bands running the length of the large intestine and
consisting of the longitudinal muscle fibers.

teniacide (tē/-ni-a-sīd): An agent that destroys tapeworms.—teniacidal, adj.

teniafuge (tē/-ni-a-fūj): An agent that
causes the expulsion of tapeworms.

teniasis (tē/-ni-a-sis): Infestation with Taenia (*q.v.*). Also taeniasis.

tennis elbow: Pain and tenderness at the
outer side of the elbow due to injury of the
lateral epicondyle of the humerus and resulting from violent twisting of the hand
as often occurs in playing tennis.

teno-: Denotes tendon.

tenodynia (ten-ō-din/-i-a): Pain in a tendon.

tenonitis (ten-ō-nī/-tis): 1. Inflammation of
Tenon's capsule (*q.v.*). 2. Inflammation of
a tendon.

tenonometer (ten-ō-nom/-e-ter): An instrument for measuring the amount of pressure exerted by the substances within the
eyeball. Also tonometer.

Tenon's capsule: The thin membrane that
envelopes the eyeball from the optic nerve
to the ciliary region and which forms a
capsule or socket within which the eyeball
moves. [Jacques R. Tenon, French anatomist and oculist. 1724-1816.]

tenoplasty (ten/-ō-plas-ti): A plastic operation on a tendon.—tenoplastic, adj.

tenorrhaphy (ten-or′-a-fi): Suturing together the cut or torn ends of a tendon.

tenosynovitis (ten-ō-sin-ō-vī′-tis): Inflammation of the thin synovial lining of a tendon sheath, as distinct from its outer fibrous sheath. It may be caused by mechanical irritation or by bacterial infection.

tenotomy (ten-ot′-o-mi): Division or cutting of a tendon; usually done to correct a deformity caused by a too short muscle, *e.g.*, strabismus.

tense: Tight; strained.

tension: 1. The act of stretching. 2. The state of being stretched. 3. In psychology, a condition of inner unrest, striving or turmoil with a feeling of psychological stress, often manifested in increased muscular tone and other physiological signs of emotional imbalance. ARTERIAL T., that exerted by the blood on the arterial walls. INTRAOCULAR T., that exerted by the contents of the eyeball on the tunics of the eye.

tensor: Any muscle that stretches or causes tension in a part.

tent: 1. A conical cylinder of sponge, cotton or similar material to be introduced into a canal or sinus to dilate it or keep it open. 2. A canopy of material arranged like a tent over a bed or part of a bed. CROUP T., a canopy arranged over the head of the bed in such a way as to maintain a high degree of moisture within it; used in treatment of croup. OXYGEN T., a covering arranged over the bed or head of it so as to maintain a high degree of oxygen when this is being used in therapy.

tentorium (ten-tō′-ri-um): An anatomical part that resembles a tent in shape. T. CEREBELLI, that part of the dura mater which lies between the cerebellum and the cerebrum.—tentorial, adj.

tepid (tep′-id): Lukewarm.

ter-: Denotes three, threefold, three times.

teras (ter′-as): A monster; a fetus with grossly malformed parts.

terat-, terato-: Denotes a teras (monster).

teratism (ter′-a-tizm): The condition of being a monster.

teratogen (ter′-a-tō-jen): Anything capable of disrupting fetal growth and producing malformation. Classified as drugs, poisons, radiation, physical agents such as ECT, infections—*e.g.*, rubella, and rhesus and thyroid antibodies.—teratogenic, teratogenetic, adj.; teratogenicity, teratogenesis, n.

teratoid (ter′-a-toid): Resembling a monster.

teratology (ter-a-tol′-o-ji): The scientific study of monstrosities, malformations and other deviations from normal development.—teratologist, n.; teratological, adj.; teratologically, adv.

teratoma (ter-a-tō′-ma): A tumor of embryonic origin and composed of various kinds of tissues, none of which are native to the part where the tumor occurs and including both epithelial and connective tissues; most commonly found in ovaries and testes.—teratomata, pl.; teratomatous, adj.

teres (tē′-rēz): Round, smooth and long; usually denotes certain muscles and ligaments.

ter in die (ter in dē′-a): Three times a day. Abbreviated t.i.d.

term: A period of time. In obstetrics, the end of the normal period of gestation.

terminal (ter′-min-al): 1. Situated at or forming an end or extremity. 2. Related to the end; final, as the T. stage of a disease. T. INFECTION, infection with a pathogenic organism that occurs during the course of a chronic disease and causes death. T. DISINFECTION, that which is done following a patient's illness, discharge from the hospital, or death; involves disinfecting any substance or object that has been used by the patient or been in contact with him.

terminology (ter-mi-nol′-o-ji): The particular words or expressions used in a special field of endeavor or science.

terror (ter′-er): Excessive fear; fright. NIGHT T., that which occurs in sleep, especially of children; nightmare.

tertian (ter′-shun): Occurring every third day (inclusive); actually every 48 hours. See **malaria.**

tertiary (ter′-shi-ar-i): 1. Third in order. 2. Recurring every third day. 3. Pertinent to a third stage or order.

tertigravida (ter-ti-grav′-i-da): A woman who is pregnant for the third time.

tertipara (ter-tip′-a-ra): A woman who has had three pregnancies resulting in live offspring.

test: 1. A means of examination. 2. A procedure done to determine the presence or absence of a substance. 3. To analyze a substance by the use of chemical reagents. 4. A trial. T. MEAL, one given for later removal from the stomach for gastric analysis. T. TUBE, a thin tube, usually of glass, closed at one end; used in various procedures in chemical and other laboratories. For special tests see under name of the test.

testalgia (tes-tal′-ji-a): Pain in the testes.

testectomy

352

testectomy (tes-tek'-to-mi): Removal of a testis. Also orchidectomy.

testicle (tes'-tik-l): Testis.—testicular, adj.

testis (tes'-tis): One of two glandular bodies contained in the scrotum of the male; they produce spermatozoa and also the male sex hormones.—testes, pl.; testicular, adj. UNDESCENDED T., the organ remains in the pelvis or inguinal canal. Cryptorchism (q.v.).

testitis (tes-ti'-tis): Inflammation of the testes; orchitis.

testosterone (tes-tos'-ter-ōn): The hormone derived from the testes and responsible for the development of the secondary male characteristics. Used in carcinoma of the breast, to control uterine bleeding, and in male underdevelopment.

test tube baby: One that results from impregnation of the mother by artificial insemination. See **insemination.**

test type: Letters of various sizes on cards used in testing visual acuity. SNELLEN'S T.T., square black letters on cards, commonly used for testing distance vision.

tetanic (tet-an'-ik): 1. Characterized by or relating to tetanus. 2. Producing tonic muscle spasm. 3. An agent that produces tonic muscle spasm.

tetanus (tet'-an-us): 1. Lockjaw. An acute infectious disease induced by the toxin of *Clostridium tetani,* an anaerobic organism growing at the site of injury to body tissues; because the organism is present sometimes in road dust, manure, and cultivated soil, accidental wounds, particularly penetrating wounds, may become infected by it. T. is characterized by painful muscular contractions, chiefly of the face and neck, hence the appellation 'lockjaw.' Muscles of the back may become involved and result in opisthotonos (q.v.). 2. Sustained tonic spasm of a muscle or muscles, produced by repetition of stimuli so often that the muscle does not have a chance to relax between their application. PUERPERAL T., that resulting from infection of the obstetric wound. T. ANTITOXIN injection produces passive immunity. DRUG T., that produced by a drug such as strychnine. T. TOXOID injection produces active immunity.—tetanic, tetanoid, adj.

tetany (tet'-a-ni): Condition of muscular hyperexcitability, due to abnormal calcium metabolism, in which mild stimuli produce cramps and spasms (cf. **carpopedal spasm**). Found in parathyroid deficiency, potassium deficiency, alkalosis, vitamin D deficiency, sprue. In infants it is associated with gastrointestinal upset and rickets.

tetr-,tetra-: Denotes four; having four parts.

tetradactyly (tet-ra-dak'-ti-li): The condition of having only four digits on a hand or foot.—tetradactylous, adj.

tetralogy of Fallot: A form of congenital heart defect which includes four abnormalities—narrowing of the pulmonary artery, a septal defect between the ventricles, hypertrophy of the right ventricle, and displacement of the aorta to the right. The condition results in deficient oxygenation of the blood with cyanosis, dyspnea, polycythemia, clubbing of the fingers. [Etienne Louis Arthur Fallot, French physician. 1850-1911.]

tetramastia (tet-ra-mas'-ti-a): The condition of having four breasts.

tetraplegia (tet-ra-plē'-ji-a): Paralysis of all four limbs. Also quadriplegia.

tetravaccine (tet-ra-vak'-sēn): A vaccine containing dead cultures of the organisms of typhoid, paratyphoid A, paratyphoid B and cholera.

tetter (tet'-er): A lay term often used for such skin diseases as eczema, herpes, ringworm, or other eruptions, or for a blister or pimple.

thalamotomy (thal-a-mot'-o-mi): Usually operative (stereotaxic) destruction of a portion of the thalamus, sometimes done in treatment of psychotic disorders that have an emotional basis, or for relief of intractable pain.

thalamus (thal'-a-mus): A collection of grey matter at the base of the cerebrum. Sensory impulses from the whole body (except olfactory) pass through on their way to the cerebral cortex.—thalami, pl.; thalamic, adj.

thalassemia (thal-a-sēm'-i-a): An hereditary, genetically transmitted hemolytic anemia in which there is interference with synthesis of hemoglobin; several types are recognized, according to the symptoms. Also Cooley's anemia, Mediterranean anemia, familial erythroblastic anemia. [Name derived from the Greek word *thalassa,* meaning sea; the disease was first described in people in the Mediterranean Sea area.]

thanat-, thanato-: Denotes death.

thanatopsia (than-a-top'-si-a): Examination of the body after death; autopsy.

Thayer-Martin culture medium: A selective medium for isolation of the pathogenic *Neiserria gonorrhoeae* and *meningitides.*

theca (the'-ka): An enveloping sheath, *e.g.,*

the synovial sheath of a tendon.—thecal, adj. T.VERTEBRALIS, the dura mater of the spinal cord.

thecitis (thē-sī'-tis): Inflammation of the sheath of a tendon.

thelalgia (thē-lal'-ji-a): Pain in the nipple.

thelitis (thē-lī'-tis): Inflammation of a nipple.

thelium (thē'-li-um): 1. Nipple. 2. A papilla.

thenar (thē'-nar): 1. Pertinent to the palm of the hand or the thumb. 2. The fleshy mound at the base of the thumb, called the thenar eminence.

theomania (thē-ō-mā'-ni-a): A type of religious insanity, especially one in which the individual imagines himself to be God or to have divine attributes.

theotherapy (thē-ō-ther'-a-pi): Treatment of disease by prayer or other religious expression.

therapeutic (ther-a-pū'-tik): 1. Pertaining to the treatment of disease. 2. Curative. 3. Descriptive of an agent that is capable of healing or curing. T. ABORTION, one induced because of poor health of the mother. T. COMMUNITY, a specially structured hospital milieu in which patients are encouraged to assume responsibility for their own behavior and to behave in a way that is socially acceptable. Term is applied particularly to mental hospitals.

therapeutics (ther-a-pū'-tiks): The branch of medical science dealing with the treatment of disease.—therapeutic, adj.; therapeutically, adv.

therapist (ther'-a-pist): A person who is trained and skilled in the treatment of a disease or the effects of disease. The word is often used in combination with another that names the disorder being treated or the type of treatment employed, e.g., speech T., physical T.

therapy (ther'-a-pi): The treatment of disease. Term is often used in combination with another which defines it specifically, e.g., drug therapy. DIET T., treatment through management of diet. ELECTROCONVULSIVE T., electric shock treatment. EMPIRIC T., that based on practical experience rather than scientific reasons. ENDOCRINE T., treatment with hormones or glandular secretions. FAMILY T., may be group psychotherapy with a family or individual therapy applied to all family members simultaneously. FEVER T., treatment with artificially produced fever. GROUP T., patients discuss their feelings and problems openly in a group with other patients; the psychiatrist acts as listener and engineer of the discussion. HEAT T., treatment with some form of heat. MILIEU T., treatment, usually psychiatric, in a carefully structured environment in which all elements such as furnishings, equipment, staff, etc. enhance the medical therapy and help the patient toward rehabilitation. OCCUPATIONAL T., the use of some occupation, usually hand crafts, for remedial effects. OXYGEN T., treatment that makes an increased amount of oxygen available to the patient. PHYSICAL T., use of such physical agents as massage, exercise, etc. in treatment. PLAY T., a method of psychiatric treatment in which the child expresses himself through play and thus enables the psychiatrist to establish communication with him. ROENTGEN T., treatment by x-rays or other radioactive substances. SHOCK T., treatment by electric current to produce convulsions; insulin and drugs are also used. SPECIFIC T., that which is directed toward the eradication of the specific cause of a disease. SUBSTITUTION T., supplying a substance that is deficient or lacking in the body. SYMPTOMATIC T., is directed toward the relief of symptoms rather than the basic cause of the disease.

therm: An indefinite term for a unit of heat. It may represent a small calorie, a large calorie, 1000 large calories, or 100,000 British thermal units.

therm-, thermo-: Denotes heat.

thermal (ther'-mal): Pertaining to heat.

thermalgia (ther-mal'-ji-a): Burning pain.

thermoanesthesia (therm-ō-an-es-thē'-zi-a): Loss or lack of the ability to recognize the sensations of heat and cold, or to distinguish between them; often due to spinal cord injury. Also thermanesthesia.

thermocautery (ther-mō-kaw'-ter-i): Destruction of tissue by means of heat, e.g., an electrically heated wire. See **cautery**.

thermoesthesia (ther-mō-es-thē'-zi-a): The ability to recognize sensations of heat and cold and to distinguish between them. Also thermesthesia.

thermogenesis (ther-mo-jen'-e-sis): The production of heat, specifically in the body. —thermogenetic, adj.

thermolabile (ther-mō-lā'-bil): Capable of being altered or destroyed by heat.

thermolysis (ther-mol'-i-sis): 1. The loss of body heat through evaporation, radiation, etc. 2. Chemical decomposition of a substance by use of heat.—thermolytic, adj.

thermometer (ther-mom′-e-ter): A device for determining temperature; consists of a substance such as mercury which expands and contracts with changes in temperature and which is enclosed in a sealed tube, usually glass, that is marked with a graduated scale. BATH T., one used for determining temperature of bath water; usually protected by a wooden case. CENTIGRADE T., one marked with a 100-unit scale in which 0° is the freezing point and 100° the boiling point. CLINICAL T., one used for determining the temperature of the body. FAHRENHEIT T., one marked with a 180-unit scale in which 32° is the freezing point and 212° the boiling point. FEVER T., a clinical T. ORAL T., one used for taking temperature of the body by mouth. RECTAL T., one used for taking temperature of the body by rectum. ROOM T.,one used for determining the temperature of the air in a room.

CLINICAL   BATH   LOTION   WALL

Thermometers

thermophile (ther′-mō-fil): A microorganism that thrives best at a relatively high temperature.—thermophilic, adj.

thermoreceptor (ther-mō-rē-sep′/tor): A nerve ending that is sensitive to heat.

thermostable (ther-mō-stā′b′l): Remaining unaltered at a high temperature, which is usually specified.—thermostability, n.

thermotaxis (ther-mō-tak′-sis): 1. The normal regulation of the body temperature. 2. The reaction that occurs in an organism when stimulated by heat.

thermotherapy (ther-mō-ther′-a-pi): Treatment by the application of heat.

thiamin (thī-a′-min): Aneurine hydrochloride; one of the members of the vitamin B complex; is slowly destroyed by heating. The antineuritic, antiberiberi vitamin. Essential for growth, good appetite and healthy nerves. Found in whole grain cereals and flour, wheat germ, nuts, yeast, liver, lean pork, heart, kidney, milk, egg yolk, leafy vegetables, fruit; also synthesized. Deficiency may produce retardation of growth, loss of appetite, mental apathy, various forms of neuritis and, if severe, beriberi.

thigh (thī): The part of the leg between the hip and the knee. T.BONE, the femur.

third intention: See **healing.**

thirst: A sensation of dryness in the mouth and throat accompanied by a desire for drink.

Thomas collar: A stiff high collar, usually made of metal and covered with leather, used as a support for the head in injuries of the neck or upper spine.

Thomas splint: A metal splint used for emergency treatment or transporting a patient with a fractured leg or arm; it is shaped like a hairpin, the open end being equipped with a padded ring that is placed in the groin or axilla when the splint is applied; it is so constructed that traction can be applied to the limb.

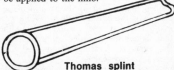

Thomas splint

thorac-, thoraci-, thoraco-: Denotes the chest or chest wall.

thoracectomy (thō-ra-sek′-to-mi): Resection of all or part of a rib.

thoracentesis (thō-ra-sen-tē′-sis): Surgical puncture of the chest wall with the insertion of a trocar and cannula into the chest cavity for the drainage of accumulated fluid; paracentesis. Also thoracocentesis.

thoracic (thō-ras′-ik): Pertaining to the thorax. T.DUCT, a channel conveying lymph (chyle) from the receptaculum chyli in the abdomen to the left subclavian vein.

thoracicoabdominal (thō-ras-i-kō-ab-dom′-

in-al): Pertaining to the thorax and abdomen. Also thoracoabdominal.

thoracodynia (thō-ra-kō-din′-i-a): Pain in the chest.

thoracolumbar (thō-ra-kō-lum′-bar): Pertaining to, arising in, or involving the thoracic and lumbar regions. Term often used in reference to the thoracic and lumbar spinal ganglia and their fibers that go to make up the sympathetic part of the autonomic nervous system.

thoracoplasty (thō′-ra-kō-plas-ti): 1. Plastic surgery on the chest. 2. An operation on the thorax in which the ribs are resected to allow the chest wall to collapse and the lung to rest; used in the treatment of pulmonary tuberculosis.

thoracoscope (thō-rak′-ō-skōp): A lighted instrument that can be inserted into the pleural cavity through a small incision in the chest wall to permit inspection of the pleural surface and treatment under visual control.

thoracostomy (thō-ra-kos′-to-mi): The establishment of a surgical opening into the chest cavity for the purpose of drainage of accumulated fluid.

thoracotomy (thō-ra-kot′-o-mi): Any surgical incision into the chest wall.

thorax (thō′-raks): The chest cavity; that part of the trunk situated below the neck and above the diaphragm and within a bony framework formed by the sternum, ribs and thoracic vertebrae. Contains the trachea, bronchi, lungs, heart and esophagus.—thoracic, adj.

threadworm: Enterobius (Oxyuris) vermicularis, a nematode parasitic in the colon of children.

thready: Describes a pulse that can barely be felt.

threshold (thresh′-old): The lowest point at which a stimulus will evoke a response. RENAL T., the point at which a substance in the blood not normally excreted by the kidneys begins to appear in the urine. T. STIMULUS, see **stimulus**.

thrill: Vibration as perceived by the sense of touch.

thrix: Hair.

-thrix: Denotes hair(s).

throat: The pharynx and fauces; the anterior part of the neck. SEPTIC SORE T., severe inflammation of the fauces and tonsils usually caused by a streptococcus organism.

throb: 1. To beat or pulsate. 2. A beating or pulsation.

throe (thrō): A severe pain or pang, by cus-

tom referring to the pains of childbirth.

thromb-, thrombo-: Denotes: (1) a blood clot; (2) the clotting of blood.

thrombectomy (throm-bek′-to-mi): Surgical removal of a thrombus from within a blood vessel.

thrombin (throm′-bin): An enzyme in shed blood that converts fibrinogen to fibrin; is formed when prothrombin combines with calcium salts. Also called thrombase.

thromboangiitis (throm-bō-an-ji-ī′-tis): Inflammation of the inner coat of a blood vessel with formation of a clot. T. OBLITERANS (syn., Beurger's disease), an uncommon disorder of unknown cause, occurring mainly in young adult males, characterized by patchy, inflammatory, obliterative, vascular disease, principally in the limbs (sometimes in the cardiac or cerebral vessels), and presenting usually as calf pains, or more severely as early gangrene of the toes and following a chronic progressive course.

thromboarteritis (throm-bō-ar-ter-ī′-tis): Inflammation of an artery with clot formation.

thromboclasis (throm-bok′-la-sis): Thrombolysis (q.v.).

thrombocyte (throm′-bō-sīt): Blood platelet; small non-nucleated disk-like body normally present in the blood in concentrations of approximately 300,000 per cu mm; its chief function is to assist in coagulation of the blood.

thrombocytolysis (throm-bō-sī-tol′-i-sis): Destruction of blood platelets.

thrombocytopenia (throm-bō-sī-tō-pē′-ni-a): A reduction in the number of platelets in the blood. Also thrombopenia.—thrombocytopenic, adj.

thrombocytopenic purpura (throm-bō-sī-tō-pē′-nik pur′-pū-ra): A syndrome characterized by a low blood platelet count, intermittent mucosal bleeding and purpura (q.v.). It can be symptomatic, i.e., secondary to known disease or to certain drugs; or idiopathic, a rare condition of unknown cause (syn., purpura hemorrhagica) occurring principally in children and young adults. In both forms the bleeding time is prolonged.

thrombocytosis (throm-bō-sī-tō′-sis): An increase in the number of blood platelets.

thromboembolism(throm-bō-em′-bō-lizm): Obstruction of a blood vessel by a thrombus that has become detached from the site where it was formed and carried to another vessel which it blocks.—thromboembolic, adj.

thromboendarterectomy (throm-bō-end-ar-ter-ek′-to-mi): Operation for removal of a thrombus that is obstructing an artery.

thromboendarteritis (throm-bō-end-ar-ter-i′-tis): Inflammation of the inner lining of an artery with clot formation.

thrombogen (throm′-bo-jen): Prothrombin (*q.v.*).

thrombogenic (throm-bō-jen′-ik): 1. Producing or capable of producing thrombi. 2. Capable of clotting blood. 3. Pertaining to thrombogen.—thrombogenicity, n.; thrombogenetic, adj.; thrombogenetically, adv.

thrombokinase (throm-bō-kin′-ās): Syn., thromboplastin (*q.v.*).

thrombolymphangitis (throm-bō-lim-fan-ji′-tis): Inflammation of a lymph vessel with the formation of a lymph clot.

thrombolysis (throm-bol′-i-sis): The dissolving of a thrombus.

thrombophilia (throm-bō-fil′-i-a): A tendency for thrombi to occur.

thrombophlebitis (throm-bō-flē-bī-tis): Inflammation of the wall of a vein with secondary thrombosis within the involved segment.—thrombophlebitic, adj.

thromboplastin (throm-bō-plas′-tin): An enzyme which converts prothrombin into thrombin. INTRINSIC T., produced by the interaction of several factors during the clotting of blood. Much more active than tissue T. TISSUE T., thromboplastic enzymes are present in many tissues, and tissue extracts are used in clotting experiments and in the estimation of prothrombin time.

thrombosed (throm′-bōs'd): 1. Clotted. 2. Describing a blood vessel that contains a clot.

thrombosis (throm-bō′-sis): The intravascular formation or presence of a clot.—thromboses, pl.; thrombotic, adj. CORONARY T., one that forms in a coronary artery and occludes it thereby depriving the coronary muscle it serves of blood and usually leading to ischemia and infarction of the myocardium.

thrombus (throm′-bus): A clot that is formed by the coagulation of blood and which remains in the location in which it was formed; it may more or less occlude a blood vessel or a heart cavity.—thrombic, thrombotic, adj.

thrush: A disease associated with white spots on the mucous membranes of the mouth and which later become ulcerous; caused by *Candida albicans*. Occurs in malnourished children who feed from unclean nipples and bottles and may involve the esophagus and napkin area. Also sometimes seen in older patients with debilitating diseases when they lack good oral hygiene.

thym-, thymo-: Denotes: (1) the thymus gland; (2) mind, soul, emotions.

thymectomy (thi-mek′-to-mi): Surgical excision of the thymus.

-thymia: Denotes mind, spirit.

thymoma (thi-mō′-ma): A tumor arising in the thymus.—thymomata, pl.

thymus (thi′-mus): A gland-like structure lying behind the manubrium of the sternum and extending upward as far as the thyroid gland. It is well developed in infancy and attains its greatest size towards puberty; then the lymphatic tissue slowly regresses and is replaced by fatty tissue. It has an immunological role. Autoimmunity is thought to result from the pathological activity of this gland.—thymic, adj.

thyr-, thyro-: Denotes the thyroid gland.

thyroadenitis (thi-rō-ad-e-ni′-tis): Inflammation of the thyroid gland.

thyrocele (thi′-rō-sēl): Enlargement of the thyroid gland; goiter.

thyroglossal (thi-rō-glos′-al): Pertaining to the thyroid gland and the tongue.

thyrohyoid (thi-rō-hi′-oid): Pertaining to the thyroid gland and the hyoid (*q.v.*) bone.

thyroid (thi′-roid): 1. Shaped like a shield. 2. The dried, powdered thyroid gland of the ox, sheep, or pig, used in the treatment of cretinism, myxedema, and other conditions caused by thyroid dysfunction. 3. The ductless gland situated in front of and on either side of the upper end of the trachea, in the front part of the neck. It secretes thyroxin(e) which controls body growth and metabolism. T. CARTILAGE, the large cartilage of the larynx, commonly called 'Adam's apple.' T. CRISIS, a serious condition resulting from the sudden increase in the basal metabolism rate due to hyperthyroidism.

thyroidectomy (thi-roid-ek′-to-mi): Surgical removal of the thyroid gland. SUBTOTAL T., removal of less than the entire thyroid gland.

thyroidism (thi′-roid-izm): A pathological condition caused either by overdoses of thyroid extract or by overactivity of the thyroid gland.

thyroiditis (thi-roid-i′-tis): Inflammation of the thyroid gland. LYMPHADENOID T. (Hashimoto's disease), a firm goiter ultimately resulting in hypothyroidism. RIEDEL'S T., a chronic fibrosis of the thyroid gland; ligneous goiter.

thyromegaly (thī-rō-meg′-a-li): Enlargement of the thyroid gland.

thyroncus (thī-rong′-kus): Goiter; thyrocele.

thyrotoxicosis (thī-rō-tok-si-kō′-sis): A condition due to excessive production of the thyroid gland hormone (thyroxine), probably in response to stimulation by an excessive production of pituitary thyrotrophic hormone, and resulting classically in anxiety, tachycardia, sweating, increased appetite with weight loss, a fine tremor of the outstretched hands, and prominence of the eyes. It is much commoner in women than in men. In older patients cardiac irregularities may be a prominent feature.—thyrotoxic, adj. Also called hyperthyroidism, thyrotoxemia, thyrotoxia.

thyrotropic (thī-rō-trō′-pik): 1. Directly affecting the secretory function of the thyroid gland. 2. A substance that stimulates the gland to activity, *e.g.*, the T. hormone secreted by the anterior pituitary gland.

thyrotropin (thī-rot′-rō-pin): A hormone originating in the anterior lobe of the pituitary gland; has the specific function of stimulating the thyroid gland. T. RELEASING FACTOR, a hormone that originates in the hypothalamus of the brain; controls release of thyrotropin by the pituitary gland which, in turn, acts upon the thyroid gland causing i t to release thyroid hormone. Isolated and synthesized in 1969; expected to become of major importance in diagnosing and treating disorders of the thyroid gland. Abbreviated TRF.

thyroxin(e) (thī-rok′-sin): An iodine-containing amino acid that is the chief active principle of the hormone secreted by the thyroid gland; essential for normal growth and metabolism. It is also prepared synthetically.

tibia (tib′-i-a): The shinbone; the inner, thicker of the two bones of the leg below the knee; it articulates with the femur, fibula and talus.—tibial, adj.

tibialgia (tib-i-al′-ji-a): Pain in the tibia.

tibiofemoral (tib-i-ō-fem′-o-ral): Pertaining to the tibia and the femur.

tibiofibular (ti-bi-ō-fib′-ū-lar): Pertaining to the tibia and the fibula.

tic (tik): Minor, purposeless, repetitious, involuntary gestures or muscular movements and twitchings, most often of the face, head, neck or shoulder, due to habit

usually but also may be associated with a psychological factor. T. DOULOUREUX, trigeminal neuralgia; severe spasms of excruciating pain in an area supplied by one of the branches of the trigeminal nerve, especially the face or mouth.

tick (tik): A mite larger than others of the same class of bloodsucking arthropods. Some of them are transmitters of diseases such as relapsing fever, Q fever, Rocky Mountain spotted fever, typhus, tularemia.

t.i.d.: Abbreviation for *ter in die*, meaning three times a day.

tidal air: See **air**.

tidal drainage: A method for continuous irrigation, most commonly used in treatment of paralyzed bladder or following surgery on the bladder; sometimes used for irrigating the chest cavity after empyema.

tinct: Abbreviation for tincture.

tincture (tink′-tūr): Solution of a drug in alcohol.

tinea (tin′-ē-a): A general term for several fungus infections of the skin; ringworm. T. BARBAE, ringworm of the beard; barber's itch. T. CAPITIS, ringworm of the scalp. T. CIRCINATA or CORPORIS, ringworm of the non-hairy surfaces of the body. T. CRURIS, ringworm of the inner sides of thigh, perineal area or groin; more common in males. T. PEDIS, chonic fungal infection of the feet, principally the areas between the toes; marked by intense itching, scaling, maceration and cracking of the skin; commonly called 'athlete's foot.' T. UNGUIUM, ringworm of the nails; see **onchomycosis**.

tinnitus (ti-nī′-tus): Subjective noises such as buzzing, thumping, ringing, roaring, clucking, or humming that accompany certain types of hearing disorders.

tissue (tish′-ū): A collection of similar cells and the intercellular tissue surrounding them that form a structure that performs a particular function in the body. The four main classes of T. are connective, epithelial, muscular and nervous. ADIPOSE T., connective T. that contains masses of fat cells. AREOLAR T., loosely arranged, widely dispersed connective tissue. CANCELLOUS T., bony tissue that is spongy in appearance. COMPACT T., bony tissue that is dense and hard. CONNECTIVE T., made up of an interlacing mass of fibers; pervades, supports and binds together tissues and organs; includes areolar, adipose, fibrous, elastic, and lymphoid tissues, cartilage and bone, blood and lymph. ENDOTHELIAL T., a single layer of flattened cells that lines serous cavities, blood vessels and lymphatics. EPITHELIAL T., one or more layers of flattened cells with little intercellular substance; lines tubes or cavities that connect with the exterior and covers the surface of the body. MUSCULAR T., made up of fibers that are capable of contracting and expanding; classified as skeletal, smooth or visceral, and cardiac. See **muscle.** NERVOUS T., made up of highly differentiated cells that compose nerves and their fibers and the tissues that support them. PARENCHYMATOUS T., the specialized tissue of an organ that makes up its functioning part as differentiated from supporting tissues. SUBCUTANEOUS T., that found directly underneath the skin; it is a type of loosely organized connective T.

tissue culture: The culture of tissue cells in the laboratory.

titer, titre (tī′-tur): A standard of strength.

titration (tī-trā′-shun): Volumetric analysis by aid of standard solutions.

TLC: Abbreviation for 'tender loving care.'

toe: One of the digits of the foot; the bones of the toes are called phalanges. HAMMER-T., a claw-like deformity caused by the permanent flexion of the joint between the second and third phalanges; most often involves the second toe; may be congenital or caused by ill-fitting shoes. PIGEON T., deformity causing toeing in or walking with the toes turned toward the center line of the body.

toilet training: The methods used to teach a child to control bowel and bladder function. Methods used, parents' attitudes about these functions, and the child's responses, are thought to have an influence on the development of his personality.

tolerance (tol′-er-ans): The ability to tolerate the application or administration of a substance, usually a drug, continuously or in large or increasing doses without ill effect. SUGAR T., the amount of sugar a diabetic person can metabolize before it begins to appear in the urine.

-tome: Denotes cutting or sectioning.

tomograph (tō′-mō-graf): A device for obtaining an x-ray photograph of a selected layer in a specified region of the body. Can be a series of films taken at different depths.—tomography,n.; tomographic, adj.; tomographically, adv.

-tomy: Denotes incision; a cutting operation.

tone (tōn): 1. A particular quality or sound of voice. 2. The normal firmness and strength of tissues. 3. The normal healthy degree of tension in resting muscles.

tongue (tung): The mobile muscular organ contained in the mouth; it is concerned with speech, mastication, swallowing and taste. STRAWBERRY T., thickly furred with projecting red papillae. As the fur disappears the T. is vividly red, like an over-ripe strawberry. Characteristic of scarlet fever. T. DEPRESSOR, a broad flat instrument, often of wood, used to depress the tongue when examining the fauces or pharynx.

tongue-tie: Limited mobility of the tongue, usually due to shortness of the frenum and resulting in interference with sucking and articulation.

tonic: 1. A state of continuous or sustained contraction, said of muscles. 2. Increasing or restoring physical or mental tone or strength. 3. A drug that invigorates or restores strength. T. SPASM, refers to a prolonged muscle spasm as differentiated from a clonic spasm; see **clonus.**

tonicity (tō-nis′-i-ti): The state of normal tension or tone of a muscle or muscles.

tono-: Denotes: (1) tone, tension; (2) pressure.

tonometer (tō-nom′-e-ter): An instrument for measuring pressure, specifically intra-ocular pressure.

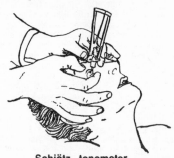

Schiötz tonometer

tonsil (ton′-sil): By custom referring to one of two small almond-shaped lymphoid bodies situated between the pillars of the fauces on either side, covered by mucous membrane and pitted with follicles. See **Waldeyer's ring.**

tonsillectomy (ton-si-lek′-to-mi): Removal of one or both of the tonsils.

tonsillitis (ton-si-lī′-tis): Inflammation of the tonsils.

tonsillolith (ton-sil′-ō-lith): Concretion arising in the body of a tonsil.

tonsillotome (ton-sil′-ō-tōm): Instrument for excision of tonsils.

tonus: The condition of normal tone.

tooth: See teeth.

top-, topo-: Denotes place, locality.

topalgia (tō-pal′-ji-a): Localized pain.

topectomy (tō-pek′-to-mi): Modified frontal lobotomy to treat a psychosis.

tophaceous (tō-fā′-shus): Gritty; sandy.

tophus (tō′-fus): A small, hard concretion forming in the earlobe, or in the tissues about the joints of the phalanges, etc., in gout.—tophi, pl.

topical (top′-ik-al): 1. Pertaining to a definite spot; local. 2. Term often used to describe a substance that is to be applied to the surface of the body for its local effect as distinguished from one that is given internally for its systemic effect.

topography (tō-pog′-ra-fi): A description of the regions of the body.—topographical, adj.; topographically, adv.

torpid (tor′-pid): Sluggish; not reacting with normal vigor or ease.

torpor (tor′-por): Sluggishness, inactivity, stupor, apathy, numbness; absence or slowness of reaction to ordinary stimuli.

torsion (tor′-shun): The act of twisting or the condition of being twisted upon an axis.

torso (tor′-sō): The trunk of the body without the head and extremities.

torticollis (tor-ti-kol′-is): Wryneck; contraction of the muscles of one side of the neck. The head is slightly flexed and drawn toward the contracted side, with the face rotated over the other shoulder.

tortuous (tor′-tū-us): Twisted; full of curves, turns and twists.

touch: 1. The special sense by which contact with objects makes one aware of their qualities. 2. To examine by touching with the finger or hand.

tourniquet (toor′-ni-ket): An apparatus for the temporary compression of the blood vessels of a limb. Designed for compression of a main artery to control bleeding. A T. is also often used to obstruct the venous return from a limb and so facilitate the withdrawal of blood from a vein. Tourniquets vary from a simple rubber band to a pneumatic cuff. ROTATING T., a system of treatment in which tourniquets are applied to all four extremities in turn, as near the trunk as possible; every 10-15 minutes, the tourniquets are rotated so that a different arm or leg is free and three tourniquets are always in place.

toxemia (toks-ē′-mi-a): A generalized poisoning of the body due to the presence of toxins in the bloodstream; usually these toxins result from bacterial action but may

also be due to other causes. T. OF PREGNANCY, a condition due to a disturbance of metabolism and characterized by hypertension, edema, albuminuria and sometimes eclampsia.

toxic (toks′-ik): 1. Poisonous. 2. Resulting from or caused by a poison. 3. Pertaining to a toxin. Syn., poisonous.

toxic-, toxico-: Denotes poison.

toxicity (toks-is′-i-ti): The quality or degree of the poisonousness of a substance.

toxicogenic (toks-ik-ō-jen′-ik): 1. Caused by a poison. 2. Producing or capable of producing a poison.

toxicologist (toks-i-kol′-o-jist): A person who specializes in the study of poisons.

toxicology (toks-i-kol′-o-ji): The science dealing with poisons.—toxicological, adj.; toxicologically, adv.

toxicomania (toks-i-kō-mā′-ni-a): WHO (*q.v.*) definition: periodic or chronic state of intoxication, produced by repeated consumption of a drug harmful to the individual or society. Characteristics are: (1) Uncontrollable desire or necessity to continue consuming the drug and to try to get it by all means. (2) Tendency to increase the dose. (3) Psychic and physical dependency as a result.

toxicosis (toks-i-kō′-sis): The condition of systemic poisoning by a toxin or poison.

toxin (toks′-in): Any poisonous substance produced by a plant or animal organism, usually referring to one produced by pathogenic bacteria.

toxin-antitoxin: A mixture of diptheria toxin and its antitoxin that was formerly used to produce immunity to diphtheria, now largely replaced by diphtheria toxoid (*q.v.*).

toxinemia (toks-in-ē′-mi-a): Toxemia (*q.v.*).

toxoid (toks′-oid): A bacterial toxin altered in such a way that it has lost its poisonous properties but retained its antigenic properties and thus is capable of producing active immunity. DIPHTHERIA T., that used to produce active immunity against diphtheria.

Toxoplasma (toks-ō-plas′-ma): A genus of protozoal parasites. *Toxoplasma gondii* causes toxoplasmosis (*q.v.*).

toxoplasmosis (toks-ō-plas-mō′-sis): Infection by Toxoplasma parasites which occur commonly in mammals and birds and may infect man. Intrauterine fetal and infant infections are often severe, producing encephalitis, convulsions, hydrocephalus and eye disease, resulting in death or, in those who recover, mental retardation and impaired sight. Infection in older children and adults may result in pneumonia, nephritis or skin rashes.

TPI test: *Treponema pallidum* immobilization test. A modern, highly specific test for syphilis in which syphilitic serum immobilizes and kills spirochetes grown in pure culture.

TPR: Abbreviation for temperature, pulse, respirations.

trabecula (tra-bek′-ū-la): In anatomy, one of the fibrous bands or septa of connective tissue that extend into the interior of an organ from its wall or the capsule that covers it, and which serve to hold the functioning cells of the organ in position.—trabeculae, pl.; trabecular, adj.

trabeculotomy (trab-ek-ū-lot′-o-mi): Operation recently devised for the relief of glaucoma.

trace elements: Metals and other elements that are regularly present in very small amounts in the tissues and thought to be essential for normal metabolism (*e.g.*, copper, cobalt, manganese, fluorine, etc.).

tracer (trā′-ser): A substance or instrument used to gain information. Radioactive tracers have extended knowledge in physiology; some are used in diagnosis, *e.g.*, radioactive iodine is used in investigating diseases of the thyroid gland.

trach-, trachea-, tracheo-: Denotes the trachea.

trachea (trā′-kē-a): The windpipe; the fibrocartilaginous tube lined with ciliated mucous membrane passing from the larynx to the bronchi. It is about 4.5 in. long and about 1 in. wide.—tracheal, adj.

tracheitis (trā-kē-ī′-tis): Inflammation of the mucous membrane lining the trachea.

trachel-, trachelo-: Denotes: (1) the neck; (2) a neck-like structure.

trachelismus (trā-ke-liz′-mus): 1. Spasm of the neck muscles. 2. Bending backward of the neck, a sign that sometimes signals the imminence of an epileptic attack.

trachelitis (trā-ke-lī′-tis): Inflammation of the cervix of the uterus.

trachelorrhaphy (trā-ke-lor′-a-fi): Operative repair of a lacerated uterine cervix.

tracheobronchial (trā-kē-ō-brong′-ki-al): Pertaining to the trachea and the bronchi.

tracheobronchitis (trā-kē-ō-brong-kī′-tis): Inflammation of the trachea and bronchi.

tracheobronchoscopy (trā-kē-ō-brong-kos′-ko-pi): Inspection of the interior of the trachea and one or both of the bronchi.

tracheoesophageal (trā-kē-ō-ē-sof′-a-jē-al):

Pertaining to the trachea and the esophagus.

tracheolaryngeal (trā-kē-ō-lar-in′-jē′-al): Pertaining to the trachea and the larynx.

tracheopharyngeal (trā-kē-ō-far-in′-jē-al): Pertaining to the trachea and the pharynx.

tracheoscopy (trā-kē-os′-ko-pi): Inspection of the interior of the trachea with a special instrument called a tracheoscope.

tracheostenosis (trā-kē-ō-ste-nō′-sis): Narrowing or constriction of the trachea.

tracheostomy (trā-kē-os′-to-mi): The surgical creation of a stoma or an opening into the trachea through the neck for the purpose of facilitating passage of air into the lungs or to remove secretions from the trachea; usually a tube is inserted to keep the opening patent.

tracheotomy (trā-kē-ot′-o-mi): The operation of making an incision into the trachea; may be done to remove a foreign body, secure a specimen for biopsy, or for exploratory purposes.

trachoma (tra-kō′-ma): A chronic communicable disease of the eye, caused by a filterable virus; may have sudden or insidious onset; if untreated may persist for years. Marked by inflammation and hyperplasia of the conjunctiva, vascularization of the cornea with later scar formation that results in deformities of the lids, progressive visual disability, and often blindness. Symptoms include redness of the conjunctiva, tearing, pain, photophobia. Found in many parts of the world; high prevalence usually associated with poor hygiene, poverty, crowded living conditions, especially in dry dusty regions.—trachomatous, adj.

tract: An area or region that is longer than it is wide; a path or track. May consist of bundles of nerve fibers that have the same origin, termination, and function; or it may consist of a number of separate organs arranged serially and engaged in performing a common function, *e.g.*, the digestive tract.

traction (trak′-shun): A steady drawing or pulling exerted manually or with a mechanical device to overcome muscle spasm so that a fracture may be reduced, to keep the ends of fractured bones in position until healing can take place, to prevent deformities or contractures from fractures or other conditions, or to correct or lessen deformities such as scoliosis. Many of the types of apparatus used to produce a steady pulling on a part involve the use of pulleys and weights. See **Balkan frame, Bryant's t.**

tractotomy (trak-tot′-o-mi): The operation of severing or making an incision into a nerve tract. Sometimes done for the relief of intractable pain.

trade name: Also called proprietary name. Usually refers to one registered by the U.S. Patent Office and is applied to a drug instead of the official name. Sometimes there are several trade names for the same drug since each pharmaceutical manufacturer may choose a different name for the same preparation.

tragus (trā′-gus): The small cartilaginous projection just anterior to the external auditory meatus, or one of the hairs at the entrance of the meatus.—tragi, pl.; tragal, adj.

trait (trāt): 1. A distinctive, individual pattern of behavior that is more or less permanent and which forms part of the whole personality. 2. An inherited physical or mental characteristic.

trance (trans): A condition of profound, unnatural stupor or sleep, or of partly suspended animation; induced by hysteria, catalepsy, or hypnosis; not due to organic disease.

tranquilizer (tran′-kwi-lī-zer): One of a group of drugs that act by alleviating tension and anxiety without inducing hypnosis or narcosis and thus they have the effect of calming the patient and making him more accessible to help from psychotherapy. They greatly exaggerate the effects of alcohol.

trans-: Denotes: (1) across, through; (2) to the other side.

transabdominal (trans-ab-dom′-in-al): Through the abdomen as the T. approach for nephrectomy.—transabdominally, adv.

transaminase (trans-am′-i-nās): An enzyme important in the catabolism of amino acids.

transamniotic (trans-am-ni-ot′-ik): Through the amniotic fluid as a T. transfusion of the fetus for hemolytic disease.

transection (tran-sek′-shun): A cutting made across the long axis of a structure. A cross section.

transference (trans-fer′-ens): The conveyance or shifting of something from one place to another. In psychiatry, the unconscious transfer by the patient of mental attitudes or emotions formerly directed to one object or person to some other object or person, frequently to the psychotherapist.

transfusion (trans-fū′-zhun): The introduc-

tion of a fluid such as plasma, blood, saline or other solution directly into the bloodstream of the patient. BLOOD T.,the transfer of blood, directly or indirectly, from one person into the vein of another person. EXCHANGE T., alternate withdrawal of part of the recipient's blood and replacement with donor's blood until the greater part has been exchanged; used for 'Rhesus' babies affected with erythroblastosis fetalis.—transfuse, v.t.

transillumination (trans-il-ū-mi-nā′-shun): The transmission of light through a cavity or sinus for diagnostic purposes.

translucent (trans-lū′-sent): Intermediate between opaque and transparent; describing a substance that allows the passage of light, but which diffuses the light so that objects are not clearly distinguishable through it.

transmigration (trans-mī-grā′-shun): A wandering. Diapedesis (*q.v.*). OVULAR T., the passage of an ovum from one ovary to the fallopian tube on the opposite side.

transmission (trans-mish′-un): 1. The transfer of a disease from one person to another. 2. The passing on of an inheritable quality from parent to offspring.

transmural (trans-mū′-ral): Through the wall, *e.g.*, of a cyst, organ or vessel.—transmurally, adv.

transpiration (tran-spir-ā′-shun): The discharge of air, vapor or sweat through the skin or a membrane.—transpire, v.t.

transplantation (trans-plan-tā′-shun): Grafting on to one part, tissue or an organ taken from another part or another body. —transplant, v.t.

transposition (trans-pō-zish′-un): 1. The location or displacement of an internal organ to the side of the body that is opposite its usual site. 2. An exchange of atoms within a molecule. 3 The attachment of a tissue flap to a new site without separating it from the old one until it has united with the tissues at the new location.

transsexual: Term applied to a person who has the body and generative organs of one sex, but the mind of the other sex. They distinguish themselves from homosexuals and transvestites and want to be physically changed to the opposite sex; this is sometimes accomplished through surgery and hormonal treatment.

transthoracic (trans-thō-ras′-ik): Across or through the chest wall or chest cavity.

transudate (trans′-ū-dāt): A liquid substance that has passed over a membrane or through some other permeable substance. See **transude.**

transude (trans-ūd'): To ooze or pass through a membrane or permeable substance, *e.g.*, the oozing of blood serum through intact vessel walls.—transudation, n.

transurethral (trans-ū-rē'-thral): By way of the urethra.

transvaginal (trans-vaj'-in-al): Through or across the vagina; performed through the vagina.—transvaginally, adv.

transventricular (trans-ven-trik'-ū-lar): Through a ventricle. Term used mainly in connection with surgery on cardiac valves. —transventricularly, adv.

transverse (trans-vers'): Crosswise or situated at right angles to the long axis of the body or of a part. T. PRESENTATION, a crosswise position of the fetus in utero that must be altered before the child can be born normally.

transvesical (trans-ves'-i-kal): Through the bladder, by custom referring to the urinary bladder.—transvesically, adv.

transvestism (trans-ves'-tizm): A sexual deviation in which one has the desire to wear the clothes and in other ways masquerade as a member of the opposite sex. Also transvestitism.

transvestite (trans-ves'-tīt): One who practices transvestism (*q.v.*).

trapezium (tra-pē'-zi-um): An irregular four-sided figure; specifically the first bone on the thumb side of the second row of carpal bones. Also called the greater multangular bone.

trapezius (tra-pē'-zi-us): The large flat, triangular superficial muscle on either side of the posterior part of the neck and upper thorax; it draws the head backward, raises, depresses and rotates the scapula and draws it backward toward the spine.

trapezoid (trap'-e-zoid): Resembling a trapezium (*q.v.*); specifically the second bone in the second row of carpal bones. Also called the lesser multangular bone.

trauma (traw'-ma): A wound or injury caused by external force or violence. PSYCHOLOGICAL T., an emotional shock or an experience that has a more or less permanent effect upon the mind, especially the subconscious mind. BIRTH T., injury to an infant during its delivery or, in psychology, the injury to the infant's psyche from the process of being born.—traumatic, adj.; traumatize, v.t.

traumatize (traw'-ma-tīz): To produce injury or trauma through accident or by careless or inept mishandling during surgery, examination or treatment of a patient.

treatment: Medical or surgical care of an ill person, aimed at relieving symptoms of a disease or curing the disease. CONSERVATIVE T., that in which surgery or other drastic measures are withheld if and as long as possible. CURATIVE T., that aimed at curing a disease. EMPIRIC T., that based on measures that experience has shown to be effective in the particular condition. KENNY'S T., see **Kenny.** MEDICAL T., T. by drugs, hygienic and other methods that are distinguished from surgical methods. PALLIATIVE T., that which aims to relieve pain and distress but does not attempt to cure the causative disease. PROPHYLACTIC T., that which aims to prevent a person from being attacked by a specific disease; also called PREVENTIVE T. SHOCK T., consists of induction of coma or convulsions by injection of insulin or other drug or by passing an electric current through the brain. SIPPY T., see **Sippy method.** SPECIFIC T., that which is aimed at removing the specific cause of a disease; frequently refers to diseases caused by bacteriological invasion. SURGICAL T., includes T. by cutting operations and manual procedures such as reducing fractures without making an incision. SYMPTOMATIC T., T. of symptoms as they arise in the course of a disease rather than treating the cause.—treat, v.t.

Trematoda (trem-a-tō'-da): A class of parasitic fluke-worms which includes many pathogens of man such as the Schistosoma of bilharziasis.

tremens (trē'-mens): Trembling; shaking. DELIRIUM T., a form of acute insanity caused by excessive use of alcohol and marked by hallucinations, memory disturbances, sweating, restlessness, mental confusion, tremor.

tremor (trem'-or): Involuntary trembling or quivering. COARSE T., violent trembling in which the vibrations are not over six or seven per second. CONTINUOUS T., that which occurs constantly as seen in paralysis agitans. FINE T., slight trembling in which the vibrations may be 10 or 12 per second; seen in the outstretched hand or tongue of a person suffering from thyrotoxicosis (*q.v.*). INTENTION T. occurs when voluntary movement is attempted; characteristic of disseminated sclerosis.—tremulous, adj.

trench: T. FEVER, a rickettsial infection caused by the bite of an infected body louse; a major medical problem of World War I when the soldiers were in trenches for long periods of time with no opportunity to practice personal hygiene. T. FOOT, a condition resembling frostbite, also a medical problem during World War I when men stood in trenches for long periods of time with wet, cold feet. T. MOUTH, see **angina, Vincent's.**

Trendelenburg: T'S. OPERATION, ligation of the long saphenous vein in the groin at its junction with the femoral vein. Used in cases of varicose veins. T. POSITION, the patient is placed on his back on a table with the head lowered and the knees elevated at a 45° angle; this position pushes the pelvic and abdominal organs toward the thoracic cavity. T'S. SIGN, seen in congenital dislocation of the hip; when the patient stands on the dislocated leg and flexes the hip and knee on the unaffected side, that side will sag whereas in normal conditions it would rise. [Friedrich Trendelenburg, German surgeon. 1844-1924.]

trephine (trĕ-fīn'): 1. An instrument with sawtooth-like edges used to remove a circular piece from a structure, *e.g.,* cornea or skull. 2. To perform an operation with a trephine. Also **trepan.**

Treponema (trep-ō-nē'-ma): A genus of motile, slender, spiral-shaped bacteria, some of which are pathogenic to man. T. PALLIDUM, the causative organism of syphilis (*q.v.*) in man. T. PERTENUE, the causative organism of yaws (*q.v.*).

treponematosis (trep-ō-nē-ma-tō'-sis): Infection caused by a variety of treponema. See **yaws.**

TRF: Abbreviation for thyrotropin releasing factor. See **thyrotropin.**

tri-: Denotes three, three times.

triage (trē'-ahzh): The sorting out and classification of injured persons in war or any disaster to determine priorities for care and the proper place for treatment. In war, this is done, along with giving first aid, at the front before evacuating the casualties to the rear.

triceps (trī'-seps): Three-headed; specifically the three-headed muscle on the back of the upper arm; it extends the forearm.

trich-, tricho-: Denotes: (1) hair; (2) filament.

trichiasis (trik-ī'-a-sis): Inversion or ingrowing of an eyelash causing irritation from friction on the eyeball.

trichinosis (trik-i-nō'-sis): A disease that results from eating raw or undercooked pork that is infected with a parasitic worm, *Trichinella spiralis.* The female worms live in the small bowel and produce larvae which invade the body and, in particular, form cysts in skeletal muscles; the usual symptoms are diarrhea, nausea, colic, fever, facial edema, muscular pains and stiffness.

trichobezoar (trik-ō-bē'-zōr): A hairball; a concretion found in the stomach or intestine and containing hairs.

trichoepithelioma (tri-kō-ep-i-thē-li-ō'-ma): A benign tumor that has its origin in a hair follicle.

trichoesthesia (tri-kō-es-thē'-zi-a): 1. The sensation one feels when a hair is touched. 2. A form of paresthesia in which one has a sensation as of hair being on the conjunctiva, the skin, or the mucous membrane of the mouth.

trichogen (trik'-ō-jen): An agent that promotes growth of hair.

Trichomonas (tri-kom'-ō-nas): A genus of flagellated protozoa certain of which are parasitic in the intestinal tract, mouth, vagina or urethra of humans. T. VAGINALIS, the causative agent of a common chronic disease of the genitourinary tract, trichomoniasis (*q.v.*).

trichomoniasis (trik-ō-mō-nī'-a-sis): Infection of the genitourinary tract with the protozoal parasite Trichomonas (*q.v.*). Characterized in women by vaginitis and profuse, foamy, yellowish discharge with a foul odor; in men the agent lives in the urethra, prostate, and seminal vesicles, and seldom causes objective symptoms. Transmitted through sexual intercourse.

trichomycosis (trik-ō-mī-kō'-sis): Any disease of the hair that is caused by a fungus.

trichophagy (trik-kof'-a-ji): The nervous habit of biting or eating hair.

Trichophyton (tri-kof'-i-ton): A genus of fungi found on the skin, hair, and nails; often a cause of allergy; a causative agent in ringworm or tinea.

trichophytosis (trik-ō-fī-tō'-sis): Infection with a Trichophyton fungus, *e.g.,* ringworm of the hair or skin.

trichorrhea (trik-ō-rē'-a): Rapid or excessive falling of the hair.

trichorrhexis (trik-ō-reks'-is): A condition in which the hair splits or breaks off easily.

trichosis (trī-kō'-sis): Any disease or abnormal condition of the hair.

trichotillomania (trik'-ō-til-lō-mā'-ni-a): An

uncontrollable compulsion to pull out one's own hair.

trichuriasis (trik-ū-rī′-a-sis): Infestation with *Trichuris trichiura,* a whipworm; a syndrome occurring most frequently in the tropics and often causing no symptoms. In some cases there is diarrhea, vomiting, nervous disorders, and loss of weight.

Trichuris trichiura: A genus of whipworms; filiform with a coiled head end. Found only in man.

tricuspid (trī-kus′-pid): Having three cusps. T. VALVE, that between the right atrium and ventricle of the heart.

trifacial (trī-fā′-shal): Denoting the 5th pair of cranial nerves. See **trigeminal.**

trigeminal (trī-jem′-in-al): Triple; separating into three sections, *e.g.,* the T. NERVES, the 5th pair of cranial nerves, which have three branches and supply the skin of the face, tongue and teeth. T. NEURALGIA, see **tic douloureux.**

trigger finger: A condition in which the finger can be bent but cannot be straightened without help; usually due to a thickening on the tendon which prevents free gliding.

trigone (trī′gōn): A triangular area, especially applied to the bladder base bounded by the ureteral openings at the back, and the urethral opening at the front.—trigonal, adj.

trimester (trī-mes′-ter): A period of 3 months. Usually refers to one-third of the length of a pregnancy.

tripara (trip′-a-ra): A woman who has had three pregnancies resulting in three live offspring. Also written Para III.

triplegia (trī-plē′-ji-a): Paralysis of three of the extremities, or of the face and an upper and lower extremity.

triplet: One of three children born at the same birth.

triplopia (trip-lō′-pi-a): A defect of vision in which one sees three images of a single object.

trismus (triz′-mus): Spasm in the muscles of mastication; lockjaw.

trisomy (trī′-sō-mi): The occurrence of three chromosomes in a cell that normally has but two. TRISOMY 21 (Down's syndrome, *q.v.*) is of two types; in one type there is a total of 46 chromosomes in cells, but within chromosome 21 there has been an interchange of a portion from another chromosome; children having this type of cell are usually born to younger mothers. In the second type, the cells have 47 chromosomes; the child develops slowly and reaches an intellectual level of 7 or 8 years, may

have cardiac abnormalities, and has a short life expectancy; children having this type of cell are usually born to older mothers. TRISOMY 18 occurs less often than trisomy 21; is the result of nondisjunction of a chromosome in Group E (16-18); usually occurs in children of parents over 30; infant has low birth weight for gestational age, may have low-set ears, congenital heart defect, micrognathia, abnormalities of fingers and feet, may be mentally retarded, and has poor prognosis for life. TRISOMY 13-15 occurs rarely; those affected have some of the characteristics of children with trisomy 18 plus abnormalities of brain and head structure; usually death occurs during the first year of life.

trocar (trō′-kar): A pointed rod which fits inside a cannula that is used for withdrawing fluid from a cavity; after the instrument is inserted, the rod is withdrawn. The term is sometimes used to designate both the cannula and the trocar. Also trochar.

trochanter (trō-kan′-ter): One of two processes,the larger one (T. major) on the outer, the other (T. minor) on the inner side of the femur between the shaft and neck; they serve for the attachment of muscles.—trochanteric, adj.

troche (trō′-ke): A medicated disk, tablet or lozenge that is held under the tongue or in the cheek until it is dissolved.

trochlea (trok′-lē-a): An anatomical term used to describe a part or structure which is like a pulley in function or appearance; usually a tendon or projection on a bone. —trochlear, adj.

troph-, tropho-, -trophy: Denotes nutrition, nourishment, growth.

trophic (trō′-fik): Pertaining to nutrition.

-trophic: Denotes relationship to nutrition.

trophoblast (trōf′-ō-blast): A layer of ectodermal tissue that serves to attach the ovum to the wall of the uterus and supply nourishment to the embryo.—trophoblastic, adj.

trophoneurosis (trōf′-ō-nū-rō′-sis): Any trophic disorder such as atrophy or hypertrophy, caused by failure of nutrition resulting from disease or injury to the nerves of a part. See **Raynaud's disease.**

tropia (trō′-pi-a): An abnormal turning or deviation of the eye; strabismus (*q.v.*).

-tropic: Denotes: (1) turning, changing; (2) attraction to a specific tissue, organ or system.

tropical: Pertaining to or common to tropic areas. T. DISEASE, one which occurs with greater frequency and/or severity in tropical parts of the world.

Trousseau's sign: See **carpopedal spasm.** [Armand Trousseau, French physician. 1801-1867.]

truncal (trung'-kal): Pertaining to the trunk of the body or of a nerve, artery, etc.

truncate (trung'-kāt): To cut off; amputate. To cut off at right angles to the long axis of the part.

trunk: 1. The torso or main part of the body to which the head and extremities are attached. 2. The main, undivided part of a nerve, blood vessel or duct. NERVE T., a collection of nerve fibers closely bound together and enclosed within a sheath of epineurium.

truss: An apparatus consisting usually of a belt and a pressure pad, worn over a hernia to keep it in place after it has been reduced.

truth serum: Common name for a drug that acts to inhibit the nervous system and which is given to a person from whom it is desirable to obtain information he would not otherwise reveal.

Trypanosoma (trī-pan-ō-sō'-ma): A genus of parasitic protozoa; a limited number of species are pathogenic to man. The species that is the vector of trypanosomiasis (q.v.) in Africa, live part of their life cycle in the tsetse fly (q.v.) and are transferred to new hosts, including man, in the salivary juices when the fly bites for a blood meal.

trypanosomiasis (trī-pan-ō-sō-mī'-a-sis): Disease produced by infection with Trypanosoma. In man this may be with *T. rhodesiense* in East Africa or *T. gambiense* in West Africa; both are transmitted by the tsetse fly and produce the illness known as African sleeping sickness, a severe often fatal disease marked by fever, intense headache, lymph node enlargement, anemia, wasting, and somnolence. Not found in the U.S., but Chagas' disease, caused by *T. cruzi* that is transmitted by bites of bloodsucking insects, is found in certain parts of South America.

trypsin (trip'-sin): A proteolytic enzyme formed in the intestine when the trypsinogen from the pancreatic juice is acted upon by the enterokinase of the intestinal juice; it is the chief protein-digesting enzyme in the human.

trypsinogen (trip-sin'-o-jen): The precursor of trypsin (q.v.), secreted by the pancreas; it is converted into trypsin when it comes into contact with enterokinase in the small intestine.

tryptophan (trip'-tō-făn): One of the essential amino acids; necessary for optimal

growth and for tissue repair; found in varying amounts in many proteins.

tsetse fly (tset'-sē): A blood-sucking fly found in Africa; the vector of Trypanosoma (q.v.). Also tzetze.

tsp: Abbreviation for teaspoon or teaspoonful.

tubal: Pertaining to a tube. T. ABORTION, one in which an extrauterine pregnancy is terminated by rupture of the fallopian tube. T. PREGNANCY, see **ectopic pregnancy.** T. FEEDING, see **feeding.**

tube: An elongated, cylindrical structure or apparatus. For special tubes see: **auditory, bronchial, digestive, drainage, eustachian, fallopian, feeding, intubation, Levin, Rehfuss, Southey's, stomach, test, tracheostomy, uterine, Wangensteen.**

tubectomy (tū-bek'-to-mi): Salpingectomy (q.v.).

tuber: A localized swelling, knob, protuberance.

tubercle (tū'-ber-k'l): 1. A small solid elevation or nodule on the skin, mucous membrane, or surface of an organ. 2. A small rounded eminence on a bone. 3. The specific lesion produced by the *Mycobacterium tuberculosis.*—tubercular, adj. See **Ghon's focus.**

tubercular (tū-ber'-kū-lar): Characterized by the presence of or pertaining to tubercles. (Some authorities hold that the term should not be used in connection with the disease tuberculosis specifically, or with one who has the disease.)

tuberculid (tū-ber'-cū-lid): A skin lesion occurring in association with tuberculosis and caused by the toxins of the *Mycobacterium tuberculosis.*

tuberculin: A sterile extract of either the crude (old T.) or refined (Purified Protein Derivative; P.P.D.) complex protein constituents of the tubercle bacillus. Its commonest use is in determining whether a person has or has not previously been infected with the tubercle bacillus, by injecting a small amount into the skin and reading the reaction, if any, in 48 to 72 hours; negative reactors have escaped previous infection. See **Mantoux.**

tuberculoid (tū-ber'-kū-loid): Resembling tuberculosis or a tubercle.

tuberculoma (tū-ber-kū-lō'-ma): 1. A large caseous tubercle, its size suggesting a tumor. 2. A tuberculous abscess. 3. Any new growth or nodule of tuberculous origin.

tuberculosis (tū-ber-kū-lō'-sis): A specific, chronic, infectious disease caused by the

tuberculostatic

tuberculostatic

tuberculostatic 366

Mycobacterium tuberculosis, characterized by the formation of tubercles in the tissues. Often asymptomatic at first; later the local symptoms depend upon the part affected and general symptoms are those of sepsis, *i.e.,* fever, sweats, emaciation. In man the disease most commonly affects the lungs but may also affect the meninges, joints, bones, lymph nodes, kidney, intestine, larynx, or skin. AVIAN T., endemic in birds and rarely seen in man. BOVINE T., endemic in cattle and transmitted to man via cow's milk, causing T. of the glands but rarely of the lungs; less common than formerly. MILIARY T., a generalized acute form of T. in which, as a result of blood stream dissemination, minute, multiple tuberculous foci are scattered throughout many organs of the body; it is often rapidly fatal. PRIMARY T., infection with *Mycobacterium tuberculosis* for the first time; characterized by the formation, usually in the lung, of a local lesion that is most often benign, self-limited, and heals spontaneously; also called childhood T. PULMONARY T., T. of the lung; the most common site of the disease in man; also called consumption, phthisis. SECONDARY T., the adult type as distinguished from the primary or childhood type.—tuberculous, adj.

tuberculostatic (tū-ber-kū-lō-stat'-ik): Inhibiting the growth of *Mycobacterium tuberculosis,* the causative agent of tuberculosis.

tuberculous (tū-ber'-kū-lus): Pertaining to or affected by tuberculosis, or caused by the *Mycobacterium tuberculosis.*

tuberculum (tū-ber'-kū-lum): The anatomical term for a small eminence, nodule, knot or tubercle.

tuberosity (tū-ber-os'-i-ti): A small, rounded elevation or protuberance, particularly one from the surface of a bone.

tuberous (tū'-ber-us): Knotty, knobby, covered with tubers.

tubo-: Denotes a tube.

tubo-ovarian: Pertaining to or involving both a fallopian tube and an ovary, *e.g.,* a tubo-ovarian abscess.

tubo-ovariotomy (tū-bō-ō-var-i-ot'-o-mi): Surgical removal of a fallopian tube and an ovary; usually refers to both right and left tube and ovary.

tubule (tū'-būl): A small tube. COLLECTING T., straight tube in the kidney medulla conveying urine to the kidney pelvis. CONVOLUTED T., coiled tube in the kidney

cortex. SEMINIFEROUS T., coiled tube in the testis. URINIFEROUS T., syn., nephron (*q.v.*).

tularemia (too-la-rē'-mi-a): Syn., deer-fly fever; tick fever; rabbit fever, etc. An endemic disease of rodents, caused by *Pasteurella tularensis;* transmitted by biting insects and acquired by man either in handling infected animal carcasses or by the bite of an infected insect. Suppuration at the inoculation site is followed by inflammation of the draining lymph glands and by severe constitutional upset with symptoms resembling those of undulant fever or plague.—tularemic, adj.

tumefacient (tū-me-fā'-shent): 1. Swollen or swelling. 2. Causing swelling.

tumefaction (tū-me-fak'-shun): 1. A swelling. 2. The condition of being swollen, puffy, or edematous.

tumescence (tū-mes'-ens): A state of swelling; turgidity.—tumescent, adj.

tumid: Swollen.

tumor: 1. A swelling. 2. A mass of abnormal tissue which resembles the normal tissue in structure, but which fulfills no useful function and grows at the expense of the body. Many types are described, often being named for the tissues from which they originate. BENIGN T., a simple, innocent, encapsulated T., that does not infiltrate adjacent tissue or cause metastases and is unlikely to recur if removed. MALIGNANT T., one that is not encapsulated, is likely to infiltrate adjoining tissue and to cause metastases, to progress, and ultimately to destroy life. See **cancer.**—tumorous, adj.

tumorigenic (tū-mor-i-jen'-ik): Causing or producing tumors.—tumorigenesis, n.

tunic: A covering, coat, or lining, particularly of a hollow or tubelike structure. See **tunica.**

tunica (tū'-ni-ka): Anatomical term for a lining membrane or a coat, especially of a tubular structure; usually named for the structure of which it is a part or for its location in that structure. The three tunicae of the arteries are: T. ADVENTITIA, the outer coat; T. INTIMA, the lining; T. MEDIA, the middle muscular coat.

tuning fork: A two-pronged forklike instrument, usually of steel, that gives off a musical note when struck. Used in some hearing tests.

turbid: Cloudy; unclear.

turbidity (tur-bid'-i-ti): Cloudiness; usually

refers to a solution in which the solid solutes have been disturbed.

turbinate (tur′-bin-āt): Shaped like a top or inverted cone. T. BONE, one on either side forming the lateral nasal walls.

turbinated (tur′-bin-ā-ted): Scroll-shaped, as the three ethmoidal T. processes which project from the lateral nasal walls.

turbinectomy (tur-bin-ek′-to-mi): Removal of a turbinate bone.

turgescence (tur-jes′-ens): Swelling; distention; inflation.—turgescent, adj.

turgid (tur′-jid): Swollen; firmly distended, as with blood by congestion.—turgescence, n.; turgidity, n.

turgor (tur′-gor): Fullness; tension.

Turk's saddle: Sella turcica (q.v.).

Turner's syndrome: Gonadal dysgenesis. Can be identified at birth. 45 chromosomes instead of 46. One sex chromosome missing. Brought up as girl though genetic male. Such an individual has small female genitalia, scanty pubic hair, atrophic ovaries, webbed neck and valgus of the elbows. [Henry H. Turner, American endocrinologist. 1892- .]

tussis (tus′-sis): A cough.

twilight sleep: A state induced by the injection of morphine and scopolamine in which awareness to pain is dulled and memory of it is dimmed or effaced; used chiefly in childbirth.

twin: One of two children produced in the same pregnancy resulting from the fertilization of one ovum or two ova at the same time.

twinge (twinj): A sudden sharp fleeting pain.

twitch: A brief spasmodic contraction of a muscle or muscle fiber. A spasm or tic.

tylosis (tī-lō′-sis): See **keratosis.**

tympanectomy (tim-pan-ek′-to-mi): Surgical removal of the tympanic membrane.

tympanic (tim-pan′-ik): Pertaining to the tympanum. T. MEMBRANE (membrana tympani), the eardrum.

tympanites (tim-pa·nī′-tēz): Abdominal distension due to accumulation of gas in the intestine. Also called 'tympanism.'

tympanitis (tim-pa-nī′-tis): Inflammation of the tympanum.

tympanoplasty (tim-pan-ō-plas′-ti): A plastic operation involving the hearing mechanism of the middle ear and the tympanum. —tympanoplastic, adj.

tympanotomy (tim-pan-ot′-o-mi): Incision of the tympanic membrane.

tympanum (tim′-pan-um): The cavity of the middle ear.

tympany (tim′-pa-ni): The drum-like resonant sound heard when a cavity containing air is percussed, e.g., an abdomen distended with gas.

typhl-, typhlo-: Denotes: (1) the cecum; (2) blindness.

typhlomegaly (tif-lō-meg′-a-li): Enlargement of the cecum.

typhlon (tif′-lon): The cecum.

typhlosis (tif-lō′-sis): Blindness.

typhoid fever (tī′-foid): A worldwide, often epidemic, systemic infectious disease caused by the *Salmonella typhi* which is transmitted by direct or indirect contact with a patient or carrier. Usual vehicles for spread of the disease are contaminated water or food, milk, milk products, or shellfish; flies are sometimes vectors. Average incubation period is 10-14 days. A progressive febrile illness marks the onset of the disease; there is anorexia, malaise, slow pulse and rose spots (q.v.) on the abdomen and back. As the organism invades the lymphoid tissue, ulceration of Peyer's patches (q.v.) and enlargement of the spleen occur. Constipation is more often a symptom than diarrhea, but when the latter occurs it is profuse with 'pea soup' stools which may become frankly hemorrhagic. Recovery usually begins at about the end of the third week. Protection is secured through scrupulous personal hygiene when in contact with patients or carriers and by inoculation with the appropriate vaccine. Community control is secured through public health measures concerning the disposal of sewage, purification of water supply, inspection and control of food handlers and discovery of carriers. See **TAB.**

typhus (tī′-fus): An acute, infectious disease caused by a rickettsial organism; characterized by high fever, a skin eruption that may be macular or papular, severe headache, mental depression; lasts about two weeks. Spread by lice, fleas, and ticks and is a disease of war, famine, and catastrophe when large groups of people are concentrated in one area and facilities for personal hygiene are lacking. Protection is secured by immunization with the appropriate vaccine. Community control during epidemics is secured through vigilant public health measures.

typing (tīp′-ing): Classifying an individual, microorganism, object, or substance in the category in which it belongs. BLOOD T., see **blood groups.**

tyremesis (tī-rem′-e-sis): The vomiting of curdy, cheesy material by infants.

tyriasis (ti-rī′-a-sis): 1. Elephantiasis (*q.v.*). 2. Alopecia (*q.v.*).

tyrosine (tī-rō′-sin): An amino acid that is concerned with growth and is an essential element in any diet. T. IODINASE, an enzyme in the thyroid; important in the production of thyroxine.

tyrosinosis (tī-rō-sin-ō′-sis): A condition due to abnormal metabolism of tyrosine; p-hydroxyphenylpyruvic acid, an intermediate product of this metabolism; is excreted in the urine.

U

U: Abbreviation for unit, units.

ula (ū'-la): The gums.

ulcer (ul'-ser): An open, circumscribed lesion on the surface of the skin, or serous or mucous membrane; characterized by necrosis, sometimes suppuration, and slow healing. CURLING'S U., a peptic U., associated with extensive burns and scalds or severe bodily injury. DECUBITUS U., bedsore (*q.v.*). DUODENAL U., one on the mucous membrane lining of the duodenum; peptic U. GASTRIC U., one on the mucous membrane lining of the stomach; peptic U. HARD U., chancre (*q.v.*). INDOLENT U., one with hard elevated edges and little or no granulation; occurs most frequently on the leg; very hard to heal. PENETRATING U., one which is locally invasive; may involve the wall of an organ or erode a blood vessel; in the latter case may result in hematemesis if the U. is in the stomach or duodenum. PEPTIC U., one which occurs in the mucous membrane lining of the stomach or duodenum; caused by the action of the acid gastric juice. PERFORATING U., one which erodes through the wall of an organ. RODENT U., one which grows slowly and is locally invasive of the skin, usually of the face. SYPHILITIC U., chancre (*q.v.*). VARICOSE U., an indolent U. in which there is loss of skin surface in the area of a varicose vein; usually occurs on the lower third of the leg; also called GRAVITATIONAL U. VENEREAL U., chancroid (*q.v.*).—ulcerative, ulcerous, adj.; ulcerate, v.; ulceration, n.

ulcerate (ul'-ser-āt): 1. To undergo ulceration. 2. To form an ulcer.

ulceration (ul-ser-ā'-shun): 1. The process of forming and developing an ulcer. 2. An ulcer or ulcers.

ulcerative (ul'-ser-ā-tiv): Pertaining to, or of the nature of an ulcer. U. COLITIS, see **colitis.**

ulcerogenic (ul-ser-ō-jen'-ik): Ulcer-producing or capable of producing an ulcer.

ulcerous (ul'-ser-us): Affected with, resembling, or pertaining to an ulcer.

-ule, -ula: Denotes small, small one.

ulectomy (ū-lek'-to-mi): 1. The surgical removal of scar tissue. 2. The surgical removal of diseased gingival (gum) tissue.

ulitis (ū-lī'-tis): Inflammation of the gums; gingivitis.

ulna (ul'-na): The bone on the inner side of the forearm extending from elbow to wrist. —ulnar, adj.

ulo-: Denotes: (1) a scar; (2) the gums.

uloncus (ū-long'-kus): A tumor or swelling on the gums.

ulorrhea (ū-lō-rē'-a): Bleeding from the gums.

ultra-: Denotes: (1) excess, excessive; (2) beyond in space, range or limits; (3) beyond what is normal, ordinary or natural.

ultramicrobe (ul-tra-mī'-krōb): An organism or object too small to be seen with an ordinary microscope.

ultramicroscope (ul-tra-mī'-krō-skōp): A microscope for viewing objects too small to be seen with an ordinary microscope; it utilizes refracted instead of direct light.—ultramicroscopic, adj.

ultrasonic (ul-tra-son'-ik): Relating to energy waves that are similar to sound waves but which have such a high frequency that they are inaudible to the human ear (above 20,000 cycles per second). When they strike living tissue their energy is changed into heat, a principle that is made use of therapeutically and in making diagnoses. In DIAGNOSTIC ultrasound, information is derived from echoes which occur when a controlled beam of this energy crosses the boundary between adjacent tissues of differing physical properties. POWER ultrasound has a destructive effect and has been used in the treatment of frostbite, Ménière's disease and in brain surgery. See **echoencephalography.** U. STERILIZATION, a method of destroying bacteria by exposing articles or materials to be sterilized to a transmitter that emanates ultrasonic waves which shatter the bacteria; used in certain industries and laboratories.

ultrasonography (ul-tra-so-nog'-ra-fi): The use of ultrasonic energy for delineating deep body structures, or for determining the size and location of tissues of differing density or of foreign objects, *e.g.*, tumors or foreign objects in the eye.

ultrasound: Ultrasonic vibrations. See **ultrasonic.**

ultraviolet: Denoting the radiant energy waves that are beyond the violet end of the spectrum. They are a natural component of sunlight but may also be produced artificially by a special lamp. They are important in the synthesis of vitamin D in the body and are also used in treatment of certain skin diseases and for their indirect effects in treatment of rickets and anemia. Since they have a bacteriostatic action they are useful in reducing the bacterial content of the air in an enclosed area.

ultravirus: An extremely small pathogenic agent. See **virus.**

ululation (ŭl-ū-lā′-shun): The loud, inarticulate wailing or crying of hysterical or emotionally disturbed persons.

umbilicated (um-bil′-i-kāt-ed): Having a central depression, *e.g.,* a smallpox vesicle.

umbilicus (um-bil′-i-kus): The scar or pit in the center of the abdominal wall left by the separation of the umbilical cord after birth; the navel. See **cord.**—umbilical, adj.

un-: Denotes: (1) not, in-, non-; (2) contrary to, opposite of; (3) to remove, release or free from.

unciform (un′-si-form): Shaped like a hook. U. BONE, the hamate bone, one of the eight bones of the carpus.

Uncinaria (un-si-na′-ri-a): A genus of nematodes including one of the causative agents of hookworm disease.

uncinariasis (un-sin-a-rī′-as-is): Hookworm disease (*q. v.*).

uncinate (un′-sin-āt): Hook-shaped. Unciform.

unconditioned reflex: A reflex that is inborn; *e.g.,* salivation at the sight of food.

unconscious (un-kon′-shus): 1. Insensible; not aware of or perceiving factors in the environment. 2. State of being unable to receive stimuli or to have subjective experiences. 3. A freudian term for that part of the mind that consists of personality factors and physiological drives of which one is unaware and which are not accessible to one's memory although they may be studied by psychoanalytical techniques.

unconsciousness (un-kon′-shus-nes): Physiological and psychological state of being unconscious (*q. v.*); lack of awareness and ability to perceive; insensibility.

unction (ung′-shun): 1. The application of a soothing ointment, salve or oil. 2. An ointment.

unctuous (ungk′-tū-us): Fatty, oily, greasy.

uncus (ung′-kus): A hook-shaped structure or process, specifically the hooked process of the anterior end of the hippocampal gyrus.

undescended: Not descended; refers specifically to a testis that does not descend into the scrotum but remains within the abdomen.

undine (un′-dīn): A small, thin glass flask used for irrigating the eyes.

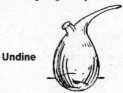

Undine

undulant (un′-dū-lant): Characterized by rising and falling, or wave-like motion. U. FEVER, brucellosis (*q. v.*).

ung: Abbreviation for *unguent* (ointment).

ungual (ung′-gwal): Pertaining to the fingernails or toenails.

unguent (ung′-gwent): Ointment. Also unguentum.

unguis (ung′-gwis): A fingernail or toenail. —ungues, pl.; ungual, adj.

uni-: Denotes one, single.

uniarticular (ū-ni-ar-tik′-ū-lar): Involving only one joint.

unicellular (ū-ni-sel′-ū-lar): Consisting of only one cell.

unilateral (ū-ni-lat′-er-al): Related to, or involving only one side of a structure or of the body.—unilaterally, adv.

uniocular (ū-ni-ok′-ū-lar): Pertaining to, affecting, or involving only one eye.

union (ūn′-yun): The process of healing or growing together as occurs between the edges of a wound or the ends of fractured bones. See **intention.**

uniovular (ū-ni-ov′-ū-lar): Pertaining to, or arising from one ovum; descriptive of certain twin pregnancies that result in identical twins. Cf. **binovular.**

unipara (ū-nip′-a-ra): A woman who has borne only one child.—uniparous, adj.

unit: 1. A single person or thing. 2. A measurement of quantity, weight, or other quality that has been adopted as standard for that particular substance.

United States Pharmacopeia: See **pharmacopeia.**

univalent (ū-ni-vā′-lent): Having a valence (chemical combining power) of one.

universal: Without limit; including or covering every one of the class, genus, or group being considered. U. ANTIDOTE, one given when the specific cause of poisoning is not known; consists of one part each of tannic acid and magnesium oxide and two parts of powdered charcoal. U. DONOR; U. RECIPIENT, see **blood groups.**

unmedullated (un-med′-ū-lāt-ed): Descriptive of a nerve fiber that has no myelin sheath.

untoward (un-tward'): Undesirable, adverse, unexpected, unfortunate; descriptive of effects of a drug or treatment.

uptake: In medicine, a term used to describe the absorption of some substance by a tissue, *e.g.*, iodine by the thyroid gland.

ur-, uro-: Denotes: (1) urine, urination; (2) the urinary tract; (3) urea; (4) uric acid.

urachus (ū'-rak-us): The stem-like structure connecting the bladder with the umbilicus in the fetus; in postnatal life it is represented by a fibrous cord situated between the apex of the bladder and the umbilicus, known as the median umbilical ligament. —urachal, adj.

uragogue (ū'-ra-gog): Diuretic (*q.v.*).

uran-, urano-: Denotes the palate or roof of the mouth.

uraniscoplasty (ū-ran-is'-kō-plas-ti): Plastic surgery of a cleft palate. Also uranoplasty.

uranoschisis (ū-ran-os'-ki-sis): Cleft palate.

urate (ū'-rāt): A salt of uric acid; such compounds are present in the blood and urine. They are also constituents of stones or concretions formed in the body, *e.g.*, the tophi formed in patients with gout.

uraturia (ū-ra-tū-ri'-a): Excess of urates in the urine.—uraturic, adj.

urea (ū-rē'-a): A white, crystalline substance, the end waste product of protein metabolism; it is synthesized in the liver and carried to the kidneys by the blood, thus is a normal constituent of blood, lymph and urine. The chief nitrogenous constituent of urine. Used in medicine as a diuretic. U. clearance, U. concentration, and U. range tests are all procedures for measuring the efficiency of kidney function.

uremia (ū-rē'-mi-a): A clinical syndrome due to renal failure resulting from either disease of the kidneys themselves, or from disorder or disease elsewhere in the body which induces kidney dysfunction, and which results in gross biochemical disturbance in the body, including retention of urea and other nitrogenous substances in the blood. Depending on the cause it may or may not be reversible. The fully developed syndrome is characterized by nausea, vomiting, headache, hiccough, weakness, dimness of vision, convulsions and coma. —uremic, adj.

uresis (ū-rē'-sis): Urination.

ureter (u-rē-ter, u'-rē-ter) The tube passing from each kidney to the bladder for the conveyance of urine; its average length is from 10 to 12 in.—ureteric, ureteral, adj.

ureterectasia (ū-rē-ter-ek-tā'-si-a): Distension of a ureter.

ureterectomy (ū-rē-ter-ek'-to-mi): Excision of a segment or all of a ureter.

ureteritis (ū-rē-ter-ī'-tis): Inflammation of a ureter.

uretero-: Denotes a ureter.

ureterocolic (ū-rē-ter-ō-kol'-ik): Pertaining to the ureter and colon, especially to an anastomosis between the two structures when there is a pathological condition of the lower urinary system.

ureterocolostomy (ū-rē-ter-ō-kō-los'-to-mi): Surgical transplantation of the ureters from the bladder to the colon so that urine is passed by the bowel.

uretero-ileostomy (ū-rē-ter-ō-il-ē-os'-to-mi): Surgical implantation of a ureter into the ileum. More often ileoureterostomy.

ureterolith (ū-rē'-ter-ō-lith): A stone in a ureter.

ureterolithotomy (ū-rē-ter-ō-lith-ot'-o-mi): Surgical removal of a stone from a ureter.

ureteronephrectomy (ū-rē-ter-ō-nef-rek'-to-mi): Removal of a kidney and its ureter.

ureteropelvic (ū-rē-ter-ō-pel'-vik): Pertaining to a ureter and the pelvis of the kidney to which it is attached.

ureteropyelonephritis (ū-rē-ter-ō-pī-e-lō-ne-fri'-tis): Inflammation of a ureter, the pelvis of the kidney and the kidney substance.

ureterosigmoidostomy (ū-rēt'-er-ō-sig-moid-os'-to-mi): The surgical implantation of a ureter into the sigmoid flexure.

ureterostenosis (ū-rēt'-er-ō-sten-ō'-sis): Stricture or narrowing of a ureter.

ureterostomy (ū-rē-ter-os'-tō-mi): The formation of a permanent fistula through which the ureter discharges urine. CUTANEOUS U., transplantation of the ureter to the skin.

ureterovaginal (ū-rē-ter-ō-vaj'-i-nal): Pertaining to a ureter and the vagina. U. FISTULA, one between the ureter and the vagina; may be congenital or the result of a pathological condition such as cancer of the cervix.

ureterovesical (ū-rē-ter-ō-ves'-ik-al): Pertaining to a ureter and the urinary bladder.

urethr-, urethro-: Denotes the urethra.

urethra (ū-rē'-thra): The channel leading from the bladder through which urine is excreted; in the female it measures about 1½ inches; in the male 8 to 9 inches.—urethral, adj.

urethralgia (ū-rē-thral'-ji-a): Pain in the urethra.

urethritis (ū-rē-thrī′-tis): Inflammation of the urethra.

urethrocystitis (ū-rē-thrō′-sis-tī′-tis): Inflammation of the urethra and urinary bladder.

urethrography (ū-rē-throg′-ra-fi): X-ray examination of the urethra. See **urography.**

urethroplasty (ū-rē′-thrō-plas-ti): Any plastic operation on the urethra.—urethroplastic, adj.

urethrorrhea (ū-rē-thrō-rē′-a): Any abnormal discharge from the urethra.

urethroscope (ū-rē′-thrō-skōp): An instrument designed to allow visualization of the interior of the urethra.—urethroscopic, adj.; urethroscopically, adv.; urethroscopy, n.

urethrostenosis (ū-rē-thrō-sten-ō′-sis): Urethral stricture.

urethrotomy (ū-rē-throt′-o-mi): Incision into the urethra; usually part of an operation for stricture.

urethrotrigonitis (ū-rē-thrō-trı-gon-ī′-tis): Inflammation of the urethra and base of bladder. See **trigone.**

urethrovaginal (ū-rē-thrō-vaj′-i-nal): Pertaining to the urethra and the vagina.

urethrovesical (ū-rē-thrō-ves′-ik-al): Pertaining to the urethra and the urinary bladder.

urhidrosis (ūr-hid-rō′-sis): The presence of urinous substances such as urea or uric acid in the sweat. The crystals of uric acid may be deposited on the skin as fine white particles.

-uria: Denotes: (1) urine; (2) some characteristic or condition of urine.

uric acid (ū′-rik as′-id): An acid formed in the breakdown of nucleoproteins in the tissues, and excreted in the urine. It is relatively insoluble and liable to give rise to stones. Present in excess in the blood in gout.

uricaciduria (ū-rik-as-i-dū′-ri-a): The presence of more than the normal amount of uric acid in the urine. Also uricemia.

uricosuria (ū-rik-ō-sū′-ri-a): The presence of more than the normal amount of uric acid in the urine.

uricosuric (ū-rik-ō-sū′-rik): An agent that enhances the excretion of uric acid in the urine; such substances are often used in treatment of chronic gout.

uridrosis (ū-ri-drō′-sis): Urhidrosis (q.v.).

urin-, urino-: Denotes urine.

urinal (ū′-rin-al): A vessel or container for receiving urine.

urinalysis (ū-rin-al′-i-sis): Examination of the urine.

urinary (ū′-rin-ar-i): Relating to, containing, or secreting urine.

urinate (ū′-rin-āt): To discharge urine from the body.

urination (ū-rin-ā′-shun): The discharge or passing of urine from the body; micturition.

urine (ū′-rin): The amber-colored fluid which is secreted by the kidneys, conveyed to the bladder by the two ureters and stored there until it is discharged from the body, usually voluntarily, via the urethra. It is slightly acid, has a specific gravity of 1.005 to 1.030, consists of 96% water and 4% solids the most important of which are urea and uric acid. Other solids normally found in urine include sodium chloride, potassium chloride, ammonia, hippuric acid, sulfuric acid, phosphoric acid, creatine. Solids that may be found in the urine of patients with various pathological conditions include bacteria, bile, blood, fat, glucose, ketone bodies, pus. The daily output varies, depending on various environmental factors, but the average is about 3 pints.

uriniferous (ū-rin-if′-er-us): Conveying urine; denoting particularly the tubules of the kidney.

urinogenital (ū-rin-ō-jen′-it-al): See **urogenital.**

urinometer (ū-rin-om′-e-ter): An instrument for estimating the specific gravity of urine.

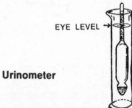

EYE LEVEL

Urinometer

urobilin (ū-rō-bīl′-in): A pigment formed by the oxidation of urobilinogen and excreted in the urine and feces.

urobilinogen (ū-ro-bī-lin′-ō-jen): A pigment formed from bilirubin in the intestine by the action of bacteria. It may be reabsorbed into the circulation and converted back to bilirubin in the liver. Small amounts are excreted in the urine and large amounts in the feces.

urobilinuria (ū-rō-bil-in-ūr′-i-a): The presence of increased amounts of urobilin in the urine.

urochrome (ū'-rō-chrōm): The brownish or yellowish pigment that is thought to give the urine its normal color.

urodynia (ū-rō-din'-i-a): Pain on urination; dysuria.

urogenital (ū-rō-jen'-it-al): Pertaining to the urinary and the genital organs.

urogram (ū'-rō-gram): Radiograph of urinary tract, or any part of it, after injection of contrast medium.

urography (ū-rog'-ra-fi): X-ray examination of any part of the urinary tract by means of contrast media, *e.g.,* pyelography (which may be intravenous, intramuscular, subcutaneous, or retrograde), cystography, cysto-urethrography, urethrography.

urokinase (ū-rō-kī'-nās): An enzyme normally found in the urine; important in the conversion of plasminogen to plasmin.

urolith (ū'-rō-lith): A stone in the urinary tract, or one passed in the urine.

urolithiasis (ū-rō-li-thī'-a-sis): A state in which there is marked tendency toward the formation of urinary stones.

urologist (ū-rol'-ō-jist): A physician who specializes in urology (*q.v.*).

urology (ū-rol'-o-ji): That branch of medical science that deals with disorders of the female urinary tract and the male genitourinary tract.—urologic, urological, adj.; urologically, adv.

urosepsis (ū-rō-sep'-sis): Septicemia resulting from the retention and absorption by the tissues of substances normally excreted in the urine.

urticaria (ur-ti-kā'-ri-a): A skin eruption characterized by circumscribed, smooth, itchy, raised wheals that are either redder or paler than the surrounding skin, developing very suddenly, usually lasting a few days, and leaving no visible trace. Common provocative agents in susceptible subjects are ingested foods such as shellfish, injected sera, and contact with, or injection of, antibiotics such as penicillin and streptomycin. See **angioneurotic edema.** Syn., nettle rash or hives.

USP: Abbreviation for United States Pharmacopeia. See **pharmacopeia.**

USPHS: Abbreviation for United States Public Health Service.

uter-, utero-: Denotes the uterus.

uteralgia (ū-ter-al'-ji-a): Pain in the uterus.

uterectomy (ū-ter-ek'-to-mi): Excision of the uterus; hysterectomy.

uterine (ū'-ter-in): Pertaining to the uterus. U. TUBE, fallopian tube (*q.v.*).

uteritis (ū-ter-ī'-tis): Inflammation of the uterus.

uterofixation (ū-ter-ō-fik-sā'-shun): Hysteropexy (*q.v.*).

uteropexy (ū-ter-ō-pek'-si): Hysteropexy (*q.v.*).

uteroplacental (ū-ter-ō-pla-sen'-tal): Pertaining to the uterus and placenta.

uteroplasty (ū'-ter-ō-plas-ti): Any plastic operation on the uterus.

uterorectal (ū-ter-ō-rek'-tal): Pertaining to the uterus and the rectum. See **Douglas' pouch.**

uterosacral (ū-ter-ō-sā'-kral): Pertaining to the uterus and sacrum.

uterosalpingography (ū-ter-ō-sal-ping-og'-raf-i): X-ray examination of the uterus and fallopian tubes after injection of a contrast medium.

uterotonic (ū-ter-ō-ton'-ik): Giving tone to the muscles of the uterus, or an agent that gives tone to uterine muscles.

uterovaginal (ū-ter-ō-vaj'-i-nal): Pertaining to the uterus and the vagina.

uterovesical (ū-ter-ō-ves'-ik-al): Pertaining to the uterus and the bladder.

uterus (ū'-ter-us): The womb; a hollow, pear-shaped muscular organ into which the ovum is received through the uterine tubes, and where it is retained during development, and from which the fetus is expelled through the vagina. Situated in the pelvic cavity, between the bladder and the rectum, it is about 3 in. long and 2 in. wide at the widest part; is divided into 3 parts, the *fundus* or upper broad part, the cavity or *body,* and the neck or *cervix;* it opens into the vagina below and the fallopian tubes above; it is maintained in position by ligaments and lined with mucous membrane called endometrium. BICORNUATE U., a uterus with two horns. GRAVID U., a pregnant uterus. —uterine, adj.; uteri, pl.

utricle (ū'-trik-l): 1. A little sac or pouch. 2. The small, delicate sac in the bony vestibule of the ear; the semicircular canals open into it.

uvea (ū'-vē-a): The pigmented middle coat of the eye, including the iris, ciliary body and choroid.—uveal, adj.

uveitis (ū-vē-ī'-tis): Inflammation of the uvea or any part of it.

uvula (ū-vū-la): Any dependent fleshy mass; term usually refers to the central tag-like structure hanging down from the posterior of the soft palate.—uvular, adj.

uvulectomy (ū-vū-lek′-to-mi): Excision of the uvula.

uvulitis (ū′-vū-lī′-tis): Inflammation of the uvula.

uvuloptosis (ū-vū-lop-tō′-sis): A falling or relaxed condition of the palate.

uvulotomy (ū-vū-lot′-o-mi): The operation of cutting off all or part of the uvula. Staphylotomy.

V

vaccinate (vak′-sin-āt): 1. To inoculate with a vaccine to produce immunity to smallpox. 2. To inoculate with a vaccine to produce immunity to the corresponding infectious disease.

vaccination (vak-sin-ā′-shun): Originally described the process of inoculating persons with discharge from cowpox to protect them from smallpox. Now applied to the inoculation of any antigenic material for the purpose of producing active artificial immunity.

vaccine (vak-sēn′): A suspension or extract of the organisms that cause a disease, either killed or modified so as to reduce their power to cause the disease while retaining their power to cause the body to form antibodies against the disease. Used chiefly in prophylactic treatment of certain infections by producing active immunity; sometimes used for amelioration or treatment of certain infectious diseases. TRIPLE V., protects against diphtheria, tetanus and whooping cough; QUADRUPLE V., protects against poliomyelitis as well. AUTOGENOUS V., one prepared from a culture of bacteria taken from the patient who is to receive the vaccine. MIXED V., one prepared from two species of bacteria. POLYVALENT V., one prepared from more than two species of bacteria. See **Sabin's v.; Salk's v.; TAB; BCG.**

vaccinia (vak-sin′-i-a): 1. Cowpox; a contagious disease of cattle, transmissible to man. 2. A disease of man that is usually limited to the site of inoculation with the virus of cowpox, either accidentally or with the purpose of conferring immunity to smallpox.

vacciniola (vak-sin-i-ō′-la): A secondary vesicular eruption that sometimes occurs after vaccination; it resembles the eruption of smallpox.

vaccinotherapy (vak-sin-ō-ther′-a-pi): The use of a vaccine for the treatment of disease. Most often this is non-specific, as in the use of TAB vaccine for producing artificial pyrexia.

vacuole (vak′-ū-ōl): A very small space formed in the protoplasm of a cell and containing air or fluid.—vacuolar, adj.

vagal (vā′-gal): Pertaining to the vagus nerve (q.v.).

vagectomy (vā-jek′-to-mi): Excision of a portion of the vagus nerve.

vagin-, vagini-, vagino-: Denotes the vagina.

vagina (va-jī′-na): 1. A sheath or sheath-like structure. 2. The musculomembranous passage extending from the cervix uteri to the vulva; it measures about 3 in. along the anterior wall and 3½ in. along the posterior wall.—vaginal, adj.

vaginal (vaj′-i-nal): 1. Like a sheath. 2. Pertaining to the vagina. V. HYSTERECTOMY, surgical removal of the uterus by way of the vagina. V. SPECULUM, an instrument used to open the vagina so as to facilitate inspection of it.

vaginate (vaj′-in-āt): To ensheath, or to be enclosed in a sheath. See **invagination.**

vaginismus (vaj-in-iz′-mus): Painful spasm of the muscular wall of the vagina preventing satisfactory sexual intercourse.

vaginitis (vaj-in-ī′-tis): Inflammation of the vagina. TRICHOMONAS V., characterized by an intensely irritating discharge; due to a ciliated protozoon which normally inhabits the bowel. See **Trichomonas vaginalis.**

vaginocele (vaj′-in-ō-sēl): Colpocele (q.v.).

vaginofixation (vaj-in-ō-fik-sā′-shun): Surgical fixation of the vagina to the abdominal wall to correct vaginal relaxation.

vaginomycosis (vaj-in-ō-mī-kō′-sis): Infection of the vagina caused by a fungus.

vaginoperineal (vaj-in-ō-per-in-ē′-al): Pertaining to both the vagina and perineum.

vaginoperineorrhaphy (vaj-in-ō-per-i-nē-or′-a-fi): Surgical repair of a lacerated or ruptured vagina and perineum.

vaginopexy (vaj-īn′-ō-pek-si): Vaginofixation (q.v.).

vaginoplasty (vaj-īn′-ō-plas-ti): Reparative plastic surgery on the vagina.

vaginovesical (vaj-i-nō-ves′-i-kal): Pertaining to the vagina and the urinary bladder.

vagolysis (vā-gol′-i-sis): Surgical destruction of the vagus nerve.

vagolytic (vā-gō-lit′-ik): 1. Pertaining to or causing vagolysis. 2. An agent that neutralizes the effect of a stimulated vagus nerve.

vagotomy (vā-got′-o-mi): 1. Surgical division of the vagus nerve. 2. Interruption of the impulses carried by the vagus nerve.

vagotonia (vā-gō-tō′-ni-a): A condition of hyperexcitability of the vagus nerve; may result in vasomotor instability, sweating, constipation.

vagus (vā′-gus): The parasympathetic pneumogastric nerve; the tenth cranial nerve, composed of both motor and sensory fibers, with a wide distribution in the neck, thorax and abdomen, sending important branches to the heart, lungs, stomach, etc. —vagal, adj.; vagi, pl.

valence (vā′-lens): The degree of combining power of one atom of an element or a radical, the combining power of one atom of hydrogen being the unit of comparison.

valgus (val′-gus): Twisted or bent outward, denoting a displacement or angulation away from the midline of the body; term is used in connection with the noun it describes, *e.g.,* hallux valgus.

valine (vā′-lēn): One of the essential amino acids (*q.v.*).

vallate (val′-āt): Cupped; a depression that is surrounded by an elevated rim. V. PAPILLAE, the papillae that occur in a V-shaped arrangement on the surface of the posterior part of the tongue.

valve (valv): A fold of membrane in a passage or tube permitting the flow of contents in one direction only.—valvular, adj.

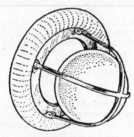

Prosthetic heart valve

valvoplasty (val′-vō-plas-ti): A plastic operation on a valve, usually reserved for the heart; includes valve replacement and valvulotomy (*q.v.*).

valvotomy (val-vot′-om-i): See **valvulotomy.**

valvulae conniventes (val′-vū-lē kon-i-ven′-tez): Circular membranous folds projecting into the lumen of the small intestine; they persist even during distension of the bowel, and act by retarding the passage of food along the bowel, and by providing a greater absorbing area.

valvulitis (val-vū-lī′-tis): Inflammation of a valve, particularly in the heart.

valvulotomy (val-vū-lot′-o-mi): Incision of a valve, by custom referring to the heart; specifically the operation of enlarging a narrowed heart valve.

vapor: The gaseous state of a liquid or solid, *e.g.,* steam, mist, gas, or an exhalation.

vaporizer (vā′-por-ī-zer): An apparatus for converting a liquid, particularly a medicated liquid, into a vapor that can be inhaled; frequently used in treatment of bronchial conditions.

vapors: A more or less obsolete term applied to hysterical nervousness, thought to be caused by bodily exhalations.

Vaquez's disease: Polycythemia vera (*q.v.*). [Louis Henri Vaquez, French physician. 1860-1936.]

varic-, varico-: Denotes varix (a twisted, tortuous vein, sometimes dilated).

varicella (var-i-sel′-la): Chickenpox (*q.v.*).—varicelliform, adj.

varices (var′-i-sēz): Pl. of varix (*q.v.*).

varicocele (var′-i-kō-sēl): Varicosity of the veins of the spermatic cord.

varicophlebitis (var-i-kō-flē-bī′-tis): Inflammation of a varicose vein.

varicose (var′-i-kōs): 1. Unnaturally swollen or distended. 2.Related to or exhibiting varices (*q.v.*). V. VEINS, dilated veins, the valves of which become incompetent so that blood flow may be reversed. Most commonly found in the lower limbs, rectum (hemorrhoids) or lower esophagus (esophageal varices).

varicosity (var-i-kos′-i-ti): 1. The state or condition of being varicose. 2.A varix (*q.v.*).

varicotomy (var-i-kot′-o-mi): Excision of a varicose vein.

variola (var′-i-ō-la): Smallpox (*q.v.*).

varioloid (var′-i-ō-loid): 1. Attack of smallpox modified by previous vaccination or attack of the disease. 2. Resembling smallpox.

varix (var′-iks): A dilated, tortuous (or varicose) vein; less often an artery or lymphatic vessel.—varices, pl.

varus (vār′-us): Bent inward; denoting a displacement or angulation toward the midline of the body; term is used in connection with the noun it modifies, *e.g.,* talipes varus (*q.v.*).

vas: A vessel or canal for carrying a fluid.—vasa, pl. V. DEFERENS, the excretory duct of the testes; it unites with the excretory duct of the seminal vesicle to form the ejaculatory duct.

vas-, vasi-, vaso-: Denotes a channel or vessel, especially a blood vessel.

vasa vasorum (vā′-za vāz-or′-um): The minute nutrient vessels of the artery and vein walls.

vascular (vas′-kū-lar): Related to or supplied with vessels, especially referring to blood vessels.

vascularization (vas-kū-lar-ĭ-zā′-shun): The acquisition of a blood supply through the formation of new blood vessels in a part. The process of becoming vascular.

vasculitis (vas-kū-lī′-tis): Inflammation of a blood vessel. Angiitis.

vasectomy (vas-ek′-to-mi): Surgical excision of the vas deferens or a part of it.

vasitis (vas-ī′-tis): Inflammation of the vas deferens.

vasoconstriction (vas-ō-kon-strik′-shun): Narrowing of the blood vessels.—vasoconstrictive, adj.

vasoconstrictor (vas-ō-kon-strik′-tor): Any agent which causes a narrowing of the lumen of blood vessels.

vasodilation (vas-ō-dī-lā′-shun): Dilation of the blood vessels.

vasodilator (vas-ō-dī-lā′-tor): Any agent which causes a widening of the lumen of blood vessels.

vasoepididymostomy (vas-ō-ep-i-did-i-mos′-to-mi): Anastomosis of the vas deferens to the epididymis.

vasoinhibitor (vas-ō-in-hib′-i-tor): Any agent that interferes with or depresses the action of vasomotor nerves thus causing dilation of the blood vessels.

vasoligation (vas-ō-lī-gā′-shun): Ligation of the vas deferens.

vasomotor (vas-ō-mō′-tor):Causing changes in the caliber of blood vessels, denoting especially nerves that have this action.

vasopressin (vas-ō-pres′-in): The antidiuretic hormone (ADH) formed in the hypothalamus; it passes down the nerves in the pituitary stalk to be stored in the posterior lobe of the pituitary. It stimulates contraction of the muscular coat of small blood vessels, thus raising the blood pressure; stimulates contraction of the intestinal muscles thus increasing peristalsis; and has some effect on muscles of the uterus. Used in treatment of diabetes insipidus.

vasopressor (vas-ō-pres′-sor): Stimulating contraction of the musculature of the smaller blood vessels, or an agent that has this effect.

vasoresection (vas-ō-rē-sek′-shun): Resection of the vas deferens.

vasospasm (vas′-ō-spazm): Constricting spasm of vessel walls.—vasospastic, adj.

vasostomy (vas-os′-to-mi): The operation of making an opening into the vas deferens.

vasovagal (vas-ō-vā′-gal): Referring to the vagus nerve and its action on the blood vessels. V. SYNDROME, an attack marked by faintness, pallor, sweating, anxiety, epigastric distress, feeling of impending death, respiratory difficulty. When part of the post-gastrectomy syndrome, it occurs a few minutes after a meal.

VD: Abbreviation for venereal disease.

VDRL test: [Veneral disease research laboratories.] A widely used serological test for syphilis.

vection (vek′-shun): The carrying of the organisms of a disease from an infected to an uninfected person; the transmission may be direct or through an intermediate host.

vector: A living carrier of disease that transmits the organisms causing the disease from one host to another; often an arthropod, e.g., mosquito, fly, flea, louse.

vegetation: A growth or accretion of any kind, especially a clot made up of fibrin and platelets occurring on the edge of the cardiac valves in endocarditis.

vegetative (veg′-e-tā-tiv): 1. Pertaining to growth or nutrition. 2. Pertaining to the non-sporing stage of a bacterium. 3. Functioning involuntarily or unconsciously. 4. In psychiatry, describes a state of inactivity or sluggishness.

vehicle: An inert or inactive substance, e.g., water or syrup, used as a carrier for a drug that is active therapeutically.

veil: 1. Any veil-like covering structure. 2. A caul (q. v.).

vein (vān): A vessel carrying blood back to the heart. It has the same three coats as an artery, i.e., inner, middle, and outer, but they are not as thick and they collapse when cut. Many v′s. have valves that prevent backflow of blood. All except the pulmonary v. carry dark, venous, deoxygenated blood.

Velpeau bandage: See **bandage.**

velum (vē′-lum): In anatomy, any structure that resembles a veil or curtain.

ven-, veni-, veno-: Denotes: (1) vein(s); (2) the vena cava.

vena (vēn′-a): The Latin word for vein.—venae, pl. V. CAVA, one of the two large veins which empty their contents into the right atrium of the heart. INFERIOR V. C., the vein which receives blood from the trunk of the body and lower extremities; it is formed by the union of the two common iliac veins. SUPERIOR V. C., the large vein which collects blood from the head, chest, and upper extremities; it is formed by the junction of the two innominate veins.

veneniferous (ven-e-nif′-er-us): Carrying or conveying poison.

venenous (ven′-e-nus): Poisonous.

venepuncture(vĕn-e-pungk′-tūr): Venipuncture (*q. v.*).

venereal (vē-nē′-rē-al): Pertaining to or caused by sexual intercourse. V. DISEASE, gonorrhea, non-specific urethritis, syphilis and soft sore.

venereology (vē-nē-rē-ol′-o-ji): The branch of medical science that deals with venereal diseases.

venery (ven′-er-i): Excessive sexual intercourse, especially that which is illicit.

venesection (ven-e-sek′-shun): Phlebotomy; a clinical procedure, formerly by opening the cubital vein with a scalpel, for the purpose of letting blood.

venin (ven′-in): Any one of the various toxic substances in snake venom (*q. v.*).

venin-antivenin (ven-in-an-ti-ven′-in): A mixture of venin and antivenin, used as a vaccine in the treatment of bites by venomous snakes.

venipuncture (ven-i-pungk′-tūr): The puncture of a vein, usually with a needle, for any purpose.

venoclysis (vē-nok′-li-sis): The slow, continuous introduction of nutrient or medicinal fluids into a vein. See **clysis.**

venogram (vē′-nō-gram): A radiograph of veins after opaque medium injection.

venography (vē-nog′-ra-fi): X-ray visualization of a vein or veins after injection with an opaque medium.—venographic, adj.; venographically, adv.

venom: A poison, particularly the substance secreted by certain snakes, insects, or animals and that is transmitted by their bite or sting.

venomous (ven′-ō-mus): Poisonous. Secreting or containing venom.

venostasis (vē-nō-stā′-sis): 1. Slowing of the blood flow in the venous system. 2. A procedure for temporarily checking the return flow of blood by applying compression to the veins of the four extremities.

venotomy (vē-not′-o-mi): Surgical incision into a vein. Phlebotomy.

venous (vē′-nus): Pertaining to the veins or the circulation within the veins.

ventilate: 1. To remove stale air and supply fresh air to take its place; may be done artificially by mechanically propelling and extracting the air or naturally by opening windows, doors, etc. 2. To oxygenate the blood and remove the carbon dioxide from it; a function carried out by the capillaries in the lungs. 3. In psychiatry, to discuss problems and grievances.—ventilation, n.

ventr-, ventri-, ventro-: Denotes: (1) the belly; (2) the anterior aspect of the body.

ventral (ven′-tral): Pertaining to the abdomen or the anterior surface of the body. Opp., dorsal.—ventrally, adv.

ventricle (ven′-trik-l): A small belly-like cavity. V.'S OF THE BRAIN, four cavities filled with cerebrospinal fluid within the brain. V.'S OF THE HEART, the two lower muscular chambers of the heart.—ventricular, adj.

ventriculitis (ven-trik-ū-lī′-tis): Inflammation of a ventricle, particularly one in the brain.

ventriculo-: Denotes a ventricle.

ventriculocisternostomy (ven-trik′-ū-lō-sis-tern-os′-to-mi): Artificial communication between cerebral ventricles and subarachnoid space. One of the drainage operations for hydrocephalus.

ventriculography (ven-trik-ū-log′-ra-fi): X-ray examination of ventricles after injection of an opaque medium.—ventriculographic, adj.

ventriculostomy (ven-trik-ū-los′-to-mi): An artificial opening into a ventricle. Usually refers to a drainage operation for hydrocephalus.

ventriculotomy (ven-trik-ū-lot′-o-mi): Surgical incision into a ventricle, *e.g.,* into a ventricle of the heart for repair of a cardiac defect or into the third ventricle of the brain for the relief of hydrocephalus.

ventrofixation (ven-trō-fik-sā′-shun): Surgical fixation of a displaced organ to the abdominal wall.

ventrohysteropexy (ven-trō-his′-ter-ō-peks-i): Surgical fixation of a displaced uterus to the abdominal wall.

ventrolateral (ven-trō-lat′-er-al): Situated or occurring both ventrally and somewhat laterally.

ventrosuspension (ven-trō-sus-pen′-shun): Surgical fixation of retroplaced uterus to the abdominal wall.

venule (vĕn′-ūl): A minute vein; the smallest division or branch of a vein, continuous at one end with the vein and at the other end with a capillary.—venulae, pl.; venular, adj.

verbigeration (ver-bij-er-ā′-shun): The constant repetition of meaningless words, phrases or sentences as seen in states of mental disorientation.

verbomania (ver-bō-mā′-ni-a): A mania for words or for talking.

vergence (ver′-jens): A turning; usually said of one eye which turns vertically or horizontally as compared with the other eye.

vermicide (ver′-mi-sĭd): An agent which kills intestinal worms.—vermicidal, adj.

vermiform (ver′-mi-form): Worm-like in form. V. APPENDIX, the vestigial, hollow, worm-like structure that is attached to the cecum, commonly called 'the appendix.'

vermifuge (ver′-mi-fūj): An agent that causes intestinal worms or parasites to be expelled.

vermin: External parasites; usually refers to insects such as lice or bedbugs. Broadly speaking, noxious, disgusting small animals or insects that are hard to control, *e.g.,* mice, rats, fleas, flies.

vermis (ver′-mis): 1. A worm. 2. The narrow middle part of the cerebellum; it lies between and connects the two hemispheres of the cerebellum.

vernix (ver′-niks): A covering. V. CASEOSA, the fatty substance which covers the skin of the fetus at birth and keeps it from becoming sodden by the liquor amnii.

verruca (ve-roo′-ka): Wart. Non-venereal warts of the genitals are called 'condylomata acuminata' (*q.v.*). V. NECROGENICA, postmortem wart,develops as result of accidental inoculation with tuberculosis. V. PLANA JUVENILIS, the common, multiple, flat, tiny warts often seen on children's hands and knees. V. PLANTARIS, a flat wart on the sole of the foot. Highly contagious. V. SEBORRHEICA, the brown, greasy wart seen in seborrheic subjects commonly on chest or back. V. VULGARIS, the common wart of the hands, of brown color and rough pitted surface.—verrucous, verrucose, adj.; verrucae, pl

version: A change of direction or turning. In obstetrics, applies to the maneuver of altering the position of the fetus in utero from an abnormal or disadvantageous to a normal or more favorable position. CEPHALIC V., turning the child so that the head presents. EXTERNAL V. is turning the child by manipulation through the abdominal wall. INTERNAL V. is turning the child by one hand in the uterus, and the other on the patient's abdomen. PODALIC V., turning the child to a breech presentation; the V. may be external or internal.

vertebr- vertebro-: Denotes a vertebra(e), vertebral column.

vertebra (ver′-te-bra): One of the 33 small bones forming the vertebral (spinal) column. There are seven cervical, 12 thoracic, five lumbar, five sacral and four coccy-

geal. The sacral and the coccygeal groups are fused in the adult.—vertebrae, pl.; vertebral, adj.

vertebrate (ver′-te-brāt): Having a vertebral column or referring to an animal that has a vertebral column.

vertebrobasilar insufficiency (ver-te-brō-bas′-i-lar): Syndrome caused by lack of blood to the hindbrain. May be progressive, episodic, or both. Clinical manifestations include vertigo, giddiness, nausea, ataxia, drop attacks, and such signs of cerebellar disorder as nystagmus.

vertebrocostal (ver-te-brō-kos′-tal): Pertaining to a vertebra and a rib.

vertex: A summit or top. In anatomy, refers usually to the top of the head.

vertigo (ver′-ti-gō): A sensation as of whirling, either of oneself in space or of the world around one; may be a symptom of disease of the inner ear, eyes, stomach, heart or brain, or of toxemia. Also often a precursor to an epileptic seizure.—vertiginous, adj.

vesical (ves′-i-kal): Pertaining to the bladder.

vesicant (ves′-i-kant): 1. Causing blisters. 2. An agent that produces blisters.

vesication (ves-i-kā′-shun): A blister or blisters, or the production of a blister or blisters.

vesicle (ves′-ik-l): 1. A small bladder, cell or hollow structure. 2. A small, circumscribed blister on the skin containing clear or nonpurulent fluid.—vesicular, adj.; vesiculation, n. SEMINAL V., one of two small sacs that store the seminal fluid until it is ejaculated.

vesico-: Denotes: (1) a bladder; (2) a blister.

vesicocele (ves′-i-kō-sēl): Hernia of the bladder.

vesicocervical (ves-i-kō-ser′-vi-kal): Pertaining to the urinary bladder and the cervix. V. FISTULA, one between the bladder and the cervix.

vesicocolonic (ves-i-kō-kō-lon′-ik): Pertaining to the urinary bladder and the colon. V. FISTULA, one between the bladder and the colon.

vesicofixation (ves-i-kō-fiks-ā′-shun): Surgical fixation of (1) the bladder to the abdominal wall; (2) the uterus to the bladder.

vesicorectal (ves-i-kō-rek′-tal): Pertaining to the bladder and the rectum. V. FISTULA, one between the bladder and the rectum.

vesicostomy (ves-i-kos′-to-mi): Syn., cystostomy. CUTANEOUS V., the bladder is drained onto the anterior abdominal wall to which an ileostomy bag is attached.

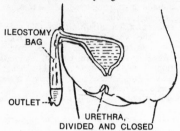

ILEOSTOMY
BAG

OUTLET

URETHRA,
DIVIDED AND CLOSED

Vesicostomy

vesicoureteral (ves-i-kō-ū-rē′-ter-al): Pertaining to the urinary bladder and the ureters.

vesicourethral (ves-i-kō-ū-rē′-thral): Pertaining to the urinary bladder and the urethra.

vesicovaginal (ves-i-kō-vag′-i-nal): Pertaining to the urinary bladder and the vagina.

vesiculectomy (ves-ik-ū-lek′-to-mi): Resection of all or part of both seminal vesicles; produces sterility.

vesiculitis (ves-ik-ū-lī′-tis): Inflammation of a vesicle, particularly a seminal vesicle.

vesiculopapular (ves-ik-ū-lō-pap′-ū-lar): Pertaining to or exhibiting both vesicles and papules.

vesiculoprostatitis (ves-ik-ū-lō-pros-ta-tī′-tis): Inflammation of the urinary bladder and the prostate gland.

vesiculopustular (ves-ik-ū-lō-pus′-tū-lar): Pertaining to or exhibiting both vesicles and pustules.

vessel (ves′-el): A tube, duct or canal, holding or conveying fluid, especially blood and lymph.

vestibule (ves′-ti-būl): 1. The middle part of the internal ear, lying between the semicircular canals and the cochlea. 2. The triangular area between the labia minora.—vestibular, adj.

vestibulotomy (ves-tib-ū-lot′-o-mi): Operation of opening into the vestibule of the inner ear.

vestigial (ves-tij′-i-al): Rudimentary; indicating a remnant of something formerly present.

viable (vī′-a-b′l): Capable of living a separate existence, said particularly of the ability of a fetus to live after birth.

vial: A small bottle for medicines or drugs. Also phial.

Vibrio (vib′-ri-ō): A genus of curved, motile microorganisms. V. CHOLERAE or COMMA causes cholera.

vicarious (vī-kār′-i-us): 1. Acting as a substitute for something. 2. Occurring in an unexpected or abnormal situation. V. MENSTRUATION, bleeding from the nose or other part of the body when menstruation is abnormally suppressed.

villus (vil′-us): A microscopic finger-like projection, such as is found in the mucous membrane of the small intestine, or on the outside of the chorion of the embryonic sac.—villi, pl.; villous, adj.

Vincent's angina: See **angina.**

viral (vī′-ral): Pertaining to, caused by, or resembling a virus (*q.v.*).

viremia (vi-rēm′-i-a): The presence of virus in the bloodstream.—viremic, adj.

viricidal (vir-i-sī′-dal): Virucidal (*q.v.*).

virile (vir′-il): Masculine. Possessing the energy, drive, and other characteristics usually considered as belonging to males.

virilism (vir′-i-lizm): The appearance of secondary male characteristics in the female.

virility (vi-ril′-i-ti): The state of being a male; having the nature and characteristics of an adult male.

virology (vi-rol′-o-ji): The study of viruses and the diseases caused by them.—virological, adj.

virucidal (vir-ū-sī′-dal): 1. Destructive or lethal to a virus. 2 Capable of destroying a virus.

virulence (vir′-ū-lens): Infectiousness; th⁀ disease-producing power of a microorganism; the relative degree of the power of a microorganism to overcome host resistance and produce disease.—virulent, adj.

virulent (vir′-ū-lent): 1. Extremely harmful or poisonous. 2. Having the power to overcome the host's defenses and produce disease.

virus (vī′-rus): Any one of a group of microorganisms so small they cannot be seen with an ordinary microscope, are capable of passing through a filter that would hold back ordinary bacteria, can live and propagate only in the presence of living tissue, and produce a variety of diseases. Classified according to anatomic area affected, viruses may be listed as dermatropic (smallpox, chickenpox, measles); pneumotropic (common cold, influenza, atypical pneumonia); neurotropic (rabies, poliomyelitis, encephalitis); and viscerotropic (yellow fever, mumps). Classified according to source, viruses may be listed as enteroviruses (those isolated from the alimentary tract; polioviruses, Coxsackie and ECHO viruses), adenoviruses (those isolated from the respiratory tract; influenza viruses); 'arbor' viruses (those isolated from biting insects; yellow fever and some other fevers). Viruses are also classified as (1) mantle viruses (fairly large; cause psittiaocis, trachoma); (2) pox viruses (smallpox); (3) pox-like viruses (herpes, varicella); (4) polioviruses (poliomyelitis); (5) myxoviruses (mumps).

viscera (vis'-er-a): Plural of viscus (*q.v.*).

visceral (vis'-er-al): Pertaining to the viscera.

visceroptosis (vis-er-op-tō'-sis): Downward displacement or falling of the abdominal organs.

viscid (vis'-id): Glutinous or sticky.

viscosity (vis-kos'-i-ti): The quality of being glutinous, sticky, viscous.

viscous (vis'-cus): Having a glutinous or ropy consistency and the quality of sticking or adhering.

viscus (vis'-kus): Any one of the internal organs, especially those in the trunk of the body.—viscera, pl.

vision: Sight; the special sense concerned with the perception of the particular qualities of an object, *e.g.,* color, size, shape. ACHROMATIC V., colorblindness. BINOCULAR V., the perception of a single image when viewed with both eyes. DOUBLE V., diplopia (*q.v.*). NIGHT V., ability to see in dim light.

visiting nurse: A trained nurse who cares for the ill in their homes; usually employed by a community agency, either private or governmental.

visual: Pertaining to vision. V. ACUITY, acuteness of sight. V. CELLS, usually refers to the rods and cones of the retina. V. FIELD, the area within which objects can be seen. V. PURPLE, the light-sensitive purple substance contained in the rods of the retina; syn., rhodopsin (*q.v.*).

vital: Pertaining to or necessary to the maintenance of life. V. CAPACITY, the amount of air expelled from the lungs after a deep inspiration. V. FUNCTIONS, those necessary for the maintenance of life. V. SIGNS, temperature, pulse, respiration. V. STATISTICS, record of births, deaths, marriages and diseases in a specific area.

vitality (vī-tal'-i-ti): 1. Vigor, liveliness, energy. 2. The power of surviving, living and growing.

Vitallium (vī-tal'-li-um): An alloy which

can be left in the tissues in the form of nails, plates, tubes, etc.

vitals (vī'-tals): Name sometimes given to the viscera.

vitamin (vī'-ta-min): Any one of several complex chemical substances found in minute quantities in certain foodstuffs. As a group, V. are essential to life, growth, reproduction, good health, and resistance to infection. Sometimes classified as fat soluble and water soluble. Some can now be synthesized. Their absence or deficiency in the diet causes a variety of deficiency diseases. (See individual vitamin listings.)

vitamin A: Fat soluble; anti-infective. Necessary for growth, reproduction, health of skin and mucous membrane, and for normal light perception. Deficiency results in night blindness, xerophthalmia, keratinization of skin and mucous membrane, predisposition to infections of skin, bladder and bronchi. Found in all animal fats, fish liver oils, egg yolk, liver, milk, butter, some green and yellow vegetables, some fruits. See **carotene.** Overdosage is possible, resulting in headache, anorexia, sparsity of hair, and certain bone changes as seen on x-ray.

vitamin B complex: An important group of water soluble vitamins. B_1 is aneurine hydrochloride or thiamine (*q.v.*); B_2 is riboflavin (*q.v.*). B_6 is pyridoxin (*q.v.*); B_{12} is cyanocobalamin (*q.v.*). The complex also includes folacin, choline, biotin, niacin, pantothenic acid, para-aminobenzoic acid.

vitamin B_1: Thiamine (*q.v.*).

vitamin B_2: Riboflavin (*q.v.*).

vitamin B_6: Pyridoxine (*q.v.*).

vitamin B_{12}: Cyanocobalamin. One of the members of the vitamin B complex. Prevents pernicious anemia and sprue, and promotes growth. Richest sources are liver, kidney, eggs, milk, muscle meats.

vitamin C: Water soluble. Necessary for building strong teeth and gums, strengthening small blood vessels, muscles, connective tissue and bones, and for formation of intercellular cement. Found in citrus and other fruits, many vegetables especially tomatoes, broccoli, spinach, sweet potatoes. Deficiency or lack results in sore bleeding gums, sore joints, tendency to bruise easily, scurvy. See **ascorbic acid.**

vitamin D: Fat soluble V.; called 'sunshine V.' because it can be produced by irradiation of ergosterol, as occurs when the skin is exposed to sunlight; also called the 'antirachitic V.' because it prevents rickets. It assists in the absorption of calcium and phosphorous and is essential for proper bone and tooth development. Found in fish liver oils, eggs, butter and milk, especially milk that has been irradiated. Overdosage is possible, producing anorexia, vomiting, diarrhea, headache, drowsiness, high blood calcium, calcification of walls of blood vessels, heart and certain soft tissues; death may ensue.

vitamin E: Tocopherol. Thought to be necessary for normal reproduction; functions still being studied. Very widely distributed in foods; wheat germ, some seeds, cereals, egg yolk, vegetable oils, fats, fat and lean meats, all leafy vegetables.

vitamin K: Necessary for the formation of prothrombin and the clotting of blood; antihemorrhagic. Absorbed only in the presence of bile. Found in fish liver and meal, animal liver, alfalfa, cabbage, spinach, tomatoes, all leafy vegetables, green vegetables, soybean oil, egg yolk.

vitamin P: A group of pigments and related compounds occurring in citrus fruits and other plants have been given this name, although there is no evidence today that these substances have activities similar to those of a true vitamin. (Has been thought to be associated with vitamin C in prevention of scurvy and considered necessary for stability of capillary walls.)

vitellin (vi-tel′-in): The chief protein in egg yolk.

vitiation (vish-ē-ā′-shun): 1. Contamination or injury. 2. Lessening of efficiency or impairment of usefulness.

vitiligo (vit-i-lī′-gō): A skin disease characterized by formation of smooth, white, circumscribed irregular patches, with normal or increased pigmentation of the surrounding skin. Leukoderma (*q.v.*).

vitreous (vit′-rē-us): Resembling jelly. v. BODY, the semifluid, transparent, jelly-like substance filling the posterior cavity of the eye.

vivi-: Denotes alive, living.

vivisection (viv-i-sek′-shun): The act of cutting or performing surgery on a living animal for purposes of research or experimentation; often extended to mean any form of animal experimentation.

vocal: Pertaining to the voice or the organs that produce voice. v.CORDS, membranous folds stretched anteroposteriorly across the larynx. Sound is produced by their vibration as air from the lungs passes between them.

void: 1. To cast off or out, as waste matter from the body. 2. To urinate.

volar (vō′-lar): Pertaining to the palm of the hand or the sole of the foot.

volatile (vol′-a-til): Evaporating rapidly.

volition (vō-lish′-un): The act or power of adopting or refraining from a certain line of action.—volitional, adj.

volitional (vō-lish′-un-al): Voluntary; describing an act of will.

Volkmann's contracture: A rapidly developing flexion deformity of the wrist and fingers, with loss of power, resulting from fixed contracture of the flexor muscles of the forearm. The cause is ischemia of the muscles by injury or obstruction to the brachial artery near the elbow. Sometimes follows improper use of a tourniquet. [Richard von Volkmann, German surgeon. 1830-1889.]

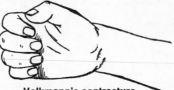

Volkmann's contracture

volume: 1. The measure of the quantity of a substance. 2. The space occupied by a substance; mass, bulk. BLOOD V., the total amount of blood circulating in the body. STROKE V., the amount of blood that leaves a ventricle during one contraction. TIDAL V., the amount of air that is breathed in and out in a normal respiration.

voluntary (vol′-un-ter i): Under the control of the will; free and unrestricted; as opposed to reflex or involuntary.

volvulus (vol′-vū-lus): A twisting of a section of bowel, so as to occlude the lumen. It causes obstruction of the bowel.

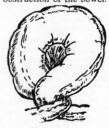

Volvulus

vomer (vō'-mer): The thin ploughshare-shaped bone that forms the inferior and posterior part of the nasal septum.

vomit (vom'-it): 1. To forcibly eject the stomach contents through the mouth. 2. Stomach contents ejected forcibly through the mouth. 3. An agent that produces vomiting; an emetic.

vomiting (vom'-i-ting): Forcible ejection of stomach contents through the mouth. CY-CLIC V., recurrent spasms of vomiting. DRY V., retching and attempting to vomit without being able to do so. FECAL V., vomiting of matter that contains feces. PERNICIOUS V., uncontrollable V.; severe V. of pregnancy. PROJECTILE V., ejection of stomach contents with great force. STERCORACEOUS V., fecal V. V. OF PREGNANCY, see **hyperemesis.**

vomitus (vom'-i-tus): Vomited matter. COFFEE-GROUND V., that which contains broken down blood mixed with matter from the stomach; occurs in malignancy and some other diseases of the stomach.

von Pirquet test: A skin test for tuberculosis.

voyeur (vwah'-yer): One who derives sexual satisfaction from seeing the sexual organs of another or from watching sexual acts. A 'Peeping Tom.'

voyeurism (vwah'-yer-izm): The characteristics, tendencies or acts of a voyeur (*q.v.*).

vulgaris (vul-gar'-is): Ordinary.

vulva (vul'-va): 1. The labia majora and minora. 2. The external female genitalia including the labia majora and minora, mons pubis, clitoris, vestibule of the vagina, perineum, and the vulvovaginal glands.

vulvectomy (vul-vek'-to-mi): Excision of the vulva.

vulvismus (vul-viz'-mus): Vaginismus (*q.v.*).

vulvitis (vul-vī'-tis): Inflammation of the vulva.

vulvorectal (vul-vō-rek'-tal): Pertaining to the vulva and the rectum, as a V. fistula.

vulvovaginal (vul-vō-vag'-in-nal): Pertaining to the vulva and the vagina. V. GLANDS, see **Bartholin's glands.**

vulvovaginitis (vul-vō-vaj-in-ī'-tis): Inflammation of the vulva and vagina or of the vulvovaginal glands.

W

waddle: To walk with short steps and a swinging side-to-side movement of the upper part of the body, seen in certain neurological disorders.

WAIS: Abbreviation for Wechsler Adult Intelligence Scale (*q.v.*).

Waldeyer's ring: A circle of lymphoid tissue that encircles the pharynx, the part above being called the pharyngeal tonsil, that on the sides the palatine tonsils, and that on the lower part the lingual tonsil. [Wilhelm von Waldeyer-Hartz, German anatomist. 1836-1921.]

wale (wāl): A linear wheal, especially one produced by a stick or whip.

walker: A metal framework, sometimes on wheels, used to aid a patient in walking.

wall: The structures that cover an anatomical unit such as a cell or an organ, or that enclose a cavity, *e.g.,* the chest cavity or the abdominal cavity.

walleye: 1. Opacity of the cornea. 2. A condition in which the iris is white or pale colored. 3. A strabismus in which the eye turns outward.

Wangensteen suction: A widely used method of continuous siphonage by suction, for the purpose of draining fluid from a body cavity, *e.g.,* the stomach, employing an apparatus that operates on the principle of negative pressure. It is most commonly used for evacuating gas and fluids from the stomach and upper intestine via a tube that is inserted through the nose into the stomach. [Owen H. Wangensteen, American surgeon. 1898- .]

wart: A benign horny projection on the skin caused by hypertrophy of the papillae of the corium. Also may occur on mucous membrane. Believed to be caused by a virus; usually painless. Many varieties are described. See **verruca.**

wash: A lotion for application to the skin or mucous membrane.

Wassermann test: Carried out in the diagnosis of syphilis. It is a complement-fixation test and is not entirely specific. See also **TPI test.** [August von Wassermann, German bacteriologist. 1866-1925.]

wasting: Emaciation; pronounced loss of body weight.

water: A colorless, odorless and almost tasteless liquid; makes up large part of the body substance; boils at 212° F (100° C) and freezes at 32° F (0° C). W. BALANCE, the condition that exists when the intake of water equals the output. W. BED, a sealed rubber sack filled with water and used as a mattress for such purposes as preventing decubiti. W. BRASH, see **pyrosis.** DISTILLED W., that which has been purified by distilling it. LIME W., calcium hydroxide. MINERAL W., contains minerals in sufficient quantity to be tasted. POLLUTED W., that which is unfit for human consumption. POTABLE W., suitable for drinking.

water-borne: Said of diseases that are spread largely by drinking-water, *e.g.,* cholera, typhoid fever.

water-hammer pulse: The full, bounding pulse felt in patients with aortic insufficiency. Also called Corrigan's pulse.

waters: Usually refers to the amniotic fluid (liquor amnii, *q.v.*). BAG OF W., the closed sac that encloses the amniotic fluid.

wave: A continuous uniformly advancing undulating rhythmic motion or series of movements that pass along a surface or through the air. BRAIN W., the fluctuating electrical potential in the brain, recorded during encephalography. PULSE W., the pulse beat as felt with the finger over an artery or shown on a sphygmograph (*q.v.*).

wax: A solid fatty substance secreted by insects or obtained from plants; also made synthetically. EAR WAX, cerumen (*q.v.*).

WBC: Abbreviation for white blood cell and white blood [cell] count.

wean: To discontinue feeding a child at the breast and substitute other methods of providing nourishment.

Weber's test: Tuning fork test for the diagnosis of conduction deafness. [Friedrich Eugen Weber, German otologist. 1832-1891.]

Wechsler Adult Intelligence Scale: A test involving performance and use of language, designed to test the intelligence of adults. Abbreviated WAIS.

weep: To exude, drop by drop, tears or other fluid such as serum. WEEPING ECZEMA, a type of eczema in which there is a vesicular eruption with the vesicles exuding serum.

Weil-Felix reaction: Agglutination reaction useful in diagnosis of the typhus group of fevers. [Edmund Weil, German physician in Prague. 1880-1922. Arthür Felix, Prague bacteriologist. 1887-1956.]

Weil's disease (wīlz): A type of jaundice with fever and splenic enlargement caused by a small spirochete voided in the urine of rats. A disease of miners, sewer workers, etc., who work in dirty water. Syn., Spirochetosis ictohemorrhagica, leptospiral jaundice. [Adolph Weil, German physician. 1848-1916.]

Welch's bacillus: *Clostridium perfringens,* the most common causative agent of gas gangrene.

wen: A retention cyst of a sebaceous gland of the skin. See **cyst.**

Wernicke's syndrome: Presbyophrenia (*q.v.*).

Wertheim's hysterectomy: An extensive operation for removal of carcinoma of the cervix, where the uterus, cervix, upper vagina, tubes, ovaries and regional lymph glands are removed. [Ernst Wertheim, Austrian gynecologist. 1864-1920.]

wet nurse: A woman who breast feeds a child who is not her own offspring.

Wharton: WHARTON'S DUCT, that of the submaxillary salivary gland. WHARTON'S JELLY, a jelly-like substance contained in the umbilical cord. [Thomas Wharton, English physician. 1616-1673.]

wheal (hwēl): An edematous, circumscribed raised area of the skin, more or less round in shape, redder or paler than the surrounding skin, usually accompanied by intense itching and usually transitory. The characteristic lesion of urticaria but may also follow insect bites or stings, or exposure to substances to which the person may be allergic.

wheeze: 1. To breathe noisily and with difficulty. 2. The hoarse whistling sound heard in conditions in which one breathes with difficulty; caused by partial obstruction of one or more of the air passages, may result from inflammation, trauma, presence of a foreign body, tumor.

whiplash injury: A popular term for injury of one or more of the cervical vertebrae resulting from sudden jerking of the head. Symptoms are pain, swelling and limitation of motion.

whipworm: See **Trichuris trichiura.**

white blood cell: A blood cell that does not contain hemoglobin. A leukocyte (*q.v.*).

whiteleg: See **thrombophlebitis.**

white matter: Nervous tissue that is whitish in color as opposed to the gray matter. Consists of myelinated nerve fibers of the neurons and makes up the conducting matter of the brain and spinal cord.

'whites': A popular term for leukorrhea (*q.v.*).

whitlow (hwĭt'-low): A felon (*q.v.*). MELANOTIC W., a malignant tumor that is characterized by changes about the border of the nail and in the nail bed. See **paronychia.**

WHO: Abbreviation for World Health Organization (*q.v.*).

whoop: The characteristic crowing intake of breath following a paroxysm of coughing in whooping cough. See **pertussis.**

whooping-cough: Pertussis (*q.v.*).

whorl (hworl): A twist or spiral turn such as in the cochlea of the ear, in the muscle fibers at the apex of the heart, in the arrangement of the ridges in a fingerprint, or in an area in which the hairs grow in a radial manner.

Widal test: An agglutination test used for diagnosing typhoid fever. [Fernand Widal, French physician. 1862-1929.]

will: The faculty of conscious and deliberate action; the power of choosing one's own actions.

Willis: See **circle of Willis.**

Wilms' tumor: A congenital, highly malignant tumor of the kidney, chiefly of children. [Max Wilms, German surgeon. 1867-1918.]

window: An opening in a structure or a wall, especially a window in the inner ear (oval window, round window).

windpipe: The trachea.

wiring: Fastening the ends of a fractured bone together with wire sutures.

wisdom tooth: The third molar on each side of the lower and upper jaws; wisdom teeth are the last to erupt, usually between the 17th and 21st years of age.

withdrawal (with-draw'-al): In medicine, the discontinuance of a medication or therapy. In psychiatry, the process by which a person retreats physically and/or psychologically to escape an emotionally disturbing situation. W. SYMPTOMS, follow the sudden deprival or withdrawal of an addictive substance, particularly a drug, from one addicted to it.

womb (woom): The uterus.

wood alcohol: Methyl alcohol.

wood tick: Any one of several varieties of ticks that cling to bushes and fasten themselves to the body of an animal or person touching them; the place of attachment often becomes an infected lesion. One variety is the vector for Rocky Mountain spotted fever.

woolsorter's disease: Pulmonary anthrax; an occupational disease that occurs in persons who handle wool of animals that have had anthrax.

wool test: A test for detecting color blindness. The person is asked to select skeins of wool of matching colors.

word blindness: A type of speech disturbance in which one is unable to perceive or understand certain sounds, syllables or phrases.

word salad: Term used to describe speech in which words and phrases are combined so that they have no logical coherence or comprehensive meaning; frequently seen in schizophrenic individuals.

World Health Organization: A specialized agent of the United Nations with headquarters in Geneva, Switzerland. Formed in 1948. Concerned with such public health and environmental problems as the control of malaria, tuberculosis, and venereal disease; maternal and child health; public sanitation and hygiene; public health administration.

wormian bones (wur′-mi-an): Small, isolated irregular bones found along the sutures of the skull.

worms: See Ascarides, Taenia, Trichuris trichuria.

wound (woond): An injury to the body that involves a break in the continuity of tissues or of body structures; results from trauma or from a surgical procedure. CONTUSED

w., one made with a blunt object and in which the skin is not broken. GUNSHOT w., one made by a bullet from a gun or small firearm. INCISED W. one made by a sharp cutting instrument. INFECTED w., one contaminated by microorganisms such as debris, bits of clothing, etc. LACERATED w., one in which the tissues are torn. OPEN w., one that opens to the surface. PENETRATING W., one that causes damage to subcutaneous tissues; has a w. of entrance but no w. of exit. PUNCTURE W., deep, narrow w. caused by penetration with a pointed object. SEPTIC W., one infected with pus-producing organisms.

wrench (rench): 1. To twist something suddenly and forcibly. 2. A painful sudden violent twist, as of an ankle or wrist.

wrist (rist): The area between the forearm and the hand; the wrist joint. Made up of the eight carpal bones. Syn., carpus.—carpal, adj. W. DROP or WRISTDROP, paralysis of the extensor muscles of the hand and fingers causing the hand to hang down at the wrist.

writer's cramp: An occupational neurosis characterized by painful spasmodic cramps of the muscles of the fingers, hand or forearm whenever an attempt is made to write.

wryneck (wrī′-nek): Torticollis (q.v.).

Wuchereria (voo-ker-ē′-ri-a): A genus of filarial worms that are parasitic in man, inhabitating chiefly the lymphatic vessels; includes the causative parasite of tropical elephantiasis (q.v.).

X

xanth-, xantho-: Denotes yellow.

xanthelasma (zan-thel-az'-ma): A variety of xanthoma. X. PALPEBRARUM, small yellowish plaques appear on the eyelids. Occurs most frequently in elderly persons.

xanthine (zan'-thēn): Dioxypurine found in liver, muscle, pancreas and urine. Present in some renal calculi.

xanthinuria (zan-thin-ū'-ri-a): The presence of abnormally large amounts of xanthine in the urine.

xanthochromatic (zan-thō-krō-mat'-ik): Having a yellow or yellowish color.

xanthocyanopia (zan-thō-sī-an-ō'-pi-a): A type of color blindness in which the person cannot distinguish red and green but is able to discern yellow and blue. Also xanthocyanopsia.

xanthoderma (zan-thō-der'-ma): Yellow colored skin.

xanthodontous (zan-thō-don'-tus): Having yellowish colored teeth.

xanthogranuloma (zan-thō-gran-ū-lō'-ma): A tumor that has characteristics of both granuloma and xanthoma (q.v.).

xanthogranulomatosis (zan-thō-gran-ū-lō-ma-tō'-sis): A form of xanthomatosis (q.v.). in which the lipid deposits are granulomatous and are found chiefly in the skull bones. Also called Hand-Schuller-Christian disease (q.v.).

xanthoma (zan-thō'-ma): A collection of cholesterol under the skin producing a yellow discoloration.—xanthomata, pl.

xanthomatosis (zan-thō-ma-tō'-sis): A condition of faulty metabolism of cholesterol, characterized by yellowish or brownish discoloration of skin and other tissues and sometimes by formation of fatty tumors; may affect general health. See **Gaucher's disease, Niemann-Pick disease.**

xanthopia (zan-thō'-pi-a): A condition in which all objects seen appear yellow or yellowish. Also xanthopsia.

xanthosis (zan-thō'-sis): Yellowish discoloration, seen especially in degenerating tissues or malignant neoplasms.

xanthous (zan'-thus): Of a yellow or yellowish color.

xanthuria(zan-thū'-ri-a): Xanthinuria (q.v.).

X chromosome: A sex chromosome that appears paired (XX) in each female human zygote and singly in each male zygote; carries the factors for femaleness.

xeno-: Denotes: (1) strange; (2) foreign material.

xenophobia (zen-ō-fō'-bi-a): Morbid fear of strangers.

xenophthalmia (zen-of-thal'-mi-a): Conjunctivitis caused by a foreign body or trauma.

Xenopsylla cheopis (zen-op-sil'-a che-op'-is): The rat flea that transmits bubonic plague.

Xenopus toad: Used in laboratory tests for pregnancy.

xer-, xero-: Denotes dry, dryness.

xerocheilia (zē-rō-kī'-li-a): Dryness of the lips. Also xerochilia.

xeroderma (zē-rō-der'-ma): Also **xerodermia.** Dryness of the skin. See **ichthyosis.** X. PIGMENTOSUM, Kaposi's disease, is a familial dermatosis probably caused by photosensitization. Pathological freckle formation (ephelides) may give rise to keratosis, neoplastic growth and a fatal termination. [Moritz Kaposi, Hungarian dermatologist. 1837-1902.]

xerophagia (zē-rō-fā'-ji-a): Subsisting on dry foods only.

xerophthalmia (zē-rof-thal'-mi-a): A serious disease of the eyeball, associated with vitamin A deficiency. The eyelids become inflamed, the conjunctiva dry and marked by appearance of yellow spots; the cornea becomes dry and ulcerated; night blindness develops and total blindness may develop in untreated cases.

xerosis (zē-rō'-sis): Dryness. X. CONJUNCTIVAE, see **Bitot's spots.**

xerostomia (zē-rō-stō'-mi-a): Dryness of the mouth from lack of saliva.

xerotocia (zē-rō-tō'-si-a): Dry labor.

xiphisternum (zif-i-ster'-num): The ensiform cartilage or process; the end section of the sternum. It is subject to much variety as to direction, shape and degree of ossification.

xiphoid (zī'-foid): Shaped like a sword. X. PROCESS, the xiphisternum.

xylene (zī'-lēn): A clear inflammable liquid resembling benzene. Has been used as an ointment in pediculosis.

xylol (zī'-lol): A hydrocarbon, derived from coal tar; used as a clarifier in microscopy. Also xylene.

x-rays: Electromagnetic rays of short length and high frequency. Produce a photographic effect and so useful in diagnosis; also penetrate deeply so useful in therapy. So called because their nature was not known at the time of their discovery (1895). Also roentgen rays.

Y

yaws: An infectious, non-veneral disease of the tropics, caused by the spirochete *Treponema pertenue* and marked by fever, rheumatic pains and a characteristic lesion called a yaw. Lesions appear on hands, face, feet, and external genitalia and are described as raspberrylike tubercles with a caseous crust; they may run together in fungus-like masses, form pustules and ulcerate. The organism enters through a break in the skin. Penicillin is the treatment of choice. Syn., frambesia tropica, pian, bouba, parangi.

This and other diseases caused by the same organism closely resemble syphilis and give a positive Wasserman reaction. The general name for this group of diseases is 'treponematosis.'

Y chromosome (krō′-mō-sōm): One of a pair of chromosomes (X and Y) carried in one-half of the male gametes, important in the determination of the sex of the offspring.

yeast (yēst): Saccharomyces. A unicellular fungus which reproduces by budding only. Used to produce alcoholic fermentation, leaven bread, and in some cases as a remedy. Some yeasts are pathogenic to man, *e.g.*, the species causing thrush. BREWER'S YEAST, a by-product from the brewing of beer; a crude but adequate and complete source of vitamin B complex.

yellow fever An acute, specific, infectious, febrile illness of the tropics, of short duration and varying intensity, caused by a virus and spread by the bite of a mosquito (*Aedes aegypti*). Characteristic features are jaundice, black vomit and anuria. Mortality rate about 5% among victims who are native to areas of the world where the disease is endemic, but much higher for those from other areas. Vaccination with 17D strain of the virus produces immunity for several years.

yellow spot: Macula lutea (*q.v.*).

yoghurt, yogurt (yōg′-hert): A form of curdled milk produced by the action of *Lactobacillus bulgaricus.*

Young's rule: A formula for determining the fraction of an adult dose of a drug which is the correct dose for a child;

$$\frac{\text{age of the child}}{\text{age of the child} + 12} =$$

the fraction of the adult dose that should be given. [Thomas Young, English physician, physicist, mathematician and philologist. 1773–1829.]

yttrium 90 (Y⁹⁰): A rare metallic substance emitting beta particles with a half-life of 64 hours.

Z

Zephiran: Benzalkonium. A soluble powder used in solutions of 1:1000 to 1:20,000 as a surface detergent and antiseptic. Its effectiveness is neutralized by soap but since it is an effective cleansing agent it can be used as both a detergent and antiseptic. Effective against most bacteria.

Ziehl-Neelsen's stain: Used in the laboratory to detect *Mycobacterium tuberculosis* (tubercle bacillus). [Franz Ziehl, German bacteriologist. 1857-1926. Friedrich Karl Adolf Neelsen. 1854-1894.]

zinc (zink): A bluish-white metallic element; many of its salts are used for their antiseptic and astringent action on skin and mucous membranes; made up in powder, solution and ointment forms.

zo-, zoo-: Denotes: (1) animal; (2) the animal kingdom.

Zollinger-Ellison syndrome: Ulcerogenic tumor of the pancreatic islets of Langerhans, hypersecretion of gastric acid, fulminating ulceration of esophagus, stomach, duodenum and jejunum. Frequently accompanied by diarrhea. Diagnosed by peroral biopsy. [Robert M. Zollinger, American surgeon. 1903- . E. H. Ellison, American physician. 1918- .]

zona (zō′-na), **zone** (zōn): In anatomy, a delimited area of the body having characteristic structure or properties. EROGENOUS or EROTOGENIC ZONES, areas of the body which produce sexual response when stimulated, *e.g.*, lips, breasts, anal and genital areas. ZONA PELLUCIDA, the vitelline membrane surrounding the ovum.

Zondek-Aschheim test: See Aschheim-Zondek test.

zonesthesia (zō-nes-thē′-zē-a): A sensation of constriction about the body resembling that produced by a tight girdle or cord.

zonula (zōn′-ū-la): Small zone, belt, or girdle. ZONULA CILIARIS, suspensory ligament attaching periphery of lens to ciliary body (*q.v.*). Also zonule.

zonulolysis (zon-ū-lol′-is-is): Breaking down the zonula ciliaris—sometimes necessary before intracapsular extraction of the lens. —zonulolytic, adj.

zoograft (zō′-ō-graft): A graft of tissue from a lower animal to man.

zoolagnia (zō-ō-lag′-ni-a)): Sexual attraction of an individual for animals.

zoology (zō-ol′-ō-ji): The science that deals with the study of animals.

zoomania (zō-ō-mā′-ni-a): Excessive love of animals.

zoonosis (zō-ō-nō′-sis): A disease that may be transmitted from animal to animal or from animal to man, *e.g.*, rabies.—zoonoses, pl.; zoonotic, adj.

zoophilism (zō-of′-i-lizm): Excessive fondness for animals, often expressed in opposition to use of animals for experimental purposes; antivivisectionism.

zoophobia (zō-ō-fō′-bi-a): Abnormal fear of animals.

zooplasty (zō′-ō-plas-ti): Transplantation of skin or other tissue from one of the lower animals to man.

zoopsia (zō-op′-si-a): A hallucination or delusion in which the individual thinks he sees animals.

zoster (zos′-ter): An acute inflammatory disease characterized by formation of vesicles which follow the course of a nerve and which are accompanied by pain and a burning sensation. Sometimes called shingles. Herpes zoster (*q.v.*).

Z-plasty: A plastic operation for relieving the contraction of scar tissue; a Z incision is made over the scar.

zygoma (zī-gō′-ma): The cheek-bone.—zygomatic, adj.

zygomatic bone (zī-gō-mat′-ik): Same as zygoma.

zygote (zī′-gōt): 1. The fertilized ovum. 2. The individual which develops as a result of the union of two gametes (*q.v.*).

zymase (zī′-mās): 1. An enzyme. 2. The enzyme in yeast that causes alcoholic fermentation.

zymogen (zī′-mō-jen): The inactive granular precursor, with the secretory cell, of enzymes.

zymolysis (zī-mōl-ī′-sis): Digestion or fermentation brought about by an enzyme.

zymosis (zī-mō′-sis): 1. Fermentation. 2. The process by which infectious diseases are thought to develop. 3. Any infectious disease.

zymotic (zī-mot′-ik): 1. Relating to zymosis. 2. A general term sometimes used to designate endemic or epidemic infectious diseases which are caused by microorganisms.